HANDBOOK OF PEER INTERACTIONS, RELATIONSHIPS, AND GROUPS

Social, Emotional, and Personality Development in Context
Kenneth H. Rubin, Series Editor

Handbook of Peer Interactions, Relationships, and Groups
Edited by Kenneth H. Rubin, William M. Bukowski, and Brett Laursen

Handbook of Peer Interactions, Relationships, and Groups

EDITED BY

Kenneth H. Rubin
William M. Bukowski
Brett Laursen

THE GUILFORD PRESS
New York   London

© 2009 The Guilford Press
A Division of Guilford Publications, Inc.
72 Spring Street, New York, NY 10012
www.guilford.com

Printed in the United States of America

This book is printed on acid-free paper.

Last digit is print number: 9   8   7   6   5   4   3   2   1

Library of Congress Cataloging-in-Publication Data is available from the Publisher.
ISBN 978-1-59385-441-6

About the Editors

Kenneth H. Rubin, PhD, is Professor of Human Development and Director of the Center for Children, Relationships, and Culture at the University of Maryland. His research interests include children's peer and family relationships and their social and emotional development. Dr. Rubin is the recipient of a Killam Research Fellowship (Canada Council) and an Ontario Mental Health Senior Research Fellowship, is past president of the International Society for the Study of Behavioral Development, and has published 11 books and over 240 peer-reviewed chapters and articles. He has twice served as an associate editor of *Child Development* and has been on the editorial boards of numerous professional journals. He has also been a member of the National Institute of Child Health and Human Development (NICHD) study section on Human Development and Aging, as well as the National Institute of Mental Health's (NIMH) study section on Risk and Prevention. Dr. Rubin is currently principal investigator for an NIMH-funded longitudinal research project on friendship and psychosocial adjustment in middle childhood and adolescence, and is co-principal investigator for an NICHD-funded project, "Social Outcomes in Pediatric Traumatic Brain Injury." He is a Fellow of the Canadian and American Psychological Associations and the Association for Psychological Science.

William M. Bukowski, PhD, is Professor and University Research Chair in the Department of Psychology at Concordia University in Montreal, Quebec, Canada. He is also the Director of the interuniversity Centre for Research in Human Development, based in Quebec. His research program focuses on the factors that influence the features and effects of peer relations in early adolescence. Dr. Bukowski is past editor of the *International Journal of Behavioral Development*.

Brett Laursen, PhD, is Professor of Psychology and Director of Graduate Training at Florida Atlantic University. His research focuses on parent–child and peer relationships during childhood and adolescence and the influence of these relationships on individual social and academic adjustment. Dr. Laursen is a Fellow of the American Psychological Association (Division 7, Developmental) and a Fellow and Charter Member of the Association for Psychological Science. He is currently editor of the Methods and Measures section of the *International Journal of Behavioral Development*. A Docent Professor of Social Developmental Psychology at the University of Jyväskylä, Finland, he is also a member of the Finnish Center of Excellence in Learning and Motivation Research.

Contributors

Kimberley A. Arbeau, MA, Department of Psychology, Carleton University, Ottawa, Ontario, Canada

Steven R. Asher, PhD, Department of Psychology and Neuroscience, Duke University, Durham, North Carolina

Thomas J. Berndt, PhD, Department of Psychological Sciences, Purdue University, West Lafayette, Indiana

Karen L. Bierman, PhD, Department of Psychology, Penn State University, University Park, Pennsylvania

Michel Boivin, PhD, School of Psychology, Laval University, Ste-Foy, Quebec, Canada

Cathryn Booth-LaForce, PhD, Department of Family and Child Nursing, University of Washington, Seattle, Washington

Julie C. Bowker, PhD, Department of Psychology, University at Buffalo, The State University of New York, Buffalo, New York

Mara Brendgen, PhD, Department of Psychology, University of Quebec at Montreal, Montreal, Quebec, Canada

B. Bradford Brown, PhD, Department of Educational Psychology, University of Wisconsin–Madison, Madison, Wisconsin

Caroline B. Browne, BA, Department of Psychology, University of North Carolina at Chapel Hill, Chapel Hill, North Carolina

William M. Bukowski, PhD, Department of Psychology and Centre for Research in Human Development, Concordia University, Montreal, Quebec, Canada

Marlene Caplan, PhD, Helen Arkell Dyslexia Centre, London, United Kingdom

Xinyin Chen, PhD, Department of Psychology, University of Western Ontario, London, Ontario, Canada

Janet Chung, MS, Department of Psychology, University of Western Ontario, London, Ontario, Canada

Antonius H. N. Cillessen, PhD, Department of Psychology, University of Connecticut, Storrs, Connecticut, and Behavioral Science Institute, Radboud Universiteit Nijmegen, Nijmegen, The Netherlands

W. Andrew Collins, PhD, Institute of Child Development, University of Minnesota, Minneapolis, Minnesota

Robert J. Coplan, PhD, Department of Psychology, Carleton University, Ottawa, Ontario, Canada

Nicki R. Crick, PhD, Institute of Child Development, University of Minnesota, Minneapolis, Minnesota

Susanne Denham, PhD, Department of Psychology, George Mason University, Fairfax, Virginia

Erin L. Dietz, BA, Department of Educational Psychology, University of Wisconsin–Madison, Madison, Wisconsin

Thomas J. Dishion, PhD, Child and Family Center, Department of Psychology, and Department of School Psychology, University of Oregon, Eugene, Oregon

Nancy Eisenberg, PhD, Department of Psychology, Arizona State University, Tempe, Arizona

Richard A. Fabes, PhD, School of Social and Family Dynamics, Program in Family and Human Development, Arizona State University, Tempe, Arizona

Wyndol Furman, PhD, Department of Psychology, University of Denver, Denver, Colorado

Scott D. Gest, PhD, Department of Human Development and Family Studies, Penn State University, University Park, Pennsylvania

Sandra Graham, PhD, Department of Education, University of California–Los Angeles, Los Angeles, California

John D. Guerry, BA, Department of Psychology, University of North Carolina at Chapel Hill, Chapel Hill, North Carolina

Laura D. Hanish, PhD, School of Social and Family Dynamics, Program in Family and Human Development, Arizona State University, Tempe, Arizona

Willard W. Hartup, EdD, Institute of Child Development, University of Minnesota, Minneapolis, Minnesota

Dale F. Hay, PhD, School of Psychology, Cardiff University, Cardiff, Wales, United Kingdom

Alice Y. Ho, MA, Department of Education, University of California–Los Angeles, Los Angeles, California

Claire Hofer, PhD, Department of Psychology, Arizona State University, Tempe, Arizona

Nina Howe, PhD, Department of Education, Concordia University, Montreal, Quebec, Canada

Carollee Howes, PhD, Psychological Studies in Education, University of California–Los Angeles, Los Angeles, California

Celia Hsiao, MS, Department of Psychology, University of Western Ontario, London, Ontario, Canada

Noah Simon Jampol, BA, Department of Human Development, University of Maryland, College Park, Maryland

Amy E. Kennedy, PhD, Department of Human Development, University of Maryland, College Park, Maryland

Kathryn A. Kerns, PhD, Department of Psychology, Kent State University, Kent, Ohio

Margaret Kerr, PhD, Department of Behavioural, Social, and Legal Sciences, Örebro University, Örebro, Sweden

Melanie Killen, PhD, Department of Human Development, University of Maryland, College Park, Maryland

Thomas A. Kindermann, PhD, Department of Psychology, Portland State University, Portland, Oregon

Gary W. Ladd, EdD, School of Social and Family Dynamics, Department of Psychology, Arizona State University, Tempe, Arizona

Brett Laursen, PhD, Department of Psychology, Florida Atlantic University, Fort Lauderdale, Florida

Peter E. L. Marks, MA, Institute of Child Development, University of Minnesota, Minneapolis, Minnesota

Carol Lynn Martin, PhD, School of Social and Family Dynamics, Program in Family and Human Development, Arizona State University, Tempe, Arizona

Melissa A. McCandless, BA, Department of Psychological Sciences, Purdue University, West Lafayette, Indiana

Kristina L. McDonald, PhD, Department of Human Development, University of Maryland, College Park, Maryland

Felicia Meyer, MA, Department of Psychology and Centre for Research in Human Development, Concordia University, Montreal, Quebec, Canada

Nazanin Mohajeri-Nelson, PhD, Institute of Child Development, University of Minnesota, Minneapolis, Minnesota

Clairneige Motzoi, MA, Department of Psychology and Centre for Research in Human Development, Concordia University, Montreal, Quebec, Canada

Dianna Murray-Close, PhD, Department of Psychology, University of Vermont, Burlington, Vermont

Alison Nash, PhD, Department of Psychology, State University of New York at New Paltz, New Paltz, New York

Kätlin Peets, PhD, Department of Psychology, University of Turku, Turku, Finland

Timothy F. Piehler, MS, Child and Family Center, Department of Psychology, University of Oregon, Eugene, Oregon

C. J. Powers, MS, Department of Psychology, Penn State University, University Park, Pennsylvania

Mitchell J. Prinstein, PhD, Department of Psychology, University of North Carolina at Chapel Hill, Chapel Hill, North Carolina

Gwen Pursell, MA, Department of Psychology, Florida Atlantic University, Fort Lauderdale, Florida

Diana Rancourt, MS, Department of Psychology, University of North Carolina at Chapel Hill, Chapel Hill, North Carolina

Amanda J. Rose, PhD, Department of Psychological Sciences, University of Missouri, Columbia, Missouri

Linda Rose-Krasnor, PhD, Department of Psychology, Brock University, St. Catharines, Ontario, Canada

Hildy Ross, PhD, Department of Psychology, University of Waterloo, Waterloo, Ontario, Canada

Kenneth H. Rubin, PhD, Department of Human Development, University of Maryland, College Park, Maryland

Adam Rutland, PhD, Centre for the Study of Group Processes, Department of Psychology, University of Kent, Canterbury, United Kingdom

Christina Salmivalli, PhD, Department of Psychology, University of Turku, Turku, Finland, and Centre for Behavioural Research, University of Stavanger, Stavanger, Norway

António José Santos, PhD, Institute of Applied Psychology, Unit for the Study of Developmental and Educational Psychology, Lisbon, Portugal

Rhiannon L. Smith, BA, Department of Psychological Sciences, University of Missouri, Columbia, Missouri

Håkan Stattin, PhD, Department of Behavioural, Social, and Legal Sciences, Örebro University, Örebro, Sweden

April Z. Taylor, PhD, Department of Child and Adolescent Development, California State University–North Ridge, North Ridge, California

Julie Vaughan, MA, Department of Psychology, Arizona State University, Tempe, Arizona

Brian E. Vaughn, PhD, Department of Human Development and Family Studies, Auburn University, Auburn, Alabama

Frank Vitaro, PhD, School of Psychoeducation, University of Montreal, Montreal, Quebec, Canada

Kathryn R. Wentzel, PhD, Department of Human Development, University of Maryland, College Park, Maryland

Preface

The typical child and adolescent spends significant periods of time each day in the company of peers. As children and adolescents, in particular, grow older, the periods of time they spend with peers lengthen and extend beyond formal settings such as school and adult-led extracurricular activities. Significantly, it is within these various peer contexts that children and adolescents acquire a wide range of skills, attitudes, and experiences that influence their adaptation across the lifespan. Accordingly, peers are viewed as powerful socialization "agents," contributing well beyond the collective influences of family, school, and neighborhood to child and adolescent social, emotional, and cognitive well-being and adjustment.

Given these empirically supported realities, it is surprising that, until the publication of this *Handbook*, there was not a previous collection of reviews discussing the history of research and theory and describing contemporary research and methods pertaining to child and adolescent peer interactions, relationships, and groups. Fortunately, this book provides such a collection. Its chapters can be viewed as both historical accounts and state-of-the-art descriptions—outlining the remarkable progress of research on peer interactions, relationships, and groups during the past five decades, and discussing what we know to date about the features, processes, and effects of children's and adolescents' experiences with their peers.

Research on the child's world of peers was initially motivated by four distinct ideas. One idea derived from social learning theory. Studies in the 1960s used the concepts of reward and imitation to understand how peers could shape each other's behavior and act as agents of socialization. Researchers typically used laboratory contexts or controlled observations in preschools to demonstrate that peers could influence each other through their experiences in, or observations of, basic forms of social interaction. These effects could be seen on such broad and disparate behaviors as cooperation, altruism, and aggression.

The central concept of the second idea, sociometry, is that in order to fully understand group membership and individual placement or status within groups, one has to recognize the attractions and repulsions between individuals. Sociometry is both an idea and a technique, as it provides researchers with ways of thinking about groups and ways of developing measures of groups per se as well as the individuals comprising a group. Most often, the groups that were of interest to the practitioners of sociometry comprised children.

A third idea is that *relationships* are significant for normal and abnormal development. This idea is apparent in the writings of (1) Blatz (1966), a pediatrician who emphasized the value of security in relationships as a critical determinant of well-being (see also
Ainsworth, Blehar, Waters, & Wall, 1978, and Bowlby, 1969/1982); (2) Hinde (1987), an
ethologist who recognized that in order to fully understand animal (and human) development one must understand how animals (humans) interact with one another and form
(and dissolve) relationships with one another, and how the groups within which animals
(and humans) are members can influence or be influenced by the group's members and
their interactions and relationships with each other; and (3) Sullivan (1953), a psychiatrist who believed that the study of personality and the study of interpersonal relationships could not be separated.

The fourth seminal idea was drawn from the observations and research of clinical
psychologists and other behavioral scientists who found that assessments of peer relations taken in childhood could predict adjustment and maladjustment in adolescence
and adulthood (e.g., Cowen, Pedersen, Bagigian, Izzo, & Trost, 1973; Roff, 1961). They
interpreted these findings to indicate that, at the least, the assessment of problematic
experiences with peers could be regarded as risk indices for unhealthy psychological
development.

Together, the aforementioned four ideas provided researchers with significant conceptual insights for conducting research on the world of peers, new user-friendly methods
and measures to assess children's experiences with peers, and a new motivation to inspire
and guide research on peer interactions, relationships, and groups. Nearly 30 years ago
these four ideas coalesced to help create the beginnings of a vibrant and ever-expanding
literature on the features and effects of peer interactions, relationships, and groups. The
confluence of developmental scientists interested in basic developmental processes and
the child clinical psychologists interested in the origins of behavioral and affective maladjustment occurred at about the same time that the concept of psychopathology during
childhood was being reconsidered. Central to this "new" approach known as "developmental psychopathology" is the idea that the study of normal developmental processes
and the study of psychopathology are mutually enriching activities (Sroufe & Rutter,
1984). Research on peers was ideally suited to this approach, perhaps more so than for
most other developmental topics.

But 30 years ago, research on the topic of the child's world of peers was relatively
homogeneous and focused. Other than emerging work on infant and toddler peer
interaction, altruistic and agonistic behavior, young children's social pretense, and early
adolescent friendship and moral development, most research on peers that appeared
in archival journals centered on concern with sociometric rejection. Over the course
of the following decades, however, peer research has become highly differentiated in
the questions it asks, and the measures used in these studies have become increasingly
refined. Development is an issue. How does the child's social life with peers develop? What
accounts for normalcy and deviation from the norm in the expression of social behavior
and the experience of social relationships? The use of broadband measures of such constructs as social competence, aggression, and withdrawal have been replaced by the use
of nuanced and specific measures that reflect sensitivity to the distinctions between phenomena that had been bundled together within a single domain. For example, measures
of aggression were developed to distinguish between whether an act was proactively or
reactively aggressive, whether it was relational or physical, and whether it was direct or
indirect. Social withdrawal was reconceptualized as reflecting the child's emotion-based

withdrawal from the peer milieu or the child's isolation and rejection by peers. There was a clearer recognition of the distinction between acceptance and friendship, peer rejection and exclusion, and social and emotional competence. Not only were group acceptance and rejection or dyadic friendship considered to be of significance in typical and atypical development, so too were romantic relationships, as well as the groups and networks within which friendships and romantic relationships occurred. For all of the above, new measures and methods were developed. This relatively recent expansion in peer-related constructs and refinements in measurement have significantly broadened and enriched the study of peer interactions, relationships, and groups. And each of these refinements and expansions is highlighted in this compendium.

As measures and methods have become more articulated, and as constructs have been introduced or reconstrued, research having to do with peer interactions, relationships, and groups has become more heterogeneous and diverse. This handbook is testimony to the field's diversity. We include chapters on methods and measures. We highlight issues pertaining to development; ethnicity, race, and culture; emotional and social-cognitive processes; play and the understanding of nonliterality; the significance of conflict and peer exclusion; and influences varying from the genetic to the family to the neighborhood. These nuances allow us to better understand the antecedents and consequences of a range of peer experiences and to develop procedures for helping children and adolescents whose peer relations are problematic.

This handbook is organized topically and developmentally. It begins with two chapters outlining historical and theoretical underpinnings to contemporary research on peer interactions, relationships, and groups. This is followed by a section on methods and measures centered on peer interactions, relationships, and groups. Thereafter, there are separate chapters focused on peer interactions, relationships, and groups within infancy and early childhood, followed by chapters focused on these same general constructs in middle childhood and adolescence. Beyond these developmentally oriented sections, we arrive at separate sections on such topics as the distal (race/ethnicity, culture, neighborhood) and the proximal (genes, temperament, parents, and family) factors influencing peer interactions, relationships, and groups in childhood and adolescence. We end with two sections—one in which the varied consequences (school and psychological adjustment) of children's peer experiences are described and the other in which policy and translational issues are noted.

Overall, this handbook marks a historical step in the field of developmental science. Thirty years ago, the field remained generally consumed by the notion that the primary influence on socioemotional development emanated from the quality of children's and adolescents' parent–child interactions and relationships. Today, however, we are more aware of the significance influence of peer interactions, relationships, and groups on development. Thirty years later, the contents of this handbook are testimony to the distance the field of developmental science has traveled.

References

Ainsworth, M. D. S., Blehar, M. C., Waters, E., & Wall, S. (1978). *Patterns of attachment*. Hillsdale, NJ: Erlbaum.

Blatz, W. (1966). *Human security: Some reflections*. Toronto: University of Toronto Press.

Bowlby, J. (1982). *Attachment and loss: Vol. 1. Attachment*. New York: Basic Books. (Original work published 1969)

Cowen, E. L., Pedersen, A., Bagigian, H., Izzo, L. D., & Trost, M. A. (1973). Long-term follow-up of early detected vulnerable children. *Journal of Consulting and Clinical Psychology, 41,* 438–446.

Hinde, R. A. (1987). *Individuals, relationships and culture.* Cambridge, UK: Cambridge University Press.

Roff, M. (1961). Childhood social interactions and young adult bad conduct. *Journal of Abnormal Social Psychology, 63,* 333–337.

Sroufe, L. A., & Rutter, M. (1984). The domain of developmental psychopathology. *Child Development, 55,* 17–29.

Sullivan, H. S. (1953). *The interpersonal theory of psychiatry.* New York: Norton.

Contents

xv

PART I
Introduction
History and Theory

CHAPTER 1

Critical Issues
and Theoretical Viewpoints

WILLARD W. HARTUP

Contemporary wisdom holds that children contribute significantly to one another's development. Beginning in the earliest years, the development of human beings seems to require input from socialization agents who are not themselves mature as well as from those who are. Whether one refers to interaction between toddlers or interaction between teenagers, the weight of the evidence suggests that "peers are necessities, not luxuries" in human development.

Parents are aware of these necessities. Relatively few adults discourage contact between their offspring and agemates except, of course, in instances they believe to be dangerous or disadvantageous. Yet scientists have been slow to provide definitive evidence that peers are developmental necessities, because almost no children are raised in isolation from other children. Animal models (based on the Rhesus macaque) demonstrate that maternal rearing without peer contact produces animals that show both contemporaneous disturbances in play and long-term disturbances in emotional development (Harlow, 1969). Current evidence shows that the consequences of peer experience combine with the competencies generated in parent–child relations to produce social adaptation, so that the main goal for developmental scientists is to determine how and when cross-agent integrations occur, and in so doing, optimize outcomes.

In this chapter, theories relating to three main issues are discussed:

1. What is the nature of peer influence, and what are the best ways to describe the processes that contribute to it?
2. What contributes to the formation and functioning of enduring relationships between children, and what is their impact on developmental outcome?
3. Relationships between children are nested within larger social networks, including networks of relationships. How are these networks organized, and how does behavior change derive from them?

Peer Influence

Contact with other children can alter a child's instrumental activity, the frequency and intensity of ongoing actions, and interpersonal perceptions. Anyone who has watched a group of children has seen innumerable instances of Child *B* doing something different after a social exchange with Child *A*. Infants shift their attention from their own feet to the face of another infant newly placed nearby; toddlers scream when another child takes away a toy; preschoolers put down their paints when a companion suggests playing house; a school-age child refuses to go to school because of a run-in with a bully; and an adolescent notes that her friend is wearing black lipstick and turns up wearing it herself the next day. Such effects, known generically as "behavior contagion," involve a wide array of social-psychological processes and occur under enormously varied conditions.

Peer Reinforcement and Performance Theory

Reinforcement theories that depend on the construct of drive reduction (e.g., Hull, 1943) have not been very useful to the empirical study of peer relations. No one denies that some changes in a child's behavior may stem from peer interaction that generates drive reduction on a contingent basis. But the earlier social learning theories based on drive reduction (e.g., Dollard & Miller, 1950) proved to be limited in their utility for several reasons: (1) attentional and observational phenomena were not accounted for adequately; (2) knowing what responses are being reinforced by what kind of drive reduction in most peer interactions is difficult to determine; and (3) connecting the acquisition of discrete responses to the complex planning and executive behavior employed by older children in their interactions with one another is difficult. Thus, the limited usefulness of these theories in peer relations research is due partly to limitations in the theories themselves and partly to difficulties in application.

Theories of operant learning (behavior modification) have been more useful in studying peer relations, because such models of behavior change depend only on the observer's ability to identify positive and negative reinforcing events in the interactional sequence (i.e., stimuli associated with response acceleration or deceleration). Over the years, Gerald Patterson and his associates have explored such events in both peer interaction and family interaction, beginning with a series of studies in which acceleration and deceleration in the aggressive behavior of nursery school children were shown to be linked either to positive or negative reinforcing reactions by the other children (Patterson, Littman, & Bricker, 1967). These studies required clearly operationalized aggression constructs, a demonstrable catalog of reinforcing events, and reliable measures of the occurrence of these stimuli and the relevant reinforcers. Positive reinforcers for aggression occurring within peer interaction turn out *not* to be approval or attention but, rather, crying, passivity, and defensiveness by the victim. Punishments consist of the victim's tattling or counterattacks.

Subsequent investigation of these notions stresses the social disadvantages that aggressive children encounter in making friends and in social activity. Escalating aggression, based on coercive socialization in both the family and the peer group (Patterson, Reid, & Dishion, 1992), limits the aggressive child in his or her attempts to acquire friends, so that close associates are likely to be aggressive and antisocial themselves. Within these contexts, talk with friends is likely to emphasize deviant behavior (Poulin, Dishion, &

Haas, 1999) and interaction to involve conflict and assertiveness (Dishion, Andrews, & Crosby, 1995), both of which lead to acceleration of troublesome, antisocial behavior. Deviant talk, then, figures centrally in the development of aggressive individuals. The extent to which these theoretical viewpoints are useful in studying the development of prosocial behavior and peer interaction, for example, or socially withdrawn behavior, are not well established.

Social Learning and Imitation: The Case of Observational Learning

Social learning theory originated with applications of drive reduction theories of reinforcement to imitation and aggression (Miller & Dollard, 1941; Dollard, Miller, Doob, Mowrer & Sears, 1939). Modern social learning theory, however, derives mostly from the work of Albert Bandura (1977) and his associates. Observational learning stands at the center of this system of ideas, along with the demonstration that contiguity between modeling cues and the observer's perceptions appears to be mainly responsible for laying down representations of the model's behavior in the observer's memory. Reinforcement of the observer is unnecessary; repeated trials are frequently unnecessary; and it appears that the information contained in modeling cues lies at the heart of the observational learning process. Modeling of specific acts may be synthesized by the observer to form regularized sequences, and these "scripts" become represented in memory. Broad categories (e.g., sympathy) may also be internalized, including information about elicitors and consequences; these categories have been called "schemas" (Schank & Abelson, 1977) and furnish the context for guiding, interpreting, and performing the modeled actions.

Reproduction of modeling cues depends on a variety of conditions. Among the most salient are observed consequences of the model's actions. Those that lead to favorable outcomes rather than unfavorable ones (as noted by the observer) are more likely to be reproduced. Empirical studies have established other conditions that determine whether a child will or will not replicate the actions of another person; for example, models who are nurturant, adept, and socially powerful are more likely to be imitated than those who do not possess these characteristics (Bandura, 1977).

But nearly everything that has been learned about such matters derives from experiments in which adult models were used with child observers. A small but significant literature exists to show that children also imitate other children. Observational effects are particularly strong in certain instances (e.g., situations involving disinhibition accompanied by vicarious reinforcement) (Masters, Ford, Arend, Grotevant, & Clark, 1979). Documentation remains poor, however, with respect to manifestations of observational peer learning in everyday life, especially when there is a delay between the modeling event and its replication by the observer. Finally, developmental studies are lacking.

Cognitive Theories

Piaget, Cooperation, and Conflict

According to Jean Piaget (1926), cognitive development depends on activity in which the individual coordinates perceptions and ideas and overcomes contradictions. Many experiences contribute to these developments, including those that occur during cooperation between the child and other children. Cooperation, however, inevitably exposes the child to views that differ from his or her own, forcing a cognitive rapprochement. Cooperative and other social interactions with children, in contrast to those with adults, involve declarations, asking questions, exchanging information, working together, argument, objection, persuasion, and comparison. In order for cognitive development to occur through collaboration, "partners [must] have a common language and system of ideas and use reciprocity in examining and adjusting for differences in their opinions" (Rogoff, 1998, p. 685).

Children's reflections on these interpersonal conflicts produce cognitive conflict within each individual. These conflicts, in turn, motivate a "coordination of understandings." Most important, these new views or ideas are produced by the children as individuals, and are not shared or consensual cognitions. Conflicts with adults, according to these ideas, are resolved differently—usually with the child yielding to the adult's point of view, simply because children recognize that adults have greater knowledge about the world than they do. Peer interaction, in contrast, forces children to coordinate or restructure their own views, an activity that is necessary to the permanence of the cognitive advance (Piaget, 1932).

Cognitive development through social exchanges with other children is constrained in the early years by limitations in both language and thought: Both their linguistic limitations and egocentric views of the world mean that young children are not often susceptible to social influence. So, the conflict-induced changes deriving from "equilibration" (as described here) occur most readily among children who can sustain logical argument and discussion with others whose viewpoints differ from their own.

Vygotsky, Mead, and Internalization

Attempting to develop a psychological theory based on dialectical materialism, L. S. Vygotsky (1978) also assumed that cognitive advances are rooted in social interaction. The central process was described as "internalization," through which the child acquires both equipment for thinking and the social rules governing the use of this equipment. For social interaction to lead to cognitive development, conversation and modeling must occur within the "zone of proximal development," defined as the difference between what the child can accomplish independently and what can be achieved with the help of others, and must involve problem-solving attempts tuned to a level just beyond the child's own. These exchanges initially induce cognitive change at an external (social) level that gradually becomes "interiorized." The child is an active participant in these events, so that internalized skills are not necessarily identical to what the socializing agent represents. Moreover, they are generalized and abstract, not situation specific (Rogoff, 1998).

Across the world's cultures, the social interaction needed for cognitive development occurs with individuals of many different ages. While expert collaborators are usually needed for the social interactions that lead to internalization, effective collaborators are not always adults. In fact, experience with peers is significant in social and cognitive development, because play and child-caretaking offer many learning opportunities rarely found in interaction with adults.

George Herbert Mead (1934) shared the idea that cognitive attributes originate in social interaction. Most readers associate this writer with his notions about the social origins of the self, but these notions were actually part of a more general theory, whereby social interaction is understood to be the main vehicle driving cognitive development. Within conversations and gestures (a broader construct than hand waving) lies the basis for the construction of symbolic thought. Linguistic and other symbols occurring in interaction gradually become internalized through their use in cooperative exchanges. "The probable beginning of human communication was in cooperation, not in imitation, where the conduct differed and yet where the act of the one answered to and called out the act of the other" (Mead, 1909, p. 406). Actions of individuals toward one another become significant symbols when, over time, they function in the same way with one individual as with others. Mind and self, according to this view, are constructed through the interiorization of symbols and linguistic behaviors originating in social interaction. One assumes that peer relations advance symbolic interiorization as well as do adult–child relations.

Attribution Theory

When children observe other children or interact with them, successive actions depend on the way children perceive, understand, and explain behavioral outcomes. The notion that an understanding of the connection between "cause" and "effect" bears on ongoing behavior comes originally from Heider (1958) and has become a major tenet in social-cognitive thought. Children's attributions have been studied most extensively in relation to cause and effect in aggressive interaction and noncompliance, and to some extent in prosocial and cooperative behavior.

Making attributions is a complex activity: It involves understanding the correlation between cause and effect, deciding among alternative attributions, understanding events in terms of their distinctiveness and consistency over time, and determining whether knowledge other than causal information is needed to make relevant attributions (Kelley, 1973). Immediately, then, questions arise as to whether attributional processes are evident in the social interactions of the very young. Young children's understanding of intentionality is constrained in many ways (Shultz, 1980), but 4-year-olds nevertheless believe it appropriate to respond to hostile provocation with aggressive retaliation, especially when provocation is unambiguous (cf. Ferguson & Rule, 1988).

Information Processing

Information-processing models of social behavior involving children and their peers were designed to account for the manner in which cognitive processes mediate social behavior. Based on the scripts and schemas derived from prior experience and biological dispositions, children are thought to respond to social events by encoding selected information from the ongoing event, representing it in memory, accessing one or several potential responses from memory, deciding among them, and activating a behavioral response utilizing their linguistic and motor repertoires (Dodge, 1986; Rubin & Krasnor, 1986). The information-processing sequence can include both emotional and cognitive elements; these cycles are supposedly iterative, and more than one sequence can occur at a time (Crick & Dodge, 1994).

Although the social information-processing model is presumed to apply broadly to interaction in every social domain, its features have been tested most extensively with aggression. This literature demonstrates, by and large, that aggressive children encode and utilize information relating to aggression differently from nonaggressive children and possess different processing "styles" that are correlated with measures of aggressive behavior (Crick & Dodge, 1994).

Context

Peer influences are contextualized to a greater extent than this account indicates. The extent to which conversation or modeling affects a child depends on the setting in which it occurs, the child being influenced, the child who is the influence source, their relationship to one another, behaviors at issue, group norms, and many other cultural and social conditions. Peer interaction always involves specific children with unique socialization histories, differing histories of interaction with one another, specific content (what the interaction is about), and a unique setting (a situation in time and place). The idea that these conditions moderate social influences is an ecological notion, one that bears a strong relation to the ideas of writers who have demonstrated the close relation between behavior and the settings and social situations in which it occurs (Barker & Wright, 1955; Bronfenbrenner, 1979). Not every contextual characteristic moderates every kind of social influence, but the issue is knowing when to incorporate relevant ones into a research or intervention model.

Peer Relationships

Socialization does not consist of myriad influence attempts scattered helter-skelter across millions of transactions with innumerable partners. Rather, the social encounters of human beings occur within organized frameworks that comprise interlocking relationships embedded in interlocking social networks. Most writers regard this design for living as having evolved with the species to protect individuals from environmental danger and increase chances of reproductive success.

"Relationships," defined as aggregations of interactions that endure over time and that form the basis for reciprocal interpersonal expectations (Hinde, 1997), are thus basic social contexts. Competence in communication, impulse regulation, getting along with others, and knowledge about the world emerge mostly from early relationships and are refined continuously within them. Relationships are resources that buffer one from stress and are instruments for both cooperative and competitive problem solving. Relationships are also forerunners of other relationships. No wonder, then, that well-functioning relationships have a bearing on mental and physical health, mortality, and well-being. Moreover, these synergies "do not appear to be artifacts of personality, temperament, behavior, or lifestyles but instead reflect the direct influence of relationship events on biological processes" (Reis & Collins, 2004, p. 233).

Psychodynamic Theories

The theory of psychosexual development enunciated by Sigmund Freud (1905/1953) aroused both contemporary controversy and continued discomfort among younger psychoanalysts and students of personality development. Most analysts did not question the importance of biological drives in behavioral functioning but, at the same time, many believed that interpersonal relations rather than vicissitudes of the libido are the major vectors of personality development. Even among those analysts who were comfortable with libido theory were some who thought that insufficient attention had been given to psychosocial experiences in personality development. Indeed, several psychoanalysts made the case that although mother–child relationships seem to be responsible for early individuation, ego development reflects relationships with other children (compeers) as well.

Harry Stack Sullivan (1953) constructed a general theory known as the "interpersonal theory" of psychiatry. According to these views, biological needs drive the individual toward satisfaction (absence of tension), whereas interpersonal relations are aimed at achieving security. In the earliest stages of development, a self "dynamism" comes to be organized around the "good me" and the "bad me," a differentiation that emerges largely from mother–child interaction. Parental approval and disapproval remain paramount in early childhood, resulting in the acquisition of basic norms and knowledge about one's culture. Beginning with the juvenile era, which follows, children make sharper self–other distinctions and become preoccupied with comparisons involving compeers. Social skills necessary for cooperation and competition, and a sense of "reputation" emerge based on interaction with other children. But it is only during preadolescence that most children locate a chum (usually of the same sex), and it is this event that produces real sensitivity to what matters to another person (empathy) and abandonment of the egocentric orientations of earlier childhood.

Preadolescent chumships were likened to love, recognizing that this is "isophilic" love, that is, love of one's own kind. These "integrating tendencies," as Sullivan called them, give children new expansiveness in interpersonal relations; they can express themselves freely to their companions, experience intimacy without fear of rebuff or humiliation, and discover "consensual validation" (agreement with their friends) on many aspects of normative behavior and attitudes. Still buffered by institutions such as the family and the school, preadolescents now have the chance, with friends, to explore interpersonal relations in ways that will be needed in adulthood. Development during adolescence itself is marked by the emergence of what Sullivan called the "lust dynamism," which transforms the adolescent's social networks so as to center on opposite-sex peers but with intimacy and empathic needs intact.

Other than the relationship between mother and child in infancy, close relationships do not appear in Erik Erikson's (1968) theory of personality development until young adulthood. Best known for the formulation of "psychosocial stages" that parallel the well-known stages of psychosexual development (even going beyond them into old age), this theory expands on libido theory rather than replaces it, postulating a series of crises, tensions, or polarities that the child must resolve during each stage to confront and assimilate the demands of succeeding stages.

Erikson regarded preadolescence as dominated by work, mastering the cognitive and social skills needed in the real world and school, acquiring competence in self-regulation, and developing talents that are gratifying and useful in one's culture. Preadolescents learn much from peers and may develop close affiliations with them, but these relationships and the accompanying challenges are not the main developmental tasks: Those remain "industry" required for mastery in home, school, and community, and, subsequently, "identity." In his volume, *Identity: Youth and Crisis* (1968), Erikson asserted that close relationships with others are not possible until identity development is complete, because intimacy requires knowing and sharing the self. Thus, relationships with friends and romantic partners during this period are ultimately in the service of identity exploration. Once again, the needs for intimacy and reciprocity are linked to success in close relationships. Note, however, that Erikson believed that the relevant events occur a decade later in the individual's development than was thought to be the case by Harry Stack Sullivan.

Other psychoanalytic theorists, such as Freud, gave little attention to peer relationships as a significant feature of personality development. One exception was Peter Blos (1979), who regarded peer relationships as critical in promoting the individual's "second individuation" from parents. In early childhood, children acquire a basis for separating "self from other" in the anxieties, approval–disapproval, and tangled elements of attraction to mothers and fathers. In adolescence, however, driven by erotic drives and the desire to affiliate with compeers, children begin a second restructuring of their relationships with their parents, in which self-regulation begins to supplant the regulation of the child's life by parents. In the course of this restructuring, adolescents turn to peers for belongingness and empathy.

Although these three psychoanalytic writers believed in a somewhat different timetable as to when peer relationships become transcendent in social life, there is agreement that intimacy, empathy, and loyalty in peer relationships emerge mainly in the second decade of life. Each of these writers took pains to argue that social epigenesis is not complete without a description of how close relationships with compeers (including romantic partners) enter the picture and what functions they serve.

Attachment Theory and the Organizational View of Adaptation

Present-day attachment theory is the work of many individuals. Sigmund Freud (1914/1957) began this work by outlining the anaclitic relationship that develops between infant and mother on the basis of the need gratification she provides. John Bowlby (1958) reconceptualized the attachment relationship as a feedback system not dependent on primary gratification and outlined its functions in evolutionary terms; early attachments were believed to protect the infant from danger, as well as to orient it toward caregiving sources that can provide nourishment, a basis for emotional regulation, and knowledge about language and the world. Bowlby (1969) also formulated the construct "inner working models" to describe the cognitive residuals provided by these early relationships and the notion that individuals carry these models forward using them later in close relationships with other persons. Mary Ainsworth (see Ainsworth, Blehar, Waters, & Wall, 1978) advanced two notions, namely, that among the most important functions of early attachments is the provision of "security," a construct tracing back through William Blatz (1966) to Harry Stack Sullivan and others, and that security in the child's adaptation is promoted by "sensitive caregiving."

Building upon these contributions, Alan Sroufe and Everett Waters (1977) advocated an organizational perspective on social development that considers the "organization" of emotion, cognition, and social behavior exhibited anywhere in development to be central to defining individual differences. Such organization derives from early relationships, especially with the primary caregiver (Sroufe, Egeland, Carlson, & Collins, 2005). Early attachments set the stage for peer relationships by not only providing the child with a secure base for expanding his or her social experience beyond the family but also by carrying forward a working model of relationships. Early relationships between child and caregiver continue to bear a direct relation to later relationships within the family and to peer competence outside it. Social development, however, is better described as a series of intertwined or complementary influences in which the quality of early family relationships has a bearing on some aspects of peer relationships (e.g., whether the child has a friend), whereas peer competence bears on others (e.g., the quality of the child's friendships). Empirical demonstration shows that these linkages extend through early adulthood and also involve romantic relationships (see Collins & Madsen, 2005).

Cognitive Viewpoints

Robert Selman (1980) suggests that developmental transformations occur in children's thinking about friendships in a more or less invariant order that is linked to the development of perspective taking in early and middle childhood. These developments begin when "friends" are regarded only as "playmates" (Stage 0); change when children regard one another as supplying primary gratification (Stage 1); regard themselves as involved in reciprocal relationships (Stage 2), then see these relationships as reciprocal ones (Stage 3), and finally conceive relationships as encompassing both dependence on one another and independence (Stage 4).

One must also note that the described developmental progression may not consist of the emergence of new and unrelated notions about friendship but rather reflect transformations in the child's understanding of reciprocity. Direct reciprocity (as opposed to complementary reciprocity) seems to underlie friendship expectations at all ages. James Youniss (1980) argued that, early in middle childhood, children expect friendship interaction to involve matched contributions by the children; during preadolescence, the reciprocities of friendship extend to cooperation and equal treatment of one another. Early adolescence extends these reciprocities even further to include a sense that friends share identities: "I" and "You" become "We." Once again, the conclusion seems warranted that reciprocities define friendship expectations—at all ages. Willard Hartup (1996) goes on to use a linguistic metaphor to describe these circumstances, namely, that whereas reciprocity constitutes the deep structure of friendship at all ages, the social behaviors exemplifying this construct change with age.

Behavior Systems Theory

Combining elements derived from Sullivan's interpersonal theory, attachment theory, and cognitive theory, Wyndol Furman uses a behavior systems orientation in research involving peer and romantic relationships (e.g., Furman & Wehner, 1994). A "behavior system" is a goal-corrected partnership functioning to maintain a tie between the individual and his or her partners. Four such systems are believed to dominate interpersonal relationships—attachment, caretaking, affiliative, and sexual/reproductive—each having a different degree of importance in different developmental epochs. The attachment system, for example, dominates parent–child relations during the early years but functions in reconfigured and less prominent ways in peer and romantic relationships during adolescence. The affiliative system, encompassing play, cooperation, collaboration, and reciprocity, appears initially in parent–child relations but comes to dominate relations with compeers in childhood (Weiss, 1986). Romantic relationships during adolescence incorporate both of these systems, but caretaking and sexual/reproductive systems are added. The individual's cognitive representations or "views" of these systems parallel behavioral functioning and reflect the developmental changes across childhood and adolescence that mark the systems themselves (see Furman & Collins, Chapter 19, this volume).

Social Exchange Theory

The various ideas that constitute social exchange theory are based on the observation that human beings survive and reproduce only by exchanging resources. The term "social exchange" does not mean "social interaction"; rather, it refers to resource-based exchanges that occur between individuals. One key assumption is that human beings attempt to maximize benefits and rewards (actually rewards minus costs) by engaging in interactions with others.

The nature of the social exchange begins to affect individuals during their first encounters in terms of expectations and behavior toward one another. Should ensuing interactions be mutually rewarding, the tendency for partners to seek out one another grows stronger and the likelihood of future interactions greater. "Interdependence" is the state of affairs that exists when individuals become dependent on one another for numerous and significant rewards (Kelley et al., 1983). The rewards and costs relevant to close relationships are varied, and some are unique to specific relationships. Social rewards, such as the experience of intimacy and closeness, are major supports for the emergence and maintenance of relationships, whereas competition, aggression, and conflict are major costs. When interdependencies are strong, encompass diverse situations and activities, and recur over substantial periods, one can consider the individuals as being in a "close" relationship (Berscheid, Snyder, & Omoto, 1989).

Two kinds of relationships may be identified depending on the equities involved: "Communal relationships" involve mutual recognition of one another's needs, and the assumption that rewards and costs will be equitable over time without close monitoring; "exchange relationships," on the other hand, depend on giving benefits, with the expectation that one will receive comparable benefits in return (Clark & Mills, 1979). Communal relationships can be symmetrical or asymmetrical in terms of the responsibility that individuals take for one another. Friendships and romantic relationships are mostly symmetrical, whereas parent–child relationships and some sibling relationships mostly are not.

Social exchange theories seem rigid and materialistic to many critics, but the interdependencies that come with these exchanges occur in many everyday contexts. As an investigator, one may prefer to regard relationships as resting on security, empathy, or the need for intimacy (see earlier discussion). But there can be little doubt that interpersonal exchanges based on social equity are evident in all cultures and facilitate coordinated social behavior (Laursen & Graziano, 2002). Given that nearly every theory relating to the formation and functioning of children's friendships stresses reciprocity, it is surprising that exchange theory has not been exploited more extensively in relevant research. Increasingly, however, this theory drives research on romantic relationships in adolescence (Furman & Collins, Chapter 19, this volume).

Peer Groups

Social experience for most children and adolescents includes banding together in collectives with two or three other children, sometimes many more. Friendships and other dyadic relationships are sometimes embedded or nested in groups, sometimes not. In any event, children's groups are more than the sum of the dyadic relationships existing within them. Groups have unique characteristics; they vary in size, cohesiveness, density, and structure in ways that relationships do not. Collectives become groups when social interaction among the members occurs regularly; values are shared, beyond those common to every child or adolescent in the culture; members have a sense of belonging; and a structure exists that supports the norms that brought the members together in the first place.

Children belong to some groups even though they do not seek membership; families and classrooms are examples. Membership in other groups is more volitional. Either way, social functioning depends on whether the group serves "reference" functions, that is, whether members are identified with it and want to continue being members.

Groups are conceived differently by younger and older children, and concepts continue to change during adolescence. Preschool-age children have little sense of group awareness and even young school-age children identify their play groups as collections of interlocking twosomes. Conceptions of peer groups as homogenous communities or cultures is largely a phenomenon of adolescence, and the idea that these groups are also pluralistic entities is an advanced notion (Jacquette, 1976).

Sociometrics and Social Networks

Sociometrics

"Sociometry" refers to the sociological thought of Jacob L. Moreno, whose work was published largely between 1925 and 1960, as well as that of other investigators working in the same tradition. The best-known element in this system is the sociometric test, which is used to measure attraction and repulsion existing between two persons. First introduced in the monograph *Who Shall Survive?* (Moreno, 1934), the theoretical system encompasses "experimental sociometrics" and its use to study individual adaptation within the peer context, group psychotherapy, and the psychodrama. The monograph contains data from several kinds of participants: Most were adult inmates of either prisons or psychiatric hospitals, but some work was also done with children and adolescents (e.g., girls incarcerated in a training school). Helen Jennings (1937–1938) was probably responsible for popularization of sociometry with children, an application that was then taken up by many others, including Mary Northway, Norman Gronlund, and Urie Bronfenbrenner, who contributed important methodological and quantitative innovations (Cillessen & Bukowski, 2000).

Several assumptions marked Moreno's theorizing: First, individuals are conceived as "social atoms," that is, the person considered together with other individuals who want to be associated with him or her. Second, assessment of the individual's social adaptation is based on the assumption that attraction and repulsion are orthogonal processes in social relations (subsequent studies have shown this assumption to be true; see Cillessen, Chapter 5, this volume). Third, sociometric assessment refers both to how the individual perceives others, in terms of liking and repulsion, and how others perceive the individual. Fourth, sociometric tests can be based on a range of information, including who wants to associate with whom; who wants to engage in certain activities with someone else; and who likes someone, dislikes someone, or does not want to associate with the other person. Fifth, quantification can take either of two basic directions: (1) Information about attraction and repulsion can be used to construct "sociograms" revealing social networks existing within a collective, as well as the individual's centrality within them; or (2) respondents' nominations can be used to calculate "sociometric scores," that is, aggregated assessments of attraction and repulsion toward the individual that are expressed by the other members of the group.

Many persons contributed to sociometric methodology over the years and no "gold standard" exists even today (Cillessen, Chapter 5, this volume). Scores based on the number of children who like or dislike an associate are used in some investigations, but in others, more elaborate derivations are used to classify children as popular, rejected, neglected, and controversial (Coie, Dodge, & Coppotelli, 1982; Newcomb & Bukowski, 1983). A conceptual change suggested by Craig Peery (1979) was important in the development of these latter assessments, to wit, that the dimensionality of sociometric status should be based in "social preference" and "social impact" rather than attraction and repulsion.

Social Networks

Social network analysis now comprises a large body of research within sociology. Its aims are to describe the manner in which individual lives are embedded in networks involving many different people, ways of thinking about these networks both qualitatively and quantitatively, the social processes involved in their creation, and their impact on individuals.

Sociograms are the basis for certain kinds of network analysis. Sociometric tests, of course, require the assessment of attraction or rejection of every member of the group by every other member, making network analysis difficult in situations involving large groups that extend beyond classrooms and schools. Children and adolescents, however, are knowledgeable informants about "who hangs out with whom," making it possible through "social-cognitive mapping" (Kindermann & Gest, Chapter 6, this volume) to identify members of social networks, the centrality of individual members to the network, the cohesiveness of the network, and various other characteristics. Robert and Beverly Cairns (1994) believe that these networks figure importantly in working out individual adaptations during preadolescence and adolescence, constituting "lifelines" when they are supportive and consonant with children's conventional norms but "risks" when composed of aggressive and antisocial children. Social networks gain this significance, in their view, owing to the homophilies (similarities) that exist within them.

Group Dynamics

"Group dynamics" is a term associated with a large body of theory and research on the character and functioning of (small) groups of adults. Some of the issues that have been central to adult studies have elicited similar work with children; scattered studies can be found dealing with cohesiveness, leadership, dominance, and other topics that supplement the adult literature. Although one would expect group dynamics to differ across ages, a developmental body of work on group dynamics has not emerged. Several issues, however, have been explored imaginatively with children.

Cooperation and Competition

Children's performance is generally enhanced under equitable goal structures (i.e., rules that provide for the equal sharing of rewards regardless of variations in individual performance; see Hartup, 1983). Cooperation and its twin, reciprocity, figure centrally in relationship formation and functioning, as described earlier, so it is not surprising that cooperative norms have pervasive influence on the functioning of small groups.

Kurt Lewin and his students provided evidence early on (Lewin, Lippitt, & White, 1938) that the type of adult leadership greatly influences the "group atmosphere" of small, ad hoc groups of children working on various tasks. Building on the ideas that he called "field theory," Lewin proposed that groups with democratic leaders who promote cooperation, the expression of ideas, and consensus would interact differently and be more productive than groups with authoritarian or laissez-faire leaders. This classic work was applied to both classrooms and to politics, and was widely interpreted as demonstrating the superiority of democratic working conditions at all ages. The results are consistent with a large body of evidence supporting the idea that cooperation and participation among group members create cohesive and friendly relations within groups and increase their output (under most conditions).

Norms and Social Identity Theory

Cooperation and competition were also targeted by Muzafer and Carolyn Sherif in a series of classic studies dealing with goal structures and their effects on both intra- and intergroup relations (Sherif & Sherif, 1953; Sherif, Harvey, White, Hood, & Sherif, 1961). The theoretical basis for this work was built, first, on an understanding of "norms" in social relations. Collectives, including twosomes, become groups only when norms that are generated distinguish group members from others and promote solidarity in members' social relations with one another. A series of field experiments, completed in the 1940s and 1950s, demonstrated vividly how norms govern informal peer groups, and how cooperation and competition affect both group members' relationships with one another and with other groups.

Social identity theory (Tajfel, 1981) also deals with group formation, intragroup relations, and intergroup relations. Some of the best known ideas within this theoretical framework include the notions that once groups are established, members accentuate differences between themselves and other groups, exaggerating their own positive attributes but overstating the negative characteristics of other groups and their members. Members reinforce these characterizations during interaction within groups, and these validations enhance group identity and solidarity.

Reference Groups

Groups with which the individual identifies or to which he or she aspires to belong are called "reference groups." Numerous individuals have contributed to current ideas about the structure and functioning of reference groups. Dexter Dunphy (1969), who was a participant observer in many adolescent reference groups, outlined five stages in their organization, beginning with unisex cliques and extending to the time when heterosexual couples pair off, crowds begin to disintegrate, and members interact in loosely associated groups of couples. Based on their intensive studies of a dozen adolescent reference groups, Muzafer and Carolyn Sherif (1964) made a particularly powerful argument that both the functioning of these groups and their impact on individuals is directly related to the cultural context in which they are embedded.

Reference groups are sometimes differentiated according to whether they are cliques or crowds, even though the distinction is a blurry one. Crowds are the larger entities and are usually based in reputations and relationships. Bradford Brown (Brown, Mory, & Kinney, 1994) believes crowds serve two major functions: fostering the individual's sense of identity and providing structure for social interaction. Adolescents carry out these functions (1) by characterizing their own and other crowds in terms of perceived traits and stereotypes; (2) by channeling members so that relationships are formed between some individuals and not others; and (3) by serving as contexts for interpersonal relationships, so that these relationships reflect crowd norms, social orientation, and social status.

One other entity deserves comment—the peer culture. This construct refers to values and orientations characteristic of children or adolescents as a whole. Whether one can meaningfully refer to the peer culture in early childhood is questionable, even though children form themselves into informal groups at very early ages. But whether the "moods and message" of a generation (Brown, 1999) are understood by preschool-age children in any meaningful sense in unlikely. Gradually, though, in middle childhood, one can identify an ethos that represents the peer culture to most children. This "youth culture" figures importantly in many writings about adolescence and is assumed to have socializing effects—mostly through the crowds and other small groups to which adolescents belong (see Brown & Dietz, Chapter 20, this volume).

Conclusion

Theoretical views in peer relations research remain diverse. Investigators must pick and chose from a theoretical smorgasbord (as well as develop their own variations) to match their research questions. Nevertheless, certain commonalities mark the viewpoints surveyed in this chapter. First, every theoretical notion mentioned assumes that the significance of peer relations in human development derives from the equal status of the participants. Whether considered in terms of chronological age, cognitive capacities, or social experience, peer relations are unique forces in human development because the individuals involved are equals. Second, most of these notions suggest that the special significance of peer relations for children and adolescents derives from the fact that the individuals involved are not mature adults. Third, most of these viewpoints recognize some construct such as reciprocity is responsible for the creation of sustained relations among children and consequences for them as individuals.

The word "reciprocity" is not always mentioned in these formulations. Cooperation may be the construct of choice, or equity, intimacy, or attraction. Even so, the one intrinsic element to all of these constructs is mutual exchange. Whether it be the direct exchange of resources or complementary exchanges does not matter. Sustained interactions, influences, relationships, and group structures only become recognizable in child–child relations when reciprocity is somewhere in the picture. Finally, one needs to observe how human adaptation seems to require that individuals experience a range of these reciprocities during the first two decades of life for optimum outcomes to be achieved.

These arguments do not deny the enormous developmental contributions made by social relations involving children with older or younger associates, especially adults. They assert only that during the first two decades of life, certain reciprocities are most easily achieved with agemates and are therefore most likely to be the ones that provide the cooperation, intimacy, and collaborative problem solving that mature adaptation requires.

References

Ainsworth, M. D. S., Blehar, M. C., Waters, E., & Wall, S. (1978). *Patterns of attachment: A psychological study of the Strange Situation*. Hillsdale, NJ: Erlbaum.

Bandura, A. (1977). *Social learning theory*. Morristown, NJ: General Learning Press.

Barker, R. G., & Wright, H. F. (1955). *Midwest and its children*. New York: Harper & Row.

Berscheid, E., Snyder, M., & Omoto, A. M. (1989). The Relationship Closeness Inventory: Assessing the closeness of interpersonal relationships. *Journal of Personality and Social Psychology, 57*, 792–807.

Blatz, W. (1966). *Human security*. Toronto: University of Toronto Press.

Blos, P. (1979). *The adolescent passage*. New York: International Universities Press.

Bowlby, J. (1958). The nature of the child's tie to his mother. *International Journal of Psycho-Analysis, 39*, 350–373.

Bowlby, J. (1969). *Attachment and loss: Vol. 1. Attachment*. New York: Basic Books.

Bronfenbrenner, U. (1979). *The ecology of human development*. Cambridge, MA: Harvard University Press.

Brown, B. B. (1999). Measuring the peer environment of American adolescents. In S. L. Friedman & T. D. Wachs (Eds.), *Measuring environment across the life span* (pp. 59–90). Washington, DC: American Psychological Association.

Brown, B. B., Mory, M. S., & Kinney, D. (1994). Casting adolescent crowds in a relational perspective: Caricature, channel, and context. In R. Montemayor, G. R. Adams, & T. P. Gullotta (Eds.), *Personal relationships during adolescence* (pp. 133–167). Thousand Oaks, CA: Sage.

Cairns, R. B., & Cairns, B. D. (1994). *Lifelines and risks*. Cambridge, UK: Cambridge University Press.

Cillessen, A. H. N., & Bukowski, W. M. (Eds.). (2000). Recent advances in the measurement of acceptance and rejection in the peer system. *New Directions for Child and Adolescent Development* (No. 88). San Francisco: Jossey-Bass.

Clark, M. S., & Mills, J. (1979). Interpersonal attraction in exchange and communal relationships. *Journal of Personality and Social Psychology, 37*, 12–24.

Coie, J. D., Dodge, K. A., & Coppotelli, H. (1982). Dimensions and types of social status: A cross-age perspective. *Developmental Psychology, 18*, 557–570.

Collins, W. A., & Madsen, S. D. (2005). Personal relationships in adolescence and early adulthood. In A. L. Vangelisti & D. Perlman (Eds.), *The Cambridge handbook of personal relationships* (pp. 191–209). New York: Cambridge University Press.

Crick, N. R., & Dodge, K. A. (1994). A review and reformulation of social information processing mechanisms in children's social adjustment. *Psychological Bulletin, 115*, 74–101.

Dishion, T. J., Andrews, D. W., & Crosby, L. (1995). Anti-social boys and their friends in early adolescence: Relationship characteristics, quality, and interactional processes. *Child Development, 66*, 139–151.

Dodge, K. A. (1986). A social information processing model of social competence in children. In M. Perlmutter (Ed.), *The Minnesota Symposia on Child Psychology: Cognitive perspectives on children's social and behavioral development* (Vol. 18, pp. 77–125). Hillsdale, NJ: Erlbaum.

Dollard, J., & Miller, N. E. (1950). *Personality and psychotherapy*. New York: McGraw-Hill.

Dollard, J., Miller, N. E., Doob, L. W., Mowrer, O. H., & Sears, R. R., with Ford, C. S., Hovland, C. L., & Sollenberger, R. T. (1939). *Frustration and aggression*. New Haven, CT: Yale University Press.

Dunphy, D. C. (1969). *Cliques, crowds, and gangs*. Melbourne: Cheshire.

Erikson, E. H. (1968). *Identity: Youth and crisis*. New York: Norton.

Ferguson, T. J., & Rule, B. G. (1988). Children's evaluations of retaliatory aggression. *Child Development, 59*, 961–968.

Freud, S. (1953). Three essays on the theory of sexuality. In J. Strachey (Ed.), *The standard edition of the complete psychological works of Sigmund Freud* (Vol. 7, pp. 125–245). London: Hogarth Press. (Original work published in 1905)

Freud, S. (1957). On narcissism. In J. Strachey (Ed.), *The standard edition of the complete psychological works of Sigmund Freud* (Vol. 14, pp. 67–102). London: Hogarth Press. (Original work published 1914)

Furman, W., & Wehner, E. A. (1994). Romantic views: Toward a theory of adolescent romantic relationships. In R. Montemayor, G. R. Adams, & T. P. Gullotta (Eds.), *Personal relationships during adolescence* (pp. 168–195). Thousand Oaks, CA: Sage.

Harlow, H. F. (1969). Age-mate or peer affectional system. *Advances in the Study of Behavior, 2,* 333–383.

Hartup, W. W. (1983). Peer relations. In P. H. Mussen (Series Ed.) & E. M. Hetherington (Vol. Ed.), *Handbook of child psychology* (4th ed.): *Vol. 4. Socialization, personality, and social development* (pp. 103–196). New York: Wiley.

Hartup, W. W. (1996). The company they keep: Friendships and their developmental significance. *Child Development, 67,* 1–13.

Heider, F. (1958). *The psychology of interpersonal relations.* New York: Wiley.

Hinde, R. A. (1997). *Relationships.* Hove, UK: Psychology Press.

Hull, C. L. (1943). *Principles of behavior.* New York: Appleton–Century–Crofts.

Jacquette, D. (1976). *Developmental stages in peer group organization: A cognitive developmental analysis of peer group concepts in childhood and adolescence.* Unpublished manuscript, Harvard University, Cambridge, MA.

Jennings, H. H. (1937–1938). Structure of leadership: Development and sphere of influence. *Sociometry, 1,* 99–143.

Kelley, H. H. (1973). The processes of causal attribution. *American Psychologist, 28,* 107–128.

Kelley, H. H., Berscheid, E., Christensen, A., Harvey, J. H., Huston, T. L., Levinger, G., et al. (1983). *Close relationships.* New York: Freeman.

Laursen, B., & Graziano, W. G. (Eds.). (2002). Social exchange in development. *New Directions for Child and Adolescent Development* (No. 95). San Francisco: Jossey-Bass.

Lewin, K., Lippitt, R., & White, R. K. (1938). Patterns of aggressive behavior in experimentally created "social climates." *Journal of Social Psychology, 10,* 271–299.

Masters, J. C., Ford, M. E., Arend, R., Grotevant, H. D., & Clark, L. V. (1979). Modeling and labeling as integrated determinants of children's sex-typed imitative behavior. *Child Development, 50,* 364–371.

Mead, G. H. (1909). Social psychology as counterpart to physiological psychology. *Psychological Bulletin, 6,* 401–408.

Mead, G. H. (1934). *Mind, self and society.* Chicago: University of Chicago Press.

Miller, N. E., & Dollard, J. (1941). *Social learning and imitation.* New Haven, CT: Yale University Press.

Moreno, J. L. (1934). *Who shall survive?* Washington, DC: Nervous and Mental Disease Publishing Company.

Newcomb, A. F., & Bukowski, W. M. (1983). Social impact and social preference as determinants of childrens' group status. *Developmental Psychology, 19,* 856–867.

Patterson, G. R., Littman, R. A., & Bricker, W. (1967). Assertive behavior in children: A step toward a theory of aggression. *Monographs of the Society for Research in Child Development, 32*(5, Serial No. 113).

Patterson, G. R., Reid, J. B., & Dishion, T. J. (1992). *Antisocial boys.* Eugene, OR: Castalia.

Peery, J. C. (1979). Popular, amiable, isolated, rejected: A reconceptualization of sociometric status in preschool children. *Child Development, 50,* 1231–1234.

Piaget, J. (1926). *The language and thought of the child.* New York: Harcourt Brace.

Piaget, J. (1932). *The moral judgment of the child.* Glencoe, IL: Free Press.

Poulin, F., Dishion, T. J., & Haas, E. (1999). The peer influence paradox: Friendship quality and deviancy training within male adolescent friendships. *Merrill–Palmer Quarterly, 45,* 42–61.

Reis, H. T., & Collins, W. A. (2004). Relationships, human behavior, and psychological science. *Current Directions in Psychological Science, 13*, 233–237.

Rogoff, B. (1998). Cognition as a collaborative process. In W. Damon (Series Ed.), D. Kuhn & R. S. Sigler (Vol. Eds.), *Handbook of child psychology* (5th ed., Vol. 2, pp. 679–744). New York: Wiley.

Rubin, K. H., & Krasnor, L. R. (1986). Social-cognitive and social behavioral perspectives on problem solving. In M. Perlmutter (Ed.), *The Minnesota Symposia on Child Psychology: Vol. 18. Cognitive perspectives on children's social and behavioral development* (pp. 1–68). Hillsdale, NJ: Erlbaum.

Schank, R. C., & Abelson, R. P. (1977). *Scripts, plan, goals and understanding.* Hillsdale, NJ: Erlbaum.

Selman, R. (1980). *The growth of interpersonal understanding.* New York: Academic Press.

Sherif, M., Harvey, O. J., White, B.J., Hood, W. R., & Sherif, C. W. (1961). *Intergroup conflict and cooperation: The Robbers Cave experiment.* Norman, OK: University Book Exchange.

Sherif, M., & Sherif, C. W. (1953). *Groups in harmony and tension.* New York: Harper.

Sherif, M., & Sherif, C. W. (1964). *Reference groups.* New York: Harper & Row.

Shultz, T. R. (1980). Development of the concept of intention. In W. A. Collins (Ed.), *The Minnesota Symposia on Child Psychology: Vol. 13. Development of cognition, affect, and social relations* (pp. 131–164). Hillsdale, NJ: Erlbaum.

Sroufe, L. A., Egeland, B., Carlson, E. A., & Collins, W. A. (2005). *The development of the person.* New York: Guilford Press.

Sroufe, L. A., & Waters, E. (1977). Attachment as an organizational construct. *Child Development, 48*, 1184–1199.

Sullivan, H. S. (1953). *The interpersonal theory of psychiatry.* New York: Norton.

Tajfel, H. (1981). *Human groups and social categories: Studies in social psychology.* Cambridge, UK: Cambridge University Press.

Vygotsky, L. S. (1978). *Mind in society: The development of higher psychological processes.* Cambridge, MA: Harvard University Press.

Weiss, R. S. (1986). Continuities and transformations in social relationships from childhood to adulthood. In W. W. Hartup & Rubin, Z. (Eds.), *Relationships and development* (pp. 95–111). Hillsdale, NJ: Erlbaum.

Youniss, J. (1980). *Parents and peers in social development.* Chicago: University of Chicago Press.

CHAPTER 2

Trends, Travails, and Turning Points in Early Research on Children's Peer Relationships

Legacies and Lessons for Our Time?

GARY W. LADD

History is instructive. Often the study of history is justified on the grounds that knowledge of the past offers people a better understanding of the present (i.e., insight into how things came to be) and a better vantage from which to solve current and future problems (i.e., perspectives that eschew past mistakes). Given that scientific research has been conducted on children's peer relations for more than 100 years (see Ladd, 2005), sufficient time has passed for the discipline to have a history. Thus, it may be instructive to examine the discipline's past to see whether it contains lessons that are pertinent to present-day and future research objectives.

Overview of Chapter Objectives

The purpose of this chapter is to consider whether some of the trends, travails, and turning points that occurred in early research on children's peer relationships might be instructive for modern-day peer relations researchers. Accordingly, the substantive focus of this chapter is children's *relationships* with peers—specifically, friendship and peer group rejection. The historical frame is an interval that began in the late 1800s and ended in the late 1940s—an epoch in the history of the peer relations discipline that I have previously termed "the first generation of research on children's peer relations" (Ladd, 2005). My specific goals in undertaking this analysis were to consider whether developments that occurred in the discipline more than 60 years ago (1) created legacies that—for better or worse—continue to affect modern-day research, and (2) offer "lessons" that might help to guide, or perhaps change, the course of future peer relations research.

Trends, Travails, and Turning Points: Definitions and Analytic Utility

Imagine for a moment that, as a scientist, you were among the first to investigate children's peer relations. Suppose that no one had previously investigated children's peer relations, and there are no preexisting theories, research agendas, or bodies of evidence to guide your decisions about what to investigate. How would you begin your work? What would you choose to investigate? After arriving at a decision, how would you conceptualize the aspects of peer relations you chose to investigate, and how would you go about gathering relevant information (empirical data) on those phenomena? Finally, would your decisions have consequences? That is, might each of these decisions affect what you would learn about children's peer relations and, if you were to publish your findings, influence the way that other researchers thought about and studied the phenomena you chose to investigate?

Most likely, the scholars who first investigated children's peer relations were confronted by these same challenges; for our purposes, it might prove instructive to consider how they addressed them. To accomplish this aim, I have attempted to identify some of the trends, travails, and turning points that occurred in early research on children's friendships and peer group relations. The term "trend," as used herein, refers to a sequence of studies undertaken by one or more investigators to address a specific question about children's peer relations. Investigative trends, then, can be seen as indicators of the types of questions that early researchers chose to study and thought were important enough to pursue repeatedly across studies and over time. The identification of early trends, therefore, provides some insight into early peer relations researchers' investigative priorities.

"Travails" refer to the dilemmas and controversies that developed as early peer relations researchers attempted to address their questions empirically. This aspect of early peer relations research is illuminating, because it highlights the conceptual and methodological dilemmas that early researchers encountered as they investigated specific questions; it provides a context for understanding the approaches they took, or the "solutions" they devised to address these problems. Travails occur because natural phenomena—including aspects of children's peer relations—are inherently difficult to define and measure, especially in an investigative context in which no prior frameworks or methods exist for this purpose. For example, among other tasks, early peer relations researchers had to define the phenomena they wished to study (e.g., formulate constructs, such as "friendship"), specify referents for constructs (e.g., stipulate empirical indicators; create operational definitions), and devise ways of measuring constructs (e.g., invent reliable and valid ways to index a construct's empirical referents).

The term "turning point" is used to describe a significant shift in the way that investigators address a specific travail or problem within an investigative trend or line of research. Turning points occur when researchers respond to travails with innovation—that is, devise new ways of addressing or overcoming existing conceptual or methodological problems. Some turning points may produce lasting "solutions" to research problems—that is, innovations that become dominant or enduring ways of addressing particular problems (e.g., accepted definitions, standard practices). Enduring innovations, especially those that perseverate over multiple generations of researchers, essentially become investigative paradigms or legacies. Other turning points may produce novel but short-lived solutions to conceptual and methodological problems. In some cases, the worth of these transient innovations is known—for example, early investigative efforts may have proven them to be ineffective or unproductive "solutions" for particular research questions or problems.

In other cases, however, transient innovations may have been abandoned before their worth was sufficiently estimated or realized. In the sections that follow, I take the position that some of the short-lived innovations introduced during early turning points deserve further consideration by modern-day peer relations researchers.

Defining and Describing Friendships and Friendship Relations

Friendship was one of the first aspects of children's peer relations that early researchers chose to investigate. The impetus for initial investigations appears to have been a desire to understand the origins of friendship, and investigators chose to address this question by researching factors that might guide children's and adolescent's friendship selection. Monroe (1898), for example, asked 2,336 children between the ages of 7 and 16 to write an essay in response to the question "What kind of a chum do you like the best?", then tabulated the frequency with which respondents mentioned the following six types of attributes in their papers: "age, sex, size, physical traits, habits, mental and moral traits" (p. 68). The findings suggested that most children wanted friends who were kind and agreeable, and of the same age, sex, and size. Expanding on this methodology, Bonser (1902) had 2,035 adolescents (12- to 22-year-olds) write compositions in which they were to provide several types of information about an "intimate" friendship, including age of onset, causes or precipitating factors, time spent with the friend, and similarity–differences in interests and dispositions. Based on frequency counts of respondent's replies, Bonser concluded that friendships began as early as infancy and, in young children, grew out of chance associations. Older children and adolescents, he inferred, were more likely to form friendships "for sympathy, for closer companionship, and for mutual confidence" (p. 226). Other conclusions were that adolescents tended to be friends with persons of the same age and gender, saw their friends regularly, and formed lasting relationships.

It is important to note that in these earliest of studies, researchers did not define "friendship" precisely but equated it with concepts such as "chum," "the intimate friend-ships of childhood and youth," and one's closest or constant "companions" (Monroe, 1898; Bonser, 1902). Little in these early writings suggests that researchers wrestled with the definition of "friendship" or deliberated over the validity of specific empirical indica-tors. Apparently, early researchers spared themselves these travails. Rather than propos-ing relatively objective, empirical indicators of friendship and gathering data on these indicators, investigators assumed that children's verbal reports were veridical and could be used to identify and gather information about their friendships. This approach to the study of friendships introduced by Monroe and Bonser was utilized by subsequent inves-tigators until the late 1920s and early 1930s (e.g., Jenkins, 1931; Warner, 1923), making it the principal way that friendships were defined and studied during the early 1900s.

It was during the early 1930s that investigators began to question whether friendships could be reliably identified and studied using only self-report data from children. At the heart of this travail was the concern that prior researchers had investigated children's and youth's friendships without looking at "actual" friendships. Hagman (1933), for example, criticized the way children's friendships had been studied by noting that investigators had "gone no further than the subject's verbally expressed choices to determine who [their] friends were," and that there had been no attempt "to correlate verbally expressed pref-erences with actual choices in work and play situations" (pp. 10–11). Similarly, Green

(1933) argued that investigators had attempted to understand friendships by gathering data from children who were *assumed to have friends*, without actually examining their relationships or the types of social exchanges that occurred in these relationships. A related concern was that the findings assembled on the origins and selection of friendships were invalid, because children and youth lacked an awareness of the "real reasons" for their friendship choices (see Challman, 1932, p. 146).

The solution or innovation that was proposed for this travail was to "determine which children really associate with each other" (Hagman, 1933; p. 12) and to develop empirical indicators of companionship or friendship (see Challman, 1932; Hagman, 1933). Hagman, in particular, argued that these objectives could best be achieved with newly developed observational techniques, such as those developed by Wellman (1926), Hubbard (1929) and Challman (1932). Wellman (1926), for example, created an "objective method ... for determining who were close friends within the school situation" (p. 126) and used it to identify friendships in a sample of 113 seventh, eighth, and ninth graders. Daily observations were conducted in school settings over a 5-month period, and pairs of children who were "seen together" most often were considered "friends." Unfortunately, the criterion used to determine when particular pairs of children had been "seen together" was not explicated. Similarly, Challman (1932) observed 33 preschoolers in a nursery school setting and noted the number of times that children were in the presence of each of their classmates. Estimates were made of the "strength" of friendships by dividing the number of times a pair of children had been seen together by the amount of time both members had been present in the classroom. Thus, pairs of children who were often observed together were considered to be "stronger" friends than pairs who were seldom in each other's company.

One of the more extensive observational studies of friendships was conducted with samples of 2- and 4-year-olds (Hagman, 1933). Unlike prior investigators, Hagman required that two conditions be met before a child could be coded as having a "friend." Not only was it necessary for the child to be in close proximity to the peer (i.e., spatially contiguous), but also the child had to exhibit certain forms of social responsiveness while in the presence of the peer. This child–partner responsiveness criterion ensured that peers who were simply standing nearby were not confused with actual companions or "friends." Children were observed during free-play periods, and a set of "companionship indices" was created for each child, indicating the frequency with which he or she associated with specific peers. Statistical analyses revealed that "a number of children associated with one, two, or three individuals and only infrequently with the remaining children in their group" (Hagman, 1933, p. 23). Thus, preschoolers' companionships, on average, did not appear to be evenly distributed across classmates but tended to be concentrated among a few peers. These findings were interpreted as evidence of "selectivity" in children's choice of "friends."

Green (1933) went a step further than Hagman by arguing that researchers needed to understand the *quality* of children's social exchanges before they could infer that pairs of peers were in fact friends. Accordingly, Green observed 40 preschoolers and recorded not only the number of times a child was near other classmates but also the extent to which the child interacted with these peers in a cooperative (friendly) or conflictual (quarrelsome) way. Every time a child interacted with a different classmate he or she was assigned a friendliness and a quarrelsomeness score for that peer. Each child's friendliness and quarrelsomeness scores were then summed across peers to create a total friendliness and a total quarrelsomeness score. Results showed that quarreling occurred in friendships, that preschoolers tended to form same-sex friendships, and that girls and older children were more likely to have friends.

The use of observation to study "actual" friendships during the late 1920s and early 1930s can be seen as a turning point, because investigators changed the way children's friendships were defined and investigated to overcome past conceptual and methodological problems. Conceptually, the assumption that friendships were self-evident was replaced with the proposition that "frequent association or companionship" was a defining feature of friendship. Over time, this operational definition was refined to include conditions such as child–partner responsiveness (i.e., making dyads the unit of analysis) and certain qualitative features of the dyad's interactions (e.g., friendly or quarrelsome exchanges). Methodologically, researchers abandoned (or, in some cases, supplemented; see Hagman, 1933) children's self-reports of friendship and instead used observed proximity between children as a marker for association or companionship. Based on this convention, metrics were created (e.g., frequency with which pairs of children were seen together) for the purpose of identifying friendships (i.e., friends were pairs of children who were seen together most often). As definitions of "friendship" changed to incorporate "process variables" (e.g., child–partner responsiveness, features of the dyad's interactions), the observational procedures and empirical criteria used to identify friendships became more complex. For example, in addition to noting a child's spatially contiguous companions, it became necessary for observers to differentiate specific dyads (i.e., identify potential friendship pairs), monitor the partner's behavior (e.g., capture the partner's reactions; Hagman, 1933), or characterize or code the nature of the interactions that occurred between dyad members (e.g., friendly vs. quarrelsome exchanges; Green 1933).

Defining and Describing Peer-Group Rejection

In addition to friendship, early researchers also investigated children's relations with members of their peer groups in contexts such as classrooms. In large part, researchers were interested in profiling the "structure" of children's peer groups and delineating the types of roles or relations that individual children developed with members of their group. One of the trends that emerged in early research on peer-group relations was driven by questions about how individuals "fit" into their peer groups and, in particular, whether some children developed poor relations with the majority of their groupmates or were relegated to low-status positions within their peer groups. Among researchers who sought to answer these questions, an enduring objective was to characterize (i.e., define and describe) the conditions under which it could be said that a child had poor peer-group relations. For many researchers, this task became one of stipulating relevant constructs and describing the intragroup dynamics that were indicative an individual's lack of fit with members of his or her peer group.

To address these questions, researchers turned to sociometry, which was originally developed by J. Moreno (1932, 1934) to learn about patterns of social preference among group members within settings such as juvenile detention centers and prisons. In these studies, individuals were asked to name members of their group with whom they would prefer to associate in real-life situations. When sociometry was adapted for research on children's peer-group relations in classrooms, investigators asked children to identify classmates that they liked or preferred for specific activities.

Koch (1933) was among the first to utilize sociometry as a means of describing children's peer-group relations (but see Hsia, 1928). She developed an index of "the success with which an individual has taken his place in a social group" (Koch, 1933, p. 164), and used a paired-comparison sociometric method to quantify this phenomenon. According to Koch (1933), successful group relations were indicated by the "extent to which [a child's] associates like to work and play with him" (p. 164). Accordingly, Koch's criterion for determining whether children fit into their social groups was whether they were *liked* by peers as play- and workmates in the classroom. To measure this criterion, Koch met individually with 17 preschoolers who attended the same classroom and presented them with pairs of classmates' names. For each pair of names presented, children were asked to indicate the classmate they liked best ("Which do you like best—Mary or Ann?" p. 165). Koch looked for patterns in children's sociometric choices as a means of understanding their peer preferences, and used the terms "popular" and "unpopular" to designate children who were most versus least liked by a majority of their classmates, respectively. Thus, within Koch's method of mapping intragroup relations, children who had poor peer-group relations (i.e., those who fit least well into their peer groups) were those whose classmates professed little liking toward them (i.e., desire to associate with them) as play- or workmates.

Following Koch, investigators continued to rely on sociometry to describe the interpersonal dynamics of peer groups and to characterize the social relations of children who were unsuccessful at "taking their place" among groupmates. Although there was some methodological consistency in the assessment of children's peer-group relations, changes occurred in way that investigators conceptualized poor or problematic peer-group relations. Unlike Koch, who construed children's group relations in terms of how much they were liked or preferred by peers, Lippitt (1941) was concerned about preschoolers whose social overtures were frequently "rejected" by peers. As the precipitating concern for her investigation, Lippitt noted that "some children continually appear to meet with rejection" (p. 305) and, in support of this point, she presented a case study that illustrated how one child's attempts to join play activities were consistently rebuffed by members of the child's peer group.

Even though persistent rejection appeared to be the facet of children's peer-group relations that concerned Lippitt (1941), she did not define this concept or incorporate it into her assessment scheme. Rather, she used Koch's paired-comparison method to assess the nature of children's peer-group relations. Individual sociometric interviews were conducted with 45 preschoolers who were enrolled in one of three different classrooms and, as in the Koch study, children were presented with pairs of classmates' names and asked to indicate which member of each pair they liked best. Children who fell in the lowest one-third of the distribution of aggregated liking scores were designated as "unpopular" among their peers. Thus, Lippitt assessed classmates' liking preferences rather than the extent to which they rejected other children's social overtures when she attempted to identify individuals who had poor peer-group relations.

Lippitt's suggestion that researchers examine children who were rejected by peers was followed by F. Moreno's (1942) proposition that it is essential to understand both "attraction and repulsion patterns" (p. 395) within peer groups. F. Moreno's study represented a turning point in the way children's intragroup relations were conceptualized and measured. She documented patterns of "acceptance" and "rejection" in peer groups using both sociometry and direct observations of children's social interactions. Essentially, F. Moreno's study departed from past work in not only the way intragroup relations were conceptualized but also the way these dynamics were measured.

F. Moreno (1942) took the position that it is important to investigate the social structure of peer groups as a means of understanding not only group processes (e.g., principles that "bind and separate children" [p. 395]), but also the group's effects on individual children. This investigator speculated, for example, that children who occupy certain social positions in peer groups (e.g., being disliked or rejected) might develop particular behavior problems, such as hostility or submissiveness. These observations served as a foundation for two general hypotheses. The first was that a group's interpersonal structure influences each member of the group. The second was that patterns of acceptance or rejection in peer groups become stable over time.

In an investigation designed to explore these hypotheses, observations were made of 12 preschoolers who had not yet formed a stable group structure, because they were newly enrolled in nursery school. F. Moreno (1942) gathered sociometric data by asking children to name classmates with whom they would like to do a painting activity, and used direct observation to document children's initiations toward classmates and peers' responses to children's initiations. Using these observational data, F. Moreno emulated Bott (1928) by constructing a matrix in which every child's interactions were arrayed against those of all classmates. For each pair of classmates, a list was made of the number of contacts that each member initiated toward another member, and the frequency of responses that each member gave to the other's initiations. Unlike Bott, however, F. Moreno was interested in documenting specific types of peer responses—those that were indicative of interpersonal acceptance or rejection. The types of responses that children received from peers were coded as positive, rejecting, or indifferent. F. Moreno also drew sociograms that graphically depicted both the initiation and response patterns that were characteristic for particular children. These sociograms illustrated disparities in peers' responses to particular children. Of specific interest were children whose initiations toward particular classmates were often met with *indifference* or *rejection.*

By focusing on the concept of interpersonal rejection, F. Moreno (1942) drew attention to an aspect of children's peer-group relations that was potentially distinct from gradations in liking and that was more negative in character (e.g., dislike, disdain, spurning). Thus, instead of conceptualizing peer-group relations only in terms of differences in the degree to which children were liked or preferred by groupmates (i.e., greater or lesser peer acceptance), F. Moreno made it possible for researchers to define and measure the extent to which children were "rejected" by members of their peer group.

Bonney (1943) conducted a subsequent study that in part was aimed at explicating children's peer-group relations. Like F. Moreno, this investigator took the position that grade-schoolers' relations with each member of their peer group varied along a continuum that ranged from "mutual attraction" to "mutual rejection," and he proposed that the totality of an individual's relations with group members (e.g., the average amount of attraction or rejection present in the child's relationships with group members) could be construed as "general social acceptance." Even though Bonney conceived of intragroup dynamics in a way that incorporated the concept of rejection, he did not measure children's peer-group relations in a way that tapped this construct. Like Koch (1933) and Lippitt (1941), Bonney (1943) used sociometry to assess children's peer-group relations. Unlike his predecessors, however, Bonney did not ask children to choose between pairs of classmates solely on the basis of a "liking" criterion. Instead, he devised a method that enabled children to nominate an unlimited number of classmates (i.e., unlimited nominations) for each of several criteria (persons preferred as workmates, as companions for arithmetic and reading tasks, as officers for a class club, as recipients of a Valentine or a Christmas present, etc.). General social acceptance scores were created by assigning weights to the nominations that children received from peers, then averaging the weights to form an overall composite. Children with poor peer-group relations were identified by dividing the distribution of general social acceptance scores into quartiles, and designating those who fell in the lowest quartile as "unpopular."

Thus, within Bonney's (1943) assessment method, children with poor peer-group relations (i.e., unpopular children) were individuals whom peers had seldom selected for some form of recognition or type of positive social role, task, or activity. Unfortunately, this form of evidence did not fully operationalize Bonney's conception of general social acceptance because the nominations were solicited only for positive criteria; thus, they did not provide an unequivocal indicator of interpersonal rejection. The children who were designated as unpopular might have, for example, received few "positive" nominations from peers because they were overlooked or forgotten rather than because they were "rejected" (i.e., viewed or treated negatively) by their classmates. Empirically, then, Bonney's assessments did not provide a way of depicting poor or problematic peer-group relations that was substantially different from those offered by Koch (1933) or Lippitt (1941); he succeeded only in identifying individuals who were least preferred by their classmates.

Northway, a contemporary of Bonney, also incorporated the concepts of peer acceptance and rejection into her writings about peer-group dynamics (Northway, 1943, 1946) and was particularly interested in "outsiders"—that is, children who were least acceptable to agemates (Northway, 1944, p. 10). From an assessment perspective, however, Northway continued the tradition of measuring children's "social acceptance" on the basis of peers' sociometrically defined liking preferences alone. For example, in one investigation, Northway (1944) followed a sample of 80 fifth- and sixth-graders over a 2-year period and assessed peer-group relations by asking children to indicate their peer preferences for several different school activities. The nominations that children received from peers were weighted and aggregated using algorithms similar to those of Bonney (1943); children whose scores fell in the lowest quartile of the social acceptance scores were labeled "outsiders." Although Northway introduced a novel term (i.e., "outsiders") to describe children who had poor peer-group relations, the methodology she used to identify these children was similar to that used by Koch, Lippitt, or Bonney, in that essentially she identified children that they had termed "unpopular"—that is, children who were low in social acceptance (i.e., least preferred) but not necessarily "rejected" by their classmates.

Implications of Early Turning Points for Contemporary Research on Friendship and Peer Rejection

Two pivotal turning points within the first generation of peer relations research have been identified and described. I now consider the significance of these turning points and whether the introduction of these innovations have implications for present-day investigators.

Significance of the Turning Point in Research on Friendships and Friendship Processes

Understanding the interpersonal determinants of children's and adolescent's friendships appears to have been the inaugural challenge of the peer relations discipline. Of the investigative trends that emerged during the discipline's earliest years, the most prominent was the explication of the personal and interpersonal factors (e.g., attributes such as age, gender, personality, behavior) that motivated children's and adolescent's friendship selections.

Although it appears that one of the first investigative trends in research on peer relations was driven by questions about the origins of friendship, it was not accompanied by efforts to define friendship or substantiate its occurrence. Rather, in the course of addressing these questions, it appears that early investigators took the meaning of friendship to be self-evident and assumed that the relationships that children reported about were in fact friendships. Perhaps it should not be surprising, then, that one of the next investigative trends to evolve within early peer relations research was concerned with empirically identifying and describing children's friendships. The cadre of investigators who instituted this trend (e.g., Challman [1932], Hagman [1933], and Green [1933]) was critical of the then dominant research paradigm and had the foresight to contemplate questions such as "What is friendship?" and "What signifies the presence of friendship?"

The collective conceptual and empirical contributions of these early researchers can be seen as a turning point in research on children's friendships that provoked a conceptual shift away from naive or unexamined views of friendship and ushered in an era in which investigators attempted to define the construct of friendship and to establish its empirical referents. Observational rather than self-report methodology became the preferred tool for identifying "actual" friendships, and criteria, such as frequent peer companionship, were established as the principal indicators of friendship.

Also, these innovations brought researchers closer to the phenomenon that they were investigating—children's friendships. Prior to this turning point, the strategy of having children report about their friendships kept investigators several steps removed from children's actual peer relationships, and provided a view of friendships that was filtered through one child's (the respondent's) perspective. By making frequent peer companionship a marker of friendship and attempting to document this attribute observationally, researchers made it more likely that friendship would be defined and investigated as a dyadic relationship. Implicit in this approach was the presumption that friendships comprised two persons, and that one could not infer the existence of a friendship unless it was possible to identify a child's consistent partner or frequent companion.

The establishment of companionship frequency, child–partner responsiveness, and interaction quality as markers of friendship not only made the dyad a unit of analysis in friendship research but also was a precursor for the study of friendship *relations*. The assessment of companionship frequency, for example, provided information about the amount of time children spent in the presence of "friends" versus other peer associates, the identities of their friendship partners (age, gender, etc.), and the locations and activities where friendship interactions occurred (e.g., classrooms, gymnasiums, school hallways, playgrounds). Companionship indices also provided a foundation for inferences about the number of friends children possessed and the uniformity or diversity of their friendship "choices" (e.g., selectivity by age, gender). Thus, research on friendship dynamics essentially began when investigators examined how children distributed their interactions across multiple friendship partners, and documented dyadic processes, such as child–partner responsiveness and the nature of the interactions that occurred between friends (e.g., friendly or quarrelsome exchanges).

Profiting from a Prior Turning Point: Considering the Implications of Early Friendship Studies

Some of the methodological and conceptual precedents that were introduced during the 1930s have considerable implications for today's investigators. These implications stem from Hagman's (1933) criticism that early researchers' failed to see the distinction between reports about friendships and the friendship itself, and from Hagman's and Green's (1933) solution to this travail—which was to go to natural settings, look for *relationships* that could be construed as friendships (i.e., identify and study dyads that fit their definition/criteria for friendship), then study these relationships.

Although the criticisms that Hagman (1933) and Green (1933) raised are not as relevant today as they were 75 years ago, their insights retain some currency in contemporary peer relations research, because children's reports about their friendships continue to be widely used and remain one of the predominate sources of information on which researchers rely to identify friendships (e.g., friendship nominations) and study friendship relations (e.g., children's reports of friendship features).

To some extent, the limitations of child reports as a means of identifying friendships have been reduced or eliminated by advances in the way these data are gathered and utilized. For example, the use of mutual rather than unilateral friendship nominations as a means of identifying friendships, and the success of researchers' efforts to validate these reports against other (including behavioral) indicators of friendship, has in large part diminished concerns about monoinformant biases, and discredited the allegation that children lack awareness of their friendships.

It is not as clear, however, that the discipline has progressed to the point of overcoming some of the limitations associated with the use of child report data to study friendship relations, dynamics, or processes. In recent years, use of child report data as a means of investigating friendship features or qualities has proliferated (for a recent review, see Rubin, Bukowski, & Parker, 2006). It has become far less common for researchers to study friendship processes, including those fundamental to friendship formation, maintenance, and termination, the way that Challman (1932), Hagman (1933), and Green (1933) did—by observing the patterns of association and interaction that transpire between friendship partners.

There are notable exceptions to the trend toward relying on children's reports as a means of investigating friendship relations, and these include several classic studies during the 1970s and 1980s—the epoch that I have termed the second generation of research on peer relations (Ladd, 2005). Among these exceptions are Gottman's (1983) study of conversational processes leading to friendship in young children, and Berndt's (1981) observational studies of cooperation and competition in friendship dyads. Unfortunately, however, investment in observational research appears to have faltered; rather than becoming the principal paradigm for research on friendship dynamics and processes, this approach has become the exception rather than the rule. This is evidenced by the fact that the vast majority of studies on friendship features and processes has involved interviewing or providing children with questionnaires about who their friends are, how they relate with their friends, how they are treated by their friends, what functions their friends serve, and so on.

Implication 1: There Are Limits to What Children's Reports Can Teach Us about "Actual" Friendships

Investigators' continued dependence on children's reports of friendship relations and processes raises the question of whether the discipline has become too reliant on child-report data. If child-report methodology has become standard practice, will this approach limit our knowledge about friendship?

In raising this issue, it seems reasonable to consider whether children's reports are optimal for capturing and understanding pivotal friendship processes (e.g., friendship features, dynamics). First, it is not clear that researchers have designed child-report questionnaires and interviews in a way that accurately portrays and solicits information about the types of exchanges that actually occur in friendships, and whether the content of these measures is equally valid for children of different ages. It is not evident that the types of friendship features or processes that researchers have incorporated within their questionnaires have their basis in actual friendship interactions, and are sensitive to differences in children's ages or level of development. Another potential shortcoming is that the processes about which children are queried tend to be framed quite broadly, or described at a fairly molar level of analysis. Moreover, we do not know much about the veridicality of children's reports/perceptions of friendship processes, or the extent to which each dyad member's perceptions square with actual quality of the interactions that transpire within their friendship. Together, these issues raise the prospect that current characterizations of friendship processes lack precision and ecological validity.

Second, within much of the research today, researchers learn about children's friendships by querying only one member of the relationship. This approach yields monoinformant data that are essentially perceptual in nature (i.e., subjective appraisals). This is not to say that we should abandon research on children's perceptions of their friendships. On the contrary, understanding how children see their friends, how they evaluate the support they receive from their friends, how satisfied they are with their friendships, and so on, are important questions in their own right. Finding out how children see their friendships likely is the best way to study relationship provisions, or how children see their friendships as affecting them (e.g., the psychological impact of friendships on children; perceived benefits and costs, such as support, harm, satisfaction or dissatisfaction with the relationship). However, were this strategy to become the predominant way that researchers investigate friendship *processes* or *dynamics*, the discipline would risk skewing the knowledge base in the direction of creating a psychology of perceived rather than actual friendship relations.

Another way to evaluate this implication is to count the potential costs of investigative myopia or misdirection. Is it likely that certain aspects of friendship relations will be overlooked or misunderstood if investigators rely largely on child-report data? By asking individuals to report about their friendships, will certain aspects of children's friendships be ignored or receive too little investigative attention? If we contrast today's preferred paradigm against that instituted by Challman, Hagman and Green, some underexplored areas of investigation are revealed.

The observational approach used by these early investigators lends itself to creating a more in-depth, descriptive analysis of children's friendships. By observing friendship dyads in natural contexts, investigators are in a position to document which friends children associate with, how children distribute their time among friends, what children do with each of their friends (e.g., activities, and variations in activities by type of friend), and the types of interactions that transpire within specific friendships and across relationships and relationship contexts. I would submit that this kind of information is currently in short supply, and that the psychology of children's friendships would profit from a richer, more naturalistic descriptive foundation. Too little is known about what children do with friends, and we lack basic descriptive data on the activities that friends pursue during childhood and adolescence, the amount of time children and adolescents spend with friends (although "beeper" studies help), and where friendship interactions and activities tend to occur (principal settings).

If friendships are dynamic entities and we wish to understand friendship *development* (i.e., formation, trajectories, transitions), then there is no good substitute for basic process-oriented research. A compelling example is Gottman's (1983) study of friendship formation in preschoolers. A principal objective was to determine whether pairs of unacquainted preschoolers differed in the way they communicated with each other during play, and whether some conversational processes culminated in their "hitting it off" in ways that led to friendship. To examine these aims, "host" children were paired with an unfamiliar peer for play sessions that occurred in the host's home. Conversations were audiotaped each time children played together, and the tapes were coded to create measures of conversational processes (e.g., types, sequences of communicative exchanges) and the extent to which children "hit it off," or progressed toward friendship. Based on the findings, Gottman arrived at a novel description of the *processes* through which young children became friends. He concluded that it was essential that dyad members begin their association by establishing clear and connected forms of communication. Once this process is established, the partners must successfully exchange information about themselves and their play, formulate common-ground activities, and manage conflict. Other processes, such as self-disclosure and exploring similarities and differences, played a greater role in friendship formation after children had become acquainted. Ultimately, the probability that a pair of children progressed toward friendship depended on their ability to manage challenges that threatened established patterns of play continuity and conversational "agreeableness." It seems unlikely that any investigator would have been able to describe this sequence, and to determine the predictive value of particular types of dyadic interactions, by interviewing children about their friendships.

The fact that this study was conducted more than 30 years ago and, in the intervening years, has not produced an enduring and prolific investigative legacy is unfortunate. Because of this, we do not have a rich description of the processes that contribute to friendship formation at other ages (e.g., middle and later childhood, adolescence, young adulthood). Equally regrettable is the fact that little process data have been gathered on other friendship developments, including the antecedents of relationship maintenance, relationship problems, and friendship dissolution (see Parker & Seal, 1996).

Implication 2: There Are Advantages to Making Dyads the Unit of Analysis in Friendship Research

Certainly there is worth in learning about children's perceptions of their friendships, and their perspectives on its functions and value. Nevertheless, such data neither provide a complete picture of the friendship dyad nor capture relationship processes from a dyadic perspective.

Hagman's (1933) recognition of child–partner responsiveness, and Green's (1933) attempts to document the types and quality of interactions that occurred within friendships (conflict, etc.) highlight the importance of studying friendships as dyadic relation-ships. Consider, for example, that much of the extant database on friendship processes (because it based on one partner's reports) may not only be imbued with that partner's perspective but may also characterize in unilateral terms what is (in reality) a dyadic pro-cess. Thus, it is arguable that what is learned about friendship by relying only on child reports is "biased," because the phenomenon of interest (a dyadic entity) is portrayed from only one participant's perspective. Attempts to assess friendship features or pro-cesses from one partner's perspective prevent investigators from describing friendship features or processes in dyadic terms.

Furthermore, children's reports about friendship processes and provisions may be biased toward providing static rather than dynamic or developmental views of friendship processes. When children respond to interviews or questionnaires, researchers obtain a temporally situated appraisal of specific friendship features (i.e., a child's perception of a friend's supportiveness at or near the time of testing) but do not gain much insight into ongoing support processes, continuity or change in support over time (i.e., trajectories), or shifts in support by task, context, or problem. Thus, prevailing paradigms risk fostering a view of friendship that is devoid of dyadic, developmental data about naturally occur-ring processes that are common to friendship, and that may be influential in directing the course of friendship relationships. These include variations in the synchrony and connectedness of friends' interactions and communications—processes that have been theorized (and in some cases found; see Gottman, 1983) to be instrumental in the forma-tion, maintenance, termination of friendships.

It would also be difficult to address questions about the role of reciprocity or equity in friendship processes without gathering dyadic data. For example, we know little about how partners balance support needs and provisions within friendships. Dyadic data would be needed to assess the extent to which support is reciprocated in friendships, and to determine whether the exchange of support becomes more or less equitable over the life of a friendship or among older versus younger friends. A dyadic perspective may be important for research on many other types of friendships processes as well (e.g., affirma-tion, aid, trust, intimacy).

Finally, much remains to be learned about how friends adjust to each other—that is, the role of partner accommodations—within friendship (see Ross & Lollis, 1989), espe-cially among older children and adolescents. Relationships likely differ in how mutual versus one-sided friendship processes are, and we know little about individual differences in such dynamics or about the potential consequences of specific asymmetries. Dysfunc-tion may be more likely within friendships in which one partner benefits more than the other, or one partner does most of the adjusting. It is also conceivable that relationship differences of this type could be used to create typologies of friendships, or to character-ize ways in which friendships are in or out of balance on key processes or provisions (see Shulman, 1993).

Significance of the Turning Point in Research on Peer-Group Rejection

Describing children's relations with members of their peer groups was another challenge that early researchers addressed. One investigative trend that emerged from this work was concerned with characterizing the intragroup associations (e.g., social roles, positions) of children who did not fit well within their peer groups. In retrospect, it is apparent that a critical step toward describing individuals' relations within peer groups was to stipulate relevant constructs and devise ways to measure them. It is not surprising that research-ers turned to sociometry for this purpose, because it was a new and innovative tool for describing patterns of social preference and attraction among individuals within group contexts. This paradigm, as it was applied to the study of children's peer groups, gave rise to a tradition in which researchers conceptualized and measured children's rela-tions within peer groups in terms of group members' sentiments (i.e., liking preferences) toward individuals.

As it was initially applied, sociometry provided more information about children who were most versus least preferred by peers (i.e., differentially liked) than about children who were rejected or disliked by members of their peer group. Thus, it would appear that one of the first constructs to be investigated as a relational feature of children's peer groups was peer-group *acceptance*, because the only criterion that was used to map intra-group dynamics was group members' feelings of liking or attraction toward individuals. Use of this criterion made it possible to characterize individual differences in peer-group relations only in terms of how well liked particular children were by group members. Children who received many liking nominations (weighted liking nominations) were seen as better accepted by peers than those who received fewer liking nominations. As we have seen, the terms that early researchers (e.g., Koch, Lippitt, Bonney) used to describe children at the extremes of this continuum were "popular" versus "unpopular" or "outsid-ers."

Although not fully appreciated at the time, the limitations of this approach became apparent as researchers recognized that peer rejection was another indicator of poor peer-group relations, and that little had been learned about this intragroup dynamic by investigating only on peers' liking preferences. F. Moreno called attention to this limita-tion by arguing that it was important to understand not only patterns of "attraction" but also "repulsion" within peer groups. Moreover, Moreno's solution to this travail was a turn-ing point because it generated knowledge about the previously undefined and unstudied construct of peer group rejection.

F. Moreno (1942) set a precedent by defining and assessing peer-group rejection in the context of children's peer interactions. Essentially, F. Moreno broke with tradition by conceptualizing rejection in terms of peers' behaviors (i.e., rejecting behaviors) rather than peers' sentiments (i.e., liking preferences) toward individuals within the group. As F. Moreno put it, there was a need for "tests based on action rather than on words" (p. 397). Thus, instead of focusing on peers' reports of how much they liked individuals within their group, F. Moreno not only observed peers' behaviors toward individuals but also tracked their reactions to individuals' social initiations.

From an assessment perspective, F. Moreno's (1942) observational scheme repre-sented a breakthrough, because it provided researchers with novel ways to operationalize and measure the construct of peer-group rejection. Although not fully explicated in her article, it appears that F. Moreno's method made it possible to derive at least two mea-sures of peer-group rejection. One was the extent to which peers directed negative or rejecting behaviors toward a child, regardless of whether these behaviors were contingent on the child's social overtures, and the other was the extent to which peers' responded to a child's social initiations with negative or rejecting behaviors. It could be argued that the latter index constituted the most innovative and informative indicator, because it approximated most closely the construct of peer-group rejection; that is, it was an empiri-cal indicator of the extent to which peers *rejected* children's attempts to connect with members of their group.

Another way this assessment strategy was an advance over prior work was that it provided researchers with a way to document the types of rejection experiences that children encountered and to make qualitative distinctions about the form and severity of these experiences. Indifference and rejection were seen by F. Moreno (1942) as two different ways that peers could deny or "repulse" a child's initiations, and the code she used for the former type of peer reaction—that is, ignoring or indifferent reactions—represented a milder form of rejection than did the latter. Thus, by coding whether peers responded to children's initiations with indifference versus more negative forms of rejection, it became possible to describe differences in the types of rejecting behaviors that individuals experienced. The scheme also made it possible to estimate the regularity with which mild versus severe forms of rejection were perpetrated against specific children, and how extensively a child was rejected by members of his or her peer group. The latter index, for example, could be obtained by determining how many peers (e.g., the number or proportion of peer-group members) regularly directed negative or rejecting behaviors toward the child, or routinely rebuffed the child's social overtures. Although F. Moreno did not construct all of these indices, or systematically explore questions related to the extensivity of a child's rejection within peer groups, or the homogeneity or heterogeneity of children's rejection experiences across group members, her work was remarkable in that she was the first to provide the tools needed to accomplish these ends.

Profiting from a Prior Turning Point:
Considering the Implications of F. Moreno's Work on Peer Rejection

Although conducted more than 60 years ago, F. Moreno's innovations and findings continue to be relevant and, in fact, have important implications for modern-day peer relations researchers. Foremost among these implications is the question of whether peer-group rejection, or rejected status, should be defined and investigated as an expression of peers' sentiments (disliking) or peers' behaviors (i.e., rejecting actions) toward individuals within the group. This question remains relevant today, because past and current research has been dominated by a sociometric paradigm in which peer-group rejection has been defined and investigated predominately as an attitude or sentiment in the minds of peers (see Buhs & Ladd, 2001). According to this view, rejection exists when a majority of a child's groupmates harbor feelings of dislike toward him or her. Rejection, therefore, is defined by intragroup attitudes or, specifically, by the feelings of dislike that peers have toward specific individuals within their peer group.

In view of F. Moreno's work as a turning point, it is worth considering whether the historical dominance of the sociometric paradigm has partially occluded our view of the concept of peer-group rejection, or has interfered with efforts to obtain direct and valid assessments of this construct. Does the traditional approach to defining and measuring peer rejection—the enduring sociometric legacy—have limitations? Might there be two viable definitional–measurement paradigms—the sociometric tradition, which is Koch's legacy, and the behavioral one that emanated from F. Moreno's work?

Even though F. Moreno's innovations represented a turning point, her innovations did not produce a robust and lasting investigative legacy. In recent years, it has been rare for investigators to define and measure peer acceptance or rejection by observing how peers respond to children's actions. If a legacy does exist, it is perhaps best exemplified by contemporary investigators' efforts to observe the success of young children's goal-directed interactions (i.e., measure peer *acceptance;* see Nelson, Rubin, & Fox, 2005;

Stewart & Rubin, 1995), or by researchers' attempts to document the rejecting behaviors that children receive at the hands of peers (see Asher, Rose, & Gabriel, 2001; Snyder et al., 2003).

To be fair, it must be recognized that instead of only measuring gradations in liking, as Koch (1933) and Lippitt (1941) did, researchers eventually revised sociometry to include indicators of disliking (e.g., negative nominations). This revised measurement strategy provided information that approximated more closely the construct of peer rejection (e.g., Coie, Dodge, & Coppetelli, 1982). But, even with this innovation, it may be risky to assume that sociometric data fully capture the construct of peer rejection and best represent the processes through which peer rejection affects children. This would be tantamount to arguing that there is only one way to investigate and acquire knowledge about peer-group rejection. Scientifically, it seems more reasonable to assume that multiple paradigms are needed to understand any social phenomenon, and that this is true for peer-group relations more generally, and for peer-group rejection specifically. Thus, rather than ignore the implications of F. Moreno's work (perhaps at our peril), it might be productive to consider whether there are lessons to be learned from her paradigm and findings. So, then, what implications of F. Moreno's innovations and findings raise important questions for modern-day peer relations researchers?

Implication 1: Peer Rejection Is Expressed by Peers and Experienced by Children Behaviorally

Does the concept of peer rejection connote more than just peers' "feelings" (i.e., dislike) toward others in their peer group? F. Moreno's work illustrates that rejection can be construed as actions performed by peers as opposed to, or in addition to, a sentiment in the minds of peers. Consider that if "reject" is construed as a verb, then its meaning implies actions of a rejecting nature. Definitions of the word "reject" include mild behaviors such as "refusing to take, agree, accede to ... " (Guralnik, 1974) and more severe actions such as "to deny, dismiss ... " (Agnes & Laird, 1996). These meanings are consistent with F. Moreno's operationalization of peer rejection—particularly her attempts to code instances in which children's overtures toward peers were ignored, refused, denied, or otherwise "repulsed."

This logic implies that the way peers *reject* others, and the way that children experience rejection, is through the actions that peers' direct toward them, or make contingent on their overtures during social interactions. If this is the case, then defining "peer rejection" as peers' collective dislike of individuals may not fully represent the meaning of this construct, and assessments that tap only peers' preferences or sentiments (attitudes/cognitions) toward individuals may not fully capture the empirical referents that correspond most closely to this construct. It may be that more direct and valid indicators of rejection are obtained when researchers assess rejecting interactions, as F. Moreno did.

Increasing the validity of peer rejection measures likely would have important implications for contemporary and future peer relations research. As one illustration, consider that a principal reason investigators have studied peer-group rejection is because it has been shown to be one of the better predictors of children's current and future adjustment. If a behavioral definition of "rejection" brought investigators closer to the presumed cause of children's adjustment problems, evidence from this approach could yield more accurate estimates of rejection's role in the development of early and later maladjustment. Although substantial benefits might be obtained by defining and measuring peer rejection behaviorally, this investigative shift would pose new conceptual and empirical challenges. For example, were investigators to take this approach, it would likely intersect and risk being confounded with contemporary efforts to define and measure other types of adverse peer relationships, such as peer victimization. Few have attempted to parse the domains of peer rejection and victimization conceptually (but see Bukowski & Sippola, 2001; Kochel, McConnell, & Ladd, 2007; Salmivalli & Issacs, 2005), yet it seems likely that the two constructs denote partially distinct phenomena, and that each has some unique behavioral referents. As an illustration, the constructs of "rejection" and "victimization" can be construed as encompassing peer behaviors that primarily serve to thwart another's overtures (e.g., peers' attempts to ignore, dismiss, refuse, or deny another's initiations) as opposed to actions that serve to inflict physical or psychological harm (e.g., peers' perpetration of direct or indirect forms of aggression, abuse, or maltreatment), respectively.

Implication 2: Peers' Rejecting Behaviors Differ in the Directness with Which They Are Expressed toward Others and in Their Severity or Potential Impact on Rejected Children

Rejection is directed against children in a variety of ways (see Asher et al., 2001), and the forms it takes and the ways it is expressed toward and/or experienced by children may determine the extent to which it affects their development. Unfortunately, when investigators define and measure peer rejection as a peer sentiment or attitude, as is done in the sociometric tradition, they fail to capture the variability that exists in children's rejection experiences, because the sociometric tradition is not well suited to describing or indexing differences in peers' rejecting behaviors or differences in children's rejection experiences. Rather, this paradigm is concerned with differences in how peers feel toward members of their group (collective liking vs. disliking) rather than differences in how peers act toward these persons. Essentially, *how* children experience rejection has been ignored by the sociometric tradition.

In contrast, F. Moreno recognized that there were differences in the way that rejection was expressed toward and experienced by children, and her assessment strategy was designed to differentiate between milder (indifference) and more severe forms of rejection (active exclusion). Although this distinction lacked precision, in the sense that it did not fully capture the vicissitudes of peer rejection, it nonetheless represented a starting point for describing qualitative differences in the types of rejecting behaviors that peers perform and children experience.

The ability to differentiate among rejecting responses on a continuum of directness or severity might benefit contemporary researchers by providing more productive ways to conceptualize rejection as construct. Basic descriptive research aimed at cataloging the ways that peers rebuff children's social overtures could help to explicate the construct of peer rejection (e.g., through the creation of categories, or taxonomies rejecting behaviors; cf. Asher et al., 2001) and to demarcate its conceptual boundaries. Greater clarity about the behaviors that fit within the conceptual domain of peer rejection (types of rejecting behaviors) would also aid in efforts to distinguish this construct from other, closely related constructs, such as peer harassment and victimization (forms of peer abuse or maltreatment).

If it became possible to differentiate among rejecting responses on a continuum of directness or severity, then it might also be feasible to formulate and test more specific premises about how rejection affects children's development and adjustment. It might be hypothesized, for example, that exposure to indirect or mild modes of rejection (e.g., peers' attempts to ignore, pretend not to see or hear, or in other ways appear indifferent to a child's overtures) harms children less (i.e., has fewer debilitating consequences) than exposure to more direct (confrontational) or severe forms of rejection (e.g., instances in which peers' unambiguously deny, dismiss, or refuse a child's overtures).

Implication 3: Children May Experience High Levels of Rejection without Being Rejected by a Majority of Their Peers

Another shortcoming of the sociometric paradigm is that it perpetuates a rather limited or inflexible way of defining and measuring the construct of peer rejection. Within this tradition, rejection is conceptualized and indexed as an aggregate of group member's sentiments toward specific individuals within the group. Children are considered to be rejected by peers when they are disliked by the *majority* of their groupmates (e.g., receive very low ratings or negative nominations from a large proportion of group members). Thus, within this tradition, unless children are roundly or consensually disliked, they are not seen as rejected or identified as individuals who are experiencing peer rejection.

F. Moreno's methods and findings suggest that some children are frequently rejected by peers or exposed to high levels of rejection, even though they are not rejected by all or even most of their groupmates. This investigator's case records raise the possibility that some children's rejection experiences occur almost entirely with one person, or with a few, rather than many, peers. Suppose that Child A interacts frequently with peers, but nearly all of his or her interactions are concentrated among a few, rather than most, of the members of his or her peer group. As a further supposition, let us assume that nearly all of Child A's interaction partners (groupmates) regularly reject his or her initiations. Now, compare this scenario to that of Child B, who interacts with similar frequency but distributes these interactions more broadly across many (most) members of his or her peer group. Let us assume that, as with Child A, Child B's interaction partners reject nearly all of his or her overtures. Would it not seem reasonable to conclude that both of these children are rejected? Is it not the case that both of these children are experiencing similar levels of peer rejection (albeit at the hands of a smaller vs. larger number of peers)? Yet within the sociometric paradigm, it is likely that *only* Child B would be identified as rejected or be designated as a child who is experiencing peer rejection (assuming that most of the peers who rejected Child B's initiations also disliked Child B).

The point of this example is that by construing peer rejection as an aggregation of group members' sentiments, the sociometric tradition risks overlooking many children who would by F. Moreno's methods and standards be identified as rejected or as experiencing substantial levels of peer rejection. This is because the sociometric tradition largely has ignored the possibility that peer rejection, or children's rejection experiences, may be concentrated within specific interaction partners (or among a few group members) rather than being distributed across most group members. In contrast, observationally based assessments, particularly those that track both the identities and actions of peers who perpetrate rejecting behaviors, or those that index the failure (vs. success) rate of children's overtures toward peers (e.g., Nelson et al., 2005), seem less prone to this kind of underestimation.

This alternative to defining and measuring peer rejection has implications for contemporary peer relations research. For example, if rejecting experiences are theorized to be a fundamental cause of child dysfunction, then it may be possible to learn more about the effects of peer rejection on children's adjustment by tracking not only the number of peers with whom they have rejecting interactions but also the number of interactions that occur with specific interaction partners that are rejecting in nature. Perhaps the absolute frequency, proportion, or chronicity of children's rejecting interactions rather than the number of different peers who reject them (i.e., that dislike them) are more powerful determinants of children's adjustment. Alternatively, both of these factors may be important; rejection's effects may be more serious when children attempt to interact with many, rather than a few, peers, and their overtures are rejected by a larger, rather than a smaller, proportion of their groupmates. It may also be the case that these aspects of rejection are exacerbated or compounded by the directness or severity of the rejection experiences that children encounter in their interactions with few versus many peers.

Summary and Conclusions

The purpose of this chapter was to consider whether early developments in the peer relations discipline—particularly turning points in research on friendship and peer-group rejection during the first generation of peer relations research—created legacies that continue to affect modern-day research, and to offer "lessons" that might help to guide the course of future research. Accordingly, an analysis was made of two early investigative trends—the study of children's friendships and the study of children's acceptance and rejection in peer groups. In both lines of investigation, pivotal investigative travails and associated turning points were identified.

The turning point that was identified in early research on children's friendships occurred when a cadre of researchers—principally Challman, Hagman, and Green—supplanted the prevailing investigative paradigm with an innovative way of defining friendship and a novel methodology for investigating friendship relations. The studies and findings conducted during this turning point advanced the discipline by making it apparent that (1) it was possible to define and operationalize the construct of friendship; (2) friendships were observable phenomena and could be studied directly through observation rather than indirectly through one participant's reports or perceptions; and (3) friendships were dyadic relationships, and insight into the nature of friendships could be obtained by observing the types of exchanges that occurred between both members of the dyad.

Clearly, the innovations introduced at this turning point were not ephemeral, because they foreshadowed further efforts to define friendship, to identify actual friendship relationships empirically, and to explicate friendship processes by observing the interactions between friendship partners. However, it appears that Challman's, Hagman's, and Green's commitment to understanding friendship processes through direct observation of friends' interactions has been the least robust or productive component of their legacy. Judging from the number of studies that have exemplified or extended this approach to explicating friendship processes over the last several decades, it appears that researchers' commitment to this paradigm has been sporadic rather than constant. Nonetheless, as I have argued in this chapter, there are many reasons why this early innovation remains relevant to modern-day peer relations research, and numerous ways in which observational research on friendship processes could advance what we know about children's and adolescents' friendships.

The second of the turning points considered in this chapter marked a shift in the way that early researchers conceptualized and assessed children's peer-group relations. This turning point was triggered by early researchers' realization that although peer rejection was a critical indicator of children's failure to fit into peer groups, the dominant method for assessing children's peer-group relations (i.e., early sociometry) provided insufficient information about this construct. F. Moreno's investigative strategy not only provided a way of tapping construct of rejection empirically but also offered unprecedented insight into the process and nature of the rejection experiences that children received at the hands of peers. Her methods, measures, and findings made it clear that (1) rejection is a multifaceted construct; (2) variability is present in children's rejection experiences; and (3) individual differences exist in how extensively children are rejected by members of their peer groups.

As novel as these discoveries were, it is hard to understand why they have had so little impact on subsequent research. It is not apparent that F. Moreno's work has a legacy, unless it is possible to consider recent efforts to index children's peer acceptance observationally (e.g., see Nelson et al., 2005), or to map the quality of rejected children's peer interactions and experiences (e.g., see Asher et al., 2001) as part of this tradition. In recent years, investigators such as Rubin and colleagues (2006) have demonstrated that observational indices of children's peer acceptance are feasible and prognostic of important developmental processes and outcomes (Nelson et al., 2005; Stewart & Rubin, 1995). Likewise, Asher et al. (2001) and Sandstrom and Zakriski (2004) have advocated for describing the social lives of rejected children, including the types of interactions that rejected children have with peers. In large part, however, the empirical work completed thus far (e.g., see Asher et al., 2001; Sandstrom & Cillessen, 2003) does not appear to be inspired by F. Moreno's study, and its principal purpose has not been to define the construct of peer *rejection*, or to identify rejected children on the basis of peers' "rejecting" responses to their social overtures. Thus, it would appear that the implications of F. Moreno's discoveries remain important and are even more compelling in light of recent efforts to describe the forms and features of rejected children's peer interactions. For this reason, I have argued that F. Moreno's innovations merit consideration. Her discoveries were important 65 years ago, and I have suggested several ways in which they remain so today.

Acknowledgment

This chapter was prepared while I was supported by a grant from the National Institutes of Health (No. R01HD-045906).

References

Agnes, M., & Laird, C. (1996). *Webster's new world dictionary and thesaurus.* New York: Macmillan.

Asher, S. R., Rose, A. J., & Gabriel, S. W. (2001). Peer rejection in everyday life. In M. R. Leary (Ed.), *Interpersonal rejection* (pp. 105–142). Oxford, UK: Oxford University Press.

Berndt, T. J. (1981). Effects of friendship on prosocial intentions and behavior. *Child Development, 52,* 636–643.

Bonney, M. (1943). Personality traits of socially successful and socially unsuccessful children. *Journal of Educational Psychology, 34,* 449–472.

Bonser, F. G. (1902). Chums: A study of youthful friendships. *Pedagogical Seminary, 9*, 221–256.

Bott, H. (1928). Observations of play activities in a nursery school. *Genetic Psychology Monographs, 4*, 44–88.

Buhs, E. S., & Ladd, G. W. (2001). Peer rejection as antecedent of young children's school adjustment: An examination of mediating processes. *Developmental Psychology, 37*, 550–560.

Bukowski, W. M., & Sippola, L. K. (2001). Groups, individuals, and victimization: A view of the peer system. In J. Juvonen & S. Graham (Eds.), *Peer harassment in school: The plight of the vulnerable and victimized* (pp. 355–377). New York: Guilford Press.

Challman, R. C. (1932). Factors influencing friendship among preschool children. *Child Development, 3*, 146–158.

Coie, J. D., Dodge, K. A., & Coppotelli, H. (1982). Dimensions and types of social status: A cross-age perspective. *Developmental Psychology, 18*, 557–570.

Gottman, J. M. (1983). How children become friends. *Monographs of the Society for Research in Child Development, 48*(3, Serial No. 201).

Green, E. (1933). Friendships and quarrels among preschool children. *Child Development, 4*, 237–252.

Guralnik, D. B. (1974). *Webster's new world dictionary.* New York: William Collins & World Publishing.

Hagman, E. P. (1933). The companionships of preschool children. *University of Iowa Studies in Child Welfare, 7*, 4.

Hsia, J. C. (1928). A study of sociability of elementary school children. *Teachers College of Columbia University Contributions to Education, 322*, 1–64.

Hubbard, R. M. (1929). A method of studying spontaneous group formation. In D. S. Thomas (Ed.), *Child development monographs* (pp. 76–85). New York: Teacher's College, Columbia University.

Jenkins, G. G. (1931). Factors involved in children's friendships. *Journal of Educational Psychology, 22*, 440–448.

Koch, H. L. (1933). Popularity among preschool children: Some related factors and a technique for its measurement. *Child Development, 4*, 164–175.

Kochel, K. P., McConnell, E. M., & Ladd, G. W. (2007). *Do negative peer relationships provoke other peer adversities?* Paper presented at the biennial meetings of the Society for Research in Child Development, Boston, MA.

Ladd, G. W. (2005). *Children's peer relationships and social competence: A century of progress.* New Haven, CT: Yale University Press.

Lippitt, R. (1941). Popularity among preschool children. *Child Development, 12*, 305–332.

Monroe, W. F. (1898). Social consciousness in children. *Psychological Review, 5*, 68–70.

Moreno, F. (1942). Sociometric status of children in a nursery school group. *Sociometry, 5*, 395–411.

Moreno, J. L. (1932). *Applications of the group method to classification.* New York: National Committee on Prisons and Prison Labor.

Moreno, J. L. (1934). *Who shall survive?: A new approach to the problem of human interrelations.* Washington, DC: Nervous and Mental Disease Publishing Company.

Nelson, L. J., Rubin, K. H., & Fox, N. A. (2005). Social withdrawal, observed peer acceptance, and the development of self-perceptions in children ages 4 to 7 years. *Early Childhood Research Quarterly, 20*, 185–200.

Northway, M. L. (1943). Social relationships among preschool children: Abstracts and interpretations of three studies. *Sociometry, 6*, 429–433.

Northway, M. L. (1944). Outsiders: A study of the personality patterns of children least acceptable to their age mates. *Sociometry, 7*, 10–25.

Northway, M. L. (1946). Personality and sociometric status: A review of the Toronto studies. *Sociometry, 9*, 233–241.

Parker, J. G., & Seal, J. (1996). Forming, losing, renewing, and replacing friendships: Applying temporal parameters to the assessment of children's friendship experiences. *Child Development, 67*, 2248–2268.

Ross, H. S., & Lollis, S. P. (1989). A social relations analysis of toddler peer relationships. *Child Development, 60*, 1082–1091.

Rubin, K. H., Bukowski, W. M., & Parker, J. G. (2006). Peer interactions, relationships, and groups. In W. Damon & R. M. Lerner (Editors-in-chief), N. Eisenberg (Vol. Ed.), *Handbook of child psychology* (6th ed.): Vol. 3. *Social, emotional, and personality development* (pp. 571–645). New York: Wiley.

Salmivalli, C., & Isaacs, J. (2005). Prospective relations among victimization, rejection, friendlessness, and children's self- and peer-perceptions. *Child Development, 76*, 1161–1171.

Sandstrom, M. J., & Cillessen, A. H. N. (2003). Sociometric status and children's peer experiences: Use of the daily diary method. *Merrill–Palmer Quarterly, 49*, 427–452.

Sandstrom, M. J., & Zakriski, A. L. (2004). Understanding the experience of peer rejection. In J. B. Kupersmidt & K. A. Dodge (Eds.), *Children's peer relations: From development to intervention* (pp. 101–118). Washington, DC: American Psychological Association.

Shulman, S. (1993). Close friendships in early and middle adolescence: Typology and friendship reasoning. In B. Laursen (Ed.), *Close friendships in adolescence* (pp. 55–72). San Francisco: Jossey-Bass.

Snyder, J., Brooker, M., Patrick, M. R., Snyder, A., Schrepferman, L., & Stoolmiller, M. (2003). Observed peer victimization during early elementary school: Continuity, growth, and relation to risk for child antisocial and depressive behavior. *Child Development, 74*, 1881–1898.

Stewart, S. L., & Rubin, K. H. (1995). The social problem-solving skills of anxious–withdrawn children. *Development and Psychopathology, 7*, 323–336.

Warner, L. M. (1923). Influence of mental level in the formation of boys' gangs. *Journal of Applied Psychology, 7*, 224–236.

Wellman, B. (1926). The school child's choice of companions. *Journal of Educational Research, 14*, 126–132.

PART II

Social Behaviors, Interactions, Relationships, and Groups
What Should Be Measured, How, and Why?

CHAPTER 3

Children's Behaviors
and Interactions with Peers

RICHARD A. FABES
CAROL LYNN MARTIN
LAURA D. HANISH

From the time that children begin interacting with other children, they exhibit a wide range of behaviors. These behaviors vary from child to child, from interaction to interaction, and from context to context. At the same time, the behaviors children engage in with their peers have some continuity—reflecting meaningful patterns over time. Moreover, these interactional patterns are important to those who study children's development, because they are thought to have significant short- and long-term consequences for both the child and his or her interactional partner(s) (Ladd, 2005). The importance of studying children's peer behaviors and interactions was recognized early in the history of research on children's development (e.g., Barnes, 1896–1897, 1902–1903; Monroe, 1899) and remains an important area of study today. But exactly what is to be studied and how best to study children's peer behaviors and interactions continue to be critical questions for the field. The purpose of this chapter is to focus broadly on issues related to what and how best to assess them, particularly in childhood and early adolescence. We also identify important developmental, historical, and future trends in these efforts.

Because of space limitations, it is impossible both to cover all the forms of children's behaviors and interactions with peers, and to review in detail the many ways these behaviors and interactions can be measured. For these reasons, we focus primarily on overt behavioral interactions and do not provide much discussion on internal processes (e.g., social-cognitive processes such as attitudes, attributions, perceptions, and reasoning), although internal and external processes can be studied together (e.g., see Fabes, Eisenberg, McCormick, & Wilson, 1988). In addition, given our constraints, we excluded the extensive literature on children's conceptions of friendships and affiliations, and on sociometric methods used to assess these aspects of peer relationships, which are covered in detail elsewhere in this volume (see Chapter 4 by Berndt & McCandless, and Chapter 5 by Cillessen, this volume). We also give more attention to the use of observational methods for the study of children's behaviors and interactions because of their potential to explicate processes involved in children's peer interactions.

Core Issues in the Study of Children's Peer Behaviors and Interaction

In the study of children's behaviors and interactions, issues of conceptualization, developmental change, contextual variation, and measurement take center stage. Importantly, these are not independent dimensions; instead, choice of one often strongly correlates with choices on other dimensions.

Conceptualizing Peer Behaviors and Interactions

Children's peer relationships can be conceptualized as comprising complex patterns of discrete interactions with peers (Hinde & Stevenson-Hinde, 1987). As noted earlier, there is considerable variability in the nature and type of children's peer interactions. For instance, interactions may be lengthy or brief in duration. They may be positive in tone—characterized by positive affect, affection, and/or prosocial behaviors; they may be negative in tone—characterized by negative affect, conflict, and/or aggression; or, as is the case for many of everyday interactions, they may be neutral and benign. Peer interactions can encompass common behaviors or novel activities. And there is substantial variability in the nature of children's interactions depending on the setting (e.g., children behave differently with peers at home vs. at school), the identity and characteristics of peers (e.g., children may interact differently with boys vs. girls), intensity (quiet and calm or active and forceful), and emotional state (e.g., peer interactions may be different when children are upset than when they are calm). Of course, individual children vary in their typical behavioral responses (e.g., some children tend to show more positive affect). Understanding how, when, and why peer behaviors and interactions vary is key to understanding the complexity of early human relationships and the consequences of these relationships for children's lives.

Developmental and Contextual Changes in Peer Interactions and Behaviors

In addition to individual variability within age, children's behaviors and interactions with peers change considerably across childhood and adolescence, and these changes affect what we can and should study. Throughout childhood, changes in children's physical, cognitive, and social skills facilitate their ability to interpret, respond to, and reason about their peer behaviors and interactions. Children's expectations about normative social behavior also become more sophisticated with age, such that the types of social behavior considered socially appropriate and likely to elicit positive peer responses differ markedly across the preschool, grade school, and adolescent years (Bierman & Montminy, 1993).

Although many of the changes that influence peer relationships occur gradually, some are relatively abrupt. For example, about the ages of 4–7 years and again at 11–14 years, children's social reasoning shows a qualitative shift that enables them to integrate information in a more complex fashion, and to construct and consider multidimensional representations of themselves and their relationships (Harris, 2006). Moreover, children often experience significant and abrupt contextual changes that affect their behaviors and interactions with peers. The transition from the open and relatively informal learning environments of the preschool classroom to the more organized elementary grade classes affects the quantity and quality of children's peer interactions (Fabes, Martin, & Hanish, 2007). Similarly, the transition from smaller, self-contained elementary school classrooms to the larger and more fluid, multiclassroom organization of secondary school also alters how children gather and interact. These changes have significant implications for the measures and methods we use to study peer relationships across childhood and into adolescence.

During the preschool years, play activities constitute the primary context for peer interactions (Power, 2000). In addition, preschool is a time when many children are first exposed to large numbers of peers outside of their family and immediate neighborhood, and first come into contact with a larger and broader array of peers than they experience at home. Preschool also is a period when children move from playing alone or alongside other children toward true interactive play, when more complex social dynamics are established. As such, preschool has been considered a particularly important period of time, possibly even a sensitive period, that may set the stage for developing the fundamental behaviors, attitudes, and preferences underlying peer interactions and relationships (C. Martin, Fabes, Hanish, & Hollenstein, 2006).

Over the course of the toddler and preschool periods, social behaviors that emerge reflect an increasing orientation toward cohesion, affiliation, and engagement with peers (Howes, 1988; Strayer, 1980). A key developmental task for preschool-age children involves the acquisition of skills necessary to sustain interactive and reciprocal play. Such skills include expressing positive affect (e.g., smiling), looking at and attending to one's play partner, acting prosocially (e.g., cooperating, sharing), being agreeable and compliant, and mastering reciprocal turn-taking play sequences. These are considered critical features of young children's successful peer interactions (Rubin, Bukowski, & Parker, 2006). Basic communication skills, including the ability to communicate clearly and to establish a common ground in play, also appear to promote peer interactions at this age (Gottman, 1986). Young children's peer interactions also are characterized by agonistic activities, such as squabbles, conflicts, and aggression, that disrupt peer interactions and activities (Bierman & Montminy, 1993; Strayer, 1992; see Vaughn & Santos, Chapter 11, this volume).

As children move into grade school, peer interactions and social behaviors become even more complex, and successful peer interactions require a wider array and diversity of skills. Children's play becomes more highly organized and elaborate, and involves complex, rule-oriented games that may include groups of children rather than the predominantly dyadic peer play seen during the preschool years. Being friendly, cooperative, helpful, assertive, and self-regulated are key qualities to successful peer interactions during elementary school. In addition, aggressiveness and agonistic behaviors decline during this period, and if they do occur, they are increasingly predictive of poor peer interactions (Ladd, 2005). Given the increased duration of peer interactions and the more frequent focus of interactions involving organized games and rules, norm-breaking behaviors such as defiance, withdrawal, and immaturity, become salient and form the basis for poor peer interactions (Coie, Dodge, & Kupersmidt, 1990).

With the onset of adolescence, play no longer accurately describes the focus of most peer interactions. Although most interactions still revolve around shared activities, these activities become more diverse (organized sports, music, shopping, etc.) and less tied to the school or classroom. Communication qualities become central features of adolescent peer interactions (Rubin et al., 2006). Although adolescents' peer interactions can be quite conflicted and destructive, their conflicts typically center on relationship issues, and physical aggression is much less likely than is the case for younger children (Hartup & Laursen, 1991). These developmental and contextual changes affect the nature of the measures and methods that can and should be used to study children's peer behaviors and interactions. We now examine these in relation to the issues discussed to this point.

Measurement Issues: What Aspects of Children's Behaviors and Interactions Should Be Measured?

Given that behaviors and interactions can vary on many dimensions within and across age, researchers are faced with the question: What should be measured? There is no strong consensus in answering this question. Instead, researchers have developed a diverse array of conceptually and empirically based constructs designed to measure what they consider to be key components of children's peer behaviors and interactions. In Table 3.1, we have summarized some (but not nearly all) representative samples of instruments used in past and contemporary research. Although there are some commonalities (e.g., aggressiveness, prosociality, and withdrawal), the particular constructs assessed vary from one measure to another, reflecting the difficulty that scholars have had in agreeing on key constructs that should be measured when studying children's peer behaviors and interactions.

To further complicate matters, researchers also have to decide which level of behavior and interaction they want to assess. Are they interested in assessing a relatively macro-level construct such as aggression, or a more micro-level construct, such as hitting? The choice of macro- versus micro-level constructs is often associated with theoretical orientation, method of assessments, analytic procedures, and the types of questions that can be asked and answered. For instance, macro-level constructs are often assessed using questionnaires, the data are typically collected at one point in time, and the focus is on understanding a broad swath of behaviors. In contrast, micro-level constructs are often assessed using observational methods that allow for assessment of detailed categories of behavior, are collected repeatedly, and are useful data for answering questions about narrower behaviors and about changes over time and context. However, these general patterns need not hold true. Broad categories of behaviors can be addressed with observational methods. For example, Smith (1978) identified developmental trends in social behavior using three relatively global behaviors: solitary behavior, parallel play, and cooperative play. Similarly, Fabes et al. (1999) had observers rate the degree of social competence shown by children in each observed peer interaction. Because every method of assessment has its advantages and disadvantages, the ideal strategy for researchers is to find the most efficient and effective method of measuring the peer behavior or interaction of interest. We now turn our attention to more detailed discussions of two of the most common types of data collected in studies of children's peer behaviors and interactions: (1) self- and other-report data, and (2) observational data.

Self- and Other-Report Data

The questionnaire instruments identified in Table 3.1, and many others not listed, have several advantages in research designed to study children's peer interactions and behav-

TABLE 3.1. Examples of Existing Scales Measuring Children's Peer Interactions and Social Behaviors

Scale	Constructs measured
Child Behavior Scale (CBS; Ladd & Profilet, 1996)	• Aggressiveness • Anxious/fearfulness • Prosociality • Asocialness • Peer exclusion
Social Competence and Behavior Evaluation (SCBE; LaFreniere & Dumas, 1996)	• Depression–joyfulness • Anxiousness–secure • Anger–tolerance • Isolation–integration • Aggressiveness–calmness • Egotistical–prosociality • Oppositional–cooperative • Dependent–autonomous
Social Skills Rating System (SSRS; Gresham & Elliott, 1990)	Social skills • Cooperative • Assertive • Responsible • Empathy • Self-control Problem behaviors • Externalizing • Internalizing • Hyperactive Academic competence
Teacher Assessment of Social Behavior (TASB; Cassidy & Asher, 1992)	• Aggressiveness • Prosociality • Social withdrawal
Teacher Social Competence (TSC; Fast Track, 2004)	• Prosocial/communication skills • Emotional regulation skills • Academic skills
Kohn Social Competence Scale (teacher rated) (Kohn & Rosman, 1972)	Factor I • Interest • Curiosity • Assertiveness Factor II • Conformity

Walker–McConnell Scale of Social Competence and School Adjustment
   Elementary (Walker & McConnell, 1988)
   Adolescent (Walker & McConnell, 1991)
	Elementary
	
	• Teacher-preferred social behavior
	• Peer-preferred social behavior
	• School adjustment
	
	Adolescent (grades 7–12)
	
	• Self-control
	• Peer relations
	• School adjustment
	• Empathy

(continued)

TABLE 3.1. *(continued)*

Scale	Constructs measured
Adaptive Social Behavior Inventory (ASBI; Hogan, Scott, & Bauer, 1992)	• Expressiveness • Compliant • Disruptive
Interpersonal Competence Scale (Cairns, Leung, Gest, & Cairns, 1995)	• Aggressive • Academic competence • Popular • Affiliative • Olympian
Matson Evaluation Scale of Social Skills with Youngsters (MESSY; Matson, Rotatori, & Helsel, 1983)	• Appropriate social skill • Inappropriate assertiveness • Impulsive/recalcitrant • Overconfident • Jealousy/withdrawal

iors. They can be quickly administered and require little to no training. Also, with computer hardware and software, the resulting data can easily be scanned into computers, minimizing data entry time and errors. Thus, these types of measures are not very costly in terms of money or resources. Another advantage is that researchers can develop items that directly address the issues of interest and ask about summaries of behavior.

Additionally, self- and other-report measures allow for, and may be the only suitable method for the assessment of *perceptions* of peer behaviors and interactions. Perceptions cannot be observed or inferred from other direct measures. These types of data are valuable to those who study behaviors/actions that depend upon people's interpretations. For instance, studies of peer victimization have shown that children's own perceptions of their victimization may diverge from peers' or teachers' perceptions and provide important insights into a child's comfort in peer settings (Graham & Juvonen, 1998). Thus, if one's interest is in perceptions of behaviors, then self- or other-reports are likely the preferred method.

Self- and other-reports are more useful for assessing stability of macro-level constructs than for assessing the variability and change in specific peer behavior and interactions. The advantage is that raters aggregate over many types, forms, and time frames of behavior to draw general conclusions about behavior. The disadvantage is that these psychological aggregations are subject to bias. Because self- and other-reports tend to be global, require reporters to abstract across multiple incidents, and often take long periods of time to make their ratings, less frequent or salient behaviors and interactions may be underreported, whereas frequent or more salient behaviors that have high impact (even if they are infrequent) may be overreported. In addition, most self- and other-report measures gather data on individual tendencies rather than on interactions per se.

Choices of measurement strategies are affected by the developmental issues we discussed previously. The normative developmental changes in the quality and quantity of peer interactions from childhood to adolescence have important implications regarding what peer behaviors and interactions to measure and how. For instance, measures that rely on children's reports of peer interactions can be problematic for young children whose verbal and cognitive comprehension and production skills are limited. Although some researchers have successfully used young children's self-reports (e.g., Vaughn & Waters, 1980), overall, the accuracy and validity of such reports of peer behaviors and interactions—whether about themselves or about others—can be questioned. For example, young children have rarely been found to play with peers they verbally report to be their friends (Foot, Chapman, & Smith, 1980).

However, for older children and teens, whose cognitive and verbal skills are more mature and advanced, these issues are less problematic. For example, Gest, Farmer, Cairns, and Xie (2003) found that the correlations of fourth and seventh graders nominations of social clusters were positive and statistically reliable with observed interaction profiles. Thus, the validity of children's reports of peer interactions potentially increases across development. Moreover, as Ladd (2005) noted, older children are in a better position to report on their own and others' behaviors, and know more about peer relationships than do the adults in their lives. As a result, researchers who study older children and teens tend to rely heavily on their reports of peer interactions and behaviors. In addition, the more specific and concrete social behaviors of preschool children may be targeted more easily in observational methods than the more complex social behaviors of older children. This, too, adds to the increased reliance on older children's reports of peer behaviors and relationships.

Despite these advantages, there are issues that should be considered when relying on older children's and adult's verbal reports of peer interactions and behaviors. Issues related to demand characteristics, self-presentational and expectational biases, as well as social desirability, can be problematic, especially for behaviors that are likely to be perceived negatively by others (e.g., aggression and jealousy) or are expected of children (e.g., being helpful to others). For example, in their meta-analysis of sex differences in children's prosocial behavior (a key component of positive peer interactions), Fabes and Eisenberg (1998) noted that the sex difference (favoring girls) was greatest when prosocial behavior was indexed by self- or other-reports but was not evident when the measure of prosocial behavior was unobtrusive observations. These findings suggest that verbal reports of prosocial behavior reflect what individuals believe boys and girls are *supposed* to be like rather than what they actually are like. Bond and Phillips (1971), for instance, found that although boys were more likely to donate than were girls, teachers tended to rate girls as more altruistic than boys. Similarly, Shigetomi, Hartmann, and Gelfand (1981) found that although girls were perceived by teachers and peers to be much more helpful than boys, the observed behavioral differences were of a lesser magnitude. Thus, when demand characteristics are clear and salient, stereotyped and socially desired responses are more likely to result.

Although teachers and parents can be in a good position to observe and report on young children's peer relationships, as children get older, more and more of their interactions with peers take place outside of the adults' sphere of influence. Even at school, as children get older, their peer interactions often take place without the presence of adults. Moreover, with a larger and more diverse group of students in later grades, it becomes more difficult for teachers to monitor all of the settings in which peer interactions occur. Teachers of older children and teens see them less often as they begin to have individualized class schedules, and to have different teachers for different classes. Thus, discrepancies can occur between adults' reports of children's peer interactions and children's behaviors or perceptions of themselves, and these discrepancies begin as early as preschool. For example, Howes (1988) found stronger congruence between teachers' ratings of children's peer relationships and observational data for infants and toddlers than for preschool children. Howes concluded that teachers may be more knowledgeable about infants' and toddlers' peer behaviors and relationships than about preschoolers' peer interactions. Gest (2006) studied teacher–peer agreement in first, third, and fifth graders, and found that teacher–peer agreement was stronger in the upper elementary grades. The reasons for these patterns of findings are unclear, because the methods used in these studies differed (observations and peer nominations). However, they do point out the need for more research focusing on discrepancies between adults' and children's assessments of peer behaviors and interactions to understand better the reasons and processes underlying them.

Additionally, researchers rarely have employed repeated measures of self- or other-reports of peer interactions to ascertain discrete, time-linked changes. When self-report measures have been used on repeated occasions, they were used across relatively long periods of time (months or years) and relatively unoften (once or twice per year). This is due in part to the relatively global nature of the measures and also due to the demands placed on children and adults when researchers try to obtain multiple reports across time. Principals, teachers, and parents are often reluctant to provide the time necessary to obtain multiple reports. Yet without such data, we are limited in our ability to study intraindividual variation in peer behaviors and interactions, as well as the dynamics of change in children's peer interactions and behavior.

Observational Data

Observational data collection methods are often considered the "gold standard" by which other methods are evaluated (Foster, Inderbitzen, & Nangle, 1993). They provide rich data about children's peer behaviors and interaction, allow for fine-grained assessments of and variability in behavior over settings and time, can be used to illustrate patterns of change, and are more likely than other methods to provide opportunities to assess specific, peer-related processes directly (e.g., influence and socialization).

Observational methods vary in their design, time frame, coding scheme, and target of observation (for a discussion of various observational methods and procedures, see Bakeman & Gottman, 1986; Sackett, 1977). We focus our discussion on the quantitative observational methods that have been used in empirical research on peer interactions and behaviors. Although alternative observational methods provide valuable information, due to space limitations we do not discuss ethnographic or participant observational methods that are qualitative in nature (e.g., see Thorne, 1993).

Historical Perspectives on Observational Research of Peer Behaviors and Interactions

Observational methods have been used to explore virtually every aspect of peer relationships, and they have a long history of use. Beginning in the 1920s, the child study movement and its emphasis on children's well-being spurred the first empirically oriented observational studies of children. During this period, researchers began to use methods that allowed for more precise studies of children, including the systematic recording of their behavior and interactions, and institute-sponsored experimental nursery schools allowed for the study of children's peer relationships under controlled conditions (Ladd, 2005).

Many of the predominant questions of this period concerned descriptions of children's peer interactions in their natural environments (Bott, Blatz, Chant, & Bott, 1928; Dawe, 1934; Goodenough, 1930). These early studies illustrated that choices of play partners were not random; instead, children showed preferences for certain partners. For example, Challman (1932) explored natural groupings of preschool children and found that "each child is apt to make a relatively weak association with almost every other child in the nursery school and to have only one or two strong friendships" (p. 150).

In classic work on children's social participation, Parten (1932, 1933) recognized that social behavior and social roles had not been carefully delineated in earlier studies of children's interactions with peers. A child who participates intensely with others was not distinguished from the child who stands by passively. Parten observed age-graded differences in various forms of social participation, for instance, identifying that solitary play decreased, while cooperative play increased from age 2 to 4 years.

The challenges associated with the use of observational methods were recognized early. Goodenough (1930, 1937) identified a number of issues, including the importance of adjusting the length of the observational interval to the complexity of the behavior being assessed, concerns about behavioral variability across situations, the types of problems best addressed by observational methods, the large numbers of samples of behavior needed to address many questions, and the difficulty of assessing reliability of observation. As we discuss shortly, these issues remain relevant today.

Early observational researchers also were interested in how behaviors changed in different settings. One of the classic observational studies was an enormous undertaking in which Barker and Wright (1955/1971) conducted a study of the habitat and behavior of people (including children's peer interactions) in a small Midwestern town. As the authors stated, "Research in psychological ecology requires the identification of units which are suitable for use in the description and analysis of the naturally occurring behavior and psychological living conditions of a community" (p. 4). It is impossible to do justice to the scope of this research; however, the range of material covered included global topics, such as the varied natures of behavioral structures and how they change over age, the social interactions of typically developing and non-typically-developing children, as well as much more detailed descriptions of percentage of time spent in every setting for children of different ages and the people with whom children interacted. Interestingly, the complexity of some of the data limited the kinds of analyses that were attempted.

It is difficult to mark the beginning of a more modern period of children's peer-related observational research. However, ethologists such as Strayer (Strayer & Strayer, 1976), and social learning theorists such as Fagot (1977; Fagot & Patterson, 1969), Patterson (Patterson & Anderson, 1964), and Hartup (Charlesworth & Hartup, 1967; Hartup, Glazer, & Charlesworth, 1967) led the way in contemporary observational studies of children's peer interactions and behaviors. Using a variety of observational methods, these researchers helped to establish that peers, even young peers, organize and shape each others' behaviors. They also helped to establish the usefulness of observational methods to study the outcomes associated with peer interactions, and they promoted the development of more sophisticated data-analytic techniques designed to answer some the challenges associated with the sequencing and patterning of the observed interactions and behaviors. For example, Patterson, Littman, and Bricker (1967) found that during everyday interactions in nursery school, child victims of aggression who counterattacked and were then positively reinforced (i.e., the perpetrator responded by being passive, crying, or being defensive) showed increasing aggressive behavior over time. Observational methods continue to be used extensively in contemporary research to study children's peer behaviors and interactions, and they are even being used in research in which peer reports have traditionally been used. For example, C. Martin et al. (2006) used observational data to conduct social network analyses, and found patterns that differed from those most often found using traditional peer nominations (e.g., consistent patterns of children who had high levels of social interactions with peers but still were not identified as members of groups).

Challenges of Observational Data Collection

As already noted, many of the same issues and concerns noted in the classic research remain evident today. For example, Goodenough (1930, 1937) lamented the difficulty associated with tapping the rich and complex nature of her observational data. She had to resort to large data aggregation—the result of which was the loss of process and change over time, and of changes over settings. Today, these issues still plague researchers who collect intensive observational data. Although there have been significant advances in data management and in analytical methods available for these purposes (e.g., sequential analyses, multilevel modeling, hierarchical longitudinal methods, social network analyses), researchers are still limited in the ability to maximize the richness of the data collected, and aggregation across data continues to be common (e.g., C. Martin & Fabes, 2001). Moreover, although the technological advances we have seen over the past 50 years (audio- and videotaping, computerization, etc.) allow researchers to gather more sophisticated and complex data on peer interactions and behaviors, the ability to visualize, to process, and to capture fully the complexity of the data is still a challenge that is likely to grow as the amount of data collected with new technologies increases.

The age-related changes in children's peer behaviors and interactions discussed earlier alter the effectiveness and appropriateness of observational methods. First, the use of observational methods has been made more difficult by the increasing complexity and sophistication of peer interactions during the grade school years. With age, peer interactions occur in more private contexts, so unobtrusive sampling of important and representative peer behavior becomes more difficult. Second, rates of many behaviors that may signify critical events for the course of peer interactions occur at low frequencies and in settings that do not include adults. Third, the peer interactions that do occur in classroom settings in which children are likely to be accessible to researchers become increasingly structured and may not be the types of peer interactions of most interest to researchers (Foster & Ritchey, 1985). These structured classroom peer settings may also become less available to researchers as school administrators, teachers, and parents restrict access for fear of distraction within the learning environment.

As children get older, the coding schemes needed to capture important elements of children's peer behaviors, and interactions become more complex and nuanced, making behavioral observations more difficult to utilize because of the increased demands on observers. For instance, there is some evidence that observations of peer responses received by disliked grade school children show greater discriminant validity than do observations of the actual behaviors initiated by these children (Bierman, 1986). Thus, with age, it appears that behavioral observation schemes need to include peer responses to children's behavior, as well as the behavior of the target children—adding more complexity to the procedures and perhaps more coders to the setting (something not appreciated by principals, teachers, and children). Additionally, the ability to negotiate one's position in a network of larger social groups and to establish alliances with peers that reflect an appropriate balance between attachment and autonomy represent important skills that are difficult to operationalize and to code with unobtrusive naturalistic observations (Bierman & Montminy, 1993).

Even in preschool, where peer behaviors and interactions are more unstructured, overt, and readily observed, implementing observational methods can be challenging. Because young children are often mobile and active, it can be challenging to observe their peer interactions unobtrusively. In addition, because young children often play alone or are involved with the teacher, it can be difficult to obtain enough observations of peer interactions and behaviors. Having a large enough sample of social behaviors becomes particularly crucial when interest is in behaviors that occur rarely. For example, in the observational data collected by Fabes, Martin, and Hanish (2003), the use of repeated 10-second scan observations of target preschool children's behavior failed to capture much in the way of negative affect, aggression, or rough-and-tumble play (fewer than 5% of observations reflected these behaviors or interactional qualities). This was true despite the fact that the researchers often obtained over 10,000 total observations per semester. Such findings point out the need to consider the type of sampling used: For low-frequency behaviors, event sampling (e.g., coding specific behaviors that occur regardless of which child emits them) rather than target child sampling may be a better approach. For instance, Fabes, Eisenberg, Smith, and Murphy (1996), used event coding to observe young children's peer conflict–related responses and obtained sufficient numbers of episodes to conduct their analyses that they could not obtain using a target child sampling procedure. Moreover, regardless of the observational procedures used, researchers should be aware of the impact of observers on children's peer interactions and behaviors. Brody, Stoneman, and Wheatley (1984) found that when observers were present in the playroom, children emitted fewer directives, engaged in less social conversation with their friends, and engaged in more task-related verbalizations than when observers were hidden.

The use of observational methods to study children's peer behaviors and interactions also leads to the question of the amount of observational data needed to establish adequate samples of behavior. Amounts of collected data vary across studies, and there is no agreed-upon protocol for determining when one has enough data (Foster et al., 1993). The issue of how much data to collect, however, can be critical. For instance, one key to understanding children's tendency to segregate their peer interactions by sex (e.g., boys play with boys, and girls play with girls) is to determine whether this sex-segregated play is a stable characteristic of children, or whether sex segregation is highly variable. Although many children frequently play with same-sex peers, there is variation in the degree to which they do so. If the degree of sex segregation is driven by stable individual characteristics of children, then researchers may want to concentrate attention on delineating the characteristics of children that influence their tendencies to segregate by sex. In contrast, if the tendency to segregate by sex varies considerably over time and situation, then researchers may want to focus attention on the situational factors that influence play patterns. Observers on a playground might notice a general tendency toward sex segregation for the group as a whole, but the children involved in sex-segregated play change from day to day and from situation to situation. As a result, variations in children's tendencies to play with same-sex playmates likely would be unstable and therefore uninformative.

Maccoby and Jacklin (1987) tested this by observing young children six times during the course of a day. One week later, an identical set of observations was collected on a subsample of the children. Based on their data, little evidence of stability in sex of play partner preference was found from one week to the next. This pattern of findings led Maccoby and Jacklin to suggest that sex segregation may not be due to individual characteristics of children. However, C. Martin and Fabes (2001), using a brief observation procedure in which children's play partner preferences were assessed repeatedly over a 6-month period, found play partner preferences to be considerably more stable over time. The differences in sampling across the two studies likely account for the different findings. In the Maccoby and Jacklin (1987) study, data were obtained in contiguous time intervals over only 2 days. In the C. Martin and Fabes (2001) study, several observations of one child were obtained during a single day, but none of the observations was contiguous in time. Moreover, C. Martin and Fabes coded behavior over a longer period of time (over 6 months). These findings suggest that decisions about the precise observational method used can have important implications for our understanding of peer behaviors and interactions. However, determining the best method is complicated and is influenced by the questions asked, the behavior to be observed, and the pragmatic aspects of the observational context (the setting, how long children are available, etc.). Clearly, more data are required for infrequent behaviors than for frequent ones and when behaviors are sampled in diverse versus similar situations, but precise guidelines regarding how much is enough remain an important research priority.

A person's behavior during a social interaction is determined by not only the person's dispositional or situational characteristics but also by his or her social relationships with interactional partners. As such, it is important to distinguish between "actor effects"—reflecting individual differences in the way one acts toward others—from "partner effects"—reflecting the consistency with which a person elicits the same behavior from others (Kenny & La Voie, 1984). Relationships are said to exist when behavior within a dyad differs from the behavior that both partners give and receive in other social contexts (Ross & Lollis, 1989). Hay and Ross (1982) observed young children's conflicts and found that past and present dyadic events, as well as dispositional factors, influenced the initiation and termination of conflicts. Thus, observational researchers studying peer interactions need to consider what individuals versus relationships contribute to the observed social interactional patterns. To do so often requires detailed data on the sequence of behaviors within the interaction—often requiring the use of videotaped interactions. Analytic methods also have been developed that allow researchers to model the statistical interdependence that naturally exists between partners in relationships. For example, the actor–partner interdependence model (Kashy & Kenny, 2000) allows one to estimate the extent to which responses are influenced by factors associated with both actors and their partners.

Thus, the challenges of collecting and using observational data are far-ranging. The process of collecting observational data typically is time-intensive, expensive, and logistically demanding. Researchers have to make significant decisions about sampling (who is observed, when, and at what level—group, dyadic, or individual) and recording methods (how behavior is coded); each of these methods has advantages and disadvantages, and produces different types of data (Bakeman & Gottman, 1986; P. Martin & Bateson, 1986). Once data are acquired, management of the data becomes challenging, although software packages and technologies have been developed to facilitate data collection and management. But the potential of observational methods has been raised to new levels by new technological and analytic procedures.

Future Directions in Studying
Children's Peer Behaviors and Interactions

As this discussion indicates, no single method is able to measure all aspects of peer behavior, and no single method is appropriate and applicable in all situations, and with all children. Since their inception, however, these methods have been the foundation for the study of children's peer behaviors and interactions and they continue to have important roles today. However, with the continuing advances made in technology, computerization, and statistical procedures, the methods available for studying children's peer behaviors and interactions are changing. With these changes come concomitant changes in the nature and type of questions that researchers are able to ask and the issues they face. We now focus our discussion on future directions in the study of children's peer behaviors and interactions, and highlight some of the key issues.

Although there are numerous examples of longitudinal analyses of children's peer relationships (e.g., Ladd, 2006), they tend to include only a few waves of measurement over relatively few points of time (e.g., measured yearly). However, in the last few decades, new methods and technologies, such as handheld computers, beepers, Web interfaces, and georeferencing hardware and software, have enhanced our ability to track, collect, manage, and organize complex data on social systems. These technologies allow researchers to collect a large amount of data on complex social patterns across different contexts and over relatively short periods of time (Eagle & Pentland, 2006).

The ability to collect dense, continuous data across different contexts should enhance and advance the study of children's peer interactions and behaviors. These data allow us to focus on *process*—something that has always been challenging to investigate (Hartup, 2005). The collection of intensive longitudinal peer interaction data gives rise to questions about the expression of time-varying characteristics that predict peer interactions, the dynamic evolution of peer groups and peer socialization, the temporal and nonlinear patterns of change in peer interactions, and the consequences of these for later functioning. These new methods, and their conceptual and analytical foundations, are not merely extensions of traditional approaches to the study of longitudinal relations. As Walls and Schafer (2006) noted, differences between intensive longitudinal data and traditional models of longitudinal data are not tied to the amount of data collected. Rather, the differences lie in the kinds of questions that can be asked: With intensive longitudinal data, researchers can ascertain complexity and variety in individual trajectories, variations within individuals over time, and differences in variances and covariances. Detailed discussion of each of these issues is beyond the scope of this chapter, but the change from data collection involving small or moderate waves of data to methods that produce intensive and large numbers (hundreds, thousands) of data points from relatively large numbers of individuals will likely produce dramatic changes in the study of children's peer interactions and behaviors.

Some of the first intensive forms of data collection on human relationships came from structured daily diary studies (Bolger, DeLongis, Kessler, & Schilling, 1989), and these have been applied to the study of children's peer behaviors and interactions (Ralph, Williams, & Campisi, 1997). Children (depending on their age) and/or their parents can be asked to complete daily (or more frequent) diary entries about their peer interactions and the qualities associated with these (e.g., who they are with, what was happening, assessments of mood). This approach was essentially the core of the "digital diary" methods, such as the experience-sampling method (Tennen & Affleck, 2002) and ecological momentary assessment (Hektner, Schmidt, & Csikszentmihalyi, 2007), in which on-the-spot information can be entered into a handheld computer regarding one's actions, thoughts, and social and relational contexts. These methods not only afford large amounts of complex social data but they also can be used in situations where direct observation is not possible, such as within romantic and intimate peer relationships (Shrier, Shih, Hacker, & de Moor, 2007). Audio- and video-recording devices are now smaller, more refined, and more capable of surreptitiously monitoring individuals' interactions with one another. These can subsequently be reviewed and coded, thereby generating high volumes of intensive social data. Additionally, coders using handheld computers can monitor and quickly enter data into preprogrammed data sheets that allow for collection of large amounts of data on the spot (see Nusser, Intille, & Maitra, 2006).

Newer technologies that are being introduced also can pave the way for the next generation of research involving intensive data on children's peer interactions. For example, collection of data using cell phones may be a particularly interesting approach to studying peer interactions. Eagle and Pentland (2006) used data collected from Bluetooth-enabled mobile phones to assess social patterns in daily user activity, to identify significant social locations, and to model social networks of college students. The application of this technology to older children and teens should be fairly straightforward and provide important information regarding "virtual" peer interactions, networks, relationship inference, and patterns of peer dynamics.

Such devices may not work so well with young children. However, new technologies also can be applied at these young ages as well. For example, "motes"—wearable computer technology that shares information via bidirectional radio links (Choi, Gouda, Kim, & Arora, 2003)—can be used with children of any age. The core of a mote is a small, low-cost, low-power computer. Motes can be programmed to gather and to provide information received from and sent to other motes in the immediate environment. The motes can be "active," such that they initiate contact with other motes based on certain conditions to identify relational patterns. Thus, young children can be provided with these easily wearable devices that record who they are in contact with, for how long, and under what conditions. And as the technology advances, these devices are continuously becoming smaller, less obtrusive, and more powerful. With some additional upgrading, other data can be recorded from these devices at the same time (e.g., physiological data, such as heart rate or respiration) and can be used in combination with peer interaction data. Of course, these new technologies bring new problems and issues (battery life, reactivity, privacy ethics, security of data, etc.). However, the development of new technologies makes it possible to expand our abilities to assess children's peer behaviors and interactions.

Conclusions

There is considerable agreement that studies of children's behaviors and peer interactions are crucial to a complete understanding of peer relationships. There is also agreement on the need to complement descriptive research with more dynamic, process-oriented designs (including experimental designs; Hartup, 2005). However, vast intra- and inter-individual differences in behaviors and peer interactions create many differences in the key constructs that we measure, and in the methods that we use to measure them. All methodologies have certain advantages and disadvantages, and the new and emerging scientific advances in methods and procedures will be no different. On the one hand, these new methods and technologies may leave us with new challenges in their use and in integrating findings across diverse studies. On the other hand, we are likely to be provided with new and exciting possibilities to expand the study of children's behaviors and interactions, and to address questions that we were not able to address adequately prior to their availability.

Acknowledgments

This research was supported in part by a research grant from the National Institute of Child Health and Human Development (No. R01 HD045816-01). Appreciation is expressed to Alicia Moss for her assistance with parts of this chapter.

References

Bakeman, R., & Gottman, J. M. (1986). *Observing interaction: An introduction to sequential analysis.* Cambridge, UK: Cambridge University Press.

Barker, R. G., & Wright, H. F. (1971). *Midwest and its children: The psychology ecology of an American town.* Hamden, CT: Archon Books. (Original work published 1955)

Barnes, E. (1896–1897, 1902–1903). *Studies in education.* Philadelphia: Author.

Bierman, K. L. (1986). The relation between social aggression and peer rejection in middle childhood. In R. J. Prinz (Ed.), *Advances in behavioral assessment of children and families* (Vol. 2, pp. 151–178). Greenwich, CT: JAI.

Bierman, K. L., & Montminy, H. P. (1993). Developmental issues in social-skills assessment and intervention with children and adolescents. *Behavior Modification, 17,* 229–254.

Bolger, N., DeLongis, A., Kessler, R. C., & Schilling, E. A. (1989). Effects of daily stress on negative mood. *Journal of Personality and Social Psychology, 57,* 808–818.

Bond, N. D., & Phillips, B. N. (1971). Personality traits associated with altruistic behavior of children. *Journal of School Psychology, 9,* 24–34.

Bott, E. A., Blatz, W. E., Chant, N., & Bott, H. (1928). Observation and training of fundamental habits in young children [Special issue]. *Genetic Psychology Monographs, 4,* 1–161.

Brody, G. H., Stoneman, Z., & Wheatley, P. (1984). Peer interaction in the presence and absence of observers. *Child Development, 55,* 1425–1428.

Cairns, R. B., Leung, M.-C., Gest, S. D., & Cairns, B. D. (1995). A brief method for assessing social development: Structure, reliability, stability, and developmental validity of the Interpersonal Competence Scale. *Behaviour Research and Therapy, 33,* 725–736.

Cassidy, J., & Asher, S. R. (1992). Loneliness and peer relations in young children. *Child Development, 63,* 350–365.

Challman, R. C. (1932). Factors influencing friendships among preschool children. *Child Development, 3,* 146–158.

Charlesworth, R., & Hartup, W. W. (1967). Positive social reinforcement in the nursery school peer group. *Child Development, 38,* 993–1002.

Choi, Y., Gouda, M. G., Kim, M. C., & Arora, A. (2003, October 20–22). *The mote connectivity protocol.* Paper presented at the 12th International Conference on Computer Communications and Networks, Dallas, TX.

Coie, J. D., Dodge, K. A., & Kupersmidt, J. (1990). Group behavior and social status. In S. R. Asher & J. D. Coie (Eds.), *Peer rejection in childhood* (pp. 17–59). Cambridge, UK: Cambridge University Press.

Dawe, H. C. (1934). An analysis of two hundred quarrels of preschool children. *Child Development, 5*, 139–157.

Eagle, N., & Pentland, A. (2006). Reality mining: Sensing complex social systems. *Personal and Ubiquitous Computing, 10*, 255–268.

Fabes, R. A., & Eisenberg, N. (1998). *Meta-analyses of age and sex differences in children's and adolescents' prosocial behavior.* Retrieved April 1, 2008, from *www.public.asu.edu/~rafabes/meta.pdf.*

Fabes, R. A., Eisenberg, N., Jones, S., Smith, M., Guthrie, I. K., Poulin, R., et al. (1999). Regulation, emotionality, and preschoolers' socially competent peer interactions. *Child Development, 70*, 432–442.

Fabes, R. A., Eisenberg, N., McCormick, S. E., & Wilson, M. S. (1988). Preschoolers' attributions of the situational determinants of others' naturally occurring emotions. *Developmental Psychology, 24*, 376–385.

Fabes, R. A., Eisenberg, N., Smith, M. C., & Murphy, B. C. (1996). Getting angry at peers: Associations with liking of the provocateur. *Child Development, 67*, 942–956.

Fabes, R. A., Martin, C. L., & Hanish, L. D. (2003). Qualities of young children's same-, other-, and mixed-sex play. *Child Development, 74*, 921–932.

Fabes, R. A., Martin, C. L., & Hanish, L. (2007). Peer interactions and the gendered social ecology of preparing young children for school. *Early Childhood Services, 1*, 205–218.

Fagot, B. I. (1977). Variations in density: Effect on task and social behaviors of preschool children. *Developmental Psychology, 13*, 166–167.

Fagot, B. I., & Patterson, G. R. (1969). An *in vivo* analysis of reinforcing contingencies for sex-role behaviors in the preschool child. *Developmental Psychology, 1*, 563–568.

Fast Track. (2004). *Teacher social competence.* Retrieved June 12, 2007, from *www.childandfamilypolicy.duke.edu/fasttrack/techrept/t/tsc/.*

Foot, H. C., Chapman, A. J., & Smith, J. R. (1980). *Friendship and social relations in children.* New York: Wiley.

Foster, S. L., Inderbitzen, H. M., & Nangle, D. W. (1993). Assessing acceptance and social skills with peers in childhood. *Behavior Modification, 17*, 255–286.

Foster, S. L., & Ritchey, W. L. (1985). Behavioral correlates of sociometric status of fourth-, fifth-, and sixth-grade children in two classroom situations. *Behavioral Assessment, 7*, 79–93.

Gest, S. D. (2006). Teacher reports of children's friendships and social groups: Agreement with peer reports and implications for studying peer similarity. *Social Development, 15*, 248–259.

Gest, S. D., Farmer, T. W., Cairns, B. D., & Xie, H. (2003). Identifying children's peer social networks in school classrooms: Links between peer reports and observed interactions. *Social Development, 12*, 513–529.

Goodenough, F. (1930). Inter-relationships in the behavior of young children. *Child Development, 1*, 29–47.

Goodenough, F. (1937). The observation of children's behaviors as a method in social psychology. *Social Forces, 15*, 476–479.

Gottman, J. M. (1986). The observation of social process. In J. M. Gottman & J. G. Parker (Eds.), *Conversations of friends. Speculations on affective development* (pp. 51–100). Cambridge, UK: Cambridge University Press.

Graham, S., & Juvonen, J. (1998). Self-blame and peer victimization in middle school: An attributional analysis. *Developmental Psychology, 34*, 587–599.

Gresham, F. M., & Elliott, S. N. (1990). *Social Skills Rating System.* Circle Pines, MN: American Guidance Service.

Harris, P. L. (2006). Social cognition. In D. Kuhn, R. S. Siegler, W. Damon, & R. M. Lerner (Eds.), *Handbook of child psychology: Vol. 2. Cognition, perception, and language* (pp. 811–858). Hoboken, NJ: Wiley.

Hartup, W. W. (2005). Peer interaction: What causes what? *Journal of Abnormal Child Psychology, 33*, 387–394.

Hartup, W. W., Glazer, J. A., & Charlesworth, R. (1967). Peer reinforcement and sociometric status. *Child Development, 38*, 1017–1024.

Hartup, W. W., & Laursen, B. (1991). Relationships as developmental contexts. In R. Cohen & A. W. Siegel (Eds.), *Context and development* (pp. 253–279). Hillsdale, NJ: Erlbaum.

Hay, D. F., & Ross, H. S. (1982). The social nature of early conflict. *Child Development, 53*, 105–113.

Hektner, J. M., Schmidt, J. A., & Csikszentmihalyi, M. (2007). *Experience sampling method: Measuring the quality of everyday life*. Thousand Oaks, CA: Sage.

Hinde, R. A., & Stevenson-Hinde, J. (1987). Interpersonal relationships and child development. *Developmental Review, 7*, 1–21.

Hogan, A. E., Scott, K. G., & Bauer, C. R. (1992). The Adaptive Social Behavior Inventory (ASBI): A new assessment of social competence in high-risk three-year-olds. *Journal of Psychoeducational Assessment, 10*, 230–239.

Howes, C. (1988). Peer interaction of young children [Special issue]. *Monographs of the Society for Research in Child Development, 53*.

Kashy, D. A., & Kenny, D. A. (2000). The analysis of data from dyads and groups. In H. T. Reis & C. M. Judd (Eds.), *Handbook of research methods in social psychology* (pp. 451–477). New York: Cambridge University Press.

Kenny, D. A., & La Voie, L. (1984). The social relations model. In L. Berkowitz (Ed.), *Advances in experimental social psychology* (Vol. 19, pp. 141–182). New York: Academic Press.

Kohn, M., & Rosman, B. L. (1972). A social competence scale and symptom checklist for the preschool child. *Developmental Psychology, 6*, 430–444.

Ladd, G. W. (2005). *Peer relationships and social competence of children and adolescents*. New Haven, CT: Yale University Press.

Ladd, G. W. (2006). Peer rejection, aggressive or withdrawn behavior, and psychological maladjustment from ages 5 to 12: An examination of four predictive models. *Child Development, 77*, 822–846.

Ladd, G. W., & Profilet, S. M. (1996). The Child Behavior Scale: A teacher report measure of young children's aggressive, withdrawn, and prosocial behaviors. *Developmental Psychology, 32*, 1008–1024.

LaFreniere, P., & Dumas, J. E. (1996). Social competence and behavior evaluation in children ages 3 to 6 years: The short form (SCBE-30). *Psychological Assessment, 8*, 369–377.

Maccoby, E. E., & Jacklin, C. N. (1987). Gender segregation in childhood. In H. W. Reese (Ed.), *Advances in child development and behavior* (Vol. 20, pp. 239–287). Orlando, FL: Academic Press.

Martin, C. L., & Fabes, R. A. (2001). The stability and consequences of young children's same-sex peer interactions. *Developmental Psychology, 37*, 431–446.

Martin, C. L., Fabes, R. A., Hanish, L., & Hollenstein, T. (2006). Social dynamics in the preschool. *Developmental Review, 25*, 299–327.

Martin, P., & Bateson, P. P. G. (1986). *Measuring behaviour*. Cambridge, UK: Cambridge University Press.

Matson, J. L., Rotatori, A. F., & Helsel, W. J. (1983). Development of a rating scale to measure social skills in children: The Matson Evaluation of Social Skills with Youngsters (MESSY). *Behaviour Research and Therapy, 21*, 335–340.

Monroe, W. S. (1899). Play interests of children. *American Educational Review, 4*, 358–365.

Nusser, S. M., Intille, S. S., & Maitra, R. (2006). Emerging technologies and next-generation intensive longitudinal data collection. In T. A. Walls & J. L. Schafer (Eds.), *Models for intensive longitudinal data* (pp. 254–278). Oxford, UK: Oxford University Press.

Parten, M. B. (1932). Social participation among pre-school children. *Journal of Abnormal and Social Psychology, 27*, 243–269.

Parten, M. B. (1933). Social play among preschool children. *Journal of Abnormal and Social Psychology, 27*, 430–440.

Patterson, G. R., & Anderson, D. (1964). Peers as social reinforcers. *Child Development, 35,* 951–960.

Patterson, G. R., Littman, R. A., & Bricker, W. (1967). Assertive behavior in children: A step toward a theory of aggression. *Monographs of the Society for Research in Child Development, 32.*

Power, T. G. (2000). *Play and exploration in children and animals.* Mahwah, NJ: Erlbaum.

Ralph, A., Williams, C., & Campisi, A. (1997). Measuring peer interactions using the Adolescent Social Interaction Profile. *Journal of Applied Developmental Psychology, 18,* 71–86.

Ross, H. S., & Lollis, S. P. (1989). A social relations analysis of toddler peer relationships. *Child Development, 60,* 1082–1091.

Rubin, K. H., Bukowski, W. M., & Parker, J. G. (2006). Peer interactions, relationships, and groups. In N. Eisenberg, W. Damon, & R. M. Lerner (Eds.), *Handbook of child psychology: Vol. 3. Social, emotional, and personality development* (pp. 571–645). Hoboken, NJ: Wiley.

Sackett, G. P. (1977). *Observing behavior: Data collection and analysis methods.* Oxford, UK: University Park Press.

Shigetomi, C. C., Hartmann, D. P., & Gelfand, D. (1981). Sex differences in children's altruistic behavior and reputations for helpfulness. *Developmental Psychology, 17,* 434–437.

Shrier, L. A., Shih, M., Hacker, L., & de Moor, C. (2007). A momentary sampling study of the affective experience following coital events in adolescents. *Journal of Adolescent Health, 40,* 1–8.

Smith, P. K. (1978). A longitudinal study of social participation in preschool children solitary and parallel play re-examined. *Developmental Psychology, 14,* 517–523.

Strayer, F. F. (1980). Social ecology of the preschool peer group. In W. A. Collins (Ed.), *Development of cognition, affect and social relations* (Vol. 13, pp. 165–196). Hillsdale, NJ: Erlbaum.

Strayer, F. F. (1992). The development of agonistic and affiliative structures in preschool play groups. In J. Silverberg & J. P. Gray (Eds.), *Aggression and peacefulness in humans and other primates* (pp. 150–188). Oxford, UK: Oxford University Press.

Strayer, F. F., & Strayer, J. (1976). An ethological analysis of social agonism and dominance relations among preschool children. *Child Development, 47,* 980–989.

Tennen, H., & Affleck, G. (2002). The challenge of capturing daily processes at the interface of social and clinical psychology. *Journal of Social and Clinical Psychology, 21,* 610–627.

Thorne, B. (1993). *Gender play: Girls and boys in school.* New Brunswick, NJ: Rutgers University.

Vaughn, B. E., & Waters, E. (1980). Social organization among preschool peers: Dominance, attention, and sociometric correlates. In D. Omark, F. Strayer, & D. Freedman (Eds.), *Dominance relations: Ethological perspectives on human conflict* (pp. 359–379). New York: Garland Press.

Walker, H. M., & McConnell, S. R. (1988). *The Walker–McConnell Scale of Social Competence and School Adjustment.* Austin, TX: Pro-Ed.

Walker, H. M., & McConnell, S. R. (1991). *The Walker–McConnell Adolescent Scale of Social Competence and School Adjustment.* Austin, TX: Pro-Ed.

Walls, T. A., & Schafer, J. L. (Eds.). (2006). *Models for intensive longitudinal data.* Oxford, UK: Oxford University Press.

CHAPTER 4

Methods for Investigating Children's Relationships with Friends

THOMAS J. BERNDT
MELISSA A. McCANDLESS

Friendships are the closest of children's relationships with peers. Friendships change dramatically with age, becoming closer and more distinctive as children grow older and move into adolescence (Newcomb & Bagwell, 1995; Rubin, Bukowski, & Parker, 2006). Moreover, the importance of friendships to children themselves strongly suggests that these relationships have important effects on children's social behavior and psychological development (Berndt, 2004; Berndt & Murphy, 2002).

Because friendships are such special relationships, a special set of measures and research methods is required to investigate their essential characteristics, their development, and their effects on children. Friendships are rooted in children's behaviors toward and interactions with their peers, so research on friendship sometimes draws upon the variety of methods used to study peer interactions in general (see Fabes, Martin, & Hanish, Chapter 3, this volume). But like other relationships, friendships involve a history of interactions, along with the interaction partners' thoughts and feelings about those interactions (Hinde, 1979). Consequently, studies of friendships go beyond studies of social behavior or social interaction.

Friendships usually form within larger groups of peers, but measures of friendships are qualitatively different from the measures of children's positions in a peer group that are obtained with sociometric techniques (see Cillessen, Chapter 5, this volume). Still, some overlap exists between measures of friendship and measures of sociometric status. We discuss this overlap and its implications for the interpretation of research findings later in this chapter.

Research on friendships also overlaps with research on children's peer groups, because pairs of friends have other friends, and these friendships become interlinked to form small groups or cliques. Researchers who study friendship groups often examine phenomena such as group size, the characteristics of the network linking group members, and a group's relationships with other groups. The same phenomena are examined in research on other types of children's groups, and a few scholars have discussed methods for exploring those phenomena (see Kindermann & Gest, Chapter 6, this volume). Consequently, our focus in this chapter is exclusively on the relationships between pairs of friends.

Many distinguished scholars have critically evaluated the various methods for research on children's friendships (Hartup, 1983; Bukowski & Hoza, 1989; Newcomb & Bagwell, 1995; Furman, 1996; Rubin et al., 2006). We seek to build on that tradition by analyzing some crucial methodological issues. Our goal is not to present a set of rules for all research on friendships, but to encourage researchers to select the methods that are most appropriate given the purposes of a specific study.

In the first section of the chapter, we explore various definitions of friendship. We suggest the usefulness of describing friendships as varying in their positions on a continuum defined by the degree to which the friends know and like each other. On this idealized continuum, "the best of friends" falls at one extreme and strangers fall at the other.

In the next section we discuss various choices that researchers must make when identifying children's friends. For example, we consider whether to limit the number of friends children can name, and whether to require reciprocity in nominations when identifying friends. In addition, we use the concept of the "friendship continuum" to illustrate how different methods affect the sample of friendships identified.

The following section focuses on the quality of children's friendships. We discuss the features of friendship that are assessed in friendship-quality measures and examine how scores on these measures relate to observations of friends' interactions. Finally, we draw together our conclusions about methods for investigating children's friendships, reiterating that researchers should choose methods that fit their research goals and strengthen the interpretation of research findings.

Definitions of Friendship

Before friendships are identified between children, the terms "friend" and "friendship" must be defined. These terms do not refer to specialized psychological constructs. On the contrary, they are part of the everyday language of children, adolescents, and adults. Consequently, their essential attributes can be gleaned from various dictionary definitions (Morris, 1981; Landau, 2001; *Webster's Encyclopedic Unabridged Dictionary*, 1989; Simpson & Weiner, 1989).

The most basic definition of a "friend" is someone whom a person knows and likes. Importantly, this knowledge and liking are assumed to be mutual; that is, a person does not call another person a friend unless he or she knows and likes that person, and assumes that the other person knows and likes him or her as well. But not all relationships that meet these criteria are labeled as friendships. Dictionary definitions match common usage in drawing distinctions between friendships on the one hand and romantic or family relationships on the other. Lovers and family members also know and like each other, but they are not normally labeled as "friends."

Other attributes of friendship are mentioned in some dictionary definitions. Friends are favored companions; that is, they usually spend many hours interacting with each other. Friends typically have feelings of benevolence toward one another, as implied by the old saying that "a friend in need is a friend indeed." Friendships may also include a high level of intimacy, a closeness that leads friends to talk freely with one another about their personal thoughts and feelings. This intimacy depends on another attribute of friendship, the trust that friends have in one another. However, friends differ in how much time they spend together, how much they help each other, and how much they share personal information and trust one another. Consequently, these attributes should probably be considered as characteristic of "friendship" but not as essential to its definition. Later in the chapter we describe these attributes as providing important information not about whether two children are friends, but about the quality of their friendship.

In one dictionary a "friend" is defined as someone whom a person *knows well and likes a lot* (Landau, 2001). By introducing the qualifiers "well" and "a lot," this definition suggests that friendships may vary in their degree of mutual knowledge and affection. By contrast, several scholars have argued that researchers who study children's friendships have too often viewed friendships as dichotomous, so that two children are judged either to be best friends or not to be friends at all (Hartup, 1996). Like these other scholars, we argue that friendships are better viewed as having different positions on a continuum that is defined simultaneously by the friends' knowledge of and liking for each other.

As Figure 4.1 suggests, the positive extreme on this continuum represents an ideal friendship. To describe such a friendship, people sometimes say that two people are "the best of friends." This comment implies that the two friends know and like each other as much as any friends could. The negative extreme on the continuum is represented by strangers, who do not know each other, so they neither like nor dislike each other.

On the continuum above the negative extreme is the range of relationships in which people refer to each other as "acquaintances," who, by definition, are people whom a person knows a little but neither likes nor dislikes very much. If two people's knowledge of each other increases to the point at which some degree of mutual liking arises, the relationship crosses the ambiguous or fuzzy boundary on the continuum to become a friendship.

Friendships cover an even broader range than acquaintanceships. This range is well understood by adults and, at least beyond a certain age (see Selman, 1980), by children. In one recent study, Simpkins, Parke, Flyr, and Wild (2006) captured this variation by asking children whether one of their peers was "a best friend, close friend, just-a-friend, or acquaintance [i.e., not a friend]" (p. 497). Other researchers seem to view best friendships and close friendships as largely synonymous. So, for example, whereas Burk and Laursen (2005) asked children to name their "three same-sex best friends," Weimer, Kerns, and

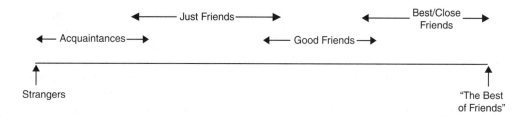

FIGURE 4.1. A schematic representation of the continuum of friendships.

Oldenburg (2004) asked adolescents to name "a close same-sex friend." Still, both sets of researchers wanted to know about relationships marked by the greatest mutual knowledge and liking. Moreover, once "best" friendships are described, it is natural to label less close relationships as "good" friendships. When relationships are even less close, two people can be described, as suggested by Simpkins et al. (2006), as "just friends." We use these labels in Figure 4.1 because they are compatible with most writings on friendships among children and adults (e.g., Hendrick & Hendrick, 2000).

Like the boundary between acquaintanceship and friendship, the boundaries between different types of friendship are ambiguous or fuzzy. For example, no specific criteria indicate when a relationship changes from a good friendship to a close friendship or vice versa. Moreover, any set of criteria is likely to identify not a single type of friendship but a range of friendships. This ambiguity or fuzziness is implied in Figure 4.1 by the overlap of the ranges on the continuum for each type of friendship.

The concept of a "friendship continuum" has important implications for research. Planning research on children's friendships always involves making decisions that, intentionally or unintentionally, affect the range of friendships that will be investigated. In particular, researchers' decisions about how to identify friends determine whether the friendships finally investigated cover a broad or a narrow range on the continuum, and how many of those friendships are near the positive extreme on the continuum, "the best of friends." Stated differently, these decisions determine whether the researchers examine mostly best/close friendships, mostly good friendships, or a mix of these two and perhaps some that are "just friendships."

In describing this consequence of methodological decisions about how to identify friends, our intention is not to say that research on "good friendships" is fatally flawed or even that it makes less of a contribution to the literature than research on best/close friendships. On the contrary, we would argue that examining different ranges on the friendship continuum can be valuable or even essential. One major reason is that not all children have a relationship that comes close to the "best of friends" ideal. If researchers insist on studying only friendships that are near this positive extreme on the continuum, children whose best friendships do not measure up to this ideal must be excluded from the final research sample. Then the final sample will be smaller and less representative of the entire population of children than are the samples of researchers who allow for a broader range of friendships. Trade-offs of this kind are emphasized in the following discussion of the choices that researchers make when identifying children's friends.

Choices in Identifying Friends

Researchers make many choices when planning a study of children's friendships. One choice that we should mention briefly is whether to identify children's friends at all. In studies of the characteristics of children's friendships, identification of their friends may not be necessary. For example, children who complete the Network of Relationships Inventory (Furman & Buhrmester, 1985) answer questions such as "How much free time do you spend with your best friend?" Even if children are asked to think of a specific friend when answering such questions, researchers need not record the friend's identity. Similarly, researchers could examine children's ideas about how best friends interact, without identifying any friends by name (but see Burgess, Wojslawowicz, Rubin, Rose-Krasnor, & Booth-LaForce, 2006).

For many other types of research, however, identification of children's friends is crucial. To accomplish this identification, researchers must answer four interrelated questions. First, who should name the child's friends? Nominations could come from children themselves, from their parents, from teachers, or from outside observers. Second, how should researchers ask for friendship nominations, and how many friends should they allow children to name? These questions go together because, for example, if children are asked about their "very, very best friend" (Rose & Asher, 2004), then they can give only one name.

Third, who can be named as a friend? Researchers rarely allow completely free nominations of friends. Often, nominations are restricted to other children who are the same sex and in the same grade, or other children who are also participating in the study. Fourth, does the peer named as a friend need to name the child in return? In other words, is reciprocity in nominations required? In discussing these four questions, we refer often to the friendship continuum. We do so not because there is only one correct answer to each question, but because different answers may lead to different interpretations of a study's results.

Who Should Be Asked to Name a Child's Friends?

The most obvious answer is that children should be asked who their friends are, and this answer seems to be the best one in most cases. Rubin et al. (2006) stated, "Normally, friendship cannot be presumed unless children have been expressly asked whether the relationship in question is a friendship" (p. 606). Thus, most researchers begin their studies of friendship by asking children to name their best friends.

Researchers have had difficulty, however, identifying the best friends of toddlers and preschool children solely from their friendship nominations (see Ladd, Kochenderfer, & Coleman, 1996). With these young children, researchers have more often relied on reports by parents and teachers, direct observations of the children's interactions with peers, or some combination of these assessments. In one study (Dunn, Cutting, & Fisher, 2002), pairs of 3- and 4-year-olds were considered as best friends if their teachers and mothers named them as friends, and observations in the preschool setting indicated that they were close to each other, showing positive affect while engaged in social play at least 30% of the time they were under observation. In short, these assessments combined the friendship nominations of knowledgeable adults with evidence that children were frequent companions and displayed other behaviors indicative of friendship.

Thus, the best answer to the question "Who should name a child's friends?" depends on the child's age. With toddlers and preschool children, the most accurate identification of friendships may be achieved with some combination of parents' and teachers' nominations, and observations of the children's peer interactions. By contrast, children in elementary and secondary school appear to be the best informants on who their friends are.

What Question Should Children Be Asked, and How Many Friends Should They Be Allowed to Name?

As mentioned earlier, children are sometimes asked to name their "very, very best friend." This question is asking about the one friendship that a child considers as closest to the positive extreme on the friendship continuum. More commonly, children are asked to name their three best or closest friends (e.g., Barry & Wentzel, 2006). Sometimes children are allowed to name up to six best friends (Malcolm, Jensen-Campbell, Rex-Lear, & Waldrip, 2006). Occasionally, children are asked to name up to 10 of their "closest friends" (Fletcher, Hunter, & Eanes, 2006). Rarely are children asked to name their closest friends without any limit on the number they can name (Parker, Low, Walker, & Gamm, 2005).

Some researchers have argued that limiting the number of nominations may lead to errors in the identification of friendships (Furman, 1996). When an interviewer asks children to name their three best friends, children with only one best friend might name nonfriends for their second and third choices to try to satisfy the interviewer's request. Conversely, children with more than three best friends would be forced to choose between those best friends in a way that distorts reporting of their friendships.

This argument depends, however, on the dichotomous view of friendships that we have rejected. Our explication of the friendship continuum suggests that when asked to name their three best friends, all children name the three peers with whom they have the closest relationship. For some children, those three are truly best friends; for others, those three may include both best and good friends. If children are asked to name 6 or 10 friends, they respond by naming some peers with whom they have less close relationships, peers whom they consider as good friends or just friends rather than best friends. In other words, allowing more nominations expands the range on the friendship continuum of the friendships finally identified.

Why would a researcher allow more nominations? Malcolm and colleagues (2006) stated, "We allowed up to six nominations in order to obtain [friendship] scores for as many students as possible" (p. 727). If fewer nominations had been allowed, more children would have lacked friendship scores and would therefore have been excluded from the final database and from the data analyses. Such exclusions reduce the final sample size and so reduce the statistical power to test hypotheses. The exclusions also make the sample less representative of the original population, because children are unlikely to be excluded randomly. Generally, the children who are excluded because they appear to have no friends also have an above-average risk of problems in social adjustment (Kiesner, Poulin, & Nicotra, 2003). In many studies these children are the subgroup of greatest interest.

To lessen these problems, we encourage researchers to think carefully about how to ask children to name their friends, and about how many friends they are allowed to name. In other words, given the goals of their studies, researchers should think carefully about where the friendships that they identify should fall on the friendship continuum. "Thinking carefully" means, in part, recognizing that aiming for very close friendships is also likely to entail excluding many children from the final sample because they do not have such close friendships or their closest friends cannot be identified by the researchers.

Who Can Be Named as a Friend?

Sometimes children's closest friends cannot be identified by researchers because the children are not given free choice in whom they name as friends. Children may be asked to name friends who attend the same school (Brendgen, Markiewicz, Doyle, & Bukowski, 2001), or friends in the same school and the same grade (Burgess et al., 2006), or in the same grade and the same class (Rose & Asher, 2004), or classmates who are also participating in the study (Adams, Bukowski, & Bagwell, 2005). Typically, children are also required to name friends of the same sex.

Children are typically required to name same-sex friends because, when friendship nominations are not restricted, peers of the opposite sex are rarely named (Hartup, 1983; Kovacs, Parker, & Hoffman, 1996). Opposite-sex nominations increase greatly during adolescence (Kuttler, La Greca, & Prinstein, 1999), but opposite-sex friendships appear to be qualitatively different from same-sex friendships and may serve different functions in development (Kovacs et al., 1996). It seems reasonable, then, to continue the usual practice of requiring same-sex nominations, unless the central purpose of a study is to compare same- and opposite-sex friendships. Even so, more research on the age changes in same- and opposite-sex friendships would be valuable.

Arguments such as those made for requiring same-sex nominations have been made for requiring that children name friends who are in their grade at their school. In particular, previous research has shown that most children name best friends in their grade at their school (Hartup, 1983). However, children name more best friends not in their grade or not attending their school than they name opposite-sex best friends. These non-school nominations demonstrate that there are multiple contexts besides the school in which children develop and maintain friendships (Fletcher et al., 2006). Moreover, a few studies have documented the importance of these nonschool relationships. Although the central measures in one study did not refer specifically to friendships, the results showed that adolescents' behavior in and out of school was significantly influenced by their close peer relationships outside of school (Kiesner et al., 2003).

Why have researchers so often reduced their ability to identify children's closest actual friendships by restricting their friendship nominations? Stated in terms of the friendship continuum, why have researchers chosen methods that increase the chances of identifying children's good friends or "just friends," rather than their best friends? The main reason for these restrictions is that they increase the number of children whose friends are also participating in the research. When both children and their friends are research participants, comparable data are available for both.

Many important research questions can only be answered by collecting comparable data for children and their friends. When peers named as friends are also participating in a study, those peers name their own friends, so reciprocity in friendship nominations can be determined. Any measures of thoughts, feelings, or behavior that are obtained for the children in a study are obtained for their friends as well, so similarities between children and their friends can be examined (e.g., Jaccard, Blanton, & Dodge, 2005). In addition, researchers sometimes identify pairs of friends who are then observed in interaction with each other (e.g., Brendgen et al., 2001; Burgess et al., 2006). These observations are possible only if children can be paired with a friend who is participating in the study.

Another point worth making is that *not* restricting children's friendship nominations does not automatically strengthen a study. When the peers named as friends are not participating in a study, crucial data about those friendships may be unavailable. Without such data, the children who nominated those peers may have to be excluded from the final sample for the study. The exclusions have the same effect as those we described in connection with decisions to limit the number of friends that children can name. When children are excluded from the final sample, the data analyses have lower statistical power, and the results are likely to be less representative of the entire population of children.

Nevertheless, the choice to restrict friendship nominations to a specific subset of peers should not be taken lightly. Not restricting friendship nominations can provide crucial data for future research. For example, Bagwell and Coie (2004) wanted to observe the interactions of aggressive boys with their best friends. These researchers did not try to pair all aggressive boys with best friends in their own grades at their schools, because previous research (Dishion, Andrews, & Crosby, 1995) indicated that aggressive boys often select their best friends not from their classmates but from other children in their neighborhoods. This example illustrates that researchers cannot know the cost of restricting friendship nominations unless they have evidence from previous research with comparable samples in which nominations were unrestricted.

To Be Identified as Friends, Does Each Peer Named by a Child Need to Reciprocate That Nomination?

The question of whether reciprocity in friendship nominations should be part of the operational definition of "friendship" has been discussed by many scholars (e.g., Furman, 1996; Newcomb & Bagwell, 1995; Rubin et al., 2006). On the one hand, dictionary definitions often refer to the mutual affection between friends. On the other hand, requiring reciprocity in friendship nominations puts researchers in the position of saying, in effect, that some peers whom children name as their friends are really *not* their friends.

Children might name as their best friends other children whom they would like to have as friends but who are not really their friends. Apparently, however, no systematic evidence of such fanciful friendship nominations exists. Moreover, fanciful nominations would have to be extremely common to explain the number of friendship nominations that are not reciprocated. In one study elementary schoolchildren received a roster with the names of their classmates, then named their three best friends in the class (Parker & Asher, 1993). Analyses revealed that more than one-fifth of the children had no reciprocated nominations, and these children were described as not having any friends.

This description is suspect partly because friendship nominations were restricted to classmates. It is also suspect because children could only name three friends (Furman, 1996). If four or more children name the same classmate as a best friend, the classmate is only able to name three of them in return. Therefore, at least one of these friendships will appear not to be reciprocal, even if the classmate considers all the other children as best friends.

Evidence that might justify the requirement of reciprocal friendship nominations was obtained in Newcomb and Bagwell's (1995) meta-analysis of research on how friends differ from nonfriends. Friendships defined by reciprocal nominations showed higher levels of positive engagement and positive relationship properties than friendships defined by unilateral nominations. Despite this finding, Newcomb and Bagwell did not strongly endorse the requirement of reciprocal nominations. They noted, first, that friend–nonfriend differences in their analyses were about as large when the friends had reciprocal nominations as when the friends had only unilateral nominations or the reciprocity in their nominations was not determined.

Second, these authors mentioned a problem already discussed twice in this chapter. Requiring reciprocal nominations leads to the exclusion of many children from the final sample for a study. The resulting reduction in sample size decreases statistical power and, most likely, decreases the representativeness of the final sample. In one study, for example, adolescents from ethnic minority groups more often appeared to be friendless than did European American adolescents when "having friends" was judged from reciprocal nominations (Barry & Wentzel, 2006). Such a difference in reciprocal nominations complicates the interpretation of ethnic differences in other aspects of friendship.

Third, Newcomb and Bagwell (1995) considered their direct comparison of reciprocal and unilateral friendships as showing that friendships defined by reciprocal nominations involve a stronger affective tie than those defined by unilateral nominations. Stated in terms of the friendship continuum, they suggested that reciprocal friendships are located nearer the positive extreme on the continuum than are unilateral friendships.

An alternative explanation of the difference between reciprocal and unilateral friendships links the concept of a friendship continuum to the concept of asymmetry in friendships. In any pair of friends, one friend may like the other more than that friend likes him or her. For example, whereas one girl may consider another girl as her second closest friend, the other girl might consider the first girl as her fourth closest friend. If both children are asked to name their three best friends, this friendship will appear to be unilateral when it is only asymmetrical. More attention to such asymmetries and their effects on friends' interactions would be worthwhile.

Despite the problems with making reciprocity in nominations a requirement for friendship, researchers sometimes need to know whether specific nominations are reciprocated. For example, researchers who want to see how children interact with their friends may first ask the children who are the primary targets of the study to name their friends. Before scheduling the interactions of the target children with any of these friends, the researchers must establish that the peers named as friends regard the target children as their friends. Thus, for practical reasons, reciprocal nominations are essential in this type of research.

Data on reciprocity in friendship nominations can also clarify exactly how friendships contribute to children's social adjustment. One little-noted consequence of defining friendship by reciprocal nominations is that the resulting measures of "having friends" or number of friendships are strongly correlated with measures of peer acceptance. In one recent study of adolescents (Demir & Urberg, 2004), the correlation between number of friends and peer acceptance was .69. Such strong correlations are inevitable, because children with more reciprocal nominations have more peers who say that those children are their best friends, and children with greater peer acceptance have more peers who say that they like those children a lot. Because friendship is based on (mutual) liking, children who receive more friendship nominations also receive more positive sociometric nominations.

In a few studies, researchers have evaluated the independent contributions of reciprocal friendship nominations and peer acceptance to indicators of social adjustment. For example, Parker and Asher (1993) showed that children with no reciprocal friendships in their classroom were lonelier than children with at least one reciprocal friendship, even after the children's peer acceptance was taken into account. In another study, children who had more reciprocal friendships were less often victims of aggression aimed at harming their social relationships, with their peer acceptance taken into account (Malcolm et al., 2006). These findings imply that children's adjustment is related not only to being liked by classmates but also to being liked by the specific classmates whom the children view as their closest friends.

Worth noting, finally, is that not all studies show that reciprocity in friendships is important. One study showed that friends influence adolescents' sexual behavior and binge drinking, and this influence was not significantly greater when the adolescents' friendship nominations were reciprocated than when they were not (Jaccard et al., 2005). These findings confirm that friendships defined by nonreciprocated nominations are far from fanciful, because they have very real consequences.

Measuring the Quality of a Friendship

A major goal of research on children's friendships is to determine how these relationships affect children's development. To achieve this goal, researchers who have identified a child's friends must then assess the quality of these relationships (Berndt, 1996, 2002). The quality of a friendship can be defined in two complementary ways. First, "quality" refers to the degree of excellence of something (Morris, 1981). The quality of an appliance, for example, may be described as high, low, or somewhere in between. Second, "quality" refers to the important features of something. These features may serve as the criteria against which the degree of excellence of a thing is measured.

The first step in assessing the quality of a friendship is defining the features that affect its degree of excellence. The second step is evaluating, for a specific friendship, whether the levels of the features are high, low, or somewhere in between. But before either of these steps is taken, it is necessary to decide *who* should define the features of a friendship and evaluate the levels of those features. In this section, we first consider who should assess the quality of children's friendships. Then we examine which features of friendship should be examined and how their levels should be evaluated. Finally, we consider whether to analyze scores for specific features or for broad dimensions of quality, how to interpret the data when two friends judge the quality of their friendship differently, and what connections exist between reports of friendship quality and direct observations of friends' interactions.

Who Should Assess the Quality of a Friendship?

Just as children's friendship nominations are the starting point for most methods of identifying friends, children's reports on their friendships are the starting point for most assessments of friendship quality (Furman, 1996). Using individual interviews or questionnaires administered to groups of children, researchers have asked children about the frequency or intensity of specific behaviors or specific types of interactions that are linked conceptually to the features of their friendships. For example, to assess the feature of companionship, researchers have asked questions such as "How true is it that you and [friend's name] go to each others' houses?" (Parker & Asher, 1993, p. 615). Children have been judged to be the best informants about the quality of their own friendships, because they are the *only* source of information on certain types of interactions between friends. For example, directly assessing the feature of friendship that deals with intimate self-disclosure during conversations with friends is difficult, because these conversations usually occur in settings (e.g., a bedroom) that researchers cannot enter without violating children's privacy and confidentiality.

In addition, some features of friendship refer to what Hinde (1979) called "multidimensional qualities" of friendship. For example, several types of interactions reflect the degree to which a relationship is "affectionate." When children report on a friendship, they can take into account all of these interactions and report the level of affection in the friendship. Hinde also noted that people think about their relationships, and their thoughts may not be directly reflected in behavior. Thus, the best way to find out how children think about their friendships is to ask them.

Many investigators have created instruments to assess friendship quality from children's reports on their friendships (e.g., Berndt & Keefe, 1995; Bukowski, Hoza, & Boivin,

1994; Furman & Buhrmester, 1985; Parker & Asher, 1993). Most measures are designed for use with children in the elementary and secondary grades, but some measures can be used with preschool and kindergarten children (Gleason, 2002; Ladd et al., 1996). However, with children under age 4, individual interviews are difficult to conduct. Therefore, most assessments of the friendships of very young children are based on adults' observations of their interactions with peers (e.g., Howes, 1996). Because the friendships of children this young also seem less close and distinctive than those among older children (Newcomb & Bagwell, 1995), we focus in this section only on the interview- and questionnaire-based measures used with older children and adolescents.

Which Features Should Be Assessed and How Should Assessments Be Done?

Some measures of friendship quality include a subscale designed to assess the feature most central to the definition of a friendship, friends' affection for one another. In this assessment children are asked to use multipoint scales to rate statements such as "How true is it that your friend would like you even if others didn't?" (Parker & Asher, 1993, p. 615). Many friendship measures include questions designed to assess the other features of friendship listed in the dictionary definitions discussed earlier in the chapter. Besides companionship, these other features include benevolence, as indicated by prosocial behavior (e.g., "How often do you depend on this person for help, advice, and sympathy?" from Furman & Buhrmester, 1985, p. 1018), intimacy (e.g., "If there is something bothering me, I can tell my friend about it even if it is something I cannot tell to other people" from Bukowski et al., 1994, p. 475), and trust (e.g., "How true is it that you can count on this friend to keep promises?" from Parker & Asher, 1993, p. 615).

All of these features are mentioned frequently when children or adolescents are asked open-ended questions about how they know that someone is their friend (see Berndt, 1986). Other positive features that children or adolescents mention in response to such questions are loyalty (e.g., a friend will stand by you when other kids pick on you) and the ease with which friends can resolve conflicts with each other. The most popular friendship quality measures include items for many or all of these positive features, which illustrates that the measures have a firm basis in children's ideas about friendship. In addition, several measures were designed to assess important features in theories of supportive social relationships (see Berndt, 1989) or theories of what social relationships provide for individuals (see Furman, 1996). In short, these measures have both empirical and theoretical foundations.

When children are asked how they can tell that someone is not their friend, they mention features that refer to various types of negative interactions between peers (Berndt, 1986). In particular, children mention the frequency of conflicts, and say that friends do not fight or argue all the time. Most measures of friendship quality include questions about conflicts between friends (e.g., "How true is it that you and your friend argue a lot?" from Parker & Asher, 1993, p. 615), but only a few measures include questions about other negative features. Berndt and Keefe (1995) asked children about the rivalry that leads to dominance attempts and unpleasant competition between friends (e.g., "How often does [friend's name] show off or brag about doing something better than you?", p. 1315). However, most friendship quality measures include many more items for positive features than for negative features. Correcting this imbalance is desirable, because negative interactions with friends appear to affect children's interactions with other peers and adults (Berndt & Keefe, 1995). Therefore, the failure to assess negative features adequately can mean failure to determine all the effects of friendships on children.

Also worth asking is whether researchers have overlooked other important features of friendship. Rose (2002) has argued that "co-rumination," which she defines as "excessively discussing and revisiting problems, speculating about problems, and focusing on negative feelings" (p. 1830), may explain why girls tend to have both higher-quality friendships and more symptoms of internalizing problems. Girls' greater self-disclosure to friends makes their friendships more intimate and therefore higher in quality. Yet this disclosure, if it leads to a focus on negative feelings, can also enhance internalizing symptoms.

Co-rumination may not be a distinct feature of friendship, however. Instead, it may be a maladaptive variant of the self-disclosure that usually has positive effects on children's adjustment. Maladaptive forms of other positive features of friendship may also exist. For example, companionship with friends may typically improve children's affect and psychological adjustment, but spending many hours in unstructured, unsupervised time with friends could contribute to antisocial behavior (Berndt & Murphy, 2002). Additional research on the adaptive and maladaptive forms of well-known friendship features may be more profitable than a search for entirely new features of friendship.

Should Researchers Analyze Individual Features of Friendship or Dimensions of Friendship Quality?

Children's evaluations of the various friendship features are not independent (Berndt, 1996; Furman, 1996). Researchers invariably report that children's scores for different positive features are strongly correlated. If more than one negative friendship feature is assessed, children's scores for those negative features are strongly correlated. Factor analyses consistently show that measures of positive features load on one factor and measures of negative features load on a second factor (Furman, 1996). The correlations between the measures of positive and negative features are weak and not always significant.

These data suggest that friendship quality should be regarded as having two broad dimensions, one for positive features and another for negative features (Berndt, 2002). Often, researchers average the scores on all positive features to create a composite score for positive friendship quality; if an instrument includes more than one subscale for negative features, scores on those subscales are averaged to create a composite score for negative friendship quality (e.g., Berndt & Keefe, 1995; Weimer et al., 2004).

By contrast, some researchers have chosen to use the scores for specific features in their data analyses rather than to create and analyze composite scores (e.g., Bagwell & Coie, 2004). This methodological decision may yield important findings. For example, the early studies of friendship quality measures often showed that ratings of the intimacy of friendships increase significantly between childhood and adolescence, whereas ratings of most other friendship features do not change consistently with age (Berndt & Perry, 1986).

Analyses of specific features are problematic, however, for both psychometric and psychological reasons. The psychometric problem is that the correlations among the scores for various positive features are nearly equal to the reliability of the measures of those features. Under these conditions, measures of different features have little discriminant validity. The measures of all features should, then, show the same correlations with any other variables that are examined in a study. Differences in the correlations for different features most likely reflect chance results.

The psychological problem is that the strong correlations among different features imply that children may not have the cognitive ability to differentiate between them. The factor analyses of friendship quality measures indicate that children can and do differentiate between two broad dimensions of friendship quality. In particular, they can report when a friendship is high both in positive features and in conflicts. Yet those analyses also suggest that children are either unable or unwilling to draw distinctions, for example, between a friend's prosocial behavior and the intimacy of their friendship with that person. To find out whether finer differentiations can be made among positive friendship features, observations of friends' interactions might be useful. But when assessments of friendship features depend on children's reports, greater differentiation among the features within each broad dimension may not be possible.

This conclusion also has implications for the investigation of novel features of friendship. If children differentiate between the broad dimensions of positive features and negative features, but do not differentiate much within each dimension, then establishing the discriminant validity of measures of new friendship features will be difficult. Consequently, researchers who want to investigate novel friendship features may need to use assessment techniques other than interviews or questionnaires.

How Should a Disagreement between Two Friends about the Quality of Their Friendship Be Interpreted?

When two children who have been identified as best friends are both asked about the quality of their friendship, they often disagree about its quality. For example, in one study of high school students (Brendgen et al., 2001), the correlations between two friends' reports of positive friendship quality and negative friendship quality were only .37 and .39, respectively.

Of course, measures of psychological constructs rarely correlate perfectly, because the reliability of their measurement is imperfect. However, the discrepancies between two friends' reports of friendship quality demonstrate important facts about friendships. First, the agreement between friends varies for different features of friendship (Simpkins et al., 2006). For example, friends agree more about their companionship (e.g., how often they go to one another's houses) than about their intimate disclosure, helpfulness toward each other, and conflict resolution. These results imply that reports of companionship, which depend mostly on the frequency of interactions between friends, are less subjective and so less open to differences in interpretation than reports of other friendship features.

Second, Simpkins and colleagues (2006) suggest that two friends may differ in their knowledge about one another. So, for example, Jane may tell Emily about everything that she thinks and feels, but Emily may not talk with Jane about many things that are important to her, and only Emily would know that she limits her intimate disclosure in this way.

Third, sometimes the items on friendship quality measures refer to a friend's behavior toward the child who is reporting on the friendship rather than to dyadic interactions. In response to a question such as "How often does your friend help you when you can't do something by yourself" (Berndt & Keefe, 1995, p. 1315), children should report how often they receive help from a friend, and that may not match the amount that they help that friend. Moreover, such unidirectional questions may be very appropriate for measures of friendship quality. If researchers want to know how a child is affected by a friendship, then it may be most reasonable to ask how the friend behaves toward him or her, rather than how both friends behave toward each other.

Differences in friends' behavior may partly explain why disagreements between friends vary with the friends' sociometric status. In one study (Brendgen, Little, & Krappmann, 2000), rejected children's reports of the quality of one of their friendships correlated with their friends' reports much less than did those of average or popular children and their friends. Moreover, rejected children judged their friendships as higher in quality than their friends did. Conversely, popular children judged their friendships as lower in quality than their friends did. Apparently, differences in the social behavior and social skills of rejected and popular children affect children's behavior toward their best friends and their other classmates.

We can summarize these points by saying that differences in reports of friendship quality partly reflect the asymmetry in friendships discussed earlier. To one child, a particular friendship may be very special. On the friendship continuum, this child may view the friendship as very close to the extreme labeled "the best of friends." But the child's friend may view their friendship as little more than an acquaintanceship. On the continuum, this child may view the friendship as somewhere in the range of "just friends." In such cases, each child's report of friendship quality is likely to depend on how close that child thinks the friendship is, not how close the friend thinks it is (Berndt, 1996). Given this asymmetry, researchers must decide which friend's perspective should be assessed, or whether assessing the perspectives of both friends would increase the interpretability of the research findings.

How Does Friendship Quality Relate to Friends' Interactions?

Many researchers have examined how children's conversations and other types of interactions differ with friends and nonfriends. The findings of this research have been summarized in various narrative reviews and a meta-analysis (Newcomb & Bagwell, 1995). Moreover, the only issues that make observations of friends' interactions markedly different from other types of observational research (e.g., the need to identify pairs of friends) have already been discussed.

Observations of friends' interaction can be a valuable supplement to studies in which friendship quality is assessed with interviews or questionnaires. As noted earlier, some friendship features are difficult or impossible to observe directly, but reports of friendship quality must be partly based on children's interactions with friends. If no connection existed between these reports and friends' interactions, researchers might wonder whether the reports have any validity.

In one study (Bagwell & Coie, 2004), children's reports of friendship quality did seem disconnected from some aspects of their interactions with friends. Aggressive fourth- and fifth-grade boys did not judge the positive features of their best friendships less positively, and did not rate conflicts with friends as more frequent, than did nonaggressive boys. When interacting with each other, aggressive boys and their friends were less positively engaged than were nonaggressive boys and their friends. On the other hand, the two groups of boys showed about the same level of enjoyment in their interactions. Aggressive boys and their friends displayed more intense negative affect during conflicts than did nonaggressive boys and their friends, but the two groups of boys did not differ in the number or duration of their conflicts. These mixed results could be interpreted as evidence that aggressive and nonaggressive boys differ in their interactions with friends, but not in their reports of friendship quality, or that aggressive and nonaggressive boys are surprisingly similar in their interactions with friends and their reports of friendship quality.

Mixed results have been found in other studies too. Adolescents in one study who reported greater conflict with friends also expressed more criticism of one another and disagreed more during their interactions, but these students' reports of positive friendship quality are not significantly related to how they interacted with each other (Weimer et al., 2004). In another study, adolescents who reported greater positive friendship quality showed more positive affect when interacting with their friends, but their reports of positive friendship quality were not related to their friends' expressions of positive affect or to their own or their friends' self-disclosure while interacting (Brendgen et al., 2001).

Two important questions can be asked about these mixed results. First, when reports of friendship quality are not significantly correlated with direct observations of friends' interactions, should researchers question the validity of the friendship quality measures or the validity of the observational measures? Of course, both types of measures could be flawed, but questions have long been raised about the ecological validity of measures derived from observations in a psychology laboratory (e.g., Bronfenbrenner, 1979), and the observations of friends' interactions have all taken place in laboratory settings. Researchers in the future need to give more attention to the issue of ecological validity when planning observational studies of friends' interactions.

Second, how *should* measures of friendship quality relate to specific aspects of friends' interactions? Answers to this question should ideally be linked to hypotheses about the types of interactions that contribute to the major dimensions of friendship quality. These hypotheses in turn should be linked to theories that explain how peer interactions lead to the development of friendships that are high or low in positive or negative features. Currently, no theories of this type exist. Formulating a theory of how interactions with friends influence children's reports of friendship quality should be a high priority for future research.

Conclusions

Studying children's relationships with friends is challenging, because research methods must be rooted in children's ideas about friendship and adapted for the purposes of specific studies. When children name a peer as a friend, they are affirming that they and the peer know and like each other. However, friends vary in their degree of mutual knowledge and liking. These variations can be represented on a continuum on which the positive extreme is for "the best of friends" and the negative extreme is for complete strangers. Overlapping ranges on the continuum can be labeled from highest to lowest as best or close friends, good friends, "just friends," or mere acquaintances (i.e., children who are not friends). However, the boundaries between these types of relationships are fuzzy.

The idea of a friendship continuum helps to clarify the implications of some methods of identifying children's friends. Except with very young children, friendships are best identified by asking children to name their friends. However, the methods used to elicit these names can vary greatly. Children may be asked to name only their "very, very best friend" or may be allowed to name any number of friends. When more nominations are allowed, researchers identify friendships that cover a greater range on the friendship continuum. Overall, then, the closeness of these friendships is lower. When fewer nominations are allowed, researchers identify closer friendships, but more children are judged not to have any friends. Often these children must be excluded from the final sample for a study, which makes the sample less representative of the population.

Researchers have often limited friendship nominations, for example, by asking children to name their closest friends in their class at school rather than their best friends overall. In addition, researchers have often required that children's nominations be reciprocated by their friends. The choices also have important implications. Imposing more restrictions and requirements leads to the identification of friendships that are nearer the "best of friends" extreme on the friendship continuum, but it increases the proportion of children for whom no friend is identified. Researchers need to recognize these trade-offs, choose the methods that are best for a specific study, and explain the reasons for their choices.

The effects of friendships on children are assumed to depend at least partly on their quality. Existing measures of friendship quality assess various positive and negative features of friendship. Children report on the level of each feature in a particular friendship by answering questions about behaviors or interactions that are indicative of that feature.

Children's reports about various positive features of friendship are strongly correlated. Similarly, children's reports about various negative features are strongly correlated. However, measures of positive features are only weakly correlated with measures of negative features. These findings suggest that children view their friendships as varying on broad dimensions of positive and negative friendship quality.

Occasionally, researchers have analyzed the scores for specific features rather than for the broad dimensions of quality. This choice is difficult to justify, because the available data suggest that children differentiate little between different positive or negative features. Previous studies have also shown that children's reports on the quality of their friendships are only moderately correlated with their friends' reports on the same friendships. These data suggest that most friendships are asymmetrical relationships, meaning that children often view friendships with specific peers as higher (or lower) in quality than the peers view the same friendships with them. Because such asymmetries are the norm, researchers need to decide whose perspective on a friendship should be assessed for a specific study.

Only a few researchers have examined how reports of friendship quality are related to observations of friends' interactions in structured laboratory settings. Those studies usually reveal some significant correlations between the friendship quality measures and the observational measures, which suggests that both types of measures have some validity. However, nonsignificant correlations between the two types of measures are also common, and the reasons for these mixed results are unclear. Additional research of this kind would be helpful in clarifying how interactions with friends contribute to children's judgments about the quality of their friendships. The additional research would also contribute to an understanding of how children's friendships might affect their psychological adjustment and development.

References

Adams, R. E., Bukowski, W. M., & Bagwell, C. (2005). Stability of aggression during early adolescence as moderated by reciprocated friendship status and friend's aggression. *International Journal of Behavioral Development, 29*, 139–145.

Bagwell, C. L., & Coie, J. D. (2004). The best friendships of aggressive boys: Relationship quality, conflict management, and rule-breaking behavior. *Journal of Experimental Child Psychology, 88*, 5–24.

Barry, C. M., & Wentzel, K. R. (2006). Friend influence on prosocial behavior: The role of motivational factors and friendship characteristics. *Developmental Psychology, 42*, 153–163.

Berndt, T. J. (1986). Children's comments about their friendships. In M. Perlmutter (Ed.), *Minnesota Symposium on Child Psychology: Vol. 18. Cognitive perspectives on children's social and behavioral development* (pp. 189–212). Hillsdale, NJ: Erlbaum.

Berndt, T. J. (1989). Obtaining support from friends in childhood and adolescence. In D. Belle (Ed.), *Children's social networks and social supports* (pp. 308–331). New York: Wiley.

Berndt, T. J. (1996). Exploring the effects of friendship quality on social development. In W. M. Bukowski, A. F. Newcomb, & W. W. Hartup (Eds.), *The company they keep: Friendship in childhood and adolescence* (pp. 346–365). New York: Cambridge University Press.

Berndt, T. J. (2002). Friendship quality and social development. *Current Directions in Psychological Science, 11*, 7–10.

Berndt, T. J. (2004). Children's friendships: Shifts over a half-century in perspectives on their development and their effects. *Merrill–Palmer Quarterly, 50*, 206–223.

Berndt, T. J., & Keefe, K. (1995). Friends' influence on adolescents' adjustment to school. *Child Development, 66*, 1312–1329.

Berndt, T. J., & Murphy, L. B. (2002). Influences of friends and friendships: Myths, truths, and research recommendations. *Advances in Child Development and Behavior, 30*, 275–310.

Berndt, T. J., & Perry, T. B. (1986). Children's perceptions of friendships as supportive relationships. *Developmental Psychology, 22*, 640–648.

Brendgen, M., Little, T. D., & Krappmann, L. (2000). Rejected children and their friends: A shared evaluation of friendship quality? *Merrill–Palmer Quarterly, 46*, 45–70.

Brendgen, M., Markiewicz, D., Doyle, A. B., & Bukowski, W. M. (2001). The relations between friendship quality, ranked-friendship preference, and adolescents' behavior with their friends. *Merrill–Palmer Quarterly, 47*, 395–415.

Bronfenbrenner, U. (1979). Contexts of child rearing: Problems and prospects. *American Psychologist, 34*, 844–850.

Bukowski, W. M., & Hoza, B. (1989). Popularity and friendship: Issues in theory, measurement and outcome. In T. J. Berndt & G. W. Ladd (Eds.), *Peer relationships in child development* (pp. 15–45). New York: Wiley.

Bukowski, W. M., Hoza, B., & Boivin, M. (1994). Measuring friendship quality during pre- and early adolescence: The development and psychometric properties of the Friendship Qualities Scale. *Journal of Social and Personal Relationships, 11*, 471–484.

Burgess, K. B., Wojslawowicz, J. C., Rubin, K. H., Rose-Krasnor, L., & Booth-LaForce, C. (2006). Social information processing and coping strategies of shy/withdrawn and aggressive children: Does friendship matter? *Child Development, 77*, 371–383.

Burk, W. J., & Laursen, B. (2005). Adolescent perceptions of friendship and their associations with individual adjustment. *International Journal of Behavioral Development, 29*, 156–164.

Demir, M., & Urberg, K. A. (2004). Friendship and adjustment among adolescents. *Journal of Experimental Child Psychology, 88*, 68–82.

Dishion, T. J., Andrews, D. W., & Crosby, L. (1995). Antisocial boys and their friends in early adolescence: Relationship characteristics, quality, and interactional process. *Child Development, 66*, 139–151.

Dunn, J., Cutting, A. L., & Fisher, N. (2002). Old friends, new friends: Predictors of children's perspective on their friends at school. *Child Development, 73*, 621–635.

Fletcher, A. C., Hunter, A. G., & Eanes, A. Y. (2006). Links between social network closure and child well-being: The organizing role of friendship context. *Developmental Psychology, 42*, 1057–1068.

Furman, W. (1996). The measurement of friendship perceptions: Conceptual and methodological issues. In W. M. Bukowski, A. F. Newcomb, & W. W. Hartup (Eds.), *The company they keep: Friendship in childhood and adolescence* (pp. 41–65). New York: Cambridge University Press.

Furman, W., & Buhrmester, D. (1985). Children's perceptions of the personal relationships in their social networks. *Developmental Psychology, 21*(6), 1016–1024.

Gleason, T. R. (2002). Social provisions of real and imaginary relationships in early childhood. *Developmental Psychology, 38*, 979–992.

Hartup, W. W. (1983). Peer relations. In P. H. Mussen (Series Ed.) & E. M. Hetherington (Vol. Ed.), *Handbook of child psychology: Vol. 4. Socialization, personality, and social development* (pp. 103–196). New York: Wiley.

Hartup, W. W. (1996). The company they keep: Friendships and their developmental significance. *Child Development, 67*, 1–13.

Hendrick, C., & Hendrick, S. S. (2000). *Close relationships: A sourcebook.* Thousand Oaks, CA: Sage.

Hinde, R. A. (1979). *Towards understanding relationships.* New York: Academic Press.

Howes, C. (1996). The earliest friendships. In W. M. Bukowski, A. F. Newcomb, & W. W. Hartup (Eds.), *The company they keep: Friendship in childhood and adolescence* (pp. 41–65). New York: Cambridge University Press.

Jaccard, J., Blanton, H., & Dodge, T. (2005). Peer influences on risk behavior: An analysis of the effects of a close friend. *Developmental Psychology, 41*, 135–147.

Kiesner, J., Poulin, F., & Nicotra, E. (2003). Peer relations across contexts: Individual-network homophily and network inclusion in and after school. *Child Development, 74*, 1328–1343.

Kovacs, D. M., Parker, J. G., & Hoffman, L. W. (1996). Behavioral, affective, and social correlates of involvement in cross-sex friendship in elementary school. *Child Development, 67*, 2269–2286.

Kuttler, A. F., La Greca, A. M., & Prinstein, M. J. (1999). Friendship qualities and social-emotional functioning of adolescents with close, cross-sex friendships. *Journal of Research of Adolescence, 9*, 339–366.

Ladd, G. W., Kochenderfer, B. J., & Coleman, C. C. (1996). Friendship quality as a predictor of young children's early school adjustment. *Child Development, 67*, 1103–1118.

Landau, S. I. (Ed.). (2001). *Cambridge dictionary of American English.* New York: Cambridge University Press.

Malcolm, K. T., Jensen-Campbell, L. A., Rex-Lear, M., & Waldrip, A. M. (2006). Divided we fall: Children's friendships and peer victimization. *Journal of Social and Personal Relationships, 23*, 721–740.

Morris, W. (Ed.). (1981). *American heritage dictionary of the English language.* Boston, MA: Houghton-Mifflin.

Newcomb, A. F., & Bagwell, C. L. (1995). Children's friendship relations: A meta-analytic review. *Psychological Bulletin, 117*, 306–347.

Parker, J. G., & Asher, S. R. (1993). Friendship and friendship quality in middle childhood: Links with peer group acceptance and feelings of loneliness and social dissatisfaction. *Developmental Psychology, 29*, 611–621.

Parker, J. G., Low, C. M., Walker, A. R., & Gamm, B. K. (2005). Friendship jealousy in young adolescents: Individual differences and links to sex, self-esteem, aggression, and social adjustment. *Developmental Psychology, 41*, 235–250.

Rose, A. J. (2002). Co-rumination in the friendships of girls and boys. *Child Development, 73*, 1830–1843.

Rose, A. J., & Asher, S. R. (2004). Children's strategies and goals in response to help-giving and help-seeking tasks within a friendship. *Child Development, 75*, 749–773.

Rubin, K. H., Bukowski, W. M., & Parker, J. G. (2006). Peer interactions, relationships, and groups. In W. Damon & R. M. Lerner (Editors-in-chief) & N. Eisenberg (Vol. Ed.), *Handbook of child psychology* (6th ed.): *Vol. 3. Social, emotional, and personality development* (pp. 571–645). New York: Wiley.

Selman, R. L. (1980). *The growth of interpersonal understanding: Developmental and clinical analyses.* New York: Academic Press.

Simpkins, S. D., Parke, R. D., Flyr, M. L., & Wild, M. N. (2006). Similarities in children's and early adolescents' perceptions of friendship qualities across development, gender, and friendship qualities. *Journal of Early Adolescence, 26,* 491–508.

Simpson, J., & Weiner, E. (Eds.). (1989). *Oxford English dictionary* (2nd ed.). New York: Oxford University Press.

Webster's encyclopedic unabridged dictionary of the English language. (1989). New York: Portland House.

Weimer, B. L., Kerns, K. A., & Oldenburg, C. M. (2004). Adolescents' interactions with a best friend: Associations with attachment style. *Journal of Experimental Child Psychology, 88,* 102–120.

CHAPTER 5

Sociometric Methods

ANTONIUS H. N. CILLESSEN

The term "sociometric methods" refers to a large class of methods that assess the positive and negative links between persons within a group. The basic principle of the sociometric method is that every group member has the capacity to evaluate every other group member on one or more criteria in a round-robin design. In the literature on peer relations, the term "sociometry" often has a narrower meaning, that is, the assessment of sociometric status in peer groups. Sociometric methods have been used extensively in the study of peer relations to assess the "attractions" and "repulsions" between children.

In this chapter, I address four aspects of sociometric research with children and adolescents. First, central issues in the use of sociometric methods to study peer relations are discussed, including the meaning of sociometric status, the basic procedure, basic elements of sociometric procedures and definitions of terms, and a detailed discussion of the methodological variations within each of the building blocks of sociometric methods. Second, theory relevant to sociometric measurement is discussed. Third, key classical and recent studies are presented that mark important milestones in the development of sociometric methods. The number of sociometric studies published during the more than 70 years since Moreno's original publication is large. The critical studies I present are selective, because of space limitations. Fourth and finally, directions for future research are discussed.

The origins of sociometric methods as applied in peer relations research are typically attributed to Jacob Moreno (1934). Moreno was indeed the founder of the methods that are still used today with children and adolescents in schools. Moreno's work was embedded in a broader movement in the social sciences at the beginning of the 20th century, aimed at measuring and determining social relationships in groups. In this way, Moreno's techniques reflect historical forces linked to changing social conditions in the 20th century and provided a common set of methods and ideas for researchers from different branches of the social sciences.

Jacob Levy Moreno (1889–1974), born Jacob Moreno Levy in Romania, was a medical student in Vienna during the heyday of Freud's psychoanalytic circle. Moreno's goal was to extend Freud's methods of individual psychotherapy to groups, making him the founder of group psychotherapy. After World War I, the Austrian government, faced with a large influx of refugees into the Vienna area, hired Moreno, by then a psychiatrist, as a consultant to design a resettlement community. Moreno decided to ask who families wanted to live next to, and his map of the attractions in the village community, represented by arrows in a graph, became the first sociogram, which was published in his 1934 book. Moreno moved to the United States in 1925, where he lived and worked in Beacon, New York. He was a colorful person, who was never really part of academic psychology, although he did interact with some of the leading social psychologists of his time. His ideas about groups and relationships quickly led to the sociometric movement, which included a large number of sociometric studies in educational, mental health, and corporate settings. For Moreno, sociometry was first a theory of social psychology, second an approach to group psychotherapy, and only third a method for the assessment of groups. Although he saw sociometric methods as merely a tool toward his grander goals, it is the methodology that Moreno is remembered for most today.

The history of sociometric methodology is long and varied (see Cillessen & Bukowski, 2000). Although Moreno initiated the method, many others worked on the application of sociometric methods for the study of child development from the beginning. This group of early child development researchers included, among others, Helen Jennings, Merl Bonney, Joan Criswell, and Mary Northway, to name just a few (for a review, see Moreno, 1960). The methodological developments since the early days of sociometry went through various stages. Variations in the methods of sociometric assessment have depended on (1) whether one chose to use peer nominations, ratings, or paired comparisons, (2) the criteria used to assess attraction (e.g., "Who do you want to work with?" vs. "Who do you want to play with?"), (3) the decision to use positive items only or to use positive and negative items (e.g., "liked most" and "liked least"), and (4) how to best quantify the scores derived from a sociometric test. Cillessen and Bukowski pointed to three critical events in the history of sociometric methods for the study of peer relations: (1) the change from one-dimensional to two-dimensional systems (co-occurring with the use of both positive and negative nominations), (2) the introduction of social impact in addition to social preference, and (3) the identification of the five sociometric status groups (popular, rejected, neglected, controversial, and average). The studies responsible for these developments are described in the section on critical studies.

The Meaning of Sociometric Status

As indicated in the Introduction of this book, peer relations can be conceptualized at three levels of social complexity: individual, dyad, and group. Information about each level can be derived from a sociometric test. For example, based on the matrix of sociometric choices within a classroom, it is possible to assign individual status scores to each child. These scores can be either continuous (e.g., acceptance or rejection), or categorical (e.g., popular, rejected, or average). It is also possible to derive dyadic information from the same sociomatrix, such as reciprocal friendship choices or mutual antipathies. Finally, it is possible to obtain social network or clique information from the same matrix of choices. This chapter focuses on the derivation of continuous or categorical scores for peer status at the individual level of analysis.

What does "individual sociometric status" mean? What does it mean to say that a child is "sociometrically accepted" or "rejected?" There is a tendency to think of sociometric status as an absolute characteristic of the individual child or adolescent (e.g., the accepted child is always socially skilled, or the rejected child is always incompetent and aggressive). However, individual status is not independent of the group, and its meaning needs to be considered relative to the group in which it is assessed. Thus, sociometric status represents the relationship between an individual and the group (Coie & Cillessen, 1993). A person who is accepted in one social context may not be accepted in another if the norms on which status evaluations are based vary by context (see Boivin, Dodge, & Coie, 1995; Stormshak et al., 1999; Wright, Giammarino, & Parad, 1986). In practice, consistency of sociometric status across settings is often expected if the determinants of social competence are universal. At the same time, there is room for inconsistency when group norms vary across different social settings.

The Basic Procedure

Throughout the 70-year history of sociometric measurement, a large variety of sociometric methods have been used. In the period before 1980, there was little consensus on what a basic procedure might look like. Today, such a consensus does exist. By combining a number of innovations by other researchers in previous years, Coie, Dodge, and Coppotelli (1982; see also Coie & Dodge, 1983) and Newcomb and Bukowski (1983, 1984) presented a sociometric method that has served as the standard since the 1980s. This standard method is for the collection of sociometric data in classrooms (rather than in entire grades).

In the Coie et al. (1982) procedure, children are asked to name three classroom peers they like most ("acceptance") and three they like least ("rejection"). Nominations received for both questions are counted for each child and standardized within classrooms to control for differences in classroom size. A continuous score for "social preference" is created by taking the difference between the standardized acceptance and rejection scores, and again standardizing the resulting scores within classrooms. A continuous score for "social impact" is created by summing the standardized acceptance and rejection scores, and restandardizing the results. Finally, with the use of detailed decision rules (see Coie et al., 1982), each child is assigned to one of five sociometric status types: *popular* (liked by many, disliked by few), *rejected* (disliked by many, liked by few), *neglected* (neither liked nor disliked), *controversial* (liked by some and disliked by others), and *average* (around the means of acceptance and rejection). In Coie and Dodge (1983), the average group comprises simply everyone who does not meet the criteria for the first four groups. Assignment to the extreme groups was based on whether a child's score on the critical variable was common or rare. Cutoffs based on standardized scores were used for this purpose.

Newcomb and Bukowski (1983, 1984) recommended a modified approach. They measured acceptance with three "best friend" nominations rather than "liked most," and proposed a probability-based criterion to identify whether a child's level of acceptance and rejection was common or rare, and to control for differences in classroom size. As a consequence, the criteria for the assignment of children to the five sociometric status groups changed as well. Terry and Coie (1991) demonstrated that there is a high concordance of sociometric status assignments between the Coie et al. (1982) and Newcomb and Bukowski (1983) methods.

There are many variations of this basic procedure. To provide a framework for the description of these variations, I first identify the basic elements of any sociometric test, using the basic procedure as an illustration, then describe the ways each basic element can vary.

Basic Elements of the Sociometric Procedure

"Sociometry" is a method to measure relationships in groups. The ideal sociometric method uses a round-robin design that, in principle, allows every group member to evaluate every other group member on one or more criteria. For example, every group member can potentially name every other group member as someone he or she likes or considers a friend. Or all group members rate each other according to their sociability or aggressiveness. The following basic elements of a sociometric procedure can be distinguished: reference group, voter population, "votee" population, sociometric criteria, data collection method, quantification method, method of standardization, sociometric dimensions, and classification method.

The "reference group" is the collection of persons (group or social network) within which status is determined. In most applications in the peer relations literature, the reference group is the classroom or grade, but other possibilities are sports teams, hobby clubs, or all children in an afterschool program. It is important to realize that peer status is always relative to the reference group in which it is assessed. Decisions about the proper reference group for a study need to be driven by considerations of ecological validity. What is the peer group within which the participants spend most of their time? Who are the peers that they know well and relative to whom their status should be considered given the goals of the study? Which peer group is developmentally most meaningful and appropriate? In North America, the reference group for kindergarten and elementary school children is typically the classroom; for early adolescents in middle school, it is all peers in their grade; and for adolescents in high school, it is also the entire grade level or even all peers in school across grades. In other cultures with a different structure of secondary education, the proper reference group may continue to be the classroom, even beyond elementary school.

The "voter population" comprises the children or adolescents who participate as evaluators in a sociometric test. The "votee population" comprises the children or adolescents who are being evaluated. Ideally, all members of the reference group (e.g., classroom or grade) participate as both voters and votees. It is recommended that, once the reference group is chosen, no restrictions be imposed on the list of voters or votees. In practice, restrictions of the voter population are almost impossible to avoid due to absenteeism on the day of testing or lack of permission to participate. However, acceptable sociometric scores can still be obtained when the voter population is incomplete. With limited nominations, a minimum participation rate of 70% is required (Crick & Ladd, 1990). With unlimited nominations, stable constructs are still obtained with a 60% participation rate (Wargo Aikins & Cillessen, 2007). Restrictions of the votee population are more easily avoidable, although some researchers intentionally ask participants to evaluate only same-sex peers, peers of one ethnicity, or randomized subsets of all peers in the reference group. Restrictions of the votee population can potentially have serious consequences. Large and not random restrictions change the nature of the reference group and, hence, the validity of status obtained relative to the reference group that was originally intended. In most studies, the voter and votee populations are subgroups of the reference group, and the former is smaller than the latter, making the voter-by-votee matrix rectangular rather than the ideal square. Although the computation of individual status is relatively robust to modest limitations of the voter and votee populations, such limitations seriously handicap the ability to identify dyadic relationships and social network structures that are built on dyadic ties.

The questions on a sociometric test are called "sociometric criteria." Moreno (1934) distinguished two types: emotional and reputational. "Emotional criteria" are subjective evaluations and personal to the voter. Items measuring acceptance and rejection (liked most, liked least, best friends) are in this category. Researchers have also used "reversed" or "meta" emotional criteria when they asked participants to nominate who they thought liked or disliked them (e.g., Bellmore & Cillessen, 2003). "Reputational criteria" measure perceived behaviors or reputations rather than personal evaluations. Nominations of peers who start fights, cooperate and share, or stay by themselves are reputational items of social behaviors. Nominations of (most) popular, least popular, good looking, good at sports, or good at school are also reputational. Reputational criteria may be called objective, whereas emotional criteria are subjective. Because reputational items measure shared rather than personal perceptions, there is a higher consensus in the peer group for reputational items than for emotional items. Today researchers often use the term "sociometric assessment" for the measurement of emotional criteria only, and the term "peer assessment" for the measurement of reputational criteria.

Data Collection

Three methods of data collection are commonly distinguished: peer nominations, ratings, and paired comparisons. Peer nominations are the most common. Technically, the peer nomination method is a method of partial rank ordering. For any given criterion, the voter ranks his or her nominees at the top of the distribution of the variable and leaves the remainder of the peer group (those who are not nominated) unranked. In the older sociometric literature, nominees were sometimes explicitly ranked as first choice, second choice, and so on, for any question. Today, this is only done for "best friend" choices.

Peer ratings continue to be used, although they are not as common as peer nominations. Maassen, van der Linden, Goossens, and Bokhorst (2000) demonstrated that ratings have certain statistical advantages over nominations, but the impracticality of collecting peer ratings in large reference groups (e.g., entire grades) often prevents researchers from using them. Bukowski, Sippola, Hoza, and Newcomb (2000) have shown that rating scale–based and nomination-based techniques can be used to create highly correlated indices of the same constructs.

In the method of paired comparisons, children are presented with all possible pairs of peers in the votee population or a random subset. For each dyad, they are asked to indicate which member best fit the criterion. This method yields highly reliable scores but is also exceptionally time consuming. It is an excellent method to collect sociometric data in small groups of very young children (e.g., kindergarten or preschool groups), although that can also be achieved with an adjusted rating method (see Asher, Singleton, Tinsley, & Hymel, 1979; Cillessen, 1991).

An issue of some importance when using peer nominations is whether to collect limited or unlimited nominations. In the first sociometric studies with children in the 1940s and 1950s, both fixed and free nominations were used. Fixed nominations were more common, but not always limited to three. Because Coie et al. (1982) and Newcomb and Bukowski (1983) solicited three nominations, this practice was followed in many studies. There are two reasons why some researchers decided to revisit this issue. First, during the practice of sociometric data collection, it is not uncommon for participants to indicate that they want to name fewer or more peers for certain questions. In those cases, letting the number of nominations be free rather than restricting them to a fixed number seems more ecologically valid. Second, researchers increasingly are collecting sociometric data in larger reference groups, such as middle and high school grades. In those contexts in particular, nominations fixed to a small number are problematic for participants. Based on these considerations, the use of unlimited nominations has increased.

There is some evidence to suggest that unlimited nominations have certain advantages. Indirect comparisons show that the stabilities of sociometric scores derived from unlimited nominations across multiple years (Cillessen & Borch, 2006; Cillessen & Mayeux, 2004) are at the high end of the distribution of stability coefficients found in a meta-analysis (Jiang & Cillessen, 2005). In a direct comparison study, unlimited nominations also yielded more stable constructs and higher correlations with measures of social behavior than did limited nominations. However, this evidence is unpublished or limited to one study (Terry, 2000). Based on the practical experience of collecting sociometric data over many years and in many settings, a reasonable hypothesis is that the relative advantage of unlimited nominations is larger at older ages (middle school or high school), or when the entire grade is the reference group, and smaller at younger ages (elementary school), or when the classroom is the reference group. In studies with elementary school children and the classroom as the reference, the correlation between sociometric scores derived from limited and unlimited nominations is expected to be high.

The use of unlimited nominations when collecting sociometric data in middle schools is now common practice (e.g., Poulin & Dishion, 2008). In some cases, unlimited nominations are restricted to a maximum to prevent students from becoming too unselective in their choices. For example, Franzoi, Davis, and Vasquez-Suson (1994) allowed high school students to name peers from any grade in their school using unlimited nominations capped at 10. When not capped, individual differences in voter selectiveness are common but not a problem. (Moreno used the term "expansion" to refer to differences between persons in the number of peers they choose as friends.) As a general rule, a vote by a less selective voter makes a smaller contribution to the data than a vote by a more selective voter. This is true even when simply counting nominations received. Differences in voter selectivity can be modeled statistically with item response theory (Terry, 2000) or other mathematical procedures (DeRosier & Thomas, 2003). I generally recommend the use of unlimited nominations, but Bukowski does not. The consensus is that more empirical data are needed to settle this issue.

A few additional logistical decisions may influence the quality of sociometric data collection. Data may be collected in individual interviews, or with the entire classroom at once (e.g., a paper-and-pencil test). de Bruyn (see de Bruyn & Cillessen, 2006a, 2006b) successfully collected sociometric data via a computerized assessment method. Sociometric data collected at the beginning of the school year may be less stable than that at the end of the school year. A good time to collect sociometric data in schools is the middle or end of the spring semester, when students have been together for the year and know each other well. There is, however, quite some variation in the timing of sociometric data collection across studies. This is generally not considered problematic as long as the data collection does not take place in the very early stages of the formation of new groups. Mayeux, Bellmore, and Cillessen (2008) found that sociometric measurement in October, February, or May of the school year in stable elementary school classrooms yielded very similar sociometric data.

Peer relations researchers agree that the unique insight obtained from peers in a sociometric test cannot easily be replaced by other sources of information. Nevertheless, the question of alternative methods of sociometric assessment comes up regularly, driven mostly by practical considerations. For example, in large-scale longitudinal studies with targeted children who distribute themselves over many schools at follow-up waves (e.g., the National Institute of Child Health and Human Development [NICDH] Study of Early Child Care and Youth Development), it is often impossible to collect sociometric data with the new peers in all the new schools. Self-reports of sociometric status, while interesting in and of themselves for researchers interested in social self-perception, cannot replace measures of status derived from peers. Teacher reports are also generally not successful replacements for peers. Cillessen, Terry, Coie, and Lochman (1992) found high agreement between teacher and peer judgments of aggression, but low overall agreement between teacher and peer judgments of status. In general, teachers overestimated the status of the children in the classrooms identifying, for example, rejected children as controversial and average children as popular. Another notable finding was the large variation among teachers: Whereas the overall concordance between teachers and peers was low, some teachers were much more accurate than others.

Another method to reduce the time needed to collect sociometric data is to ask only a subgroup of experts who can provide the information needed rather than asking all students in a classroom or grade to participate. This idea to use sociometric experts was launched by Angold et al. (1990), and is analogous to Brown's (1990) method to use expert informants to identify cliques. They identified sociometric experts with Monte Carlo simulations as the voters who most closely represented the overall pattern of sociometric data obtained from all peers. They also examined the characteristics of peers named by teachers as "students who know what is going on socially in the classroom" and found that they were likely to be girls and good academic achievers. In a recent study, Prinstein (2007) found good correspondence between judgments of perceived popularity by selected experts and the entire classroom in high school youth.

As in any research, ethical issues are important in sociometric studies. Mayeux, Underwood, and Risser (2007) provide a detailed treatise of the ethical issues involved in sociometric research. Here I cover only a few main issues. The fact that children or adolescents are asked to evaluate each other, or to evaluate each other negatively, is sometimes a concern for parents or teachers. Most peer relations researchers use careful instructions and procedures to prevent any negative consequences, such as explaining and emphasizing confidentiality, using code numbers instead of names, and creating an atmosphere of respect for privacy in the classroom. Relative to the number of sociometric studies, the number of problems is small. Most children and adolescents consider a sociometric test interesting, and the judgments they make are not very different from their judgments of each other during a regular school day. Ethical decisions also involve weighting costs and benefits. The benefits of sociometric studies, such as selecting children for intervention, evaluating the effects of intervention, and understanding basic processes of social development, may outweigh the potential risks that are generally small.

Quantification

The "quantification method" refers to the way scores are computed for each participant in a sociometric study. For peer nominations, this is first a count of the total number of peer nominations received for each sociometric criterion. For peer ratings, it is the determination of average ratings received. And for the method of paired comparisons, it is the number of times participants were chosen across all dyads in which they appeared.

An important issue in the quantification of peer nominations is that the number of votes received correlates positively with the size of the voter population. Thus, raw scores are not comparable between classrooms or grades that differ in size. The "standardization method" refers to controlling for these differences. There are three methods: standard scores, probability scores, and proportion scores. In the standard score method (Coie et al., 1982), the most common and the easiest to use, raw nominations received are standardized to z-scores within the votee population. Thus, this method is closely linked to the idea that status is relative to the group in which it is assessed. The probability score method was first proposed by Bronfenbrenner (1945) and refined by Newcomb and Bukowski (1983). This method was originally intended for limited nominations. Using the binomial distribution, calculation of the probability of occurrence of each raw number of votes received is based on the number of voters, the number of votees, and the number of nominations requested. ten Brink (1985) extended this method to unlimited nominations using the generalized binomial distribution. The proportion score method entails dividing the number of nominations received by the number of nominators, creating scores that express the proportion of all possible voters that chose the participant for each question (e.g., Hodges & Perry, 1999).

"Sociometric dimensions" are the continuous scores for peer status derived from a sociometric test. Five dimensions are distinguished: acceptance, rejection, preference, impact, and (perceived) popularity. Assuming peer nominations, acceptance is the number of "liked most" choices received, standardized with one of the three methods. Rejection is the standardized number of "liked least" votes received. Social preference is the standardized difference between acceptance and rejection, and social impact is the standardized sum. Popularity is either the standardized number of "most popular" votes, or the standardized difference between the standardized numbers of "most popular" and "least popular" votes.

Jiang and Cillessen (2005) conducted a meta-analysis of the stability of acceptance, rejection, and preference across 72 studies. The stability of these dimensions is high, as high as the stabilities of aggression and extraversion, typically the most stable constructs in the social development literature. The stabilities of acceptance, rejection, and preference also follow the pattern characteristic of a stable developmental dimension: Stability is higher over shorter time intervals, and stability over intervals of equal length is higher when assessed later in developmental time. The stability of social impact is almost never reported; therefore not enough data were available for inclusion in the meta-analysis. When reported, the stability of social impact is often low, although there are exceptions, and there seems to be much variability in the stability of impact. A hypothesis based on anecdotal observation is that social impact is more stable in adolescent groups than among children. In studies that include stabilities of both popularity and acceptance or preference, the stability of popularity is higher. This makes sense, because judgments of popularity are reputations that reflect a group consensus, whereas judgments of acceptance and preference are personal evaluations that are more likely to vary across perceivers. While everyone may agree about who is popular, there may be large individual differences in the degree to which one likes this person.

Related to this last point is the issue of the association between the continuous sociometric dimensions. Acceptance and rejection are negatively correlated; the negative correlation is typically modest (e.g., $-.20$ in Coie et al., 1982), although it is sometimes larger depending on method. The correlation between social preference and social impact is zero by definition, because of the way they are computed, which reflects a deliberate choice to conceptualize these two dimensions as orthogonal. Perceived popularity correlates positively with both preference and impact. The correlation between social preference and perceived popularity is positive in middle childhood (typically around .60) but decreases in adolescence, especially for girls. In Cillessen and Mayeux (2004), the correlation between social preference and perceived popularity decreased from .73 to .40 from grade 5 to grade 9 for boys, but from .67 to .04 for girls. After grade 9, the correlation stayed positive for boys but crossed over to become negative for girls (Cillessen & Borch, 2006). The correlation between perceived popularity and social impact is positive (Chen, 2005), which is consistent with the view of perceived popularity as a dimension of influence, visibility, or power.

Classification

The "classification method" refers to the way sociometric dimensions are used to classify children into sociometric status groups, types, or categories. Common in the older sociometric literature were one-dimensional systems in which students were classified as high, average, or low on one dimension of acceptance or popularity. Today, there is a clear consensus that classification systems should be two-dimensional. As indicated, the standards were set by Coie et al. (1982) and Newcomb and Bukowski (1983), who classified children as popular, rejected, neglected, controversial, or average based on social preference and impact. The popular and rejected groups are set apart by social preference, whereas the neglected and controversial groups are set apart by impact. In a scatterplot with social preference on the x axis and impact on the y axis, average children are near the center of the graph, whereas popular, rejected, neglected, and controversial children are at the extremities. Therefore, these groups are often referred to as the "extreme" status groups, for which the average group serves as the contrast group.

When the standard method is applied to peer nomination data limited to three nominations collected in classrooms, about 55% of the sample is average, 15% is popular or rejected, and between 5% and 10% is neglected or controversial. These percentages vary when grade is the reference group or when unlimited nominations are used. There is also a small but consistent trend for girls to be overrepresented in the popular group and boys to be overrepresented in the rejected group.

Subgroups of sociometric status types have also been identified. Most known is the distinction between aggressive and nonaggressive or withdrawn subtypes of rejection (Bierman & Wargo, 1995; Cillessen, van IJzendoorn, van Lieshout, & Hartup, 1992). Rodkin, Farmer, Pearl, and Van Acker (2000) distinguished two types of popular peers: "models" who are prosocial and kind, and "toughs" who are high in status but also aggressive. These subtypes match the distinction between sociometric and peer-perceived popularity. Both are dimensions of high status in the peer group, but whereas sociometric popularity correlates with prosocial traits and behaviors, perceived popularity correlates with a mixture of prosocial and antisocial characteristics (for a review, see Cillessen & Rose, 2005).

There are fewer studies on the stability of sociometric categories than on the stability of the underlying continuous dimensions. Cillessen, Bukowski, and Haselager (2000) conducted a meta-analysis of 12 studies reporting stabilities of sociometric categories over various time intervals, ranging from 6 months to multiple years. On average, about 50% of popular and rejected students retained their status from one year to the next. The stabilities of neglected and controversial status were lower. When using Cohen's kappa as a conservative measure of stability to control for agreement due to chance, stability was low for the overall category system, as well as for each individual status type.

Even though the stability of sociometric categories is relatively low, their concurrent validity is excellent. Newcomb, Bukowski, and Pattee (1993) conducted a meta-analysis of studies in which the five status groups were compared on measures of social behaviors and competencies derived from various sources of information. The extreme status groups are consistently distinguished from average, with moderate to large effect sizes. Thus, important behavioral differences exist between the status groups. Other studies have examined the social-cognitive (e.g., Dodge, 1986) and emotional differences (e.g., Hubbard & Coie, 1994).

Thus, while the validity of sociometric status types is excellent, their stability tends to be low, partly due to the fact that information is lost when continuous dimensions are divided into categories based on arbitrary cutoff scores. This is evidenced by the excellent stability of the continuous dimensions underlying status classification (Jiang & Cillessen, 2005). To the degree that either a continuous or a categorical measure of sociometric status is unstable, it also reflects development. Peer status is not carved in stone from one school year to the next, but varies depending on developmental factors of the individual child or adolescent (e.g., increased social competence), normative developmental changes (e.g., developmental changes in the importance attached to individual status vs. friendships or clique membership), and structural changes in social context that are correlated with development (e.g., increasing grade size at school transitions and changes in the gender and/or ethnic composition of the peer group).

The issue of whether to use continuous scores or categories of status relates to a general debate within psychology about dimensions versus types. This debate has been conducted about parenting practices (Baumrind, 1991; Maccoby & Martin, 1983), the nature of personality (Caspi, 1998), and clinical prediction (Waller & Meehl, 1998), among other things. The title of Coie et al.'s (1982) article is "Dimensions *and* Types of Peer Status," suggesting that there is room for both. This is also the position I advocate here. Sometimes types are preferred or necessary, such as when selecting children for intervention programs, or when determining the effect of intervention on the risk of peer rejection. In other cases, continuous scores are preferred, such as when research questions require the analysis of sociometric data with structural equation models (e.g., Cillessen & Mayeux, 2004) or growth curve modeling (e.g., Cillessen & Borch, 2006).

Which Method Is Best?

As the previous sections indicate, multiple choices are possible for each element of a sociometric procedure. Combining the options at each decision point creates many possible methods. Ever since the first sociometric studies, methods have varied. And even though there is more consensus about standards today, they continue to vary. This is not necessarily bad. Most methodological variations have been implemented for good reasons. A reassuring feature of sociometric research is also that despite the variation in methods, results are often consistent across studies (see Newcomb et al., 1993; Parker & Asher, 1987).

Because studies differ in more than one methodological aspect, often confounded by differences in sample characteristics, it is difficult to isolate the effects of each methodological decision from an indirect comparison of studies. Comparing methods also requires criteria for when a method is better, but such criteria are lacking. Is a method better when the status types derived from it are more stable? Sometimes instability is part of a developmental process. Is a method better when the effect sizes for contrasts between the extreme groups and the average group are larger? A lower effect size may be due to behavioral heterogeneity within a status group, which may be an important substantive phenomenon rather than a methodological artifact.

Answers to the question about which method is best should come from direct comparison studies in which one methodological decision is varied at the time. Such comparisons are doable when they involve different statistical manipulations of the same data, such as research on the effects of different standardization and classification methods (e.g., Terry & Coie, 1991). Such comparisons are more difficult when they require collecting data with different methods, but this too has been done throughout the history of sociometric measurement (e.g., Maassen et al., 2000; Witryol & Thompson, 1953). Given the limited time available for data collection in schools, it is often difficult to build multiple methodological variations into one data collection. Nevertheless, to enhance proper construct measurement, direct comparison studies of methodological aspects remain an important direction of future research.

Relevant Theory

Moreno's (1934) sociometry was a theory first, and a method second. Moreno had an idiosyncratic theory of social relationships and group dynamics. Moreno's theory is abstract and difficult to summarize, but an important premise of his theory is that the larger social system in which an individual is embedded (e.g., the group or social network), and not the individual itself, should be the unit of analysis for scholars studying social processes. Individuals are called "social atoms," elements in the social network between whom two forces operate—attractions and repulsions. Many of Moreno's writings dealt with understanding these two forces. In the sociometric method, attractions were translated into the dimension of acceptance, and repulsions into rejection. Acceptance and rejection are the remnants of Moreno's theoretical system in the sociometric method. A fairly detailed and accessible account of Moreno's philosophical system can be found in Fox (1987).

A more recent conceptualization relevant to sociometric measurement is that peer status is a reflection of underlying social competence. This was the dominant theory of social status during the 1980s and 1990s, although not always formulated explicitly (see Ladd, 2005). The idea is that peer rejection is an indicator of social incompetence, whereas peer acceptance (or sociometric popularity) is an indicator of social competence. A dominant view of the role of peers in development was also that adequate relationships with peers are essential for cognitive and social growth (e.g., Hartup, 1983; Sullivan, 1953). Translated to sociometric status, the idea here is that popular children have good relationships with peers that benefit their development, whereas rejected children have poor relationships that put them at risk. Where the neglected and controversial groups fitted on a dimension of social competence was left ambiguous.

Parker and Asher (1987) combined these two theories into two models of the role of peers in development. In the incidental model, the quality of a child's relationships with peers is a reflection of underlying dimensions of social competence, social adjustment, or psychopathology. In the causal model, the quality of a child's interactions with peers has a direct impact on the child's future competence, adjustment, and health. Today, the consensus is that both models operate at the same time, and that the associations between peer relations and social competence and adjustment are reciprocal (see Ladd, 2005).

Coie (1990) applied these ideas about reciprocal causation to peer rejection by distinguishing two phases, one in which behavior drives status, and another in which status drives behavior. In the emergence phase of peer rejection, children are primarily data-driven in their decisions about who they do and do not like. In this stage, children's behaviors and competences (or lack therefore) in interactions with peers determine their status. In the maintenance stage, status has been acquired, and children base their judgments of others on their reputations rather than their actual behaviors. Here, being rejected impairs the child's interactions with peers, who maintain their negative perceptions of the rejected child, depriving him or her of opportunities to benefit from interactions with peers even further.

Three larger theoretical systems are also relevant for understanding sociometric status in the peer group: group dynamics, ecological and social-contextual theories, and ethological approaches. Moreno's (1934) original theory of sociometry was a theory of group dynamics. Moreno's ideas were somewhat comparable to the field theory of Lewin (e.g., Lewin, Lippitt, & White, 1939), whom Moreno had met. In either theory, persons are seen as embedded in a large social network, and the roles of persons in the network depend on their position in it and the forces that impinge upon them. These ideas are still present in modern theories of group dynamics (e.g., Forsyth, 2006).

An important part of such theories is also that they do not see the role of individuals in groups as static, but as constantly changing and dynamic. Sherif and Sherif's (1964) work on group processes with children is an example of this approach. In a recent example, Light and Dishion (2007) used dynamic systems theories to understand changes in social networks over time. According to group dynamic theories, the distribution of roles within a group varies depending on a number of control parameters. This fits with sociometric measurement in which some groups have a flat distribution of social roles, with many average children and few children in the extreme types, whereas other groups have a more peaked distribution, with more extreme children and fewer average children. A challenge for future research is to identify the factors that explain this variation in the distribution of social status types within peer groups.

Ecological or social-contextual theories emphasize the role of the social context as a determinant of individual social behavior. One of the most well-known ecological theoreticians was Bronfenbrenner (1945), who, interestingly, was also a member of the first generation of sociometric researchers. Ecological theories specify how the individual is embedded in multiple layers of the social context that influence each other and the individual's social behavior over time. The peer group is a context in which status emerges. The peer group is part of larger social systems (school, neighborhood, subculture) that further influence the emergence of certain status types, for example, through the unique way in which behaviors are valenced.

Ethological approaches to social status and behavior focus to a great extent on dominance hierarchies, their functions, and the factors that explain and determine them.
Several peer relations researchers have applied ethology to understanding social status
and social behavior, and in particular the role of aggression (see Hawley, Little, & Rodkin,
2007). Group dynamic, dynamic systems, ecological, and ethological theories all have
in common their focus on the social structure of peer groups and the behaviors or contextual factors that explain this structure. These theories continue to be important for
understanding the peer system.

Key Classical and Modern Research Studies

One problem with the selection of key studies about sociometric measurement is that
there are many from which to choose. Many excellent studies have appeared over the
70-year history of sociometric measurement. Any selection is biased, and numerous excellent articles are not included in the list below. My goal in this list was to create a "Top 10
of sociometric measurement," but this turned out to be impossible, and the list includes
15 papers.

Koch's (1933) study of popularity in preschool groups was the first sociometric article to appear in *Child Development*. It exemplifies the careful conduct and application
of a sociometric study with young children. Moreno (1934) obviously set the stage for
sociometric research, while also providing a theoretical background and making the link
between sociometric status and interventions in groups. Gronlund's (1959) book was
presented as a manual for teachers on how to conduct a sociometric test in the classroom,
but it became much more. It is an excellent review of the first three decades of sociometric research in school settings and includes detailed information about the psychometric
properties of the sociometric methods used at that time.

Lemann and Solomon (1952) published an important article that was responsible
for the shift from one-dimensional systems of sociometric status to two-dimensional systems. Clifford (1963) introduced the dimension of social visibility or social impact that
later became the second dimension of sociometric status, in addition to social preference. Peery (1979) put these ideas together and was the first to propose four "extreme"
status groups in the corners of a two-dimensional space formed by social preference and
social impact.

Coie et al. (1982) provided the standard method for sociometric status assessment
that was used by others for many years to come. Newcomb and Bukowski (1983) presented the same method but extended it to include the probability method of standardization introduced earlier by Bronfenbrenner (1945). These two articles were important
because they set the stage for the now classic sociometric status types—popular, rejected,
neglected, controversial, and average—used by many researchers in subsequent years.
Newcomb et al. (1993) presented an important meta-analysis of the differences in social
behavior and competencies among the five sociometric status groups derived from this
generation of studies. Earlier, Parker and Asher (1987) had published an equally important meta-analytic review of the predictive effects of measures of sociometric status (in
particular, rejection) on later adjustment.

Following earlier ideas by Northway (1946), Parkhurst and Hopmeyer (1998) were
the first to make the distinction between sociometric and perceived popularity in the
context of one study. Noteworthy is their finding of overlap, but not redundancy, between

perceived popularity and controversial status. This article also showed that aggression correlates negatively with sociometric popularity, but positively with perceived popularity. Cillessen and Mayeux (2004) put these findings in developmental perspective by showing that the two popularity constructs increasingly diverge from middle childhood to adolescence, particularly for girls. The positive association between aggression and perceived popularity also became stronger with development.

Two final articles are important, because they demonstrate how sociometric research can benefit from advanced statistical methods. Terry (2000) showed how item response theory can be used to score sociometric data collected with unlimited nominations. DeRosier and Thomas (2003) applied principles from advanced mathematical statistics to sociometric data. This article is also important because it exemplifies the development of specific software packages for the processing and scoring of sociometric data, of which there are now several.

Future Directions

In summary, what started as a simple paper-and-pencil test some 70 years ago has grown into an increasingly sophisticated methodology for social development research. More than seven decades after its invention, sociometry is still widely used in research and applied settings. One reason for its continued use is that the procedure is relatively straightforward, yet the information obtained is powerful. Sociometric status correlates with behavioral, social-cognitive, and emotional variables in important ways. Another reason for its continued use is that peer status cannot easily be determined via methods that do not use the peer group.

In the same way that sociometric methods enjoy continued use, they also continue to evolve. New methods are invented and improvements continue to be made. At the same time, there are several important goals for future research.

A first goal is the integration of levels of analysis. As evidenced by this book, peer relations researchers distinguish individual, dyadic, and group levels of analysis. Sociometric status is at the individual level; friends, enemies, and other types of relationships are at the dyadic level; and cliques and crowds are at the group level. Although this distinction is extremely useful for research and descriptive purposes, the three levels are interwoven in the everyday social lives of children and adolescents. Despite studies that look at the intersections (e.g., friendships of rejected children, or cliques of same-status peers), there is no method to integrate all three levels or to examine their relative influence at different times in development. The integration of the three levels, specifically placing individual status clearly in the context of dyads and groups, is an important agenda for future research.

Second, although Newcomb et al. (1993) documented the correlates of peer status, these correlates may vary by gender, ethnicity, culture, and development. More research is needed to examine how these factors, and interactions among them, may moderate the associations among peer status and social behavior, cognition, and emotion. The role of development is particularly important. It is often assumed that the correlates of peer status are the same in all age groups. More attention is needed to the developmental heterogeneity of the correlates of peer status. This heterogeneity may be further moderated by gender, ethnicity, and culture.

Third, an important agenda for future research continues to be the measurement of sociometric status in social contexts other than schools. The peer relations literature now includes a large number of studies with sociometric assessments across the entire age range, from 3 to 18 years, in school settings. Much less is known about peer status in contexts outside of school, such as sports teams, afterschool programs, or neighborhoods, and the consistencies or inconsistencies of peer status across these various contexts.

The other contexts in which to examine peer status should also include the world of cyberspace. Children and adolescents spend large amounts of time in chat rooms and on the Internet, where both prosocial and antisocial interactions occur as much as they do in person. Online interactions may be used to maintain students' reputations at school. A child may also develop a certain status or reputation in the virtual peer community, and be targeted for cyberbullying. What occurs between peers on the Internet may have many repercussions for their subsequent interactions in person. For example, online threats or gossip may lead to retaliation at school. Assessing these multiple roles of online peer relations is an important goal for future research.

Furthermore, relatively little is known about peer status after age 18 in college or in the workforce. What happens to peer relations after high school graduation? Is there an equivalent of sociometric status in emerging adulthood? If so, how should it be measured, and what is the proper reference group? Can peer status be measured in college or in the workplace, and are the resulting constructs meaningful in those contexts? We know relatively little about peer status in the college environment, yet the implications for health risk behaviors are large. The corporate world is increasingly interested in bullying and social aggression in the workplace, and their implications for well-being and productivity. This research will benefit from the development of new methods to assess young adult peer relations. Cillessen and Gallus (2007) examined longitudinal associations between adolescent peer relations assessed with traditional sociometric methods in high school and self-reported peer status and workplace incivility measured after the transition from high school into the workforce. Such developmental studies would also benefit from new methods to assess young adult peer relations that are not based on self-reports.

Sociometric methods continue to evolve with a focus on, for example, different types and numbers of peer nominations, and the use of information technology to assess peer status. Sociometry may be seen as a tool toward an end. However, sociometric methodology in itself is a fascinating area of research, and a developing field with continuous improvements. Much work remains to be done for years to come in this exciting area of research.

References

Angold, A., Coie, J. D., Burns, B. J., Terry, R., Costello, E. J., Lochman, J., et al. (1990). *Methods for developmental studies of conduct problems: Assessments of service use and peer ratings of social status and behavior.* Unpublished manuscript, Department of Social and Health Sciences, Duke University, Durham, NC.

Asher, S. R., Singleton, L. C., Tinsley, B. R., & Hymel, S. (1979). A reliable sociometric measure for preschool children. *Developmental Psychology, 15,* 443–444.

Baumrind, D. (1991). The influence of parenting style on adolescent competence and substance use. *Journal of Early Adolescence, 11,* 56–95.

Bellmore, A. D., & Cillessen, A. H. N. (2003). Children's meta-perceptions and meta-accuracy of acceptance and rejection by same-sex and other-sex peers. *Personal Relationships, 10,* 217–234.

Bierman, K. L., & Wargo, J. B. (1995). Predicting the longitudinal course associated with aggressive-rejected, aggressive (non-rejected) and rejected (non-aggressive) status. *Development and Psychopathology, 7,* 669–682.

Boivin, M., Dodge, K. A., & Coie, J. D. (1995). Individual-group behavioral similarity and peer status in experimental playgroups of boys: The social misfit revisited. *Journal of Personality and Social Psychology, 69,* 269–279.

Bronfenbrenner, U. (1945). The measurement of sociometric status, structure and development. *Sociometry Monographs, 6,* 1–80.

Brown, B. B. (1990). Peer groups and peer cultures. In S. S. Feldman & G. R. Elliott (Eds.), *At the threshold: The developing adolescent* (pp. 171–196). Cambridge, MA: Harvard University Press.

Bukowski, W. M., Sippola, L., Hoza, B., & Newcomb, A. F. (2000). Pages from a sociometric notebook: An analysis of nomination and rating scale measures of acceptance, rejection, and social preference. In A. H. N. Cillessen & W. M. Bukowski (Eds.), *Recent advances in the measurement of acceptance and rejection in the peer system* (No. 88, pp. 11–26). San Francisco: Jossey-Bass.

Caspi, A. (1998). Personality development across the life course. In W. Damon (Series Ed.) & N. Eisenberg (Vol. Ed.), *Handbook of child psychology: Vol. 3. Social, emotional, and personality development* (pp. 311–388). New York: Wiley.

Chen, Q. (2005). *Convergent and discriminant validity of popularity measures in adolescence.* Unpublished master's thesis, Department of Psychology, University of Connecticut, Storrs, CT.

Cillessen, A. H. N. (1991). *The self-perpetuating nature of children's peer relationships.* Kampen, The Netherlands: Mondiss.

Cillessen, A. H. N., & Borch, C. (2006). Developmental trajectories of adolescent popularity: A growth curve modeling analysis. *Journal of Adolescence, 29,* 935–959.

Cillessen, A. H. N., & Bukowski, W. M. (Eds.). (2000). Recent advances in the measurement of acceptance and rejection in the peer system: *New Directions for Child and Adolescent Development* (No. 88). San Francisco: Jossey-Bass.

Cillessen, A. H. N., Bukowski, W. M., & Haselager, G. J. T. (2000). Stability of sociometric categories. In A. H. N. Cillessen & W. M. Bukowski (Eds.), Recent advances in the measurement of acceptance and rejection in the peer system: *New Directions for Child and Adolescent Development* (No. 88, pp. 75–93). San Francisco: Jossey-Bass.

Cillessen, A. H. N., & Gallus, J. A. (2007, April). *A longitudinal examination of workplace incivility in young adults.* Paper presented at the annual meeting of the Society for Industrial and Organizational Psychology, New York, NY.

Cillessen, A. H. N., & Mayeux, L. (2004). From censure to reinforcement: Developmental changes in the association between aggression and social status. *Child Development, 75,* 147–163.

Cillessen, A. H. N., & Rose, A. J. (2005). Understanding popularity in the peer system. *Current Directions in Psychological Science, 14,* 102–105.

Cillessen, A. H. N., Terry, R., Coie, J. D., & Lochman, J. E. (1992, April). *Accuracy of teacher-identification of children's sociometric status positions.* Paper presented at the biennial Conference on Human Development, Atlanta, GA.

Cillessen, A. H. N., van IJzendoorn, H. W., van Lieshout, C. F. M., & Hartup, W. W. (1992). Heterogeneity among peer rejected boys: Subtypes and stabilities. *Child Development, 63,* 893–905.

Clifford, E. (1963). Social visibility. *Child Development, 34,* 799–808.

Coie, J. D. (1990). Toward a theory of peer rejection. In S. R. Asher & J. D. Coie (Eds.), *Peer rejection in childhood* (pp. 365–401). New York: Cambridge University Press.

Coie, J. D., & Cillessen, A. H. N. (1993). Peer rejection: Origins and effects on children's development. *Current Directions in Psychological Science, 2,* 89–92.

Coie, J. D., & Dodge, K. A. (1983). Continuities and changes in children's social status: A five year longitudinal study. *Merrill–Palmer Quarterly, 29,* 261–282.

Coie, J. D., Dodge, K. A., & Coppotelli, H. (1982). Dimensions and types of social status: A cross-age perspective. *Developmental Psychology, 18,* 557–569.

Crick, N. R., & Ladd, G. W. (1990). Nominator attrition: Does it affect the accuracy of children's sociometric classifications? *Merrill–Palmer Quarterly, 35,* 197–207.

de Bruyn, E. H., & Cillessen, A. H. N. (2006a). Heterogeneity of girls' consensual popularity: Academic and interpersonal behavioral profiles. *Journal of Youth and Adolescence, 35*, 435–445.

de Bruyn, E. H., & Cillessen, A. H. N. (2006b). Popularity in early adolescence: Prosocial and antisocial subtypes. *Journal of Adolescent Research, 21*, 1–21.

DeRosier, M. E., & Thomas, J. M. (2003). Strengthening sociometric prediction: Scientific advances in the assessment of children's peer relations. *Child Development, 74*, 1379–1392.

Dodge, K. A. (1986). A social information processing model of social competence in children. In M. Perlmutter (Ed.), *Minnesota Symposia on Child Psychology: Cognitive perspectives on children's social and behavioral development* (Vol. 18, pp. 77–125). Hillsdale, NJ: Erlbaum.

Forsyth, D. R. (2006). *Group dynamics* (4th ed.). Pacific Grove, CA: Brooks/Cole.

Fox, J. (Ed.). (1987). *The essential Moreno: Writings on psychodrama, group method, and spontaneity by J. L. Moreno, M.D.* New York: Springer.

Franzoi, S. L., Davis, M. H., & Vasquez-Suson, K. A. (1994). Two social worlds: Social correlates and stability of adolescent status groups. *Journal of Personality and Social Psychology, 67*, 462–473.

Gronlund, N. E. (1959). *Sociometry in the classroom.* New York: Harper.

Hartup, W. W. (1983). Peer relations. In E. M. Hetherington (Vol. Ed.) & P. H. Mussen (Series Ed.), *Handbook of child psychology: Vol. 4. Socialization, personality, and social development* (pp. 103–196). New York: Wiley.

Hawley, P. H., Little, T. D., & Rodkin, P. (Eds.). (2007). *Aggression and adaptation: The bright side to bad behavior.* Hillsdale, NJ: Erlbaum.

Hodges, E. V. E., & Perry, D. G. (1999). Personal and interpersonal antecedents and consequences of victimization by peers. *Journal of Personality and Social Psychology, 76*, 677–685.

Hubbard, J. A., & Coie, J. D. (1994). Emotional correlates of social competence in children's peer relationships. *Merrill–Palmer Quarterly, 40*, 1–20.

Jiang, X. L., & Cillessen, A. H. N. (2005). Stability of continuous measures of sociometric status: A meta-analysis. *Developmental Review, 25*, 1–25.

Koch, H. L. (1933). Popularity in preschool children: Some related factors and a technique for its measurement. *Child Development, 4*, 164–175.

Ladd, G. W. (2005). *Children's peer relations and social competence. A century of progress.* New Haven, CT: Yale University Press.

Lemann, T. B., & Solomon, R. L. (1952). Group characteristics as revealed in sociometric patterns and personality ratings. *Sociometry, 15*, 7–90.

Lewin, K., Lippitt, R., & White, R. K. (1939). Patterns of aggressive behavior in experimentally created "social climates." *Journal of Social Psychology, 10*, 271–299.

Light, J. M., & Dishion, T. J. (2007). Early adolescent antisocial behavior and peer rejection: A dynamic test of a developmental process. *New Directions in Child and Adolescent Development, 118*, 77–89.

Maassen, G. H., van der Linden, J. L., Goossens, F. A., & Bokhorst, J. (2000). A ratings-based approach to two-dimensional sociometric status determination. In A. H. N. Cillessen & W. M. Bukowski (Eds.), Recent advances in the measurement of acceptance and rejection in the peer system. *New Directions for Child and Adolescent Development* (No. 88, pp. 55–73). San Francisco: Jossey-Bass.

Maccoby, E. E., & Martin, J. A. (1983). Socialization in the context of the family: Parent–child interaction. In P. H. Mussen (Series Ed.) & E. M. Hetherington (Vol. Ed.), *Handbook of child psychology: Vol. 4. Socialization, personality, and social development* (4th ed., pp. 1–101). New York: Wiley.

Mayeux, L., Bellmore, A. D., & Cillessen, A. H. N. (2008). Predicting changes in adjustment from repeated assessments of sociometric status. *Journal of Genetic Psychology, 169*.

Mayeux, L., Underwood, M. K., & Risser, S. D. (2007). Perspectives on the ethics of sociometric research with children: How children, peers, and teachers help to inform the debate. *Merrill–Palmer Quarterly, 53*, 53–78.

Moreno, J. L. (1934). *Who shall survive?* Washington, DC: Nervous and Mental Disease Publishing Company.

Moreno, J. L. (1960). *The sociometry reader.* Glencoe, IL: Free Press.

Newcomb, A. F., & Bukowski, W. M. (1983). Social impact and social preference as determinants of children's peer group status. *Developmental Psychology, 19*, 856–867.

Newcomb, A. F., & Bukowski, W. M. (1984). A longitudinal study of the utility of social preference and social impact sociometric classification schemes. *Child Development, 55*, 1434–1447.

Newcomb, A. F., Bukowski, W. M., & Pattee, L. (1993). Children's peer relations: A meta-analytic review of popular, rejected, neglected, controversial, and average sociometric status. *Psychological Bulletin, 113*, 99–128.

Northway, M. L. (1946). Personality and sociometric status: A review of the Toronto studies. *Sociometry, 9*, 233–241.

Parker, J. G., & Asher, S. R. (1987). Peer relations and later personal adjustment: Are low-accepted children "at risk"? *Psychological Bulletin, 102*, 357–389.

Parkhurst, J. T., & Hopmeyer, A. (1998). Sociometric popularity and peer-perceived popularity: Two distinct dimensions of peer status. *Journal of Early Adolescence, 18*, 125–144.

Peery, J. (1979). Popular, amiable, isolated, rejected: A reconceptualization of sociometric status in preschool children. *Child Development, 50*, 1231–1234.

Poulin, F., & Dishion, T. J. (2008). Methodological issues in the use of sociometric assessment with middle school youth. *Social Development, 17.*

Prinstein, M. J. (2007). Assessment of adolescents' preference- and reputation-based peer status using sociometric experts. *Merrill–Palmer Quarterly, 53*, 243–261.

Rodkin, P. C., Farmer, T. W., Pearl, R., & Van Acker, R. (2000). Heterogeneity of popular boys: Antisocial and prosocial configurations. *Developmental Psychology, 36*, 14–24.

Sherif, M., & Sherif, C. W. (1964). *Reference groups.* Chicago: Regnery.

Stormshak, E. A., Bierman, K. L., Bruschi, C., Dodge, K. A., Coie, J. D., & the Conduct Problems Prevention Research Group. (1999). The relation between behavior problems and peer preference in different classroom contexts. *Child Development, 70*, 169–182.

Sullivan, H. S. (1953). *The interpersonal theory of psychiatry.* New York: Norton.

ten Brink, P. W. M. (1985). *The generalized binomial distribution as an alternative for the computation of sociometric status according to the probability model.* Unpublished master's thesis, Department of Psychology, Radboud Universiteit Nijmegen.

Terry, R. (2000). Recent advances in measurement theory and the use of sociometric techniques. In A. H. N. Cillessen & W. M. Bukowski (Eds.), *Recent advances in the measurement of acceptance and rejection in the peer system: New Directions for Child Development* (No. 88, pp. 27–53). San Francisco: Jossey-Bass.

Terry, R., & Coie, J. D. (1991). A comparison of methods for defining sociometric status among children. *Developmental Psychology, 27*, 867–881.

Waller, N. G., & Meehl, P. E. (1998). *Multivariate taxometric procedures: Distinguishing types from continua.* Thousand Oaks, CA: Sage.

Wargo Aikins, J., & Cillessen, A. H. N. (2007). *Stability and correlates of sociometric status in early adolescence.* Unpublished manuscript, Department of Psychology, University of Connecticut, Storrs, CT.

Witryol, S. L., & Thompson, G. G. (1953). An experimental comparison of the stability of social acceptability scores obtained with the partial-rank-order and the paired-comparison scales. *Journal of Educational Psychology, 44*, 20–30.

Wright, J. C., Giammarino, M., & Parad, H. W. (1986). Social status in small groups: Individual-group similarity and the social "misfit." *Journal of Personality and Social Psychology, 50*, 523–536.

CHAPTER 6

Assessment of the Peer Group
Identifying Naturally Occurring Social Networks and Capturing Their Effects

THOMAS A. KINDERMANN
SCOTT D. GEST

The notion of a "group" implies a social unit that extends beyond the dyad. In developmental psychology, there are at least three distinct traditions that study peer-group effects. The first tradition, building on Moreno's (1934) work, focuses on sociometric groups of individuals who receive similar nominations of liking and disliking from peers in a setting, such as a classroom (Bukowski & Cillessen, 1998). A second tradition examines social crowds of youth who share a common reputation among peers for patterns of behavior and values (Brown, 1999). A third tradition focuses on groups of youth whose social ties (friendships or interactions) are differentially directed toward one another rather than to other peers in the setting (Cairns, Perrin, & Cairns, 1985; Hallinan, 1979). Each approach assumes that knowledge about a person's group membership has diagnostic value for assessing his or her functioning, and that group membership leads to socialization influences (for review, see Rubin, Bukowski, & Parker, 2006).

Figure 6.1 illustrates the different roles of individuals, relationships, and interactions (Hinde, 1997). The approaches differ first in how groups are created. Groups that are culturally assigned or "obligatory" (e.g., classrooms) (Laursen, 1997) are defined independently of the people under study. Sociometric research holds this perspective: The peer group is where people interact. The other groups are less well-defined, because they depend on individual preferences. The approaches also differ in the social ties that define the groups. For sociometric and crowd researchers, the goal is to identify subgroups of people who share commonalities. In sociometry, these are commonalities in social status (e.g., of rejected or popular children; individual ties are not implied). In crowds, the defining feature is social–behavioral reputation; members of a crowd (e.g., nerds, jocks) share "ideational ties" and are committed to a shared set of norms (Simmel, 1950), but they do not necessarily share ties. In contrast, friendship and interaction

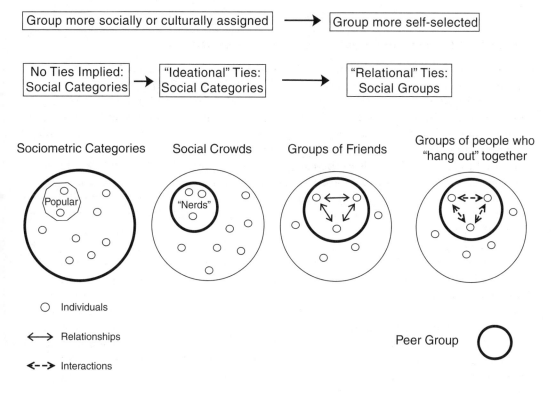

FIGURE 6.1. Schematic overview over types of peer groups, with attention to the roles of individuals, groups, relationships, and interactions.

groups are defined by "relational ties." The distinctions have implications for decisions about the social partners that need to be identified, as well as for expectations about processes within groups.

In this chapter, we focus on social crowds, friendship groups, and interaction groups. Our goal is to document the challenges that the approaches are facing and to outline suggestions for their integration in a way that supports theory building.

The study of peer groups has historically been plagued by two thorny issues: how to identify groups in natural settings and make sense of the "abstract art" of Moreno-type diagrams (Cairns, 1983); and how to conceptualize and empirically capture their effects. Many studies document correlations between the characteristics of individuals and those of their groups, but it is not clear how the correlations should be interpreted. They can imply that groups influence individuals, but it is just as likely that they denote that people who form groups are similar to one another. Experimental studies in which members are randomly assigned to groups demonstrate that influence is possible, but such studies cannot easily be generalized to the real world in which people are able to select partners based on social preferences. Both challenges are inextricably linked: Choices of methods for identifying peer groups imply a conceptualization of the processes by which groups are likely to shape development; and conceptualizations of group influences rely on methods to adequately capture the characteristics of peer groups.

Central Issues in the Assessment of Peer Groups

Sources of Information Regarding Crowds and Groups

Social crowds are defined as reputational labels assigned to individuals *by their peers* that involve stereotypes about personality and behavior (Brown, 1999). Crowds can be identified with ethnographic methods (e.g., Eckert, 1989), but by definition, peers are the ideal source of information. Brown (1999; Brown & Klute, 2003) developed a two-stage process in which (1) an overall account is obtained of the social categories upon which children agree exist in a setting (e.g., jocks, nerds), and (2) social "type" ratings of peers are used to assign individuals to the categories. Self-reports ("Which crowd would most of your classmates say you belong to?") may be sufficient, because they correlate with peer reports and are similarly related to indices of personal adjustment (Urberg, Degirmencioglu, Tolson, & Halliday-Scher, 2000), but they are also subject to concerns about self-enhancement biases.

Friendship groups are defined by feelings of liking between individuals. As with dyads (see Berndt & McCandless, Chapter 4, this volume; Hartup, 1996), self-reports give the best information. Nonetheless, there are differing perspectives on measurement operations and on the importance of reciprocity. Most researchers ask youth to identify their friends, but alternative procedures include nominations of "liked" peers or ratings of "liking." Disagreements about the value of reciprocity fall along disciplinary lines. Developmentalists see reciprocity as a requirement: A friendship exists when both individuals agree on the friendship; sociologists tend to view unreciprocated friendships as key reference groups or as links that connect larger groups (Bearman, Moody, & Stovel, 2004).

Social groups based on frequent interaction can also be identified via self-reports, but because children tend to exaggerate associations with popular peers (Leung, 1996), alternative strategies have been developed. One alternative is to observe peers (Hanish, Martin, Fabes, Leonard, & Herzog, 2005; Ladd, 1983; Strayer & Santos, 1996), but such studies are costly and often constrained by limited access to interaction settings. In contrast, peers are expert participant–observers with unique access to interactions in social settings. This led Robert Cairns to develop the *Socio-Cognitive Map* (SCM) procedure, in which peers in a school setting are asked to identify classmates who "hang around together a lot" (Cairns et al., 1985; Gest, Farmer, Cairns, & Xie, 2003; Kindermann, 1996). Respondents name or list as many groups as they can but are not required to classify all peers into groups. The reports are aggregated into a symmetrical co-occurrence (or conomination) matrix in which each off-diagonal cell contains the frequency with which a pair of youth is reported to belong to the same group. This matrix can be analyzed with various quantitative techniques; because peer reports typically show considerable consensus, not every student in a class needs to participate to arrive at a reliable map.

Approaches to Identifying Group Structures

Social Crowds

A central issue in analyzing crowd data is whether to constrain each individual to be in only one crowd or to permit membership in multiple crowds. In Brown's original two-stage peer-report approach, each student was classified into a unique crowd; but later the coding procedure was refined so that each individual received a separate score for each crowd label (the proportion of peers who assigned the individual to each crowd; Brown & Klute, 2003). Similar coding options exist for self-reports of crowd affiliations.

Social Groups

Strategies for identifying group structures fall into two approaches and are equally applicable to data on friendships and interactions (Frank, 1995; Gest, Moody, & Rulison, 2007; Moody, 2001). In one approach, individuals are grouped together when their patterns of ties are similar (i.e., correlated). For example, in the 1950s, network researchers factor-analyzed interaction matrices: Individuals with highly correlated profiles loaded on the same factor and were seen as members of the same group. Researchers using the SCM data collection method follow this tradition. Cairns and colleagues (1985) originally identified dyads whose nomination profiles were reliably correlated and then used decision rules to build groups; later they used confirmatory factor analysis (Cairns, Cairns, Neckerman, Gest, & Gariepy, 1988). More recently, SCM researchers have used a computer program that identifies groups composed of individuals whose profiles are correlated ($r > .40$) with at least 50% of the other group members (Estell, Farmer, Cairns, & Cairns, 2002; Farmer, Estell, Bishop, O'Neal, & Cairns, 2003; Rodkin, Farmer, Pearl, & Van Acker, 2006), whereas Gest and colleagues (2007) used principal component analysis. Hierarchical cluster analysis also falls in this tradition (Strayer & Santos, 1996).

A second approach is to *search directly* for groups by applying algorithms that optimize intuitive notions of internally cohesive yet distinct group structures, such as not splitting apart triads of mutual friends, or maximizing the density of friendships within groups (e.g., [UCINET; University of California at Irvine Network program] by Borgatti, Everett, & Freeman, 1999; [NEGOPY; Negative Entropy] by Richards, 1995). Other approaches directly identify groups based on graph theory features, such as degree of embeddedness (Moody & White, 2003). With the same data, different algorithms will often (but not always) yield similar group structures; there is some indication that variations may be especially consequential when friendship nominations rather than SCM groups are analyzed (Gest et al., 2007).

These approaches aim to divide a social network into largely nonoverlapping groups. A different approach is to identify groups individually for each person, preserving multiple group overlap. With friendships, this can involve identifying unreciprocated nominations. With SCM interaction groups, probabilities can be computed from the conomination matrix to determine the peers with whom an individual is conominated more often than can be expected by chance. This strategy gives up on notions that groups exist over and above the level of individuals' ties.

Assessment of Group Characteristics

The second task is to capture the groups' central characteristics. Developmentalists are highly interested in whether the *characteristics* of peer groups influence children. We take as a starting point that the measures characterizing the individual group members must be obtained independently from the perspective of any other member of the group, because individuals' descriptions of group-mates are shaped by their own characteristics (Jaccard, Blanton, & Dodge, 2005). When individuals' characteristics are defined independently (by self-, peer, or teacher report), they can be aggregated across group members to form composite group profiles.

Group profiles are typically calculated as group averages. Such scores pose different challenges in studies of nonoverlapping groups versus individually defined groups. With nonoverlapping groups, researchers commonly compute separate group profile scores for each individual in the group by excluding his or her own score from the average. So, for a group of four individuals, each individual's group average is calculated across the other three members. This has two advantages: (1) Conceptually, this accounts for the fact that a group is experienced differently by its members (e.g., a group of one girl and two boys is experienced by the girl as a group of boys, but as a mixed-sex group by each boy); and (2) statistically, it makes it possible to examine individual differences in group contexts. But this approach also has disadvantages: Conceptually, it denies the possibility that groups have shared qualities beyond the sum of their members; statistically, it does not fully take into account the nonindependence of group scores for members of the same group. An alternative is to move to the group as the unit of analysis. Hierarchical linear modeling (HLM) can be used to separate individual within-group effects from between-group effects (Ryan, 2001). This works well when groups are nonoverlapping and have low turnover over time, but to account for the realities of group dynamics, HLM approaches need to be developed further to take into account time-varying and overlapping group structures. The situation is simplified when there is group overlap and groups are identified separately for each individual (e.g., Kindermann, 2007); group profiles can be computed individually. Conceptually, this ensures that group averages include *all* partners who have ties with an individual. Statistically, there are fewer problems with nonindependence of group profiles when these include individuals' ties that bridge across groups.

Relevant Theoretical Models

When identifying natural groups, methodological choices are closely connected to underlying theoretical perspectives: We begin with a brief summary of theories of group-level dynamics, including approaches to dyadic processes that have implications for group contexts. We then discuss their implications for methodological decisions and for studying group selection and influence processes. The discussion is highly selective; we include only theoretical frameworks that pay attention to member selection (i.e., excluding groups that are not self-selected, for example, in the literatures on group dynamics and organizational psychology), and only approaches that require researchers to identify the individuals that form a group (i.e., excluding purely ideational groups, for example, social categories from an individual social perception perspective, and intrapsychic approaches to social identity and ingroup–outgroup comparisons).

Theories and Models Relevant to Group-Level Processes

Social Interaction Processes

Proximal processes that occur in frequent interactions are seen as the "engine" of development (Bronfenbrenner & Morris, 1998) and of individual differences in adjustment. With regard to groups, two key phenomena are individuals' influences on groups (e.g., member selection and group dissolution), and groups' influences on individuals. With regard to group selection, Patterson, Littman, and Bricker (1967) proposed a "shopping" model, in which adolescents seek out affiliates according to compatibility of personal characteristics and interaction patterns. Processes of group influence on individuals include evaluative feedback, persuasion, coercion, resource control, and a variety of social learning processes (Altermatt & Pomerantz, 2003; Berndt, Laychak, & Park, 1990; Dishion, Andrews, & Crosby, 1995; Hawley, Little, & Pasupathi, 2002). Social learning processes are relevant to group processes in two ways. A group can be narrowly defined as an individual's set of direct interaction partners; these constitute highly overlapping groups of ecological microsystems (Sage & Kindermann, 1999). However, groups can also be defined more broadly. It is possible that group contexts amplify the salience of dyadic exchanges that occur within them (Thibaut & Kelley, 1959); thus, groups can be defined as mesosystems that also include indirect links.

Theories of Close Relationships

Close relationship researchers focus on the broader relational context of social interactions (Hartup & Stevens, 1994; Hinde, 1997). A major focus of developmental research has been on change in the norms underlying friendship. Laursen and Hartup (2002) contend that reciprocity norms govern friendships across development, but that these norms shift over time, from a focus on material equality to a focus on needs that allows for short-term imbalances in each partner's contributions. This formulation builds upon social-psychological theories (Thibaut & Kelley, 1959) that frame dyadic and group processes in terms of the exchange of resources (information, goods). Social exchange dynamics become extremely complex in group contexts but can be expected to generate differentiated role and status structures and to generate pressure for conformity to group norms (Thibaut & Kelley, 1959).

Social Comparison Theory

According to Festinger (1954), humans have a fundamental need to compare themselves to others to evaluate their abilities and opinions. This press for social comparison motivates individuals to affiliate with similar others. Within those groups, individuals compare themselves to others who are not too different from themselves. When discrepant evaluations among members of the same group emerge, individuals will attempt to reduce the discrepancy by changing their own positions or by attempting to change the positions of other group members. Most research on social comparison has focused on adults in laboratory situations (Suls, Martin, & Wheeler, 2002), but a significant literature indicates that many adult-like comparison processes are evident in children by about fourth grade (Ruble & Dweck, 1995). Social comparison theory provides explanations for the tendency to affiliate in groups, for selection pressures that create group similarity, and for the development of shared group norms; but it does not specify the nature of the groups that are most likely to motivate social comparisons (e.g., crowds, friendship groups, interaction groups).

Influences from Outside the Group

Members of a group can differentiate themselves from other groups partly by fostering within-group conformity but also by pressuring members of other groups to adhere to different sets of norms (Brewer & Miller, 1996). Moreover, stereotypes held by outgroup members can lead to biases in the treatment of groups. Such external pressures are most applicable to crowds, which are defined as peer-assigned social categories (Brown, 1999) that represent "normative guideposts" for adolescents' behavior and give "directives on attending to and interpreting messages from the broader youth culture" (p. 76). Similar outside influences may also exist for relationship or interaction groups. Teachers can treat members of a group similarly, or members can share experiences with adults, institutions, or other groups. A key distinction, however, is that youth are free to leave both kinds of groups when external pressures are excessive. However, because crowd membership is defined by the peer culture rather than by the individual, external pressures on members of a crowd may be impossible to avoid.

Structural Balance Theory

Generalizing from Heider's (1946) work on attitude formation, Cartwright and Harary (1956) described a press for structural balance in social networks. The basic notion is that every triad in a network can be described in terms of whether the ties among members are in balance. For example, if mutual friendships exist between AB, AC, and BC, then triad ABC is in balance and there is no press for change. In contrast, if AB and AC are friends but B and C are not, a state of imbalance exists, resulting in pressure for BC to form a friendship, or for AB or AC to dissolve their friendship. Empirical studies have validated the proposition that states of structural imbalance can predict network changes over time; developmentally, it highlights that the formation and dissolution of individual ties can result from larger structural features of a network. Because structural balance is defined with respect to direct ties among individuals (friendship, interaction), it is not applicable to the study of social crowds.

Individual Status in a Network Context

Developmental researchers measure individual status with "impact"-type indices (nominations for friendship, liked most, perceived popularity, "coolness," or social group membership) that capture the number of nominations directed to an individual, but not their patterning. Alternative indices focus on the degree to which individuals occupy strategic positions of influence within the network of ties (Wasserman & Faust, 1994). For example, two individuals may receive an equal number of friendship nominations, but the one who represents the only "bridge" between two otherwise distinct groups can occupy a more important position for the transmission of ideas or behaviors across groups (Granovetter, 1983). This is related to the study of "contagion" processes, in which direct ties can mediate or amplify information from indirect affiliates (Bearman et al., 2004) Borgatti (2005) discusses several "topological" indices of network centrality and the theoretical notions they embody. Working within this tradition, Moody and White (2003) found that after controlling for the number of friendship nominations youth received, those youth whose friendships were tightly interconnected in highly cohesive subgroups reported stronger feelings of school connectedness.

Implications for Methodological Choices

The theoretical processes described differ in the types of social ties they implicate. Friendship and interaction groups emphasize close relationships and social learning processes, respectively, but both types of ties are subject to similar group-level dynamics (involving social comparisons, social exchange, structural balance, and variations in topological network position). In contrast, the lack of ties within crowds suggests that only imitation and social comparison dynamics are necessarily in play within them, and that social processes occur in interchanges with the outside. Theories also differ in whether they require the researcher to (1) identify each individual's direct interaction partners, (2) identify non-overlapping groups, or (3) consider the entire network without identifying subgroups. Contingency learning (including evaluative discourse), persuasion, and power assertion all require identification of the direct partners who exert influence. In contrast, imitation, social comparison, and social exchange theories highlight the importance of structures that entail both direct and indirect ties. Finally, concepts of structural balance and topological importance can be explored without identifying subgroups.

Implications for Studying Peer-Group Selection and Influence

The most challenging questions for peer research are about developmental processes. Historically, the main interest has focused on processes that produce similarities among group members: initial selection of members; similarities that members share with regard to their experiences outside of their group; and mutual influences among group members.

Selection is a defining feature of all natural groups and a key process by which children can influence the contexts to which they are exposed. Social learning–based "shopping" models (Patterson et al., 1967), social comparison theory (Festinger, 1954) and close relationship research (Laursen & Hartup, 2002; Thibaut & Kelley, 1959) all assume that peers form groups based on similarity. In contrast, it is the specific merit of crowd approaches and theories of between-group differentiation that they highlight group-external influences. Finally, within-group influences are conceived of as socialization processes. This concept dominated the literatures three decades ago, but research has declined because of sobering conclusions about the extent to which correlational studies allow researchers to make causal interpretations (Harris 1995). For research on peers, the concept needs to be reconceptualized. The traditional understanding was that influence was unidirectional, and that it would "make" a child similar to a socialization ideal. In peer groups, the socialization agents are also children, and influences of each member of a group extend toward all other members. This perspective has two implications.

First, conformity may not be the best indicator to study. Experimental and naturalistic studies have traditionally taken conformity as the indicator of group socialization (Asch, 1955; Sherif, Harvey, White, Hood, & Sherif, 1961). Although member convergence *can* indicate influence, it is just one of many processes. In natural groups, similarity exists in many features when groups are formed (Kandel, 1978). In addition, such groups are highly fluid, and it is hard to disentangle changes that are due to member turnover from changes due to member convergence. Analyses are typically restricted to stable groups ("after selection has occurred"; Urberg, Degirmencioglu, & Pilgrim, 1997, p. 835), but stable groups may be special groups. Finally, the focus on group convergence may lead researchers to "reify" groups as discrete units. Treating groups as segregated spheres is warranted with experimental groups and justifiable with crowds. However, because relational groups tend to be fuzzy, and people are members of many groups at the same time, there is risk in adopting group-level analytic strategies and potential value in studying individually defined groups.

Second, natural groups may not always produce uniform outcomes. Socialization implies change; a focus on change broadens the scope of peer influences and suggests consideration of a range of outcomes (in addition to convergence) and change in various directions (Kindermann, 2003; Mounts & Steinberg, 1995). In groups of friends, questions about change have been examined in terms of onset of deviant behaviors (Ennett & Bauman, 1994; Urberg et al., 1997) and in terms of academic attitudes, behavior, and motivation (Berndt & Keefe, 1995; Berndt, Hawkins, & Jiao, 1999). With interaction groups, analyses of change have been used to study school motivation (Kindermann, 2003, 2007). Group interactions were expected to make children increasingly different from one another: Students who were "rich" in terms of motivation and motivation of affiliates were expected to become "richer" over time, whereas "poor" children would decline. Theoretically, it is hard to reconcile beliefs that intimate relationships provide mutual support with expectations that they produce uniform outcomes in the form of a social "mold" (Cairns & Cairns, 1994). Instead, social groups may make children enjoy activities that they would not enjoy (as much) if they were not with a group (Furrer & Skinner, 2003), and they may also foster increasing autonomy and differentiation (Deci & Ryan, 1985; Altermatt & Pomerantz, 2003).

Key Studies

Studies Clarifying the Reliability and Validity of Group Measurement Approaches

Group Homogeneity

All approaches share an interest in the extent to which members of groups are similar to one another. This is also called "homophily" (Kandel, 1978), "mesh" (Hinde, 1997), "assortativeness" (Kindermann, 2003), or "synchrony" among members (Cairns, Neckerman, & Cairns, 1989). Often, homogeneity of a group is taken as validity information that a group exists. Virtually all studies from all approaches find homophily; the pervasive finding is that "good" groups tend to consist of well-adjusted members (and vice versa), and that membership in such groups is predictive of various kinds of positive developmental pathways (e.g., Brown, 1999; Cairns & Cairns, 1994; Epstein, 1989).

Assessments of social crowds (Brown, 1999) have been explicitly developed with the goal to detect within-group homogeneity of members' social reputation. Prinstein and LaGreca (2002) showed that adolescents' self-nominations for most kinds of crowds overlapped with peer-assigned crowd designations. Crowds of popular students have been shown to match perceptions of teachers (Rodkin, Farmer, Pearl, & van Acker, 2000). Groups of friends also tend to be homogeneous (Kandel, 1978). An important question is about aggregation of dyads into larger groups. Urberg, Degirmencioglu, Tolson, and Halliday-Scher (1995) reported that over 90% of adolescents' best friends were members of their friendship groups, but concordance dropped to 70% when all friends were considered. Questions also extend to the definitions of groups and raise caution about whether friendship groups should include isolated dyads, "loose groups" (in which not every member can be reached by every other member via a direct or indirect path), or "liaisons" (children who are not members of a group but have friends in cliques, and ties bridging across cliques). Finally, interaction networks show similar homophily in a variety of variables (Cairns & Cairns, 1994; Kindermann, 2007), and they have also been examined with regard to whether they capture "real" groups. Overall, SCM maps tend to converge with group affiliations identified in independent observations (Gest et al., 2003).

Group Stability

All peer relationships are fluid over time. Relatively little is known about the stability of crowds (Brown, 1999). Stability of individual friendships has been studied extensively, but because there is no consensus on how to quantify group stability, estimates from studies using different metrics are difficult to interpret. For example, Hallinan (1979) reported that 18 to 30% of groups in middle school kept at least three members during the year, whereas Cohen (1977) found that 76% of high school friendship groups kept 50% of their members across a school year. Estimates for interaction groups vary similarly, ranging from 40 (Kindermann, 1993) to 60% (Cairns, Leung, Buchanan, & Cairns, 1995) within a school year. The most informative studies use the same metric to examine variations in stability in different contexts. Neckerman (1996) found that interaction group stability was low when students were divided over multiple classrooms across years, but remained moderate when classrooms were kept together. However, high fluidity does not need to imply low stability of the psychological group environment: Even when member turnover is high, selection processes can occur such that the psychological composition of the groups remains fairly consistent (Kindermann, 1993).

Studies That Clarify Overlap among Crowds, Friendship Groups, and Interaction Groups

Structural Similarity

Gest and colleagues (2007) applied three group-detection algorithms (one similarity-based, two graph-theoretic) to two types of data (self-reported friendships, peer-reported interaction groups). Results indicated that the similarity of solutions varied for the different data types. For self-reported friendship data, agreement across grouping strategies was modest, suggesting that the strategies are not interchangeable. For peer-nominated interaction groups, the grouping solutions were much more concordant. A *valued conomination matrix* provided the most robust basis for identification, making the choice of algorithms less consequential. For both types of data, homophily was strongest for groups identified by principal components analysis (a similarity-of-ties algorithm).

There are also indications that members of the different kinds of groups are not the same. Kindermann (2007), in a cohort of sixth graders in a small town, found that although most students were members of interaction networks (80%), and about the same number had reciprocal friends (in class, in school, and outside school), groups of friends were not identical with interaction groups. Slightly more than half of children's friends were members of their interaction groups (others were friends that were not publicly known), but 70% of the members of interaction groups were not friends. Most children without an interaction group had reciprocal friends, and most children without friends had an interaction group. To gauge crowd structures, children were also asked to give names to nominated groups. Many names converged with crowd designations reported in the literature (e.g., popular kids, nerds, brains, jocks; Brown, 1999; Eckert,

1989), but students with large networks were typically members of several crowds. Large groups of "cool" students or "nerds" bridged between separate interaction groups; among the six separate crowds of "nerds" or "geeks," two provided the connection between the otherwise separate crowds of "popular" students (the map can be viewed at *www.psy.pdx. edu/~thomas/Research*).

Similarity in Composition

The different identification methods also converge in their findings on specific target phenomena, even across different kinds of groups. One of the main research areas is aggression. At least some aggressive children tend to affiliate with one another; some are popular as a crowd, with aggressive cliques or with their own interaction group (e.g., Cairns et al., 1988; Chen, Chang, & He, 2003; Estell et al., 2002; Farmer et al., 2002, 2003; Rodkin et al., 2006). Homophily also exists in deviant and problem behaviors (e.g., Ennett & Bauman, 1994; Urberg et al., 1995, 1997, 2000). Finally, a large body of research also indicates homophily in children's school motivation, academic aspirations, performance, and school dropout. Findings on crowds (Clasen & Brown, 1985) converge with those on friendship groups (Berndt et al., 1999; Berndt & Keefe, 1995; Hallinan & Williams, 1990) and interaction groups (Cairns & Cairns, 1994; Chen et al., 2003; Kindermann, 2007; Ryan, 2001).

Functional Differences

The consistency of findings across different kinds of groups is striking and invites suspicions that the respective assessments may be measures of the same underlying phenomenon. However, there are indications that the functions of the different kinds of groups can be different. For example, Urberg and colleagues (2000; see also Brown, 1999) argued that although friendship groups appear to be uniquely predictive of adolescents' problem behavior over and above crowd associations, relationship ties and interactions can "channel" or modify norms of the peer culture. Thus, mutual influences in relationships and social interactions may occur differently when adolescents belong to different crowds.

Studies Clarifying Peer Selection Effects

Studies of selection typically focus on a dyadic level, but the processes have implications for the development of group structures (Epstein, 1989). At the group level, peer selection has traditionally been seen as a methodological "problem" (Kandel, 1978; Urberg et al., 1997) and has not been studied extensively. This contrasts with key studies of dyadic selection of friends (Gottman, 1983; Hallinan, 1979; Parker & Seal, 1993; for review, see Hartup & Stevens, 1997). Patterson and colleagues' (1967) "shopping" model was adapted by Kindermann (1993) with the assumption that, over time, children would optimize the composition of their interaction groups. In the one classroom of fourth graders that was examined, students' levels of motivation at the beginning of a school year predicted how the motivational composition of their peer groups changed over the year when students' own scores were weighted with the number of newly gained peers. The effect was weak, but suggests that when children include many new members in their groups, they tend to do so in a way that matches their own motivation levels.

Studies Clarifying Group Influence Effects

Two research programs have examined details of group influence processes on children's school motivation. Berndt and colleagues (Berndt & Keefe, 1995; Berndt et al., 1999) studied groups of friends, and Kindermann (1993, 2007) examined interaction groups. Both programs followed similar strategies to come as close to causal interpretations as possible. In terms of design, both examined change in children's own characteristics over time as a consequence of the composition of their earlier peer groups; individuals served as their own controls with regard to selection processes. Studies from both programs indicate that groups can influence children's development. Berndt and colleagues (1999) showed that the characteristics of friendship groups predicted changes in sixth graders' adjustment over a school year. Kindermann's (2007) study focused on interaction groups and included controls for a range of selection factors (group size, stability, homogeneity), as well as involvement of parents and teachers. Despite membership changes, group motivation profiles were moderately stable, and group profiles predicted changes in students' motivation over the school year, even when selection and group-external adult influences were controlled.

Studies Clarifying Intragroup Processes

Correlational studies with rigorous controls suggest that group influences are possible, but they do not explain how they can come about. A second step is to examine whether the mechanisms theoretically postulated to cause change do actually occur in the real world. This requires natural observations. Several such studies have documented that a variety of interactions (e.g., discussions, evaluative discourse, prosocial interchanges, learning contingencies) can be mechanisms of group influence (Adler & Adler, 1995; Dishion et al., 1995; Hawley et al., 2002; Wentzel, McNamara-Barry, & Caldwell, 2004). One study (Sage & Kindermann, 1999) examined learning contingencies in a classroom of fifth graders. Sequential analyses showed that behaviors had different consequences when children were members of different interaction groups: The more engaged students were, the more they experienced contingent support for their (frequent) on-task behavior from group members, whereas nonmembers responded at random. For students with low motivation, positive responses from group members were rare. These patterns can explain differential changes in children and are consistent with the changes found in correlational studies. The study followed Bronfenbrenner's ecological model (Bronfenbrenner & Morris, 1998) for identifying the sources of peer influences in school, and used SCM assessments to identify *all* of children's interaction partners as *direct* socialization agents. Note that a group-level analysis would likely have required assignment of each child to one specific group (i.e., excluding multiple group memberships) exclusion of ties with others who were not members of this main group (i.e., liaisons or dyadic ties), and inclusion of indirect connections (in analogy to "friends of friends") even if those individuals themselves were not identified as direct interaction partners.

Future Directions

In this chapter we have reviewed and compared three approaches to peer groups that have evolved from over 70 years of research. All three aim to examine group influences.

However, each approach holds different assumptions about the nature of groups and their developmentally active ingredients, and each has developed its own assessment strategy. Nevertheless, each finds group homogeneity in many characteristics. At the same time, it is not really clear what this means. Is this diagnostic information about individuals, the functioning of social systems, or selection processes? Or is this information about the developmental effects of groups? A key problem is how to design studies that allow us to make causal inferences.

Advances in the modeling of social network dynamics should allow us to reconceptualize group experiences, so that the model of a socialization "mold" can be overcome and bidirectional models can be developed. The characteristics of self-selected groups that we can identify in natural settings can guide us toward models of their developmental functions, and free us from relying on analogies that can only be created in a lab. The social-psychological theories we have described can be elaborated, integrated, and translated into sophisticated models of network dynamics. Most promising are models of the "coevolution" of networks and individual characteristics (Handcock, Hunter, Butts, Goodreau, & Morris, 2003; Snijders, Steglich, & Schweinberger, 2007). They are not comprehensive (e.g., social ties need to become scalable; subgroup differentiations need to be incorporated), but they allow investigators to specify a range of dynamics that are linked to social-psychological theories (Espelage, Green, & Wasserman, 2007; Light & Dishion, 2007).

As a first step, we need to overcome the idea that there is only one valid representation of peer groups. This pertains both to different analysis techniques, even when studying the same kind of group, and to theorizing across approaches. There is a tension between the desire to settle on a small set of "standard" approaches and the need to document the consequences of differing measurement strategies. Given the current state of knowledge, a realistic recommendation is that researchers should be urged to provide explicit theoretical rationales for their choices, and, if possible, to compare the results of multiple measurement strategies within the same study.

A second task is to discover more about how natural peer groups emerge and about diverse patterns of socialization. The most informative studies will consider how processes of selection and socialization work together in the real world. On the one hand, the openness of natural groups can shape social influences in complex ways. For example, negative influence processes (e.g., coercion) may not be found that frequently; if such interactions dominate, people are likely to leave or the group may break up. On the other hand, if people select others similar to themselves, interaction processes do not have as great an opportunity to increase similarity. Rather, socialization may produce maintenance or even increased diversity. For example, children may select peers who like them just the way they are, and they may stay with them as long as the peers remain supportive; the role of groups may be to support or amplify preexisting characteristics. It appears possible that peer groups can create diversity: Once similar children join together in a group, the group may socialize them into different roles, or members may strive to express their individuality. Such processes would lead not to increased homogeneity but to patterns in which groups, and the individuals within them, become more different from each other over time.

The third task will be integration that remains truthful to the strengths of the theoretical assumptions about the different kinds of peer groups. A rough sketch might look like the following: For decades, peer researchers have aimed to show that relationships influence development. Because of their reliance on the experimental model, they have looked mainly at similarity among friends and convergence over time, and have largely ignored peer selection. Convergence can occur, but it is hard to detect whether friends are similar to one another at the outset. In groups of friends with high-quality relationships, it is questionable whether a social mold model (in which friends attempt to change each other) makes much sense at all. Instead, friendship may be what holds people, and perhaps societies, together; a sense of relatedness may be what helps children and adolescents make sense of the world and of themselves. Friendship groups could be the equivalent of a "safe haven" in social settings.

In contrast, social crowds (and, similarly, sociometric categories) may say more about structure, order, access to resources, and minimization of friction in a social system (e.g., Merton, 1957); crowd affiliations may help adolescents to orient themselves within the larger peer culture. Both kinds of groups and their associated processes should coexist in cultures, as well as in smaller social systems such as schools, and the patterns of overlap in affiliations that people show across both kinds of groups may denote how they define themselves. Finally, if Bronfenbrenner and Morris (1998) are correct that social interactions are the "engine" of development, interaction networks would be the place where groups of people share activities they enjoy, perhaps influence each others' behavior (directly as well as indirectly), and play an instrumental role for each other in acquiring competencies.

Decisions about the kinds of groups to be identified need to be informed by expectations about the kinds of peers who provide the arena for the characteristics under study. Groups that are publicly known tend to engage in public activities; when public behavior is of interest (e.g., in classrooms; Kindermann, 1993, 2007), public interactions with groups may be most influential. In contrast, personal relationships may have strongest effects on private characteristics that may or may not be displayed in public. If private perceptions or goals are targets of examination (e.g., academic or social goals; Berndt & Keefe, 1995; Wentzel et al., 2004), close friends, because of their intimate relationships, should be most influential. As a consequence, it may be less important to construct separate theories about the different kinds of groups that we can identify, and more important to provide theoretical accounts and models of their interconnections and combined functions for development. Empirically, it may not matter much whether the variables derived from a specific approach are more powerful in predicting a specific outcome than another approach. Instead, what may be needed most are studies exploring how multiple identifiable aspects of children's peer relationships work together over time. Empirical information about the interconnections of the different kinds of groups may be necessary before we can attempt to build theories about their individual or combined influences.

We began this chapter by highlighting the different traditions of studying social crowds, friendship groups, and interaction groups (Figure 6.1). In reviewing the methods and theories associated with these traditions, it should be clear that the study of crowds, which do not necessarily involve direct ties among crowd-mates, implicates a very distinct set of influence processes and requires a very different set of measurement strategies than the study of friendship or interaction groups. And although both friendship groups and interaction groups involve direct relational ties among their members, surprisingly little empirical research documents the degree to which they overlap in structure or function across different periods of childhood and adolescence. Research that is grounded in the rich tradition of social-psychological theorizing about groups and close relationships may play a key role in motivating studies that address such questions and contribute to broader theoretical integration in the study of peer groups.

References

Adler, P. A., & Adler, P. (1995). Dynamics of inclusion and exclusion in preadolescent cliques. *Social Psychology Quarterly, 58*(3), 145–162.

Altermatt, E. R., & Pomerantz, E. M. (2003). The development of competence-related and motivational beliefs: An investigation of similarity and influence among friends. *Journal of Educational Psychology, 95*, 111–123.

Asch, S. E. (1955). Opinions and social pressure. *Scientific American, 193*, 31–55.

Bearman, P. S., Moody, J., & Stovel, K. (2004). Chains of affection: The structure of adolescent romantic and sexual networks. *American Journal of Sociology, 110*, 44–91.

Berndt, T. J., Hawkins, J. A., & Jiao, Z. (1999). Influences of friends and friendships on adjustment to junior high school. *Merrill–Palmer Quarterly, 45*, 13–41.

Berndt, T. J., & Keefe, K. (1995). Friends' influences on adolescents' adjustment to school. *Child Development, 66*, 1312–1329.

Berndt, T. J., Laychak, A. E., & Park, K. (1990). Friends' influence on adolescents' academic achievement motivation: An experimental study. *Journal of Educational Psychology, 82*, 664–670.

Borgatti, S. M. (2005). Centrality and network flow. *Social Networks, 27*, 55–71.

Borgatti, S. M., Everett, G., & Freeman, L. C. (1999). *UCINET V for windows: Software for social network analysis, Version 5.2.0.1.* Natick, MA: Analytic Technologies.

Brewer, M. B., & Miller, N. (1996). *Intergroup relations.* Pacific Grove, CA: Brooks/Cole.

Bronfenbrenner, U., & Morris, P. A. (1998). The ecology of developmental processes. In W. Damon (Series Ed.) & R. M. Lerner (Vol. Ed.), *Handbook of child psychology: Vol. 1. Theoretical models of human development* (5th ed., pp. 993–1028). New York: Wiley.

Brown, B. B. (1999). Measuring the peer environment of American adolescents. In S. L. Friedman & T. D. Wachs (Eds.), *Measuring the environment across the life span: Emerging methods and concepts* (pp. 59–90). Washington, DC: American Psychological Association.

Brown, B. B., & Klute, C. (2003). Cliques, crowds, and friendships. In G. R. Adams & M. Berzonsky (Eds.), *Handbook of adolescent development* (pp. 330–348). London: Blackwell.

Bukowski, W. M., & Cillessen, A. H. (Eds.). (1998). *Sociometry then and now: Building on six decades of measuring children's experiences with the peer group. New Directions for Child Development* (Vol. 80). San Francisco: Jossey-Bass.

Cairns, R. B. (1983). Sociometry, psychometry, and social structure: A commentary on six recent studies of popular, rejected and neglected children. *Merrill–Palmer Quarterly, 29*, 429–438.

Cairns, R. B., & Cairns, B. D. (1994). *Lifelines and risks: Pathways of youth in our time.* New York: Cambridge University Press.

Cairns, R. B., Cairns, B. D., Neckerman, H. J., Gest, S. D., & Gariepy, J. L. (1988). Social networks and aggressive behavior: Peer support or peer rejection? *Developmental Psychology, 24*, 815–823.

Cairns, R. B., Leung, M.-C., Buchanan, L., & Cairns, B. D. (1995). Friendships and social networks in childhood and adolescence: Fluidity, reliability, and interrelations. *Child Development, 66*, 1330–1345.

Cairns, R. B., Neckerman, H. J., & Cairns, B. D. (1989). Social networks and shadows of synchrony. In G. R. Adams, R. Montemayor, & T. P. Gullota (Eds.), *Biology of adolescent behavior and development* (pp. 275–305). Beverly Hills, CA: Sage.

Cairns, R. B., Perrin, J. E., & Cairns, B. D. (1985). Social structure and social cognition in early adolescence: Affiliative patterns. *Journal of Early Adolescence, 5*, 339–355.

Cartwright, D., & Harary, F. (1956). Structural balance: A generalization of Heider's theory. *Psychological Review, 63*, 277–292.

Chen, X., Chang, L., & He, Y. (2003). The peer group as a context: Mediating and moderating effects on relations between academic achievement and social functioning in Chinese children. *Child Development, 74*, 710–727.

Clasen, D. R., & Brown, B. B. (1985). The multidimensionality of peer pressure in adolescence. *Journal of Youth and Adolescence, 14*, 451–468.

Cohen, J. M. (1977). Sources of peer group homogeneity. *Sociology of Education, 50*, 227–241.

Deci, E. L., & Ryan, R. M. (1985). *Intrinsic motivation and self-determination in human behavior.* New York: Plenum Press.

Dishion, T. J., Andrews, D. W., & Crosby, L. (1995). Antisocial boys and their friends in early adolescence. *Child Development, 66*, 139–151.

Eckert, P. (1989). *Jocks and burnouts: Social categories and identity in the high school.* New York: Teachers College Press.

Ennett, S. T., & Bauman, K. E. (1994). The contribution of influence and selection to adolescent peer group homogeneity: The case of adolescent cigarette smoking. *Journal of Personality and Social Psychology, 67*, 653–663.

Epstein, J. L. (1989). The selection of friends. In T. J. Berndt & G. W. Ladd (Eds.), *Peer relationships in child development* (pp. 158–187). New York: Wiley.

Espelage, D. L., Green, H. D., & Wasserman, S. (2007). Statistical analysis of friendship patterns and bullying behavior among youth. In P. Rodkin & L. Hanish (Eds.), *Social network analysis and children's peer relationships. New Directions for Child and Adolescent Development* (Vol. 118, pp. 61–75). San Francisco: Jossey-Bass.

Estell, D. B., Farmer, T. W., Cairns, R. B., & Cairns, B. D. (2002). Social relations and academic achievement in inner-city elementary classrooms. *International Journal of Behavioral Development, 26*, 518–528.

Farmer, T. W., Estell, D. B., Bishop, J. L., O'Neal, K., & Cairns, B. D. (2003). Rejected bullies or popular leaders?: The social relations of aggressive subtypes of rural African American early adolescents. *Developmental Psychology, 39*, 992–1004.

Farmer, T. W., Leung, M.-C., Pearl, R., Rodkin, P. C., Cadwallader, T. W., & Van Acker, R. (2002). Deviant or diverse peer groups?: The peer affiliations of aggressive elementary students. *Journal of Educational Psychology, 94*, 611–620.

Festinger, L. (1954). A theory of social comparison processes. *Human Relations, 7*, 117–140.

Frank, K. A. (1995). Identifying cohesive subgroups. *Social Networks, 17*, 27–56.

Furrer, C., & Skinner, E. A. (2003). Sense of relatedness as a factor in children's academic engagement and performance. *Journal of Educational Psychology, 95*, 148–162.

Gest, S. D., Farmer, T. W., Cairns, B. D., & Xie, H.-L. (2003). Identifying children's peer social networks in school classrooms: Links between peer reports and observed interactions. *Social Development, 12*, 513–529.

Gest, S. D., Moody, J., & Rulison, K. L. (2007). Density or distinction? The roles of data structure and group detection methods in describing adolescent peer groups. *Journal of Social Structure, 8*(1).

Gottman, J. M. (1983). How children become friends. *Monographs of the Society for Research in Child Development, 48*(Serial No. 201).

Granovetter, M. (1983). The strength of weak ties: A network theory revisited. *Sociological Theory, 1*, 201–233.

Hallinan, M. T. (1979). Structural effects on children's friendships and cliques. *Social Psychology Quarterly, 42*(1), 43–54.

Hallinan, M. T., & Williams, R. A. (1990). Students' characteristics and the peer-influence process. *Sociology of Education, 63*, 122–132.

Handcock, M. S., Hunter, D. R., Butts, C. T., Goodreau, S. M., & Morris, M. (2003). *Statnet: An R package for the modeling of social networks.* Available online at *www.csde.washington.edu/statnet.*

Hanish, L. D., Martin, C. L., Fabes, R. A., Leonard, S., & Herzog, M. (2005). Exposure to externalizing peers in early childhood: Homophily and peer contagion processes. *Journal of Abnormal Child Psychology, 33*(3), 267–281.

Harris, J. R. (1995). Where is the child's environment?: A group socialization theory of development. *Psychological Review, 102*, 458–489.

Hartup, W. W. (1996). The company they keep: Friendships and their developmental significance. *Child Development, 67,* 1–13.

Hartup, W. W., & Stevens, N. (1994). Friendships and adaptation in the life course. *Psychological Bulletin, 121,* 355–370.

Hawley, P. H., Little, T. D., & Pasupathi, M. (2002). Winning friends and influencing peers: Strategies of peer influence in late childhood. *International Journal of Behavioral Development, 26,* 466–474.

Heider, F. (1946). Attitudes and cognitive organization. *Journal of Psychology, 21,* 107–112.

Hinde, R. A. (1997). *Relationships: A dialectical perspective.* Hove, UK: Psychology Press.

Jaccard, J., Blanton, H., & Dodge, T. (2005). Peer influences on risk behavior: An analysis of the effects of a close friend. *Developmental Psychology, 41,* 135–147.

Kandel, D. B. (1978). Homophily, selection, and socialization in adolescent friendships. *American Journal of Sociology, 84,* 427–436.

Kindermann, T. A. (1993). Natural peer groups as contexts for individual development: The case of children's motivation in school. *Developmental Psychology, 29,* 970–977.

Kindermann, T. A. (1996). Strategies for the study of individual development within naturally existing peer groups. *Social Development, 5,* 158–173.

Kindermann, T. A. (2003). Development of children's social relationships. In J. Valsiner & K. Connolly (Eds.), *Handbook of developmental psychology* (pp. 407–430). Thousand Oaks, CA: Sage.

Kindermann, T. A. (2007). Effects of naturally-existing peer groups on changes in academic engagement in a cohort of sixth graders. *Child Development, 78,* 1186–1203.

Ladd, G. W. (1983). Social networks of popular, average, and rejected children in school settings. *Merrill–Palmer Quarterly, 29,* 283–307.

Laursen, B. (1997). Close relationships across the life-span: A symposium. *International Journal of Behavioral Development, 21,* 641–646.

Laursen, B., & Hartup, W. W. (2002). The origins of reciprocity and social exchange in friendships. In W. G. Graziano & B. Laursen (Eds.), *Social exchange in development. New Directions for Child and Adolescent Development* (Vol. 95, pp. 27–40). San Francisco: Jossey-Bass.

Leung, M.-C. (1996). Social networks and self enhancement in Chinese children: A comparison of self reports and peer reports of group memberships. *Social Development, 5,* 146–157.

Light, J. M., & Dishion, T. J. (2007). Early adolescent antisocial behavior and peer rejection: A dynamic test of a developmental process. In P. Rodkin & L. Hanish (Eds.), *Social network analysis and children's peer relationships. New Directions for Child and Adolescent Development* (Vol. 118, pp. 77–89). San Francisco: Jossey-Bass.

Merton, R. K. (1957). *Social theory and social structure.* New York: Free Press.

Moody, J. (2001). Peer influence groups: Identifying dense clusters in large networks. *Social Networks, 23,* 261–283.

Moody, J., & White, D. R. (2003). Social cohesion and embeddedness: A hierarchical conception of social groups. *American Sociological Review, 68,* 103–127.

Moreno, J. L. (1934). *Who shall survive?: A new approach to the problem of human interrelations.* Washington, DC: Nervous and Mental Disease Publishing.

Mounts, N. S., & Steinberg, L. (1995). An ecological analysis of peer influence on adolescent grade point average and drug use. *Developmental Psychology, 31,* 915–922.

Neckerman, H. J. (1996). The stability of social groups in childhood and adolescence: The role of the classroom social environment. *Social Development, 5,* 131–145.

Parker, J. G., & Seal, J. (1996). Forming, losing, renewing, and replacing friendships: Applying temporal parameters to the assessment of children's friendship experiences. *Child Development, 67,* 2248–2268.

Patterson, G. R., Littman, R. A., & Bricker, W. (1967). Assertive behavior in children: A step towards a theory of aggression. *Monographs of the Society for Research in Child Development, 32*(5, Serial No. 113).

Prinstein, M. J., & LaGreca, A. M. (2002). Peer crowd affiliation and internalizing distress in childhood and adolescence: A longitudinal follow-back study. *Journal of Research on Adolescence, 12,* 325–351.

Richards, W. R. (1995). *NEGOPY 4.30.* Simon Fraser University, Brunaby, BC, Canada.

Rodkin, P. C., Farmer, T. W., Pearl, R., & van Acker, R. (2000). Heterogeneity of popular boys: Antisocial and prosocial configurations. *Developmental Psychology, 36,* 14–24.

Rodkin, P. C., Farmer, T. W., Pearl, R., & van Acker, R. (2006). They're cool: Social status and peer group supports for aggressive boys and girls. *Social Development, 15,* 175–204.

Rubin, K. H., Bukowski, W., & Parker, J. G. (2006). Peer interactions, relationships, and groups. In W. Damon & R. M. Lerner (Series Eds.) & N. Eisenberg (Vol. Ed.), *Handbook of child psychology: Vol. 3. Social, emotional, and personality development* (6th ed., pp. 571–645). New York: Wiley.

Ruble, D. N., & Dweck, C. S. (1995). Self-conceptions, person conceptions, and their development. In N. Eisenberg (Ed.), *Review of personality and social psychology: Social development* (Vol. 15, pp. 109–139). Thousand Oaks, CA: Sage.

Ryan, A. M. (2001). The peer group as a context for the development of young adolescents' motivation and achievement. *Child Development, 72,* 1135–1150.

Sage, N. A., & Kindermann, T. A. (1999). Peer networks, behavior contingencies, and children's engagement in the classroom. *Merrill–Palmer Quarterly, 45,* 143–171.

Sherif, M., Harvey, O. J., White, B. J., Hood, W. E., & Sherif, C. W. (1961). *Intergroup conflict and cooperation: The Robber's Cave Experiment.* Norman: University of Oklahoma Book Exchange.

Simmel, G. (1950). *The sociology of Georg Simmel* (K. H. Wolf, Ed.). New York: Free Press.

Snijders, T. A. B., Steglich, C. E. G., & Schweinberger, M. (2007). Modeling the co-evolution of networks and behavior. In K. van Montfort, H. Oud, & A. Satorra (Eds.), *Longitudinal models in the behavioral and related sciences* (pp. 41–71). Mahwah, NJ: Erlbaum.

Strayer, F. F., & Santos, A. J. (1996). Affiliative structures in preschool peer groups. *Social Development, 5,* 117–130.

Suls, J., Martin, R., & Wheeler, L. (2002). Social comparison: Why, with whom and with what effect? *Current Directions in Psychological Science, 11,* 159–163.

Thibaut, J. W., & Kelley, H. H. (1959). *The social psychology of groups.* New York: Wiley.

Urberg, K. A., Degirmencioglu, S. M., & Pilgrim, C. (1997). Close friend and group influence on adolescent cigarette smoking and alcohol use. *Developmental Psychology, 33,* 834–844.

Urberg, K. A., Degirmencioglu, S. M., Tolson, J. M., & Halliday-Scher, K. (1995). The structure of adolescent peer networks. *Developmental Psychology, 31,* 540–547.

Urberg, K. A., Degirmencioglu, S. M., Tolson, J. M., & Halliday-Scher, K. (2000). Adolescent social crowds: Measurement and relationship to friendships. *Journal of Adolescent Research, 15,* 417–445.

Wasserman, S., & Faust, K. (1994). *Social network analysis: Methods and applications.* New York: Cambridge University Press.

Wentzel, K. R., McNamara-Barry, C., & Caldwell, K. A. (2004). Friendships in middle school: Influences on motivation and school adjustment. *Journal of Educational Psychology, 96,* 195–203.

PART III

INFANCY AND EARLY CHILDHOOD

CHAPTER 7

The Beginnings of Peer Relations

DALE F. HAY
MARLENE CAPLAN
ALISON NASH

Peer relations begin in the first weeks of life, when infants notice each other and respond to each other's cries. By the end of the first year, infants begin to communicate, share, and participate in conflict with peers, and to forge early friendships. Yet this body of evidence is not incorporated into developmental theory and does not inform most studies of older children's peer relations. In this chapter, to redress the balance, we set forth the theoretical issues that need to be addressed and review the existing evidence that bears on those issues. We conclude by recommending new directions for research that will link the study of young peers with other areas of developmental science. We believe that the serious study of early peer relations has major implications for theory and interventions designed to foster children's social competence.

Key Issues

The key developmental issues concern the meaning, origins, and consequences of early peer relations. These three issues lead to developmental questions that must be addressed by empirical investigation.

What Is the Social Meaning of Early Peer Relations?

What do early peer interactions mean for infants themselves? Are infants' interactions truly social? A positive answer to this question rests on the premise that nonverbal interaction can be social, an assumption that sets the literature on infants' peer relations apart from contemporary social psychology and cognitive science, both of which draw attention to the cognitive underpinnings of social interaction. In contrast, the literature on early peer relations draws on more general theories of development, and on the methods used to analyze nonverbal communication in other social species (e.g., Cairns, 1979).

Taking as their premise the possibility that early peer relations do have social meaning, investigators in this area pose a series of developmental questions: At what age do the nonverbal behaviors of young peers meet criteria for contingent social interaction? In what precise ways do these early interactions resemble the social interactions of older children and adults? When is it evident that infants hold cognitive representations about their peers' behavior? When do they form distinct relationships with particular peers? And when can they coordinate their behavior to interact in small groups, with more than one peer at a time?

Where Do Infants' Peer Relations Originate?

What are the developmental origins of early peer relations? Does early interaction with peers reflect a preexisting human capacity to relate to other human beings? If so, interactions with peers should arise *in parallel* with interactions with parents, siblings, and other people. Alternatively, is an earlier capacity to relate to primary caregivers a *prerequisite* for peer relationships? If the mother–infant relationship is paramount, how exactly does it influence early peer relations? Through social learning processes, such as stimulus and response generalization, and the emulation of adult models? Or at the representational level, through the construction and consultation of infants' "working models" of personal relationships (Bowlby, 1969)? What are the other sources of influence on early peer interaction?

Are Early Peer Relations Consequential for Later Development?

Is the early capacity to relate to peers an ephemeral phenomenon, unrelated to later development? Or do early peer relations have consequences for children's later lives? Does a resemblance between early peer relations and later ones imply that similar factors influence peer relations at both points in a child's life? It is certainly possible that biological and social factors influencing early peer relations are still at work in later childhood, so any correlation between early and later peer relations may be due to the operation of other variables. It is therefore important to investigate the factors within the child, the child's broader social environment, and the immediate situation that influence the frequency and quality of early peer relations.

To address this question, it is necessary to use longitudinal methods to explore both continuity and discontinuity in peer relations over time. The enterprise of tracing continuities in peer relations over time is conceptually more complex than analogous efforts to detect continuities in children's relations with their parents and siblings. Family membership remains stable, and in most cases, even if households change as a function of separation or divorce, family relationships endure. In contrast, as children move through their lives, some friendships endure, but children repeatedly are challenged by the need to meet and relate to new peers.

Theories

That there is, to our knowledge, no encompassing theory of early peer relations does not mean that this literature is atheoretical. Rather, the study of young peers is a laboratory in which most major theories are tested. No major developmental theory has explicitly predicted that young peers will interact in meaningful ways (Table 7.1), and so evidence

TABLE 7.1. Developmental Theories' Predictions about the Meaning, Origin, and Consequences of Early Peer Relations

	Psychoanalytic theory	Evolutionary theory	Attachment theory	Social learning theory	Cognitive developmental theory	Behavioral genetic theories	Social systems theories
Infants' capacities for peer interaction	Absent or limited due to emotional limitations of infants	Limited due to primacy of parent–offspring relationships	Limited due to monotropy	Limited by infants' capacities for learning	Limited by infants' egocentrism	Individual variation due to genetic basis of temperament	Fostered by infants' interest in all other humans
Origins	Mother–infant relationship	Social adaptations during hominid evolution	"Working models" of attachment	Contingency learning and observational learning	Progress to concrete operational thought	Individual temperament	Biological capacity for interaction with conspecifics
Consequences	No predicted effect of peers	No predicted effect of peers	No effect on later development	Later peer modeling consequential	Later peer relations are consequential	Peer relations consequential through gene–environment effects	All relationships have consequences
Challenging observation	A. Freud and Dann's (1951) study of attachment to peers	Protective functions of peers over social isolation (Mineka & Suomi, 1978)	Peers can serve as a secure base for exploration (Gunnar et al., 1984)	Response to peers' cries without prior learning (Sagi & Hoffman, 1976)	Peer influence on deferred imitation (Piaget, 1962)	Early peer relations more predictive than temperament (Fagot & Leve, 1998)	Infants prefer peers to unfamiliar adults (Brooks & Lewis, 1976)

for infants' social competence with peers provides a major challenge to received wisdom about development.

Classic Developmental Theory

Psychoanalytic Theory

Psychoanalytic theory emphasizes the emotional limitations of infants (the "primary process of infancy," in which the infant's actions are dominated by the id) and the primacy of the mother–infant relationship, with the father–child relationship taking on more prominence later in childhood (S. Freud, 1938). Although psychoanalytic theorists have focused some attention on children's relationships with peers (Sullivan, 1953), there is no expectation that infants' peer relations are significant for development. However, an important piece of counterevidence was presented by A. Freud's observation of emotionally significant peer relationships in very young children rescued from a concentration camp (A. Freud & Dann, 1951).

Evolutionary Theory

Theories of evolution focus on the transmission of inherited characteristics from one generation to the next, so an emphasis on the parent–offspring relationship, and on parent–offspring conflict in particular, is prominent in evolutionary theory (Trivers, 1974). Evolutionary ideas have influenced the study of children's peer relations through the discipline of *human ethology* (Blurton Jones, 1972); however, human ethologists initially focused their research on dominance relations in preschool groups (e.g., Strayer, 1980). Infants' peer relations were deemed somewhat unnatural; Konner (1976) argued that, in the early human environment, in small hunter–gatherer groups, there would have been few opportunities for infants to meet up with peers. However, experimental studies of macaques have shown that, in comparison with social isolation, being reared with peers provides a protective function for primate social development (Mineka & Suomi, 1978), although young macaques who have been reared with peers may also have some undesirable traits (Ichise et al., 2006).

Attachment Theory

The assumption that infants are immersed in their relationships with their parents, and only gradually turn their attention to peers, is made explicit in Bowlby's (1969) attachment theory, which synthesized key ideas in evolutionary theory, psychoanalysis, and cognitive science. Although Bowlby was at pains to avoid conflating the terms "primary attachment figure" and "biological mother," he proposed that evolution has biologically prepared infants to form "monotropic" attachments to primary caregivers. Although not explicitly stated, a corollary of Bowlby's concept of monotropy is that relationships with other individuals, such as peers, are formed later, through different processes (Nash, 1995).

Social Learning Theory

In the 1950s, when Bowlby was enriching psychoanalytic theory with evolutionary and ethological ideas, American social learning theorists were attempting to translate psychoanalytic concepts such as identification with parents into the language of learning theory (see Cairns, 1977). Parents were seen as important influences on their children's social development, which was underpinned by processes of modeling and social reinforcement. Attachment itself was seen as a learned attainment, through processes of contiguity learning (Cairns, 1966) or operant conditioning (Gewirtz, 1972). Peer relations were assumed to be influenced primarily by parental models, and the reinforcement and punishment that took place in the family home. In later childhood and adolescence, peer models were thought to contribute to children's subsequent development, particularly with respect to antisocial behavior (e.g., Bandura & Walters, 1963).

Cognitive Developmental Theory

Although the critical influence of peers is a core component of Piaget's theory (1932) of moral development, and a famous episode of toddler–peer interaction (Jacqueline's mimicry of a peer's tantrum) influenced his theory of imitation (Piaget, 1962), Piaget argued that peer influence begins to operate in later childhood. His depiction of infancy is one of individual discovery of the physical world, in which even parental influence is not emphasized. The quantity and quality of earlier peer relations are constrained by young children's cognitive limitations, in particular the egocentrism characteristic of the preoperational stage of cognitive development. Gradually, however, children begin to engage in verbal arguments with peers, which were thought to foster the ability to understand the views of others (Piaget, 1932).

Other cognitive-developmental theorists devoted even less attention to the possible importance of early peer relations, with young children thought to be at "Stage 0" with respect to an understanding of friendship (Damon, 1977). Sociocultural-cognitive theorists (Rogoff, 2003; Vygotsky, 1982) view cognitive development as proceeding through social interactions between novices and experts, thus focusing on infants' relationships with adult experts, not peers (e.g., Mosier & Rogoff, 1994).

Behavioral-Genetic Theories

With the explosion of new genetic technologies, theories that emphasize the role of genes and inborn temperament have come to the fore in developmental research. Strong versions of behavioral-genetic theory downplay the contribution of parents (Scarr, 1992); one such theory emphasizes the role of peers (Harris, 1999). However, in Harris's theory, as in the other major theories of development, peer influence is thought to be important at a later stage in children's lives. Other theorists who concentrate attention on the interplay between genes and environments (e.g., Moffitt, 2005) draw attention to children's unique experiences (i.e., those not shared between children in the same family) but do not focus on peer influence in particular.

An Alternative Perspective: Social Systems Theories

The preceding review shows that most major developmental theories hold that (1) infants' capacities for true social interaction are limited; (2) the ability to engage in peer relationships develops later in childhood and derives from earlier relationships with caregivers; and (3) later peer relationships are consequential for development but early ones are not (see Table 7.1 for a summary of each theory's position on these points; an example of work within each theoretical tradition that challenges these views is also noted).

In contrast, a few developmental theorists argue that the human infant is already a member of broader society and takes an active role in social interactions with siblings, peers, and other members of the communities in which they reside. Although this "social systems" perspective by no means represents a unitary school of thought, there are common elements to these theories: (1) an emphasis on the innate, active, sociable nature of infants, who are attracted to other members of their species and socialize others as they are being socialized themselves (Rheingold, 1969); (2) an emphasis on infants' abilities to engage in multiple relationships (Dunn, 1993); (3) an appreciation of the complex social networks in which infants and their families are embedded (e.g., Lewis, 2005; Rheingold & Eckerman, 1975); and (4) an analysis of the parallel development of infants' relationships with their mothers and other social partners (Dunn, 1993; Nash, 1988). For example, studies of infant–peer and infant–parent interactions reveal that infants' emerging skills with mothers and peers follow a similar timetable (Hay, 1985).

Despite differences of emphasis in these writings, they share a critical framework. The social systems approaches subscribe to the notion of an evolutionary basis of human social relations but deviate from Bowlby's (1969) assumptions about monotropy and the primacy of the mother–infant relationship (see Nash, 1988). Nash (1995) and, more recently, Van IJzendoorn (2005) have shown that a social network model fits better than the monotropic model into the contemporary evolutionary concept of inclusive fitness. In other words, infants may be biologically prepared for social relationships in general, rather than to attachments to one specific primary caregiver. Thus, similar processes may underlie infants' developing capacities to interact with a variety of individuals, including peers.

Classic and Modern Studies of Early Peer Relations

Although their capacity for social life has mostly been ignored by theorists, infants and toddlers do spend time together, under both ordinary and extraordinary circumstances. In the 1920s and 1930s, developmental psychologists and educators observed infants and toddlers in orphanages and the first university nursery schools (e.g., Bridges, 1933; Dawe, 1934; Maudry & Nekula, 1939; Murphy, 1937). A resurgence of interest in young peers occurred in the 1970s, when developmental psychologists made observations in informal parent–toddler groups (e.g., Mueller & Brenner, 1977), child care settings (e.g., Rubenstein & Howes, 1976), and laboratory playrooms (e.g., Eckerman, Whatley, & Kutz, 1975). In the 1990s, assessments of early peer relations were incorporated into longitudinal studies of children's social competence, aggression, and prosocial behavior (Calkins, Gill, Johnson, & Smith, 1999; Fagot & Leve, 1998; National Institute of Child Health and Human Development Early Child Care Research Network [NICHD], 2004; Rubin, Hastings, Chen, Stewart, & McNichol, 1998; Rubin, Burgess, Dwyer, & Hastings, 2003). There is considerable coherence across the decades of observations, so both historical and later studies can be examined for evidence bearing on the three main issues about early peer relations: their social meaning, origins, and consequences.

The Social Meaning of Early Peer Relations

Are Infants Capable of "True" Social Interaction?

The evidence suggests that a rudimentary capacity for peer interaction is present in the first months of life. Based on nonverbal criteria, social interaction can be identified when infants' encounters with peers incorporate mutual engagement of attention, explicit communicative acts, sensitivity to the behavior of the partner, and coordination of actions with those of the partner. These attainments rest on a more basic recognition of peers as conspecifics and interest in peers as potential social partners (Fogel, 1979).

The foundations of peer interaction can be traced to the earliest days of life, when infants cry in response to the cries of other infants in the nursery (Sagi & Hoffman, 1976). Research on slightly older infants demonstrated that this matching of emotion was neither coincidental nor due to an inability to discriminate between the cries of self and other (Hay, Nash, & Pedersen, 1981; Dondi, Simion, & Caltran, 1999). Rather, it is best construed as an innate sensitivity to the emotional expressions of others. Infants' responsiveness to peers' distress continues to develop during the next 2 years, when they begin to show attention, problem solving, aggression, and amusement, and not just matching of the distress (Demetriou & Hay, 2004; Lamb & Zakireh, 1997; Murphy, 1937).

As they grow older, infants show interest in one another in the first year of life, when they look at, gesture toward, and touch their peers (Eckerman et al., 1975; Vandell, 1980). Interest in peers may stem from a general attraction to other human beings seen in studies of infants' responses to faces and voices (Yale, Messinger, Cobo-Lewis, Oller, & Eilers, 1999). However, evidence shows that infants look longer at peers than at unfamiliar adults (Young & Lewis, 1979). This is not accounted for simply by height, because infants prefer to interact with other infants than with adults of restricted growth (Brooks & Lewis, 1976).

Statistically significant contingent interaction between infant peers can be detected when 6-month-olds touch each other and touch toys held by their peers (Hay, Nash, & Pedersen, 1983). During the first year, infants begin to engage in interactions that focus on objects (Adamson, Bakeman, & Deckner, 2004): Infants begin to communicate with and share the use of toys with their peers (Eckerman et al., 1975). However, infants' abilities to sustain contingent interaction with peers are most evident when toys are absent (Eckerman & Whatley, 1977; Hay et al., 1983; Vandell, 1980).

Does Early Peer Interaction Resemble Social Interaction at Older Ages?

Three important forms of social interaction are commonly studied in childhood and later life: (1) "prosocial exchanges," in which social partners work together to share resources and solve problems, or respond to each others' needs; (2) "social conflict," in which antagonists object to each other's behavior and act to defend their own territory or resources against encroachment from others; and (3) episodes of "social influence," when actors learn from, conform to, or are persuaded by their companions. Rudimentary forms of both prosocial exchanges and conflict with peers are present by the first birthday, and social learning from peers has been identified in the second year of life.

By the first birthday, infants show early forms of prosocial behavior. They share what they find of interest with their peers by pointing out, showing, and offering objects to other children (Eckerman et al., 1975). Spontaneous sharing stays at stable levels over the first 3 years of life (Hay & Cook, 2007). In contrast, in a cross-sectional study, 12-month-old infants were significantly *more* likely than 24-month-old toddlers to share an object in response to a peer's requests or designs on their possessions (Hay, Caplan, Castle, & Stimson, 1991). In older toddlers, sharing in response to a peer's request is significantly associated with sensitivity to the peer's distress (Hay, Castle, Davies, Demetriou, & Stimson, 1999).

Early signs of cooperative games can be discerned around the time of the first birthday. Observers of infants' and toddlers' interaction with peers have drawn attention to "shared meanings" held by both participants (Mueller & Brenner, 1977). Mutual engagement in a common activity and shared meaning of particular interactions is revealed in infants' spontaneous games with peers, in which each infant repeats distinctive actions (e.g., rolling a ball, or hitting two blocks together) in sequence, alternating turns in a game-like fashion (Ross, 1982). Cooperative problem solving in experimental tasks becomes evident by 24 months of age (Brownell, Ramani, & Zerwas, 2006).

Most infants engage in disputes with peers but not at high rates (Hay & Ross, 1982). Conflicts over toys and intrusions on physical space emerge in the last quarter of the first year of life (Caplan, Vespo, Pedersen, & Hay, 1991). The attractiveness of a toy appears to increase by virtue of another person simply contacting it (Eckerman, Whatley, & McGehee, 1979), even when an exact duplicate is available (Caplan et al., 1991). However, infants often avoid conflict. In a comparison of six studies of young peers ranging in age from 9 months to 4 years, in which the same operational definition of conflict was used, and a set of actions that might begin a dispute were identified, on about two of every three occasions when a conflict could have occurred, infants and toddlers remained calm and let peers do what they would without resistance, protest, or retaliation (Hay et al., 2007). In this light, toddlers' capacities for "parallel play" (Parten, 1932)—the ability to remain in the company of a peer, quietly pursuing one's own interests—may serve a conflict-reducing function in early peer groups.

In the course of conflict, infants sometimes do use force against their peers, pushing or striking their peers, and tugging on their toys. These forceful acts come into the repertoire shortly before the first birthday (Bridges, 1933; Eckerman et al., 1975), and 12- and 24-month-olds display these acts of force at equivalent rates (Caplan et al., 1991). Although parents report that most infants and toddlers hit, kick, or bite other people (Côté, Vaillancourt, LeBlanc, Nagin, & Tremblay, 2006), observed rates of force against peers are low and are shown by a minority of infants and toddlers (for a review, see Hay, 2005). Informants' reports and observations converge in identifying a peak in the use of force around 30 months of age (Hay, Castle, & Davies, 2000; Holmberg, 1980; Tremblay & Nagin, 2005); however, 2-year-olds are significantly more likely to offer toys to their peers than to grab peers' possessions (Hay et al., 2000).

Is toddlers' use of force truly aggressive? "Hard hits" are especially rare and shown by a minority of toddlers (Brownlee & Bakeman, 1981). The instrumental use of force (e.g., tugging on peers' possessions) is more common than direct physical assaults against the peer (Caplan et al., 1991; Hay & Ross, 1982). In a study of toddlers observed at home with familiar peers, instrumental force declined over 6 months, but physical assaults remained at a stable, low rate of occurrence (Hay et al., 2000). These findings suggest that in the context of familiar peer relationships, toddlers may find other, more socially acceptable ways of seeking access to peers' possessions. For example, toddlers who claimed toys by saying "Mine" were significantly less likely to use force 6 months later (Hay, 2006). Older toddlers use force less often, but, when they do use force, their aggressive behaviors are more sustained (Fagot & Hagan, 1985). Conflict provides an important arena in which infants develop, practice, and refine their strategies for negotiating the possession of toys.

Social Influence between Peers

Social influence between young peers can be detected in the context of prosocial exchanges and conflict; for example, there is evidence of reciprocity in sharing (Hay et al., 1999) and retaliation in conflict (Hay & Ross, 1982). Imitation plays an important role in early peer interactions, although infants' games with peers contain both complementary and imitative actions (Camaioni, Baumgartner, & Perucchini, 1991; Eckerman et al., 1979). Clear evidence for toddlers' abilities to learn from their peers is provided by an experiment in which infants were trained to serve as peer models, having been shown how to perform particular actions on toys (Hanna & Meltzoff, 1993). Untrained toddlers emulated the modeled actions and showed deferred imitation days after the modeling took place. This finding suggests that novices can learn from experts (Mosier & Rogoff, 1994), even when the expert is another toddler.

Do Infants and Toddlers Form Distinct Relationships with Particular Peers?

Experimental studies have shown that the interactions in which particular peer dyads engage have a distinct character. Even at 6 months of age, members of dyads are similar to each other in the extent to which they touch each other, and different from members of other dyads (Hay et al., 1983). An experimental study in which 21-month-olds were paired with particular partners for several days, then presented with a new partner on a test day, similarly identified the influence of particular peers on toddlers' behavior (Hay & Ross, 1982). Infants respond differently to familiar as opposed to unfamiliar peers (Young & Lewis, 1979).

When infants spend time together on a daily basis, they develop distinct preferences for particular companions (Bridges, 1933; Howes & Phillipsen, 1992; Zaslow, 1980). These preferences appear to be influenced by the peer's sex and individual traits (Howes & Phillipsen, 1992). These early peer relationships exert unique influence on toddlers' behavior. Ross and colleagues have applied Kenny and La Voie's (1985) social relations model to the behavior of groups of young peers in Canada and in an Israeli kibbutz (Ross, Cheyne, & Lollis, 1988; Ross & Lollis, 1989). Their analyses demonstrated effects of particular dyadic relationships on toddlers' social behavior that existed in addition to effects of individual actors and the individual partners with whom they played.

When do children begin to form cognitive representations of particular peers? Sociometric research would suggest that views about particular peers are clearly present by 3 or 4 years of age, when children can report on the peers they like and dislike (e.g., Denham, McKinley, Couchoud, & Holt, 1990). However, relatively little is known about earlier representations of peers. It is clear that when they acquire language, toddlers begin to gossip about their peers. Parents' reports of the names of children their toddlers talked about at home predicted the extent of their children's interaction with different classmates in the child care setting (Krawczyk, 1984). One-year-olds in kibbutz toddler houses can indicate toys and table places that belong to particular peers (Zaslow, 1980). By 3 years of age, children possess knowledge about ways to comfort distressed peers (Caplan & Hay, 1989) and repair friendships (Hurst & Hay, 2007) that presumably draws on representations of friendship that originate in the toddler years.

Early peer relationships have emotional significance. Toddler peers can be a source of encouragement and comfort, facilitating each others' exploration of new environments (Ispa, 1981; Gunnar, Senior, & Hartup, 1984). In extreme circumstances, as in a Nazi concentration camp, peers can serve as a focus of emotional attachment in the midst of untold horror and deprivation (A. Freud & Dann, 1951).

Are Infants and Toddlers Able to Interact in Groups?

The simplest form of group is a "triad," so it seems likely that young children's abilities to interact with more than one peer at a time are manifested in triadic settings. However, very few studies of triadic interaction have been conducted at any point in childhood, so the developmental course of triadic interaction is not known. When 2-year-olds were tested in groups of three, in two different samples, approximately one-fifth of their sequences of interaction were actively triadic, with all three toddlers making verbal or nonverbal communications in the course of the interaction (Ishikawa & Hay, 2006). Even more common was the situation with two toddlers engaged in dyadic interaction, closely monitored by the third. This interest in and capacity for triadic interaction may be detected even earlier in infants' nonverbal exchanges with other infants (Selby & Bradley, 2003).

Beyond actual instances of triadic relations, children's groups show emerging social structures that derive from transitive patterns of dyadic relationships, for example, dominance structures that emerge from patterns of initiating and yielding in peer conflict (Strayer, 1980; see also Vaughn & Santos, Chapter 11, this volume). Taken together, the available evidence suggests that the basic element of group life—the triadic relation—emerges before the age of 3, although there is considerable development thereafter.

The Origins of Peer Relations: Are Early Relations with Caregivers a Prerequisite?

Comparisons of Infants' Interactions with Mothers and Peers

In most major developmental theories, infants' skills are honed and refined in interactions with adults, and only later are used in interactions with agemates. Thus, in this perspective, the mother–infant relationship is a prerequisite to the infant's subsequent relations with other people (for a review, see Nash & Hay, 1993). In contrast, our parallel development model views infants' interaction skills as developing with adults and peers in tandem (Hay, 1985). Empirical studies that have directly compared infant-peer and infant–mother interactions found no evidence for skills emerging first with mothers and only later with peers (Bakeman & Adamson, 1984; Nash, 1986; Vandell, 1980; Vandell & Wilson, 1987). However, two recent studies on infant–peer interaction indicate that the prerequisite versus parallel development debate continues.

Brownell et al. (2006) charted the development of "true cooperation" with peers and concluded that active coordination of activities to reach a shared goal emerges at the end of the second year of life, *after* such abilities emerges in toddlers' activities with adults

(Warneken, Chen, & Tomasello, 2006). Brownell's claim was based on a comparison with the literature, as her own study did not include adults. Different tasks have been used in studies of toddler–peer and of toddler–adult cooperation.

In contrast, Selby and Bradley (2003) developed a two-step methodology that they termed "thick description" (qualitative interpretation followed by behavioral evidence) to assess intersubjectivity in young infant–peer triads, and found that shared meaning occurred in infants as young as 6 months of age. They suggested that infants are biologically prepared for group social life, and that they use their emerging social capacities with a variety of individuals, adults and peers alike.

Debates about the status of the mother–infant relationship as a prerequisite for or parallel attainment with peer relationships will continue until more researchers observe infants with caregivers and with peers, and use multiple measures of interaction with each partner, when the other is present or absent. Although most studies of young peers take place in the presence of mothers or other caregivers, mothers may actually inhibit peer interaction. For example, a comparison of playgroup infants on days when their mothers volunteered their time as caregivers and days when the mothers were absent showed that the mother's presence interfered with her infant's harmonious interaction with peers (Field, 1979).

Prediction of Peer Relations from Mother–Infant Relationships

The question of maternal influence on early peer relations goes beyond the debate about the prerequisite versus parallel development models. Individual differences in mothers may be linked to differences in their infants' peer relations. For example, the mother's mental state may influence children's peer relations; in comparison to children of depressed mothers, the 2-year-old children of well mothers showed more negative affect but also more prosocial behavior with peers (Denham, Zahn-Waxler, Cummings, & Iannotti, 1991).

In addition to its stress on the evolutionary function of the mother–infant relationship, attachment theory draws attention to individual differences in attachment relationships. The mother–infant relationship may influence peer relations in different ways depending on the quality of attachment between mother and infant. Security of infant–mother attachment has been shown to predict children's dealings with peers later in childhood (e.g., Waters, Wippman, & Sroufe, 1979); however, the evidence for a contemporaneous link between the security of attachment and early peer relations is mixed, with different patterns of association found for the different insecure groups. For example, whereas compared to secure toddlers, avoidant toddlers have fewer conflicts with peers, resistant toddlers are more likely to be ignored by peers (Pastor, 1981); in particular, the peer relations of resistant 18-month-olds compared to secure toddlers showed less reciprocity in positive behavior (Fagot, 1997). In the latter study, secure and avoidant infants did not differ in the quality of interaction with peers. Furthermore, when observed patterns of family interaction were taken into consideration, attachment no longer predicted the quality of peer interaction. Rather, in line with the predictions of social learning theory, negative interactions in the family setting were associated with negative interactions with peers. Thus, fathers and siblings, as well as mothers, influence early peer relations. Indeed, many different factors influence the behavior of young peers.

Other Sources of Influence on Early Peer Relations

Genes

To our knowledge, researchers have not employed genetically informative designs or methods to investigate the biological underpinnings of early peer relations. It is not clear whether the most commonly used genetic design, the twin study, is appropriate to the study of peer relations, insofar as twins are unique in the human population in having siblings who are also agemates. What effect this might have on the frequency and quality of peer interaction is not clear. However, twin studies have indicated genetic, as well as environmental, influence on dimensions of toddlers' behavior that feature in early peer interaction, including aggression (Dionne, Tremblay, Boivin, Laplante, & Pérusse, 2003), empathic concern (Zahn-Waxler, Robinson, & Emde, 1992), and prosocial behavior (Knafo & Plomin, 2006).

The Child's Sex

Although sex differences in activity levels and preferences for different types of toys might influence the content of play with peers, there is little evidence for striking sex differences in prosocial behavior or conflict with peers before the third birthday. In most observational studies of infants and toddlers, no significant sex differences are reported. This may be partly a function of statistical power to detect small effects; in one larger sample of primarily middle-class Canadian children, sex differences in aggression were identified (Rubin et al., 1998). However, no sex differences were detected in a similarly large, demographically representative sample of toddlers who were observed longitudinally for several months in experimentally created playgroups (Fagot, 1997).

The available evidence suggests that sex differences in aggression and conflict with peers emerge between ages 2 and 4 years, with differences emerging sooner in groups than in dyads (NICHD, 2001). Rather than showing a pattern of consistent sex differences in actual behavior with peers, the literature reveals ways in which the sex of the child is a moderating variable, influencing the impact of other factors within the child and social setting. Furthermore, there is evidence for the importance of the sex of the peer as an influence on infants' behavior; even in the first year of life, the sex composition of the dyad or triad influences infants' participation in conflict with peers (Caplan et al., 1991). It is also clear that girls and boys are socialized differently in the context of early peer interaction; girls' aggression tends to be ignored (Fagot & Hagan, 1985), and girls are more likely than boys to be asked to relinquish their possessions in response to peers' demands (Ross, Tesla, Kenyon, & Lollis, 1990).

Temperament and Emotion Regulation

Temperamental differences in infants' activity levels and ability to regulate their emotions influence early peer relations. For example, inhibited temperament in infancy predicts later shyness with peers (Rubin, Burgess, & Hastings, 2002). Proneness to anger and low tolerance of frustration influence the extent to which toddlers become involved in interaction with peers (Denham et al., 1991) and take part in aggressive conflict (Calkins, Gill, Johnson, & Smith, 1999; Rubin et al., 1998). It appears that positive ability to regulate one's negative emotions and dysregulation of emotion are not opposites; rather, they show somewhat different patterns of association with toddlers' conflict and cooperation with peers (e.g., Calkins et al., 1999; Rubin et al., 1998).

Cognition and Language

Relatively few studies have sought to determine the cognitive and linguistic underpinnings of early peer relations. The games played by toddlers with peers indicate shared meaning (Mueller & Brenner, 1977). As soon as language develops, toddlers speak to their peers and, by the time they are 2½, engage in structured conversations (Hay, 2006). Toddlers' verbal ability is correlated with prosocial behavior with peers (Ensor & Hughes, 2005), and with informants' reports of toddlers' aggressive behavioral problems (Dionne et al., 2003; Hughes & Ensor, 2006).

The degree of social understanding that toddlers acquire in the first years of life influences their dealings with peers. For example, toddlers' understanding of emotion predicts prosocial behavior with peers (Ensor & Hughes, 2005). Toddlers' awareness of peers' intentions, as evidenced by withdrawing objects out of the reach of peers who indicate interest in those objects, is associated with the use of force and with proactive aggression 6 months later (Hay et al., 2000). An emerging understanding of the relationship between people and objects, as revealed by the use of possessive pronouns and other speech that refers to possession of objects, is associated with both sharing and the use of force, but it predicts rates of sharing, not rates of aggression, 6 months later (Hay, 2006).

Other Family Members

In contrast to the emphasis on the importance of the mother–infant relationship as a precursor to peer relations, there is a paucity of research on the contribution of other family members to infants' relations with peers. We have seen that family processes influence peer relations (Fagot, 1997); however, relatively little is known about ways in which fathers influence infants' interactions with other infants. Sibling relationships influence the peer relations of older children (e.g., Herrera & Dunn, 1997); however, the literature on young peers reveals little evidence for sibling influence and many null results. There is some evidence that experience with siblings decreases the frequency of positive interaction with peers. Pairs of firstborn infants are more likely than pairs of second-born babies to interact (both positively and negatively; Vandell, Wilson, & Whalen, 1981). The more siblings infants have, the less affiliative they are with peers (Lewis, Young, Brooks, & Michalson, 1975). Toddlers with older siblings are reliably less likely to share with peers (Hay et al., 1999), and reliably more likely than other toddlers to respond negatively to peers' distress (Demetriou & Hay, 2004).

The Broader Culture

Key features of interaction between young peers are evident across cultural settings. For example, two forms of early peer interaction, cooperative games and conflict, have been documented in Western and traditional societies, for example, in studies in Britain (Hay et al., 2000), Canada (Ross, 1982), Israel (Ross, Conant, Cheyne, & Alevizos, 1992), Italy (Camaioni et al., 1991), and Papua New Guinea (Eckerman & Whitehead, 1999). The

New Guinea study suggested that themes of games may differ by culture, but the requisite skill of reciprocal imitation facilitated game playing in both the United States and in New Guinea. These data suggest that infants' and toddlers' relations with agemates reveal general capacities for social relatedness that transcend culture.

The Consequences of Early Peer Relations

There are relatively few longitudinal datasets in which to assess the consequences of early peer relations for later development. Continuities in children's styles of relating to peers are evident, although these longitudinal data do not provide firm proof of the causal status of early experiences with peers.

Continuities in the Use of Force

Longitudinal studies have shown that toddlers' aggressive and destructive behavior shows continuities over the toddler period (Hay et al., 2000). Early aggression with peers predicts later aggression and behavioral problems (e.g., Cummings, Iannotti, & Zahn-Waxler, 1989; Fagot & Leve, 1998; Rubin et al., 2003). For example, observations of toddlers' negative interactions with peers predicted teachers' ratings of externalizing problems at age 5, whereas standardized measures of temperament and Strange Situation classifications of attachment relationships did not predict the teachers' ratings (Fagot & Leve, 1998).

Some investigators have documented significant stability in aggressive behavior over time for males, but not for females (Cummings et al., 1989); others have found the reverse to be true (Hay et al., 2000; Rubin et al., 2003). Continuities in the quality of peer relations are bound up with slightly different sources of influence on the two sexes, such as the quality of maternal behavior and children's own temperament and IQ (Fagot & Leve, 1998; Rubin et al., 2003).

Continuities in Prosocial Exchanges

Infants' positive interactions with peers also have predictive power. Stable individual differences in toddlers' prosocial interactions with peers emerge between the second and third birthdays (Hay et al., 1999). Positive experiences with peers in the toddler years predict social competence with peers in middle childhood (NICHD, in press). Prosocial responses to preschool classmates, which may derive from earlier peer experiences, promote acceptance by peers in the preschool setting (Denham et al., 1990). Thus, positive interactions with peers in the first years of life have consequences for children's later development.

New Directions

The three great surges of interest in young peers have defined this literature. The classic studies of infants in orphanages and nursery schools in the 1920s and 1930s drew attention to key features of early peer relations; the experimental studies of the 1970s documented the social nature of early peer interactions and the development of distinct peer relationships; and the longitudinal studies of the 1990s revealed individual differences and drew attention to the import of early peer relations for children's subsequent development. Despite these advances, few developmental psychologists now study early peer relations, perhaps because of the practical difficulties encountered in recruiting and assessing two or more toddlers at the same time. There is considerable interest in early aggression and prosocial behavior, but most investigators rely on informants' reports (e.g., Hughes & Ensor, 2006; Knafo & Plomin, 2006), rather than direct observations of social exchanges between young peers.

We believe that it is important to study early peer relations directly in experimental and natural settings, if we are to understand the developmental processes that underlie social development. In designing such new studies, it is important to integrate the behavioral study of early peer relations with contemporary theory and evidence about early emotional and cognitive development. In particular, we need to study dimensions of early peer relations that go beyond overt behavior. In the first years of life, young children develop cognitive representations of peer relationships and emotional ties to particular peers. Several fundamental questions need to be answered.

What Cognitive and Learning Mechanisms Underlie the Capacity for Interaction with Peers?

There has been relatively little attention to the basic cognitive and learning processes that underlie early peer relations (for exceptions, see Ensor & Hughes, 2005; Hanna & Meltzoff, 1993). Hay, Payne, and Chadwick (2004) proposed a theoretical model of the requisite skills for peer interaction in the first years of life, including joint attention, imitation, causal understanding and executive function abilities. Although these processes are examined extensively in experimental studies of typically developing and atypical children, individual variation in such skills is linked to informants' reports of children's general adjustment and psychological problems, not to direct assessments of peer interaction. There is great need to integrate the methods and findings of the literatures on cognitive and social development.

When Do Infants Begin to Think about Their Peers?

A related question concerns the nature of representations about peers held by infants and toddlers. By the first birthday, infants' observable behavior suggests that they prefer some peers to others (Howes, 1988). They show distinct patterns of interaction with peers as opposed to their own mothers, peers' mothers, and unfamiliar short adults (e.g., Brooks & Lewis, 1976). Experimental studies are needed to investigate infants' representations of peers in a more systematic manner.

When Do Peer Relations Become Intentional, and What Intentions Do Young Peers Have?

Even in the first year of life, behavior with peers is socially directed, persistent, and flexible; thus, it can be defended as intentional. But what are young peers' intentions? Early investigators suggested that infants were "socially blind," seeking access to toys and treating peers as just another obstacle to desired objects (Maudry & Nekula, 1939). This view is refuted by evidence that scarcity of toys does not promote toddlers' conflict, though it is a moderator of other variables (Caplan et al., 1991), and that toddlers' interest in particular toys is sparked by peers' possession of those toys, even when duplicates are readily available (Caplan et al., 1991; Hay & Ross, 1982). Toddlers exchange objects, cooperate to solve problems, and quarrel with their peers; but do they intend to give pleasure, or inflict harm on their peers? For example, is their use of force truly aggressive, in the sense of wanting to give pain to the peer? New methods are required to investigate toddlers' intentions, which are only imperfectly conveyed by their speech.

When Do Infants Attain Intersubjectivity with Peers, and How Is That Enriched over Time?

Although evidence suggests that infants use their developing social skills with peers at the same time or soon after they first show them with their mothers (Hay, 1985), studies that directly compared infants' interactions with mothers and peers documented the nature of infants' interactive behavior (i.e., *what* overt communicative gestures and speech were being displayed). In contrast, current studies of early social development focus on the development of intersubjectivity and social understanding (i.e., the *meaning* of communication; see review by Reddy & Legerstee, 2007). Recent studies of infants' capacities for intersubjectivity concentrate attention on infant–adult interaction (e.g., Parise, Cleveland, Costabile, & Striano, 2007; Tomasello, Carpenter, Call, Behne, & Moll, 2005), despite the fact that researchers have suggested that peer interaction may be a particularly suitable context for the development of intersubjectivity and shared meaning (Brownell, Nichols, & Svetlova, 2005). Furthermore, some writers have suggested that infants' own capacities for social engagement and intersubjectivity may be overestimated in interactions with mothers, and are best demonstrated in interactions with peers (Reddy, Hay, Murray, & Trevarthen, 1997).

Evidence for shared meaning in young peers' coordinated interactions and social games has long been reported (e.g., Ross, 1982). Conflict over toys or intrusions on personal space is also an arena in which infants and toddlers make inferences about the other's intentions and desires, for example, by withdrawing objects that have only been pointed at by the peer (Hay et al., 2000). Two-year-old peers sustain sequences of symbolic play and verbal dialogue that shows response to each other's remarks, not just collective monologue (Hay, 2006). New research that extends these findings and adapts paradigms used to study intersubjectivity between infants and mothers would clarify the nature of toddlers' own skills, apart from the scaffolding provided by their mothers.

When Do Toddlers Become Aware of Their Membership in Social Groups?

We have seen that the capacity for triadic interaction and transitive relations in peer groups emerge in the early years (Ishikawa & Hay, 2006; Selby & Bradley, 2003). These findings suggest that the capacity for interaction in groups and the awareness of social categories and distinctions between ingroups and outgroups originate in toddlers' interactions with peers. However, little is known about the factors that influence toddlers' understanding of group relations. Toddlers' sensitivity to social categories is evident in the emerging gender segregation of peer groups, which is evident in the preschool years and predated by toddlers' differential treatment of same-sex and opposite-sex peers (Hay et al., 1999; Howes & Phillipsen, 1992). Although there is much debate about the effect of child care on children's social behavior (e.g., NICHD, 2002), there has been relatively little analysis of the group dynamics in toddlers' peer groups that contribute to the processes of gender segregation and peer rejection. Again, new methods that tap into young peers' representations of their social lives might illuminate these issues.

Conclusions

We have reviewed studies from the last 90 years for evidence concerning the meaning, origins, and consequences of early peer relations. The literature clearly demonstrates that even the earliest interactions of infants have social meaning. Young infants recognize their peers as fellow humans. The capacities for sharing, cooperation, sympathy, conflict, and aggression all emerge in the first years of life, as do the earliest abilities to sustain dyadic relationships and group interaction. With respect to the origins of peer relations, there is no clear proof that peer relations derive from earlier relations with the mother; rather, the literature suggests that the capacities for both types of relationships develop more or less in parallel, and there may be a number of connections across the different types of relationships in which infants engage. The longitudinal evidence shows that individual variations in behavior and responses to peers' behavior predict later aggression and social competence, even when factors such as temperament and attachment relations are taken into account.

Nonetheless, because the findings from this literature are at odds with mainstream developmental theory, this body of evidence has not been incorporated into received wisdom. Much more needs to be known about the transition from the nonverbal interactions of infants to the more complex conversations, quarrels, social structures, and opinions about peers that characterize the social lives of preschool children. In particular, much more needs to be known about the emotional and cognitive underpinnings of peer relations during the transition from infancy to childhood. Therefore, new, theoretically guided research is needed if we are to understand the processes whereby early peer relations contribute to children's later development.

References

Adamson, L. B., Bakeman, R., & Deckner, D. F. (2004). The development of symbol-infused joint engagement. *Child Development, 75*, 1171–1188.

Bakeman, R., & Adamson, L. B. (1984). Coordinating attention to people and objects in mother–infant and peer–infant interaction. *Child Development, 55*, 1278–1289.

Bandura, A., & Walters, R. H. (1963). *Social learning and personality development.* New York: Holt, Rinehart & Winston.

Blurton Jones, N. (Ed.). (1972). *Ethological studies of child behaviour.* Cambridge, UK: Cambridge University Press.

Bowlby, J. (1969). *Attachment and loss: Vol. 1. Attachment.* London: Hogarth.

Bridges, K. M. B. (1933). A study of social development in early infancy. *Child Development, 4*, 36–49.

Brooks, J., & Lewis, M. (1976). Infants' responses to strangers: Midget, adult, and child. *Child Development, 47*, 323–332.

Brownell, C. A., Nichols, S., & Svetlova, M. (2005). Early development of intentionality with peers. *Behavioral and Brain Sciences, 28*, 693–694.

Brownell, C. A., Ramani, G. B., & Zerwas, S. (2006). Becoming a social partner with peers: Cooperation and social understanding in one- and two-year-olds. *Child Development, 77*, 803–821.

Brownlee, J., & Bakeman, R. (1981). Hitting in toddler peer interaction. *Child Development, 52,* 1076–1079

Cairns, R. B. (1966). Attachment behavior of mammals. *Psychological Review, 73,* 409–426.

Cairns, R. B. (1977). *Social development: The origins of plasticity of interchanges.* San Francisco: Freeman.

Cairns, R. B. (Ed.). (1979). *The analysis of social interactions: Methods, issues, and illustrations.* Hillsdale, NJ: Erlbaum.

Calkins, S. D., Gill, K. L., Johnson, M. C., & Smith, C. L. (1999). Emotional reactivity and emotional regulation strategies as predictors of social behavior with peers during toddlerhood. *Social Development, 8,* 310–334.

Camaioni, L., Baumgartner, E., & Perucchini, P. (1991). Content and structure in toddlers' social competence with peers from 12 to 36 months of age. *Early Child Development and Care, 67,* 17–27.

Caplan, M., & Hay, D. F. (1989). Preschoolers' responses to peers' distress and beliefs about bystander intervention. *Journal of Child Psychology and Psychiatry and Allied Disciplines, 30,* 231–242.

Caplan, M., Vespo, J. E., Pedersen, J., & Hay, D. F. (1991). Conflict and its resolution in small groups of one- and two-year-olds. *Child Development, 62,* 1513–1524.

Côté, S., Vaillancourt, T., LeBlanc, J. C., Nagin, D. S., & Tremblay, R. E. (2006). The development of physical aggression from toddlerhood to pre-adolescence: A nation wide longitudinal study of Canadian children. *Journal of Abnormal Child Psychology, 34,* 71–85.

Cummings, E. M., Iannotti, R. J., & Zahn-Waxler, C. (1989). Aggression between peers in early childhood: Individual continuity and change. *Child Development, 60,* 887–895.

Damon, W. (1977). *The social world of the child.* San Francisco: Jossey-Bass.

Dawe, H. (1934). An analysis of two hundred quarrels of preschool children. *Child Development, 5,* 139–157.

Demetriou, H., & Hay, D. F. (2004). Toddlers' reactions to the distress of familiar peers: The importance of context. *Infancy, 6,* 299–319.

Denham, S. A., McKinley, M., Couchoud, E. A., & Holt, R. (1990). Emotional and behavioral predictors of preschool peer ratings. *Child Development, 61,* 1145–1152.

Denham, S. A., Zahn-Waxler, C., Cummings, E. M., & Iannotti, R. J. (1991). Social competence in young children's peer relations: Patterns of development and change. *Child Psychiatry and Human Development, 22,* 29–44.

Dionne, G., Tremblay, R. E., Boivin, M., Laplante, D., & Pérusse, D. (2003). Physical aggression and expressive vocabulary in 19-month-old twins. *Developmental Psychology, 39,* 261–273.

Dondi, M., Simion, F., & Caltran, G. (1999). Can newborns discriminate between their own cry and the cry of another newborn infant? *Developmental Psychology, 35,* 418–426.

Dunn, J. (1993). *Young children's close relationships: Beyond attachment.* London: Sage.

Eckerman, C. O., & Whatley, J. (1977). Toys and social interactions between infant peers. *Child Development, 48,* 1645–1656.

Eckerman, C. O., Whatley, J., & Kutz, S. L. (1975). Growth of social play with peers during the second year of life. *Developmental Psychology, 11,* 42–49.

Eckerman, C. O., Whatley, J., & McGehee, L. J. (1979). Approaching and contacting the object another manipulates: A social skill of the 1-year-old. *Developmental Psychology, 15,* 585–593.

Eckerman, C. O., & Whitehead, H. (1999). How toddler peers generate co-ordinated action: A cross-cultural exploration. *Early Education and Development, 10,* 226–241.

Ensor, R., & Hughes, C. (2005). More than talk: Relations between emotion understanding and positive behaviour in toddlers. *British Journal of Developmental Psychology, 23,* 343–363.

Fagot, B. I. (1997). Attachment, parenting, and peer interactions of toddler children. *Developmental Psychology, 33,* 489–499.

Fagot, B. I., & Hagan, R. (1985). Aggression in toddlers: Responses to the assertive acts of boys and girls. *Sex Roles, 12,* 341–351.

Fagot, B., & Leve, L. D. (1998). Teacher ratings of externalising behaviour at school entry for boys and girls: Similar early predictors and different correlates. *Journal of Child Psychology and Psychiatry and Allied Disciplines, 39*, 555–546.

Field, T. M. (1979). Infant behaviors directed toward peers and adults in the presence and absence of mother. *Infant Behavior and Development, 2*, 47–54.

Fogel, A. (1979). Peer- vs. mother-directed behavior in 1- to 3-month-old infants. *Infant Behavior and Development, 2*, 215–226.

Freud, A., & Dann, S. (1951). An experiment in group upbringing. *Psychoanalytic Study of the Child, 6*, 127–168.

Freud, S. (1938). *An outline of psychoanalysis.* London: Hogarth.

Gewirtz, J. L. (Ed.). (1972). *Attachment and dependency.* Washington, DC: Winston.

Gunnar, M., Senior, K., & Hartup, W. W. (1984). Peer presence and the exploratory behavior of 18- and 30-month-old children. *Child Development, 35*, 1103–1109.

Hanna, E., & Meltzoff, A. N. (1993). Peer imitation by toddlers in laboratory, home, and day care contexts: Implications for social learning and memory. *Developmental Psychology, 29*, 701–710.

Harris, J. R. (1999). *The nurture assumption: Why children turn out the way they do.* New York: Touchstone.

Hay, D. F. (1985). Learning to form relationships in infancy: Parallel attainments with parents and peers. *Developmental Review, 5*, 122–161.

Hay, D. F. (2005). The beginnings of aggression in infancy. In R. E. Tremblay, W. W. Hartup, & J. Archer (Eds.), *Developmental origins of aggression* (pp. 107–132). New York: Guilford Press.

Hay, D. F. (2006). "Yours and mine": Toddlers' talk about possession with familiar peers. *British Journal of Developmental Psychology, 24*, 39–52.

Hay, D. F., Caplan, M., Castle, J., & Stimson, C. A. (1991). Does sharing become increasingly "rational" in the second year of life? *Developmental Psychology, 27*, 987–994.

Hay, D. F., Caplan, M., Pedersen, J., Ishikawa, F., Nash, A., & Vespo, J. E. (2007). *Young girls and boys in conflict.* Manuscript under review.

Hay, D. F., Castle, J., & Davies, L. (2000). Toddlers' use of force against familiar peers: A precursor of serious aggression? *Child Development, 71*, 457–467.

Hay, D. F., Castle, J., Davies, L., Demetriou, H., & Stimson, C. A. (1999). Prosocial action in very early childhood. *Journal of Child Psychology and Psychiatry and Allied Disciplines, 40*, 905–916.

Hay, D. F., & Cook, K. V. (2007). The transformation of prosocial behavior from infancy to childhood. In C. A. Brownell & C. B. Kopp (Eds.), *Transitions in early socioemotional development: The toddler years* (pp. 100–131). New York: Guilford Press.

Hay, D. F., Nash, A., & Pedersen, J. (1981). Responses of six-month-olds to the distress of their peers. *Child Development, 52*, 1071–1076.

Hay, D. F., Nash, A., & Pedersen, J. (1983). Interaction between six-month-old peers. *Child Development, 52*, 1071–1075.

Hay, D. F., Payne, A. J., & Chadwick, A. J. (2004). Peer relations. *Journal of Child Psychology and Psychiatry and Allied Disciplines, 45*, 84–108.

Hay, D. F., & Ross, H. S. (1982). The social nature of early conflict. *Child Development, 53*, 105–111.

Herrera, C., & Dunn, J. (1997). Early experiences with family conflict: Implications for arguments with a close friend. *Developmental Psychology, 33*, 869–881.

Holmberg, M. C. (1980). The development of social interchange patterns from 12 to 42 months. *Child Development, 51*, 448–456.

Howes, C. (1988). Peer interaction of young children. *Monographs of the Society for Research in Child Development, 53*(Serial No. 217).

Howes, C., & Phillipsen, L. (1992). Gender and friendship: Relationships within peer groups of young children. *Social Development, 1*, 230–242.

Hughes, C., & Ensor, R. (2006). Behavioural problems in 2-year-olds: Links with individual differences in theory of mind, executive function and harsh parenting. *Journal of Child Psychology and Psychiatry and Allied Disciplines, 47,* 488–497.

Hurst, S. L., & Hay, D. F. (2007, April). *Preschool children's understanding of friendship.* Presented at the Biennial Meeting of the Society for Research in Child Development, Boston, MA.

Ichise, M., Vines, D. C., Gura, T., Anderson, G. M., Suomi, S. J., Higley, J. D., et al. (2006). Effects of early life stress on [11C]DASB positron emission tomography imaging of serotonin transporters in adolescent peer- and mother-reared rhesus monkeys. *Journal of Neuroscience, 26,* 4638–4643.

Ishikawa, F., & Hay, D. F. (2006). Triadic interaction between newly acquainted two-year-olds. *Social Development, 15,* 145–168.

Ispa, J. (1981). Peer support among Soviet day care toddlers. *International Journal of Behavioral Development, 4,* 255–269.

Kenny, D. A., & La Voie, L. (1985). The social relations model. In L. Berkowitz (Ed.), *Advances in experimental social psychology* (Vol. 19, pp. 141–182). New York: Academic Press.

Knafo, A., & Plomin, R. (2006). Prosocial behaviour from early to middle childhood: Genetic and environmental influences on stability and change. *Developmental Psychology, 42,* 771–786.

Konner, M. (1976). Relations among infants and juveniles in comparative perspective. *Social Science Information, 15,* 371–402.

Krawczyk, R. (1984). *Friendships in a toddler preschool.* Unpublished doctoral dissertation, State University of New York at Stony Brook.

Lamb, S., & Zakhireh, B. (1997). Toddlers' attention to the distress of peers in a day care setting. *Early Education and Development, 8,* 105–118.

Lewis, M. (2005). The child and its family: The social network model. *Human Development, 48,* 8–27.

Lewis, M., Young, G., Brooks, J., & Michalson, L. (1975). The beginning of friendship. In M. Lewis & G. Rosenblum (Eds.), *The origins of behavior: Vol. 4. Friendship and peer relations* (pp. 27–65). New York: Wiley.

Maudry, M., & Nekula, M. (1939). Social relations between children of the same age during the first two years of life. *Journal of Genetic Psychology, 54,* 193–215.

Mineka, S., & Suomi, S. J. (1978). Social separation in monkeys. *Psychological Bulletin, 85,* 1376–1400.

Moffitt, T. E. (2005). The new look of behavioral genetics in developmental psychopathology: Gene–environment interplay in antisocial behaviors. *Psychological Bulletin, 131,* 533–554.

Mosier, C., & Rogoff, B. (1994). Infants' instrumental use of their mothers to achieve their goals. *Child Development, 65,* 70–79.

Mueller, E., & Brenner, J. (1977). The origins of social skills and interaction among playgroup toddlers. *Child Development, 48,* 854–861.

Murphy, L. B. (1937). *The roots of sympathy.* New York: Columbia University Press.

Nash, A. (1986). *Infants' social competence with their mothers and a peer.* Unpublished doctoral dissertation, State University of New York at Stony Brook.

Nash, A. (1988). Ontogeny, phylogeny, and relationships. In S. W. Duck (Ed.), *Handbook of personal relationships: Theory, research and interventions* (pp. 121–141). Chichester, UK: Wiley.

Nash, A. (1995). Beyond attachments: Toward a general theory of the development of relationships in infancy. In K. E. Hood, G. Greenberg, & E. Tobach (Eds.), *Behavioral development: Concepts of approach/withdrawal and integrative levels* (pp. 287–326). New York: Garland Press.

Nash, A., & Hay, D. F. (1993). Relationships in infancy as precursors and causes of later relationships and psychopathology. In D. F. Hay & A. Angold (Eds.), *Precursors, causes, and psychopathology* (pp. 199–232). Chichester, UK: Wiley.

NICHD Early Child Care Research Network. (2001). Child care and children's peer interaction at 24 and 36 months. *Child Development, 72,* 1478–1500.

NICHD Early Child Care Research Network. (2002). The interaction of child care and family risk in relation to child development at 24 and 36 months. *Applied Developmental Science, 6,* 144–156.

NICHD Early Child Care Research Network. (2004). Trajectories of physical aggression from toddlerhood to middle childhood. *Monographs of the Society for Research in Child Development, 69*(4, No. 278), 1–146.

NICHD Early Child Care Research Network. (in press). Social competence with peers in third grade: Associations with earlier peer experiences in child care.

Parise, E., Cleveland, A., Costabile, A., & Striano, T. (2007). Influence of vocal cues on learning about objects in joint attention contexts. *Infant Behavior and Development, 30,* 380–384.

Parten, M. B. (1932). Social participation among preschool children. *Journal of Abnormal and Social Psychology, 27,* 243–269.

Pastor, D. L. (1981). The quality of mother–infant attachment and its relationship to toddlers' initial sociability with peers. *Developmental Psychology, 17,* 326–335.

Piaget, J. (1932). *The moral judgement of the child.* London: Routledge & Kegan Paul.

Piaget, J. (1962). *Play, dreams and imitation.* New York: Routledge.

Reddy, V., Hay, D. F., Murray, L., & Trevarthen, C. (1997). Communication in infancy: Mutual regulation of affect and attention. In G. Bremner, A. Slater, & G. Butterworth (Eds.), *Infant development: Recent advances.* Hove, UK: Psychology Press.

Reddy, V., & Legerstee, M. (2007). What does it mean to communicate? *Infant Behavior and Development, 30,* 177–179.

Rheingold, H. L. (1969). The social and socializing infant. In D. A. Goslin (Ed.), *Handbook of socialization theory and research.* Chicago: Rand McNally.

Rheingold, H. L., & Eckerman, C. O. (1975). Some proposals for unifying the study of social development. In M. Lewis & L. A. Rosenblum (Eds.), *Friendship and peer relations* (pp. 293–298). New York: Wiley.

Rogoff, B. (2003). *The cultural nature of human development.* New York: Oxford University Press.

Ross, H. S. (1982). Establishment of social games among toddlers. *Developmental Psychology, 18,* 509–518.

Ross, H. S., Cheyne, J. A., & Lollis, S. (1988). Defining and studying reciprocity in young children. In S. Duck, D. F. Hay, S. E. Hobfoll, W. Ickes, & B. M. Montgomery (Eds.), *Handbook of personal relationships: Theory, research, and interventions* (pp. 143–160). Chichester, UK: Wiley.

Ross, H. S., Conant, C. L., Cheyne, J. A., & Alevizos, E. (1992). Relationships and alliances in the social interaction of kibbutz toddlers. *Social Development, 1,* 1–17.

Ross, H. S., & Lollis, S. (1989). A social relations analysis of early peer relationships. *Child Development, 60,* 1082–1091.

Ross, H., Tesla, C., Kenyon, B., & Lollis, S. (1990). Maternal intervention in toddler peer conflict: The socialization of principles of justice. *Developmental Psychology, 26,* 994–1003.

Rubenstein, J. L., & Howes, C. (1976). The effects of peers on toddler interaction with mothers and toys. *Child Development, 47,* 597–605.

Rubin, K. H., Burgess, K. B., Dwyer, K. M., & Hastings, P. D. (2003). Predicting preschoolers' externalizing behaviors from toddler temperament, conflict, and maternal negativity. *Developmental Psychology, 39,* 164–176.

Rubin, K. H., Burgess, K. B., & Hastings, P. D. (2002). Stability and social–behavioral consequences of toddlers' inhibited temperament and parenting behaviors. *Child Development, 73,* 483–495.

Rubin, K. H., Hastings, P., Chen, X., Stewart, S., & McNichol, K. (1998). Intrapersonal and maternal correlates of aggression, conflict, and externalising problems in toddlers. *Child Development, 69,* 1614–1629.

Sagi, A., & Hoffman, M. L. (1976). Empathic distress in the newborn. *Developmental Psychology, 12,* 175–176.

Scarr, S. (1992). Developmental theories for the 1990s: Development and individual differences. *Child Development, 63*, 1–19.

Selby, J. M., & Bradley, B. S. (2003). Infants in groups: A paradigm for the study of early social experience. *Human Development, 46*, 197–221.

Strayer, F. F. (1980). Social ecology of the preschool peer group. *Minnesota Symposium on Child Psychology, 13*, 165–196.

Sullivan, H. S. (1953). *The interpersonal theory of psychiatry.* New York: Norton.

Tomasello, M., Carpenter, M., Call, J., Behne, T., & Moll, H. (2005). Understanding and sharing intentions: The origins of cultural cognition. *Behavioral and Brain Sciences, 28*, 675–691.

Tremblay, R. E., & Nagin, D. (2005). The developmental origins of physical aggression in humans. In R. E. Tremblay, W. W. Hartup, & J. Archer (Eds.), *Developmental origins of aggression* (pp. 83–106). New York: Guilford Press.

Trivers, R. L. (1974). Parent–offspring conflict. *American Zoologist, 14*, 249–264.

Vandell, D. L. (1980). Sociability with peer and mother during the first year. *Developmental Psychology, 16*, 335–361.

Vandell, D. L., & Wilson, K. S. (1987). Infant's interactions with mother, sibling, and peer: Contrasts and relations between interaction systems. *Child Development, 58*, 176–186.

Vandell, D. L., Wilson, K. S., & Whalen, W. T. (1981). Birth-order and social-experience differences in infant–peer interaction. *Developmental Psychology, 17*, 438–445.

van IJzendoorn, M. (2005). Attachment in social networks: Toward an evolutionary social network model. *Human Development, 48*, 85–88.

Vygotsky, L. (1982). *Mind in society: The development of higher mental processes.* Cambridge, MA: Harvard University Press.

Warneken, F., Chen, F., & Tomasello, M. (2006). Cooperative activities in young children and chimpanzees. *Child Development, 77*, 640–663.

Waters, E., Wippman, J., & Sroufe, L. A. (1979). Attachment, positive affect, and competence in the peer group: Two studies in construct validation. *Child Development, 50*, 821–829.

Yale, M. E., Messinger, D. S., Cobo-Lewis, A. B., Oller, D. K., & Eilers, R. E. (1999). An event-based analysis of the coordination of early infant vocalizations and facial actions. *Developmental Psychology, 35*, 505–513.

Young, G., & Lewis, M. (1979). Effects of familiarity and maternal attention on infant peer relations. *Merrill–Palmer Quarterly, 25*, 105–119.

Zahn-Waxler, C., Robinson, J. L., & Emde, R. N. (1992). The development of empathy in twins. *Developmental Psychology, 28*, 1038–1047.

Zaslow, M. (1980). Relationships among peers in kibbutz toddler groups. *Child Psychiatry and Human Development, 10*, 178–189.

CHAPTER 8

Peer Interactions and Play in Early Childhood

ROBERT J. COPLAN
KIMBERLEY A. ARBEAU

All work and no play makes Jack a dull boy.
—*Proverbs in English, Italian, French, and Spanish* (1659).

One way to think about play, is as the process of finding new combinations for known things—combinations that may yield new forms of expression, new inventions, new discoveries, and new solutions. ... It's exactly what children's play seems to be about and explains why so many people have come to think that children's play is so important a part of childhood and beyond.
—*Mister Rogers Talks with Parents* (1983)

The rapid advances in social, language, social-cognitive, and cognitive skills observed in preschool-age children provide the "tools" for increasingly complex social exchanges with peers. These new and developing skills sets intersect in the realm of children's play, which essentially acts as the central medium of social interaction with peers in early childhood. Young children spend much of their time engaged in play, which becomes more social in nature as children age. As children play they have the opportunity to practice and to further advance their emerging cognitive, social-cognitive, linguistic, and social skills. Children's first play partners are usually their parents and siblings (e.g., Dale, 1989). However, the preschool years typically provide young children with opportunities to play and to interact with a potentially wide range of different children. *Play* is essentially the method by which children communicate with each other in social settings.

Central Issues

In this chapter we attempt to integrate two streams of theory and research that historically have remained somewhat distinct in relation to young children's behaviors with peers. To begin with, we describe the developmental progress of peer interactions during the pre-

143

school years. Peer "interactions" are social exchanges between children, in which "participants' actions are interdependent, such that each actor's behavior is both a response to, and stimulus for, the other participant's behavior" (Rubin, Bukowski, & Parker, 2006, p. 576). This definition establishes notable "boundaries" for the scope of this chapter. For example, for a detailed discussion of children's "relationships" with peers (i.e., friendships) in early childhood, we refer readers to Howes (Chapter 10, this volume). As well, for a review of factors that contribute toward "individual differences" in preschool children's interactions and relationships, we refer readers to the chapter on social and emotional competence by Rose-Krasnor and Denham (Chapter 9, this volume).

In the second half of this chapter, we turn our attention more specifically to the construct of children's play. Rubin, Fein, and Vandenberg (1983) defined the characteristics of "play" as (1) intrinsically motivated; (2) spontaneous and involving self-imposed goals; (3) concerned with "What can I do with (as opposed to "what is") this object or person?"; (4) comprising nonliterality; (5) free from externally imposed rules; and (6) involving active engagement. In this chapter, we are primarily concerned with the unique and critical role of play in the development of young children's peer interactions. In this regard, we provide an overview of the classic theories of play, and discuss historical and recent research that explores different forms and structures of children's play as they relate to young children's social interactions. In particular, we focus here on the adaptive functions of play, its contributions toward the development of children's self-regulation, and its role as a context for children to learn about the world around them.

Peer Interactions in Early Childhood: Relevant Theory and Research Studies

In this section we review the developmental progress of peer interaction during the preschool years. It is clear that the preschool years witness a steep advancement in many aspects of interactions. The driving force behind these developmental changes is likely attributable to accompanying increases in children's self-regulatory, cognitive, social-cognitive, linguistic, and social-communicative abilities (e.g., Dunn, 1999).

Development in the Preschool Years

Quantity of Peer Interactions

Some of the earliest reports of developmental change in the quantitative patterns of preschoolers' social interactions were provided by Parten (1932), who described various categories of "social participation" that were postulated to comprise a developmental progression from nonsocial to "semi"-social, and eventually socially interactive behaviors. Nonsocial behaviors included being "unoccupied" (absence of focus or intent), "onlooking" (observation of peer activities without attempts to join in), and "solitary" play (apart from other children in terms of distance, orientation, or attention). "Parallel" play was defined as the child playing beside but not with other children. Finally, two categories of socially-interactive play were also initially proposed, including "associative" play, which involved social interaction and the use of similar play materials, but no real cooperation or division of labor; and true "cooperative" play, comprising organized group activities orchestrated to attain a common goal. These latter two categories were later combined as "social" play (Rubin, Watson, & Jambor, 1978) and have often been employed since as an observational index of preschoolers' peer interactions (for a recent review, see Coplan, Rubin, & Findlay, 2006). Parten portrayed a developmental sequence in which younger children would progress from solitary play forms during the early preschool years to the predominant display of parallel play at age 3 years, to increasing amounts of social play by age 5 years.

Subsequent empirical research has indicated that, for the most part, between the ages of 3 and 5 years there is a general decrease in unoccupied, onlooking, and parallel play, accompanied by an increase in group play and peer conversation (e.g., Blurton-Jones, 1972; for a review, see Rubin et al., 1983). Also during the preschool years, children begin to direct more speech at peers and interact with a wider range of peers (Garvey, 1974; Howes, 1983). Moreover, whereas peer interactions in younger children are primarily dyadic (e.g., Ladd, Price, & Hart, 1990), children from about age 4 years on become more likely to play in larger groups (Benenson, Apostoleris, & Parnass, 1997). However, as we report in a subsequent section related to the *cognitive* quality of children's play activities with peers, Parten's (1932) proposed developmental sequence of social participation appears to be somewhat oversimplified (Rubin et al., 1983).

Interestingly, researchers have also shifted away from the study of age-related *macro*-level changes in social participation toward a more *micro*-level focus on the role of social participation categories in the transition from solitary activities to social engagement. In particular, this has led to a reexamination of the construct of parallel play. Contrary to the early postulations of Parten (1932), parallel play does not "disappear" in older pre-schoolers, and in fact it remains a predominant play form in 4- and 5-year-old children (e.g., Rubin et al., 1978). As well, later researchers noted that older preschoolers move from "parallel-engaged" play (i.e., engaging in similar activities in the proximity of other children with little demonstrated awareness of others) to a the more mature form of "parallel-aware" play, which includes eye contact and mutual awareness of others (Howes, 1980; Howes & Matheson, 1992).

Moreover, Bakeman and Brownlee (1980) suggested that parallel play may represent an important "sequential bridge" to peer interaction in preschool-age children (see also Howes & Matheson, 1992). There is recent empirical support for this notion. Robinson, Anderson, Porter, Hart, and Wouden-Miller (2003) used lag-sequential analysis to explore sequential transition patterns in young children's social play in preschool. They found that preschoolers exhibited a three-step sequential play pattern, going from onlooker behavior into parallel-aware play, then to social interactions with peers. These behaviors formed a reciprocal "bidirectional pathway," with parallel play acting as a "bridge" (in both directions) between solitary and social activities. These findings also further illustrate the importance of parallel play in young children's group entry behaviors with peers (e.g., Dodge, Schlundt, Schocken, & Delugach, 1983).

It is also worth noting that individual differences in children's social participation also appear to have significant implications for children's peer interactions (for a recent review, see Coplan et al., 2006). For example, unoccupied and onlooking behaviors do not disappear during the preschool years and beyond. Moreover, the frequent display of such reticent behavior in the presence of preschool peers is a marker for shyness and social fear (Coplan, Prakash, O'Neil, & Armer, 2004) and has been associated with anxiety, loneliness, low self-esteem, and other internalizing problems, as well as social incompetence and peer exclusion (Coplan, Closson, & Arbeau, 2007; Coplan, Findlay, & Nelson, 2004; Coplan, Gavinski-Molina, Lagacé-Séguin, & Wichmann, 2001).

Quality and Content of Peer Interactions

The development of social interactions during this age period involves more than just increases in raw frequency. "Qualitative" differences are also observed, including more coordinated social exchanges that involve longer sequences and turns (Blurton-Jones, 1972; Eckerman, Whatley, & Kutz, 1975; Holmberg, 1980; Rubin et al., 1978). Moreover, as we explore in some detail in a later section, social exchanges during preschool increasingly include aspects of role playing and dramatic play. The ability of children to *share* their pretend play with peers (i.e., "intersubjectivity"; Goncu, 1993; Trevarthen, 1979) is a major accomplishment of the preschool period.

The preschool period also involves important advances in the social–emotional content of social exchanges. For example, preschoolers are more likely to demonstrate helping, sharing, and other prosocial behaviors with peers (Eisenberg, Fabes, & Spinrad, 2006). Moreover, even at this young age, preschoolers appear to be able to manipulate their social communications according to social context. For example, Brownell (1990) reported that preschoolers as young as 2 years of age adjusted both the behavioral content and the complexity of their social behaviors to the age of their partners. More recently, Genyue and Lee (2007) described the emergence of "flattery" behavior between 3 and 6 years of age. Older preschoolers more appropriately moderated their display of flattery based on the familiarity and actual presence or absence of the intended target. Thus, it appears that preschoolers are able to demonstrate very advanced and nuanced forms of social communication with peers.

Along with these changes in "positive" substance, preschoolers' peer interactions evolve in terms of the content of hostile and aggressive interchanges. After peaking at age 2–3 years, instances of overt "harm doing" begin to decline, particularly with regard to instrumental aggression (i.e., fights over toys and possessions; National Institute of Child Health and Human Development [NICHD] Early Child Care Research Network, 2001). Interestingly, despite the overall decrease in aggression, an increasing proportion of aggression becomes hostile in intent. Moreover, preschoolers begin to display the more socially cognitive "advanced" forms of *social* and *relational* aggression (Crick, Casas, & Mosher, 1997), likely due to an increased understanding of peers' motives and intentions (Lee & Cameron, 2000).

This is also reflected in the changing nature of preschoolers' conflicts (Laursen & Hartup, 1989). For example, Chen, Fein, and Tam (2001) observed 2- to 4-year-olds' conflicts during free play at preschool. They found a shift in the content of issues that generated conflict. Younger preschoolers were more likely to fight over the distribution of resources, whereas older preschoolers were more likely to engage in conflict initiated by differences in behaviors (i.e., play) and ideas.

Selection of Peer Interaction Partners

Given the aforementioned increases in advanced social behaviors, it should not be surprising that preschoolers also assume a markedly more active role in the selection of their interaction partners. Much of the early research in this area focused on the "gender segregation" of young children's peer interactions. From as early as 3 years of age, children demonstrate a clear preference for same-sex playmates when in mixed-sex play groups (e.g., Fabes, Martin, & Hanish, 2003; LaFreniere, Strayer, & Gauthier, 1984). Interestingly, preference for same-sex interaction in childhood appears to be culturally universal (Maccoby, 1998; Munroe & Romney, 2006; Whiting & Edwards, 1988).

Same-sex play is both implicitly and explicitly encouraged by teachers and peers (Martin, Fabes, Evans, & Wyman, 1999). For example, Colwell and Lindsey (2005) recently reported that preschool children who engage in same-sex play are viewed by both teachers and peers as more socially competent. Moreover, the implications of a high preponderance of same-sex peer interactions are magnified by qualitative differences in the same-sex interactions of boys and girls. When playing together, boys are more likely to be more active, rougher, and more hierarchical, whereas girls are more likely to converse, cooperate, and engage in role-playing and dramatic activity (Else-Quest, Hyde, Goldsmith, & Van Hulle, 2006; Neppl & Murray, 1997). This undoubtedly is a contributing factor to "the two cultures of childhood" (Maccoby, 1998, p. 32).

To a lesser extent, preschool-age children also prefer to interact with peers who are more similar to themselves in terms of other visible characteristics, such as race (e.g., Shrum, Cheek, & Hunter, 1988). Interestingly, there is also support for the notion that preschoolers' interaction preferences are also based on behavioral homophily (e.g., Farver, 1996; Hanish, Martin, Fabes, Leonard, & Herzog, 2005). For example, Rubin, Lynch, Coplan, Rose-Krasnor, and Booth, (1994) reported that 4-year-olds indicate a greater attraction to peers whose behavioral tendencies are similar to their own in terms of both their levels of social participation and the cognitive quality of their play. However, other factors also appear to be important. Gleason, Gower, Hohmann, and Gleason (2005) did *not* find any support for the notion that preschoolers would select friends who were similar to themselves in terms of temperamental traits. Instead, they reported that, regardless of their own temperamental dispositions, preschool children were more likely to select as friends children who were higher in impulsivity and soothability.

Notwithstanding, preschoolers appear to become more nuanced and selective in their *responses* to negative peer interactions. For example, Persson (2005) reported that 4-year-old children observed to display higher frequencies of prosocial behaviors are more likely to become the *recipients* of subsequent prosocial acts from peers. In contrast, peers observed to display aggression are less likely to elicit later prosocial initiations from peers. Similarly, preschool children who display other types of less attractive social traits (i.e., overactivity; Attili, 1990) also tend to receive fewer social initiations from peers. Thus, preschoolers are more likely to reward positive and prosocial behaviors with "in kind" responses. Interestingly, this effect appears to be even more pronounced with teachers, who are less inclined to respond to the *prosocial* behaviors of preschoolers who tend to be aggressive (McComas, Johnson, & Symons, 2005).

Finally, in terms of social interactions, preschoolers clearly distinguish between friends and nonfriends (Howes, Chapter 10, this volume). For example, preschoolers direct more social overtures, engage in more social interaction, play in more complex ways, and are more cooperative with friends than with nonfriends (Charlesworth & LaFreniere, 1983; Doyle, 1982; Howes, Droege, & Matheson, 1994).

To summarize, from ages 2–5 years there are clear developmental advances in young children's peer interactions. During this period, preschool children engage in increasingly frequent social interactions with peers, and these interactions become richer, more nuanced and sophisticated, and increasingly complex with age. Moreover, preschool children assert increasing agency in the selection of their peer interaction partners and friends, and display an increasingly differentiated response to positive and negative peer behaviors.

Play in Early Childhood: Relevant Theory and Research Studies

We now turn to an examination of children's play during the preschool years. It is interesting to note that despite dealing with similar themes, the study of children's *play* in early childhood has been surprisingly "separate" from the study of children's early interactions with peers. We begin this section with a description of the development of play in early childhood, followed by a detailed review of the contributions of play to early peer interactions.

Development in the Preschool Years

Similar to early research on social participation, historical research on the development of play in early childhood focused on the linear progressions of children's play forms. For example, Piaget (1962) and Smilansky (1968) categorized the development of "structural" components of play. In infancy and toddlerhood, play was most often manifested as "functional" (or sensory–motor). Functional activity involves repeating the same movements (with or without objects) with no particular purpose, and the child appears to gain pleasure from the performance of the behavior itself. Echoing aspects of an evolutionary perspective, Piaget (1962) argued that this "practice play" served to hone basic motor skills that would be helpful in later, more complex activities. "Constructive" (or object play) comes soon after, and involves the building or creation of something. Constructive play was thought to be a positive venue for children to explore objects and "how things work" (Rubin et al., 1978).

Finally, the preschool years were most noted for the rapid growth in "dramatic" (or symbolic) play, which involves nonliteral–symbolic transformation and the production of decontextualized behaviors.[1] Children soon learn to share and coordinate these decontextualized and substitutive activities with others. The ability to share symbolic meanings through social pretense is seen as the major social interactive advance in the early preschool years (Goncu, 1989; Howes & Matheson, 1992). "Sociodramatic" play becomes increasingly common from ages 3 to 6 years (Smith, 2005), and is widely viewed as a positive contributor toward cognitive, language, and social–emotional functioning (Fisher, 1992).

However, in another parallel to the historical research on social participation, the proposed notion of a strict linear developmental progression of children's play forms has turned out to be somewhat oversimplistic (Rubin & Coplan, 1994). For example, Rubin, Maioni, and Hornung (1976; Rubin et al., 1978) explored the Piagetian structural components of play in early childhood nested within different social participation categories. Their results indicated that the major developmental changes in the play of preschoolers involved specific combinations of cognitive maturity and social participation contexts.

Moreover, it has become clear that both the cognitive quality and social participatory context must be taken into consideration when exploring the meaning and implications of children's play. For example, when preschool children engage in dramatic play while playing alone in the presence of peers, this structural form of play appears to take on an entirely different meaning (Rubin, 1982). "Solitary–active" play (which includes both solitary functional and dramatic behaviors) is thought to reflect social immaturity and impulsiveness (Coplan, Wichmann, & Lagacé-Séguin, 2001). Furthermore, its frequent display in the preschool among peers has been associated with peer rejection, poor social problem solving, impulsivity, externalizing problems, and academic difficulties (Coplan, 2000; Coplan, Rubin, Fox, Calkins, & Stewart, 1994; Coplan, Gavinski-Molina, et al., 2001; Rubin, 1982).

Similar results are evident in terms of constructive activities. There is growing evidence to suggest that constructive play (in general) contributes greatly to children's learning about spatial concepts, proportion, and mathematics (Ness & Farenga, 2007). However, the social-participatory context also appears to be particularly important here. For example, although early research indicated that the frequent display of "solitary–passive" play (which includes quiet exploration and solitary constructive play) in preschool is not associated with negative outcomes (e.g., Coplan et al., 1994; Coplan & Rubin, 1998; Rubin, 1982), results from more recent studies have called into question the "benign" nature of solitary–passive play, even in early childhood (e.g., Coplan, Prakash, et al., 2004; Henderson, Marshall, Fox, & Rubin, 2004; Nelson, Rubin, & Fox, 2005). For example, Coplan, Gavinski-Molina, et al. (2001) reported that observed solitary–passive play in kindergartners is associated with temperamental shyness and indices of maladjustment for boys but not girls.

Rough-and-Tumble Play

Finally, traditional descriptions of the development of the structural forms of play in childhood have not typically included "physical activity play." Pellegrini and Smith (1998) defined "physical play" as playful context combined with a dimension of vigor. Within this larger category is "rough-and-tumble play" (RT), which refers to playful fighting behaviors such as wrestling, kicking, and tumbling in a social context. A key component of RT is that the behavior appears aggressive. RT increases during the preschool years and peaks in middle childhood.

There has been some debate as to how to best *categorize* RT (e.g., McCune, 1998), which has been considered as both a play form (Pellegrini, 2002) and a category of peer interaction (Blurton-Jones, 1972). Because both conceptualizations fit into the scope of this chapter, we include research related to RT in the following section, where we consider theory and research linking play to the development of social interactions in early childhood.

Contributions of Play to Peer Interactions

The important contributions of play to children's cognitive and emotional growth have been widely documented (for recent reviews, see Fromberg & Bergen, 2006; Singer, Golinkoff, & Hirsh-Pasek, 2006). Moreover, it has been argued that play is the primary context for fostering social interactions with peers for young children, and that it helps develop all the skills needed for social interactions (Bredekamp & Copple, 1997). Even further, we forward the notion that in many ways, play provides the adaptive *content* for a large portion of the social interactions between young children and their peers. In the following sections, we highlight three central, relevant themes that emerge from historical and modern play theories and empirical research.

Adaptive Function of Play

We begin with the relatively straightforward notion that play is important for peer interactions because it *serves an adaptive function*. The earliest evolutionary theories of play emphasized how children's play provided a context for acquiring and practicing survival skills (Groos, 1898), or that sequential development of children's play forms recapitulated behaviors demonstrated during historical epochs of the human species (Hall, 1920). Although not all these ideas are widely accepted today, there remains an increased focus on the evolutionary and sociocultural functions of different forms of play (e.g., Goncu & Gaskins, 2006). For example, Singer and Singer (2006) recently postulated that childhood imaginative play may be an important precursor for the development of adult consciousness.

One reason to contemplate an adaptive function for play is that it occurs in many other animal species (e.g., Fagen, 1981; Fry, 2005). In fact, some researchers have argued that the mammalian brain is "hardwired" for play (Panksepp, 1998). Smith (1982) postulated that for animals, play provides the adaptive opportunity to try to solve problems in a safe environment, where mistakes do not result in a threat to survival.

For example, RT allows for the practice of fighting skills and hunting behaviors. In addition, a primary function of RT also appears to be establishment of dominance (Pellegrini & Smith, 1998; Smith, 1982; see also Vaughn & Santos, Chapter 11, this volume). Teachers tend to have a negative view of RT, and often misconceive it as real aggression (Smith, Smees, Pellegrini, & Menesini, 2002). However, RT may promote social cohesion and bonding between peers (Pellegrini, 2003). For example, RT in preschool appears to promote mutual liking and the formation of friendships (Smith & Lewis, 1985).

However, subsequent research results have made it clear that not all RT is "created equal." For example, popular and socially skilled children employ RT as a playful and well-regulated form of peer interaction that often leads to games with rules and other more advanced forms of social play. In contrast, for unpopular and less socially skilled children, RT often degenerates into bouts of aggression and conflict (Pellegrini, 1988). In addition, whereas same-sex RT in preschool is associated with peer liking and teacher ratings of social competence, the same behaviors observed in opposite-sex dyads are associated with peer disliking and lower ratings of social competence (Colwell & Lindsey, 2005).

Play and Self-Regulation

Our second theme is somewhat related to the evolutionary perspective, and suggests that play *provides a critical forum for children's self-regulation*. The genesis of this notion can be seen in some of the earliest theories of play, which suggested that play serves to reestablish homeostasis by helping to deplete surplus or replenish expended energy (Patrick, 1916; Spencer, 1873). This was echoed by later theorists, who argued that play modulates arousal associated with excessively high or low levels of stimulation (e.g., Berlyne, 1960). Dating back to Freud (1961), play has also been considered a medium for children to reconstruct and gain mastery over *emotionally* arousing experiences. This notion has remained central to the study of the development of children's *emotion regulation*, a set of skills that help individuals to modify, monitor, and evaluate their emotions to produce behavior that is adaptive for situations (Walden & Smith, 1997). Self-regulation is a critical skill in the promotion of positive peer interactions (Thompson, 1994).

In particular, the context of pretend play offers children opportunities to replay, elaborate, explore, and ultimately master situations that involve intense emotional arousal (Fein, 1989). These experiences help to regulate emotions and reduce anxiety and ultimately promote the development of emotion regulation skills. Moreover, the development of social-cognitive skills during play likely enhances children's self-regulation abilities. For example, sociodramatic play appears to assist in the development of children's emotional understanding (e.g., Lindsey & Colwell, 2003; Youngblade & Dunn, 1995), which would in turn promote emotion regulation. In support of this notion, a number of researchers have reported links between pretend play and indices of "emotional health" (e.g., Berk, Mann, & Ogan, 2006; Fein, 1989; Galyer & Evans, 2001).

Similar to the development of social-cognitive skills, the *social* aspect of pretend play appears to be particularly important to the development of children's self-regulation. For example, Elias and Berk (2002) reported that preschoolers' observed display of sociodramatic play predicted improvements in self-regulation during cleanup and circle time later in the school year. In contrast, observed solitary–dramatic play was negatively related to later cleanup performance. These findings are consistent with previous research linking solitary–dramatic (and functional) play to indices of impulsivity and dysregulation (e.g., Coplan, Wichmann, et al., 2001).

Finally, although further research is required, RT may be an important context with regard to the inhibition of aggressive impulses in early childhood (Peterson & Flanders, 2005). Children appear to be quite skilled in distinguishing playful fighting from actual aggression (e.g., Smith & Boulton, 1990). Moreover, as mentioned earlier, RT play exchanges between socially competent children seldom elicit hostile responses or degrade into aggression (Boulton, 1991). In this regard, regulation of aggression may be enhanced by participation in RT play, particularly through the enhancement of executive control (Peterson & Flanders, 2005).

Play and Cognitive Development

Our final theme, which has likely received the most research attention, is that play provides a *fundamental context for children to learn about the world around them.* The notion that children gain knowledge of their *social* worlds though play can be traced back to the early writings of Piaget (1962). Piaget considered play to be the purest form of "assimilation," a process in which children incorporate events, objects, or situations into existing ways of thinking. Later, Vygotsky (1967) stressed the importance of symbolic play in children's understanding of the links between words, concepts, and objects.

It is now clear that play is an important contributor to several aspects of children's cognitive development. Early researchers focused on the links between sociodramatic play and divergent thinking skills (e.g., Clark, Griffing, & Johnson, 1989; Dansky, 1980a; Johnson, 1976). The exploration of alternate symbolic representations during shared pretense may push the child to try new things, thus encouraging cognitive flexibility and the development of creativity (Bateson, 2005; Saracho, 2002; Singer & Lythcott, 2002). Interestingly, relations between dramatic play and divergent thinking appear to be stronger when the pretense is shared (Dunn & Herwig, 1992). Thus, the *social* component again appears to be particularly important. Moreover, longitudinal associations between pretend play and divergent thinking abilities hold even when researchers control for child IQ (Russ, Robins, & Christiano, 1999). Wyver and Spence (1999) argued that there is a transactional and reciprocal relation in the development of divergent problem solving and play skills, with both constructs influencing each other over time.

Other researchers have emphasized the importance of play for the development of linguistic skills (Andresen, 2005). For example, language and communicative skills may be aided during the discussions, negotiations, and conflicts surrounding the establishment of "roles and rules" during shared pretense, in which children practice words and phrases (Ervin-Tripp, 1991). Such interactions during play are further thought to support early literacy skills (Zigler, Singer, & Bishop-Josef, 2004). Today, the cognitive benefits of play are widely accepted in terms of their general contributions toward early childhood education (e.g., Henniger, 1991; Saracho & Spodek, 1998).

Although there is little doubt that these skills also contribute to the development of children's peer interaction skills, we would also like to focus more specifically on the links between play and children's *social-cognitive* skills. For example, it has been argued that RT promotes a special sensitivity to social information that facilitates the development of social cognition (Bjorklund & Brown, 1998). Similarly, Pellegrini (2002) suggested that RT provides a forum for children to practice encoding and decoding social information, and that the changing roles taken on by children in these social exchanges promote perspective-taking skills.

A similar argument can be made with regard to role taking during sociodramatic play (Rubin 1980; Rubin & Pepler, 1980). In addition, the "give and take" of social pretense aids children with negotiation skills and is thought to encourage conflict resolution and other social problem-solving skills (Rubin et al., 1983). Moreover, when children engage in social pretend play, they develop the understanding that objects can have more than one representation. This contributes to the belief that *people* have different viewpoints and understandings of situations. In this regard, in the last 15 years there has been a growing interest in the links between play and the development of children's theory of mind (Smith, 2005).

"Theory of mind" can be defined as an understanding that other individuals may have emotions and understandings that are different from one's own, and that other people's behaviors may be as a result of their own mental states (Milligan, Astington, & Dack, 2007; Premack & Woodruff, 1978). Harking back to the early work by Selman (e.g., 1977, 1980) and others (e.g., Oppenheimer, 1978; Rubin & Krasnor, 1983; Weinheimer, 1972), the ability to take another's perspective is considered a critical task of early childhood, with important implications for children's early social interactions (e.g., Fitzgerald & White, 2003; Slaughter, Dennis, & Pritchard, 2002).

A number of studies have demonstrated empirical links between social pretend play and aspects of theory of mind development (e.g., Nielsen & Dissanayake, 2000; Youngblade & Dunn, 1995), even when controlling for age, vocabulary, and levels of solitary pretend play (Schwebel, Rosen, & Singer, 1999). Again, the social context appears to be particularly critical, as solitary–dramatic (and functional) play has been negatively related to early academic, language, and cognitive skills. Moreover, its frequent display in the preschool among peers has been associated with peer rejection, poor social problem solving, impulsivity, externalizing problems, and academic difficulties (Coplan, Gavinski-Molina, et al., 2001; Coplan, Wichmann, et al., 2001; Rubin, 1982).

To summarize, play in early childhood provides an important and unique context for children to acquire, implement, and master an array of critical skills that support and contribute to positive social interactions with peers. Particularly in early childhood, play provides the structural forms that contribute toward much of the content of peer interactions. As noted earlier play can enhance children's emotional regulation and cognitive abilities, and can serve adaptive functions, all of which can aid in children's ongoing and future peer relationships. Specifically, these functions can potentially aid in children's regulation and inhibition of negative behaviors, as well as enhance children's perspective-taking and negotiating abilities. In the context of play, children are also safe to practice these skills and try out behaviors needed in future interactions with peers. If children do not have experience interacting with their peers prior to moments of real conflict, then they may be at risk for developing deficits in their peer relationships. Play grants children the opportunity to enhance both their cognitive and social growth, properties that are beneficial throughout the lifespan.

Future Directions

It is important that future researchers continue to bridge the theoretical gap between the study of young children's play and children's peer interactions. In this regard, an increased emphasis on longitudinal studies will be required to better understand the contribution of play to the development of social competence and peer relationships.

Researchers must also continue to explore the meanings and implications of specific play forms for the peer interactions of young children. As described earlier, the same structural form of play (i.e., pretense) may "mean" something very different when it is displayed in a solitary- versus a group social-participatory context (e.g., Coplan, Gavinski-Molina, et al., 2001). Furthermore, the continued exploration of specific combinations of play and social participation is warranted. For example, although parallel play is considered one of the most common forms of social participation in preschool, very little is known about the implications of different structural play forms displayed in this context (Rubin et al., 1978). As well, although RT does not peak until middle childhood, there is still much to be learned about RT in preschool and its potential contribution to the regulation of anxiety and aggression. In addition, although there is converging evidence linking sociodramatic play and aspects of social-cognitive development (e.g., Elias & Berk, 2002), the underlying conceptual mechanisms of these relations are still not well understood. Moreover, there are aspects of children's social cognitions (particularly related to peer interactions) that warrant further investigation, including empathy, altruism, and other components of prosocial behavior.

The development of more advanced research methodologies and statistical techniques will certainly be of assistance in these pursuits (see Fabes, Martin, & Hanish, Chapter 3, this volume). For example, Martin, Fabes, Hanish, and Hollenstein (2005) employed a dynamic systems approach, state–space grid analysis (Granic & Hollenstein, 2003), to explore the role of behavioral homophily in the peer interactions of groups of preschool children. This process involves the collection of thousands of observations of preschoolers' social behaviors and peer interactions over the school year, including information about their temporal and spatial (i.e., location within the playroom) organization.

This interesting new research necessarily takes into account the role of *context* in young children's play and peer interactions. Early research on contextual factors focused on the nature of the play area (e.g., play space density, indoor vs. outdoor, availability of toys and playground equipment) and its effect on the display of different structural forms of play (e.g., McGhee, Ethridge, & Benz, 1984; Rubin, 1977; Rubin & Howe, 1985). As well, a large literature has explored the impact of the quality of child care settings on young children's interactions with peers (e.g., Howes & James, 2002; NICHD Early Child Care Research Network, 2002).

However, we know considerably less about young children's play and peer inter-actions outside of the preschool, day care, or laboratory playroom. Future researchers must increase their focus on preschoolers' social activities outside of school (e.g., Ladd & Golter, 1988), in the neighborhood, on the playground (Hart, 1993), and in orga-nized peer-group contexts, such as sports teams and clubs (Krombholz, 2006). Moreover, although play can be observed in all cultures, the *meanings* and implications of different play forms and specific peer behaviors may differ across cultures (Chen, Chung, & Hsiao, Chapter 24, this volume).

Researchers must also continue to assess the applications of play research for early intervention and prevention. The notion of "play training" has been around for a very long time (Smilansky, 1968). Early research in this area comprised having experimental groups of children witness adults engaging in play or having children gain access to props for use in pretend play (e.g., Dansky, 1980b; Saltz, Dixon, & Johnson, 1977). However, these studies have been criticized for the presence of experimenter biases (i.e., lack of blind experimenters), inadequate control groups, and "lax" statistical analyses (Rubin et al., 1983). In later studies that corrected for these flaws, results were much weaker and indicated that adult stimulation, as opposed to play tutoring, appeared to be the criti-cal component to improve children's developmental outcomes (e.g., Smith & Whitney, 1987). These programs may enjoy more success when peers, as opposed to adults, are employed (Schneider, Coplan, & DeBow, 2008).

As a final note, we call upon researchers to continue to promote the benefits of play to parents, teachers, school board officials, child care workers, and government agencies. Young children spend an increasing amount of time attending school, doing homework, engaging in structured activities, or sitting in front of the television or computer. This leaves a dwindling amount of time for *play*, and all work and no play will make Jack (and Jill) a dull boy (and girl).

Acknowledgments

This research was supported by a Social Science and Humanities Research Council of Canada research grant to Robert J. Coplan and Social Science and Humanities Research Council of Canada doctoral fellowship to Kimberley A. Arbeau.

Note

1. *Games with rules* are also typically included in this taxonomy, and involve a spontaneous accep-tance of a division of labor, prearranged rules, and the adjustment to these rules. This form of play is rarely evident during the preschool years and is therefore not a focus of this chapter.

References

Andresen, H. (2005). Role play and language development in the preschool years. *Culture and Psychology, 11*, 387–414.

Attili, G. (1990). Successful and disconfirmed children in the peer group: Indices of social compe-tence within an evolutionary perspective. *Human Development, 33*, 238–249.

Bakeman, R., & Brownlee, J. R. (1980). The strategic use of parallel play: A sequential analysis. *Child Development, 51*, 873–878.

Bateson, P. (2005). The role of play in the evolution of great apes and humans. In A. D. Pellegrini & P. K. Smith (Eds.), *The nature of play: Great apes and humans* (pp. 13–24). New York: Guilford Press.

Benenson, J. F., Apostoleris, N. H., & Parnass, J. (1997). Age and sex differences in dyadic and group interaction. *Developmental Psychology, 33*, 538–543.

Berk, L. E., Mann, T. D., & Ogan, A. T. (2006). Make-believe play: Wellspring for development of self-regulation. In D. G. Singer, R. M. Golinkoff, & K. Hirsh-Pasek (Eds.), *Play = learning: How play motivates and enhances children's cognitive and social-emotional growth* (pp. 74–100). New York: Oxford University Press.

Berlyne, D. E. (1960). *Conflict, arousal and curiosity.* New York: McGraw-Hill.

Bjorklund, D. F., & Brown, R. D. (1998). Physical play and cognitive development: Integrating activity, cognition and education. *Child Development, 69*, 604–606.

Blurton-Jones, N. G. (1972). Categories of child–child interaction. In N. G. Blurton-Jones (Ed.), *Ethological studies of child behavior* (pp. 97–127). Oxford, UK: Cambridge University Press.

Boulton, M. J. (1991). Partner preferences in school children's playful fighting and chasing: A test of some competing functional hypotheses. *Ethology and Sociobiology, 12*, 177–193.

Bredekamp, S., & Copple, C. (1997). *Developmentally appropriate practice in early childhood programs* (rev. ed.). Washington, DC: National Association for the Education of Young Children.

Brownell, C. A. (1990). Peer social skills in toddlers: Competencies and constraints illustrated by same-age and mixed-age interaction. *Child Development, 61*, 838–848.

Charlesworth, W. R., & LaFreniere, P. (1983). Dominance, friendship and resource utilization in preschool children's groups. *Ethology and Sociobiology, 4*, 175–186.

Chen, D. W., Fein, G., & Tam, H. P. (2001). Peer conflicts of preschool children: Issues, resolution, incidence, and age-related patterns. *Early Education and Development, 12*, 523–544.

Clark, P., Griffing, P., & Johnson, L. (1989). Symbolic play and ideational fluency as aspects of the evolving divergent cognitive style in young children. *Early Child Development and Care, 51*, 77–88.

Colwell, M. J., & Lindsey, E. W. (2005). Preschool children's pretend and physical play and sex of play partner: Connections to peer competence. *Sex Roles, 52*, 497–509.

Coplan, R. J. (2000). Assessing nonsocial play in early childhood: Conceptual and methodological approaches. In K. Gitlin-Weiner, A. Sandgrund, & C. Schaefer (Eds.), *Play diagnosis and assessment* (2nd ed., pp. 563–598). New York: Wiley.

Coplan, R. J., Closson, L., & Arbeau, K. A. (2007). Gender differences in the behavioral associates of loneliness and social dissatisfaction in kindergarten. *Journal of Child Psychology and Psychiatry, and Allied Disciplines, 48*, 988–995.

Coplan, R. J., Findlay, L. C., & Nelson, L. J. (2004). Characteristics of preschoolers with lower perceived competence. *Journal of Abnormal Child Psychology, 32*, 399–408.

Coplan, R. J., Gavinski-Molina, M. H., Lagacé-Séguin, D., & Wichmann, C. (2001). When girls versus boys play alone: Gender differences in the associates of nonsocial play in kindergarten. *Developmental Psychology, 37*, 464–474.

Coplan, R. J., Prakash, K., O'Neil, K., & Armer, M. (2004). Do you "want" to play? Distinguishing between conflicted-shyness and social disinterest in early childhood. *Developmental Psychology, 40*, 244–258.

Coplan, R. J., & Rubin, K. H. (1998). Exploring and assessing non-social play in the preschool: The development and validation of the Preschool Play Behavior Scale. *Social Development, 7*, 72–91.

Coplan, R. J., Rubin, K. H., & Findlay, L. C. (2006). Social and nonsocial play. In D. P. Fromberg & D. Bergen (Eds.), *Play from birth to twelve: Contexts, perspectives, and meanings* (2nd ed., pp. 75–86). New York: Garland Press.

Coplan, R. J., Rubin, K. H., Fox, N. A., Calkins, S. D., & Stewart, S. (1994). Being alone, playing alone, and acting alone: Distinguishing among reticence and passive and active solitude in young children. *Child Development, 65,* 129–137.

Coplan, R. J., Wichmann, C., & Lagacé-Séguin, D. (2001). Solitary–active play: A marker variable for maladjustment in the preschool? *Journal of Research in Childhood Education, 15,* 164–172.

Crick, N. R., Casas, J. F., & Mosher, M. (1997). Relational and overt aggression in preschool. *Developmental Psychology, 33,* 579–588.

Dale, N. (1989). Pretend play with mothers and siblings: Relations between early performance and partners. *Journal of Psychology and Psychiatry, 30,* 751–759.

Dansky, J. L. (1980a). Make-believe: A mediator of the relationship between play and associative fluency. *Child Development, 51,* 576–579.

Dansky, J. L. (1980b). Cognitive consequences of sociodramatic play and exploration training for economically disadvantaged preschoolers. *Journal of Child Psychology and Psychiatry, 21,* 47–58.

Dodge, K. A., Schlundt, D. C., Schocken, I., & Delugach, J. D. (1983). Social competence and children's sociometric status: The role of peer group entry strategies. *Merrill–Palmer Quarterly, 29,* 309–336.

Doyle, A. B. (1982). Friends, acquaintances, and strangers: The influence of familiarity and ethnolinguistic background on social interaction. In K. H. Rubin & H. S. Ross (Eds.), *Peer relationships and social skills in childhood* (pp. 229–252). New York: Springer-Verlag.

Dunn, J. (1999). Making sense of the social world: Mindreading, emotion, and relationships. In P. D. Zelazo, J. W. Astington, & D. R. Olson (Eds.), *Developing theories of intention: Social understanding and self control* (pp. 229–242). Mahwah, NJ: Erlbaum.

Dunn, L., & Herwig, J. (1992). Play behaviors and convergent and divergent thinking skills of young children attending full-day preschool. *Child Study Journal, 22,* 23–38.

Eckerman, C. O., Whatley, J. L., & Kutz, S. L. (1975). Growth of social play with peers during the second year of life. *Developmental Psychology, 11,* 42–49.

Eisenberg, N., Fabes, R. A., & Spinrad, T. L. (2006). Prosocial development. In W. Damon & R. M. Lerner (Series Ed.) & N. Eisenberg (Vol. Ed.), *Handbook of child psychology: Vol. 3. Social, emotional, and personality development* (6th ed., pp. 646–718). New York: Wiley.

Elias, C. L., & Berk, L. E. (2002). Self-regulation in young children: Is there a role for sociodramatic play. *Early Childhood Research Quarterly, 17,* 216–238.

Else-Quest, N. M., Hyde, J. S., Goldsmith, H. H., & Van Hulle, C. A. (2006). Gender differences in temperament: A meta-analysis. *Psychological Bulletin, 132,* 33–72.

Ervin-Tripp, S. (1991). Play in language development. In B. Scales, M. Almy, A. Nicolopoulou, & S. Ervin-Tripp (Eds.), *Play and the social context of development in early care and education* (pp. 84–97). New York: Teachers College Press.

Fabes, R. A., Martin, C. L., & Hanish, L. D. (2003). Young children's play qualities in same-, other-, and mixed-sex peer groups. *Child Development, 74,* 921–932.

Fagen, R. (1981). *Animal play behavior.* New York: Oxford University Press.

Farver, J. M. (1996). Aggressive behavior in preschoolers' social networks: Do birds of a feather flock together. *Early Childhood Research Quarterly, 11,* 333–350.

Fein, G. G. (1989). Mind, meaning, and affect: Proposals for a theory of pretense. *Developmental Review, 9,* 345–363.

Fisher, E. P. (1992). The impact of play on development: A meta-analysis. *Play and Culture, 5,* 159–181.

Fitzgerald, D. P., & White, K. J. (2003). Linking children's social worlds: Perspective-taking in parent–child and peer contexts. *Social Behavior and Personality, 31,* 509–522.

Freud, S. (1961). *Beyond the pleasure principle.* New York: Norton.

Fromberg, D. P., & Bergen, D. (2006). *Play from birth to twelve: Contexts, perspectives, and meanings* (2nd ed.). New York: Garland Press.

Fry, D. P. (2005). Rough-and-tumble social play in humans. In A. D. Pellegrini & P. K. Smith (Eds.), *The nature of play: Great apes and humans* (pp. 54–85). New York: Guilford Press.

Galyer, K. T., & Evans, I. M. (2001). Pretend play and the development of emotion regulation in preschool children. *Early Child Development and Care, 166,* 93–108.

Garvey, C. (1974). Some properties of social play. *Merrill–Palmer Quarterly, 20,* 163–180.

Genyue, F., & Lee, K. (2007). Social grooming in the kindergarten: The emergence of flattery behavior. *Developmental Science, 10,* 255–265.

Gleason, T. R., Gower, A. L., Hohmann, L. M., & Gleason, T. C. (2005). Temperament and friendship in preschool-aged children. *International Journal of Behavioral Development, 29,* 336–344.

Goncu, A. (1989). Models and features of pretense. *Developmental Review, 9,* 341–344.

Goncu, A. (1993). Development of intersubjectivity in the dyadic play of preschoolers. *Early Childhood Research Quarterly, 8,* 99–116.

Goncu, A., & Gaskins, S. (2006). *Play and development: Evolutionary, sociocultural, and functional perspectives* (The Jean Piaget symposium series). Mahwah, NJ: Erlbaum.

Granic, I., & Hollenstein, T. (2003). Dynamic systems methods for models of developmental psychopathology. *Development and Psychopathology, 15,* 641–669.

Groos, K. (1898). *The play of animals.* New York: Appleton.

Hall, G. S. (1920). *Youth.* New York: Appleton.

Hanish, L. D., Martin, C. L., Fabes, R. A., Leonard, S., & Herzog, M. (2005). Exposure to externalizing peers in early childhood: Homophily and peer contagion processes. *Journal of Abnormal Child Psychology, 33,* 267–281.

Hart, C. H. (1993). *Children on playgrounds: Research perspectives and applications* (SUNY Series, Children's Play in Society). Albany: State University of New York Press.

Henderson, H., Marshall, P., Fox, N. A., & Rubin, K. H. (2004). Converging psychophysiological and behavioral evidence for subtypes of social withdrawal in preschoolers. *Child Development, 75,* 251–263.

Henniger, M. L. (1991). Play revisited: A critical element of the kindergarten curriculum. *Early Child Development and Care, 70,* 63–71.

Holmberg, M. (1980). The development of social interchange patterns from 12–42 months. *Child Development, 51,* 448–456.

Howes, C. (1980). Peer play scale as an index of complexity of peer interaction. *Developmental Psychology, 16,* 371–372.

Howes, C. (1983). Patterns of friendship. *Child Development, 54,* 1041–1053.

Howes, C., Droege, K., & Matheson, C. C. (1994). Play and communicative processes within long- and short-term friendship dyads. *Journal of Social and Personal Relationships, 11,* 401–410.

Howes, C., & James, J. (2002). Children's social development within the socialization context of child care and early childhood. In P. K. Smith & C. H. Hart (Eds.), *Blackwell handbook of childhood social development* (pp. 137–155). Oxford, UK: Blackwell.

Howes, C., & Matheson, C. C. (1992). Sequences in the development of competent play with peers: Social and social-pretend play. *Developmental Psychology, 28,* 961–974.

Johnson, J. (1976). Relations of divergent thinking and intelligence test scores with social and nonsocial make-believe play of preschool children. *Child Development, 47,* 1200–1203.

Krombholz, H. (2006). Physical performance in relation to age, sex, birth order, social class, and sports activities of preschool children. *Perceptual and Motor Skills, 102,* 477–484.

Ladd, G. W., & Golter, B. S. (1988). Parents' management of preschoolers' peer relations: Is it related to children's social competence. *Developmental Psychology, 24,* 109–117.

Ladd, G. W., Price, J. M., & Hart, C. H. (1990). Preschoolers' behavioral orientations and patterns of peer contact: Predictive of peer status? In S. R. Asher & J. D. Coie (Eds.), *Peer rejection in childhood* (pp. 90–115). New York: Cambridge University Press.

LaFreniere, P., Strayer, F. F., & Gauthier, R. (1984). The emergence of same-sex preferences among preschool peers. *Child Development, 55,* 1958–1966.

Laursen, B., & Hartup, W. W. (1989). The dynamics of preschool children's conflicts. *Merrill–Palmer Quarterly, 35,* 281–297.

Lee, K., & Cameron, A. (2000). Extracting truthful information from lies: Emergence of the expression–representation distinction. *Merrill–Palmer Quarterly, 46*, 1–20.

Lindsey, E. W., & Colwell, M. J. (2003). Preschoolers' emotional competence: Links to pretend and physical play. *Child Study Journal, 33*, 39–52.

Maccoby, E. E. (1998). *The two sexes: Growing up apart, coming together.* Cambridge, MA: Belknap Press.

Martin, C. L., Fabes, R. A., Evans, S. M., & Wyman, H. (1999). Social cognition on the playground: Children's beliefs about playing with girls versus boys and their relations to sex segregated play. *Journal of Social and Personal Relationships, 16*, 751–771.

Martin, C. L., Fabes, R. A., Hanish, L. D., & Hollenstein, T. (2005). Social dynamics in the preschool. *Developmental Review, 25*, 299–327.

McComas, J. J., Johnson, L., & Symons, F. J. (2005). Teacher and peer responsivity to pro-social behaviour of high aggressors in preschool. *Educational Psychology, 25*, 223–231.

McCune, L. (1998). Immediate and ultimate functions of physical activity play. *Child Development, 69*(3), 601–603.

McGhee, P. E., Ethridge, L., & Benz, N. A. (1984). Effect of level of toy structure on preschool children's pretend play. *Journal of Genetic Psychology, 144*, 209–217.

Milligan, K., Astington, J. W., & Dack, L. A. (2007). Language and theory of mind: Meta-analysis of the relation between language ability and false-belief understanding. *Child Development, 78*, 622–646.

Munroe, R. L., & Romney, A. K. (2006). Gender and age differences in same-sex aggregation and social behavior: A four-culture study. *Journal of Cross-Cultural Psychology, 37*, 3–19.

Nelson, L. J., Rubin, K. H., & Fox, N. A. (2005). Social withdrawal, observed peer acceptance, and the development of self-perceptions in children ages 4 to 7 years. *Early Childhood Research Quarterly, 20*, 185–200.

Neppl, T. K., & Murray, A. D. (1997). Social dominance and play patterns among preschoolers: Gender comparisons. *Sex Roles, 36*, 381–393.

Ness, D., & Farenga, S. J. (2007). *Knowledge under construction: The importance of play in developing children's spatial and geometric thinking.* Lanham, MD: Rowman & Littlefield.

NICHD Early Child Care Research Network. (2001). Child care and children's peer interaction at 24 and 36 months: The NICHD study of early child care. *Child Development, 72*, 1478–1500.

NICHD Early Child Care Research Network. (2002). Child-care structure, process, outcome: Direct and indirect effects of child-care quality on young children's development. *Psychological Science, 13*, 199–206.

Nielsen, M., & Dissanayake, C. (2000). An investigation of pretend play, mental state terms and false belief understanding: In search of a metarepresentational link. *British Journal of Developmental Psychology, 18*, 609–624.

Oppenheimer, L. (1978). The development of the processing of social perspectives: A cognitive model. *International Journal of Behavioral Development, 1*, 149–171.

Panksepp, J. (1998). Attention deficit hyperactivity disorder, psychostimulants, and intolerance of childhood playfulness: A tragedy in the making? *Current Directions in Psychological Science, 7*, 91–98.

Parten, M. B. (1932). Social participation among preschool children. *Journal of Abnormal Psychology, 27*, 243–269.

Patrick, G. T. W. (1916). *The psychology of relaxation.* Boston: Houghton Mifflin.

Pellegrini, A. D. (1988). Elementary-school children's rough-and-tumble play and social competence. *Developmental Psychology, 24*, 802–806.

Pellegrini, A. D. (2002). Rough-and-tumble play from childhood through adolescence: Development and possible functions. In P. K. Smith & C. H. Hart (Eds.), *Blackwell handbook of childhood social development* (pp. 437–453). Malden, MA: Blackwell.

Pellegrini, A. D. (2003). Perceptions and functions of play and real fighting in early adolescence. *Child Development, 74*, 1522–1533.

Pellegrini, A. D., & Smith, P. K. (1998). Physical activity play: The nature and function of a neglected aspect of play. *Child Development, 69*, 577–598.

Persson, G. E. B. (2005). Young children's prosocial and aggressive behaviors and their experiences of being targeted for similar behaviors by peers. *Social Development, 14*, 206–228.

Peterson, J. B., & Flanders, J. L. (2005). Play and the regulation of aggression. In R. E. Tremblay, W. W. Hartup, & J. Archer (Eds.), *Developmental origins of aggression* (pp. 133–157). New York: Guilford Press.

Piaget, J. (1962). *Play, dreams, and imitation in childhood.* New York: Norton.

Premack, D., & Woodruff, G. (1978). Does the chimpanzee have a theory of mind? *Behavioral and Brain Sciences, 1*, 515–526.

Robinson, C. C., Anderson, G. T., Porter, C. L., Hart, C. H., & Wouden-Miller, M. (2003). Sequential transition patterns of preschoolers' social interactions during child-initiated play: Is parallel-aware play a bidirectional bridge to other play states. *Early Childhood Research Quarterly, 18*, 3–21.

Rubin, K. H. (1977). The social and cognitive value of preschool toys and activities. *Canadian Journal of Behavioural Science, 9*, 382–385.

Rubin, K. H. (1980). Fantasy play: Its role in the development of social skills and social cognition. In K. H. Rubin (Ed.), *Children's play* (pp. 69–84). San Francisco: Jossey-Bass.

Rubin, K. H. (1982). Non-social play in preschoolers: Necessary evil? *Child Development, 53*, 651–657.

Rubin, K. H., Bukowski, W. M., & Parker, J. G. (2006). Peer interactions, relationships and groups. In N. Eisenberg (Ed.), *The handbook of child psychology* (6th ed., pp. 571–645). New York: Wiley.

Rubin, K. H., & Coplan, R. J. (1994). Play: Developmental stages, functions, and educational support. In F. Weinert (Section Editor), *International encyclopedia of education*. New York: Pergamon Press.

Rubin, K. H., Fein, G. G., & Vandenberg, B. (1983). Play. In P. Mussen (Series Ed.) & E. M. Hetherington (Vol. Ed.), *Handbook of child psychology* (Vol. 4, 4th ed., pp. 693–774). New York: Wiley.

Rubin, K. H., & Howe, N. (1985). Toys and play behaviors: An overview. *Topics in Early Childhood Special Education, 5*, 1–10.

Rubin, K. H., & Krasnor, L. R. (1983). Age and gender differences in the development of a representative social problem solving skill. *Journal of Applied Developmental Psychology, 4*, 463–475.

Rubin, K. H., Lynch, D., Coplan, R. J., Rose-Krasnor, L., & Booth, C. L. (1994). "Birds of a feather . . . ": Behavioral concordances and preferential personal attraction in children. *Child Development, 65*, 1778–1785.

Rubin, K. H., Maioni, T. L., & Hornung, M. (1976). Free play behaviors in middle- and lower-class preschoolers: Parten and Piaget revisited. *Child Development, 47*, 414–419.

Rubin, K. H., & Pepler, D. J. (1980). The relationship of child's play to social-cognitive development. In H. Foot, T. Chapman, & J. Smith (Eds.), *Friendship and childhood relationships* (pp. 209–234). London: Wiley.

Rubin, K. H., Watson, K., & Jambor, T. (1978). Free play behaviors in preschool and kindergarten children. *Child Development, 49*, 534–536.

Russ, S. W., Robins, A. L., & Christiano, B. A. (1999). Pretend play: Longitudinal prediction of creativity and affect in fantasy in children. *Creativity Research Journal, 12*, 129–139.

Saltz, E., Dixon, D., & Johnson, J. (1977). Training disadvantaged preschoolers on various fantasy activities: Effects on cognitive functioning and impulse control. *Child Development, 48*, 367–380.

Saracho, O. N. (2002). Young children's creativity and pretend play. *Early Child Development and Care, 172*, 431–438.

Saracho, O. N., & Spodek, B. (1998). *Multiple perspectives on play in early childhood education. SUNY series, early childhood education: Inquiries and insights.* Albany: State University of New York Press.

Schneider, B. H., Coplan, R. J., & DeBow, A. (2008). Clinical diagnosis, prevention, and intervention. In A. LoCoco, H. Rubin, & C. Zappulla (Eds.), *L'isolamento sociale durante l'infanzia [Social withdrawal in childhood]* (pp. 121–141). Milan: Unicopli.

Schwebel, D. C., Rosen, C. S., & Singer, J. L. (1999). Preschoolers' pretend play and theory of mind: The role of jointly constructed pretence. *British Journal of Developmental Psychology, 17,* 333–348.

Selman, R. L. (1977). A structural–developmental model of social cognition: Implications for intervention research. *Counseling Psychologist, 6,* 3–6.

Selman, R. L. (1980). *The growth of interpersonal understanding: Developmental and clinical analyses.* New York: Academic Press.

Shrum, W., Cheek, N. H., & Hunter, S. M. (1988). Friendship in school: Gender and racial homophily. *Sociology of Education, 61,* 227–239.

Singer, D. G., Golinkoff, R. M., & Hirsh-Pasek, K. (2006). *Play = learning: How play motivates and enhances children's cognitive and social-emotional growth.* New York: Oxford University Press.

Singer, J. L., & Lythcott, M. (2002). Fostering school achievement and creativity through sociodramatic play in the classroom. *Research in the Schools, 9*(2), 43–52.

Singer, J. L., & Singer, D. G. (2006). Preschoolers' imaginative play as precursor of narrative consciousness. *Imagination, Cognition and Personality, 25,* 97–117.

Slaughter, V., Dennis, M. J., & Pritchard, M. (2002). Theory of mind and peer acceptance in preschool children. *British Journal of Developmental Psychology, 20,* 545–564.

Smilansky, S. (1968). *The effects of sociodramatic play on disadvantaged preschool children.* New York: Wiley.

Smith, P. K. (1982). Does play matter?: Functional and evolutionary aspects of animal and human play. *Behavioral and Brain Sciences, 5,* 139–184.

Smith, P. K. (2005). Play: Types and functions in human development. In B. J. Ellis & D. F. Bjorklund (Eds.), *Origins of the social mind* (pp. 271–291). New York: Guilford Press.

Smith, P. K., & Boulton, M. (1990). Rough-and-tumble play, aggression, and dominance: Perception and behavior in children's encounters. *Human Development, 33,* 271–282.

Smith, P. K., & Lewis, K. (1985). Rough-and-tumble play, fighting, and chasing in nursery school children. *Ethology and Sociobiology, 6,* 175–181.

Smith, P. K., Smees, R., Pellegrini, A. D., & Menesini, E. (2002). Comparing pupil and teacher perceptions for playful fighting, serious fighting, and positive peer interaction. In J. L. Roopnarine (Ed.), *Conceptual, social-cognitive, and contextual issues in the fields of play: Vol. 4. Play and culture studies* (pp. 235–245). Westport, CT: Ablex.

Smith, P. K., & Whitney, S. (1987). Play and associative fluency: Experimenter effects may be responsible for previous positive findings. *Developmental Psychology, 23,* 49–53.

Spencer, H. (1873). *Principles of psychology* (Vol. 2, 2nd ed.). New York: Appleton.

Thompson, R. A. (1994). Emotion regulation: A theme in search of definition. *Monographs of the Society for Research in Child Development, 59,* 25–52.

Trevarthen, C. (1979). Communication and cooperation in early infancy. A description of primary intersubjectivity. In M. Bullowa (Ed.), *Before speech: The beginning of human communication* (pp. 321–347). London: Cambridge University Press.

Vygotsky, L. S. (1967). Play and its role in the mental development of the child. *Soviet Psychology, 12,* 62–76.

Walden, T. A., & Smith, M. C. (1997). Emotion regulation. *Motivation and Emotion, 21,* 7–25.

Weinheimer, S. (1972). Egocentrism and social influence in and children. *Child Development, 43,* 567–578.

Whiting, B., & Edwards, C. P. (1988). A cross-cultural analysis of sex differences in the behavior of children aged 3 through 11. In G. Handel (Ed.), *Childhood socialization* (pp. 281–297). New York: Hawthorne.

Wyver, S. R., & Spence, S. H. (1999). Play and divergent problem solving: Evidence of a reciprocal relationship. *Early Education and Development, 10*, 419–444.

Youngblade, L. M., & Dunn, J. (1995). Individual differences in young children's pretend play with mother and sibling: Links to relationships and understanding of other people's feelings and beliefs. *Child Development, 66*, 1472–1492.

Zigler, E. F., Singer, D. G., & Bishop-Josef, S. J. (2004). *Children's play: The roots of reading.* Washington, DC: Zero to Three/National Center for Infants, Toddlers and Families.

CHAPTER 9

Social–Emotional Competence in Early Childhood

LINDA ROSE-KRASNOR
SUSANNE DENHAM

Four-year-old Hannah sleepily gets out of bed, rubs her eyes, and tries to convince her mother to let her wear her new "party shoes" to preschool that day. When she arrives at preschool, Hannah tries unsuccessfully to get her teacher's attention, to show him the new shoes. Later, Hannah's careful construction of a Lego spaceship is endangered by the rough-and-tumble play of her nemesis Ryan. How to keep him away?? During outside time, Hannah tries to physically "ease" Bonnie off the tricycle, until the teacher approaches, when Hannah tearfully explains to him that Bonnie isn't sharing. Hannah soon gets a turn. After snack, Hannah notices the new girl Kate looking sadly out the window. Hannah would like to help Kate but doesn't know how to approach her. So she just moves closer and starts to play. And it isn't even lunchtime yet!

The social life of a preschooler is not a simple one. Successfully navigating social challenges, such as those described here, draws on a wide range of skills and motivations, including communication abilities, emotion knowledge, self-regulation, access to a repertoire of appropriate and effective social strategies, and a sense of self-efficacy in social situations. Although preschoolers' social competencies are considerably more limited than those of adults, the early childhood period is a time of rapidly growing abilities. Indeed, young children often show remarkable skill in negotiating their social landscapes. In this chapter, we explore social–emotional competence in early childhood, from both theoretical and empirical perspectives.

Our chapter has three major sections. In the first, we discuss two major conceptual theoretical issues concerning the nature of social–emotional competence. Our second, more empirically based section focuses on several foundational skills sets underlying social–emotional competence, to illustrate relevant developmental changes during the early childhood period. We specifically focus on self-regulation, social problem solving, and prosocial behavior, because they have been widely recognized as important to competence and are not the focus of other *Handbook* chapters covering this age range. Key studies are identified and some additional relevant theory is introduced. In addition, we briefly discuss a number of other foundational skills. In the third and final section, we discuss several issues and gaps in the literature, suggest some directions for future research, and summarize our major points.

Central Issues and Relevant Theory

Defining Social–Emotional Competence

To create a solid foundation for our discussion, clear definitions of social–emotional competence, couched within developmental theory, must be put forward. First, the "developmental task" view can aid in discerning preschool-age children's most important accomplishments in this domain. In general, the young child who successfully negotiates the developmental task of *sustaining positive engagement with peers* is in a good position to continue thriving in a social world. In fact, successful, independent interaction with agemates is a crucial predictor of later mental health and well-being, beginning in preschool, continuing during the grade school years, when peer reputations solidify, and thereafter (Denham & Holt, 1993; Robins & Rutter, 1990; Rubin, Bukowski, & Parker, 2006). A second central developmental task of this period is *regulating emotional experience and expressiveness* (Parker & Gottman, 1989). Socially competent behaviors in this age period would be organized around succeeding at these all-important developmental tasks—sustained positive engagement with peers, marked by positive, regulated emotions (Howes, 1987; Waters & Sroufe, 1983).

An adaptation of Rose-Krasnor's (1997) theorizing is useful in elaborating on crucial definitional issues and helping to resolve them in a working definition of "social–emotional competence." Rose-Krasnor put forward a prism model that defines the construct, at its topmost level, as *effectiveness in interaction*, the result of organized behaviors that meet short- and long-term developmental needs. In this view, the elements of social–emotional competence are important contributors to a child's ultimate successful, effective interaction—sustained positive engagement with peers, marked by positive, regulated emotions. This definition is a good beginning point for delineating aspects of social–emotional development that would benefit from careful assessment.

Within this theoretical view, it also is necessary to decide whether to focus on the self-domain or the other-domain. Are we interested in accessing the child's success in meeting personal goals or his or her interpersonal connectedness? Differentiating the evaluators of a child's social–emotional competence is important. For example, depending on the goal that the child holds, his or her view of the effectiveness of interaction may be quite different from those of peers or adults. One child may be quite satisfied when he gets his way through aggression, and he may consider himself to be socially effective. In contrast, this child's budding peer-group status may not be as high as his own view of his social efficacy, and his teacher probably views his social–emotional competence as lacking. When social–emotional competence is described and measured, then, both the child's and others' views of social effectiveness can be useful. Furthermore, because of the different perspectives of the participants in any interactions, this middle level of Rose-Krasnor's prism model refers to success in both intra- and interpersonal goals (e.g., attachment and friendship relationship quality, group status variables such as popularity and social self-efficacy).

This differentiation between intra- and interpersonal goals parallels the distinction between autonomy and connectedness aspects of development that have long been recognized as fundamentals of human behavior (Bakan, 1966; Rose-Krasnor, 1997; Ryan & Deci, 2000). Autonomy focuses on agentic and individual development, whereas connectedness centers on relationships and interactions. Both are necessary for successful interaction and social development. The importance of achieving a *balance* between these two domains has been stressed in several theoretical discussions of competence, including those by Yeates and Selman (1989) and Baltes and Silverberg (1994), thus supporting the inclusion of both inter- and intrapersonal aspects in our competence definition (Rubin & Rose-Krasnor, 1992).

At the bottom and most concrete level of the prism model reside social, emotional, and social-cognitive abilities, behaviors, and motivations, all of which are primarily individual in nature. Actual "social–emotional content" resides at this bottom level of analysis. Here, specific behaviors, social-cognitive abilities, and motivations are categorized into "boxes" to indicate groupings of similar content. As already noted, we have chosen to focus on social problem solving, self-regulation, and prosocial behavior as representative of this level of our model (see Figure 9.1 on p. 172).

Furthermore, the "depth" dimension of the prism represents the multiple social contexts in which the child interacts (e.g., family, community activities). In this way, we recognize that the child's group status, relationship quality, and sense of self-efficacy may vary across contexts. In addition, the types of foundational skills needed to achieve competence may themselves depend on specific contexts. We return to the role of context in the last section of our chapter, in which we discuss cultural considerations and measurement concerns.

The Transactional Nature of Social–Emotional Competence

Social–emotional competence is not a trait that resides *within* the child. The transactional nature of competence is inherent in our definition of it as an individual's ability to meet self-needs while maintaining positive relationships (Rose-Krasnor, 1997). Rather than being an internal attribute, competence emerges out of interactions between individuals and their social partners. In the same way that a child's attachment security status may vary with different attachment figures (e.g., Belsky, Garduque, & Hrncir, 1984), individuals may show varying levels of competence with different partners. For example, a child interacting with a supportive and responsive partner is much more likely to have his or her needs met *and* to maintain a positive relationship than the same child interacting with a hostile and unresponsive partner. Support for this transactional view of competence comes from several sources, including Vygotsky's concepts of scaffolding and the *social relations model*, which is an analytic approach that separates individual, partner, and relationship influences on social behaviors.

Vygotsky (1978) emphasized the role of social interaction in facilitating the development of young children. This facilitation depends on the skills of an expert partner, who supports and extends children's skills to more advanced levels. Without this scaffolding, the child may "appear" to be relatively low functioning. The difference between the child's level of independent functioning and the level he or she obtains with skilled scaffolding is known as the *zone of proximal development* (ZPD). Therefore, the width of the ZPD represents the range of competencies shown by a child under varying effectiveness of support. Although Vygotsky's focus was largely on cognitive and task performance, the ZPD concept is directly relevant for describing the variation in social–emotional competence that occurs when a child interacts with others at differing levels of competence. A skilled interaction partner, for example, could support the social behaviors of a less skilled child by providing suggestions for social play, adjusting for egocentrism by explicitly explaining perspectives, helping the child think of possible alternative social strategies, and prompting ways to cope with anger or distress. With such assistance, the child may achieve the main tasks of social competence; without it, the child may fail.

Another source of support for the transactional nature of competence comes from an analytic approach that has enabled researchers to decompose variance in behavior into that attributable to *individual* characteristics, *partner* effects, and *relationship* influences. Known as the *social relations model* (SRM; Kashy & Kenny, 2000), this form of analysis can be used when individuals in a group (e.g., family, play group) interact with each of the other group members. In this way, one can estimate the extent to which an individual acts similarly across partners (actor effects), the extent to which his or her behavior varies as a function of specific interaction partners (partner effects), and the variation due to specific relationships (relationship effects). In studies using this methodology, substantial variance in social behavior has been attributed to relationship and partner effects. For example, Coie et al. (1999) used SRM to test the importance of relational factors in explaining aggression shown in quartets of school-age boys. The unique relationships between individuals explained as much variance as did specific partners or actors. Similarly, relationship effects (e.g., mother–child, father–child) have been found to be as strong as actor effects in predicting adolescent attachment security, suggesting that internal working models not be considered as purely intrapersonal concepts, independent of the identity of the attachment figure (Cook, 2000).

Next we describe several foundational skills, assess their relation to competence, briefly review empirical evidence that describes how these skills are manifested during preschool period, and introduce some theory relevant to the specific development of these abilities.

Key Research Studies

Self-Regulation

Self-regulation is generally defined as the "ability to actively control arousal and emotional responses" (Derryberry & Rothbart, 1988, p. 959). Hannah's difficulty in waiting for her turn on the tricycle and Ryan's problems keeping his exuberant rough-and-tumble play within acceptable bounds are examples of self-regulatory challenges typical of this age period. Self-regulation is a characteristic with wide individual variability and considerable stability (Rothbart & Bates, 2006; Vaughn, Kopps, & Krakow, 1984). The study of self-regulation has encompassed a variety of related components (see reviews in Kochanska, Murray, & Harlan, 2000; Kopp & Wyer, 1994; Rothbart & Bates, 2006), including conscience development, delay of gratification, "effortful control" (ability to inhibit a dominant response and substitute a less dominant one), executive function, attention, and appropriate responding in the face of conflicting options.

Such skills clearly are important for achieving social competence and avoiding social problems (e.g., Rawn & Vohs, 2006; Riggs, Jahromi, Razza, Dillworth-Bart, & Mueller, 2006). For example, a child who never subordinates his or her own needs to those of an interaction partner will have difficulty establishing and maintaining healthy friendships (Selman, Watts, & Schultz, 1997). Furthermore, uncontrolled strong emotions are likely to disrupt interactions and damage relationships. For example, unregulated behaviors (e.g., aggression) and emotions (e.g., fear) may interfere with a child's sensitivity to another's needs and desires, disrupt social information processing, and lead to impulsive and potentially hurtful actions. Sustained and successful interaction, therefore, is facilitated by children's abilities to regulate both their emotions and social behaviors (e.g., Eisenberg, Fabes, Guthrie, & Reiser, 2000).

In support of this theoretical link between self-regulation and social–emotional competence, effortful control has been related positively and longitudinally to social competence and peer popularity (e.g., Blair, Denham, Kochanoff, & Whipple, 2004; Spinrad et al., 2006). Delay of gratification also has been linked positively to subsequent parent- and peer-rated social competence (Mischel, Shoda, & Rodriguez, 1989), and greater responsivity to social demands (Kopp & Wyer, 1994). In addition, Funder, Block, and Block (1983) found that ego control is positively related to interpersonal success in preschoolers, including less victimization and more stable relationships in girls and greater cooperation in boys.

Self-regulation has been associated with preschool children's abilities to cope with potential social difficulties and has been linked to the promotion of competence. Effortful control, for example, positively predicts effective anger management (Eisenberg, Fabes, Nyman, Bernzweig, & Pinuelas, 1994). Furthermore, such control may reduce the potentially problematic social interactions of children with difficult temperaments, by making it possible for them to inhibit predispositions toward impulsive or negative actions (Kieras, Tobin, Graziano, & Rothbart, 2005). Problems in self-regulation also may underlie aggression and withdrawal (Calkins & Fox, 2002).

Children make important advances in their ability to regulate behaviors and emotions during the preschool years (Thompson, 1994; Yeates et al., 2007). External sources of control are gradually replaced by internal mechanisms, and regulatory strategies become more effective, adaptive, and stable (Rothbart & Bates, 2006; Thompson, 1994). In the following paragraphs, we briefly discuss the age-related processes considered to underlie such changes in self-regulation.

Brain development, especially in the cortical and limbic areas, has been linked to changes in several components of self-regulation (e.g., Rothbart & Bates, 2006; Yeates et al., 2007). In an extensive review of the literature on the relation between children's brain disorders and social outcomes, Yeates and his colleagues summarized evidence linking self-regulation to developments in the amygdala, ventral striatum, and orbitofrontal cortex. Effortful control and the ability to direct attention voluntarily are associated with maturation of the limbic system and prefrontal cortex during early childhood (see Riggs et al., 2006; Rothbart & Bates, 2006); both of these processes are important for resisting temptation, delaying gratification, and regulating emotions. Similarly, the development of self-control has been linked to changes in prefrontal cortex during early childhood, including a cycle of synapse production and pruning (see Thompson, 2006).

Self-regulation is further enhanced by cognitive changes that typically occur during toddlerhood and early childhood. Kopp and Wyer (1994) have proposed a comprehensive framework for understanding links between self-regulation and the development of four cognitive dimensions: (1) the ability to understand and generalize others' expectations for appropriate behavior; (2) increased memory skills, allowing the recall of guidelines for appropriate behavior; (3) representational abilities, especially increases in language and communication skills, and the ability to use language to self-direct actions; and (4) self-monitoring of activities and emotions. Kopp (1982) noted the child's increasing ability to use self-control processes flexibly, allowing adaptation to changing contexts. This is similar to Block and Block's (1980) concept of ego-resiliency, which has been related to socially important processes in preschoolers, such as egocentrism (Gjerde, Block, & Block, 1986) and subsequent shyness and extraversion (Weir & Gjerde, 2002).

Interpersonal influences affect the development of self-regulation in early childhood, in addition to primarily individual-level changes such as brain maturation. Parenting has been commonly considered a source of such social influences, in terms of both parenting style and parent–child relationships. Indeed, authoritative and responsive parenting has frequently been found to facilitate the development of self-regulation and internalization (see Grusec & Goodnow, 1994). Karreman, van Tuijl, van Aken, and Dekovic (2006) recently conducted a meta-analysis of the relation between parenting and self-regulation in preschoolers, to help them understand some of the inconsistencies in previous findings. Three components of self-regulation were included: compliance to parental directives, inhibition, and emotion regulation. Parenting also comprised three constructs: positive control (e.g., guidance, instruction); negative control (e.g., hostility, high power assertion); and responsiveness (e.g., acceptance, sensitivity). Results indicated that self-regulation was positively predicted by positive control and negatively predicted by negative control, as expected. Subsequent analyses showed that relations between regulation and parental control were driven largely by the associations between the two forms of parental control and the compliance component of regulation. Contrary to expectations, parental responsiveness was not related to self-regulation, and the authors suggested that this aspect of parenting may be related more closely to the development of autonomy than to self-regulation.

Internalization of parental values and standards provides both a motivation for self-regulation and guidelines for its direction. In their review of the literature on parenting and internalization, Grusec and Goodnow (1994) suggested that previous research had not adequately addressed the role of individual differences among children (e.g., temperament) and their families (e.g., cultural standards and practices) in investigating how parenting shapes children's internalization. Similarly, Karreman et al. (2006) noted the lack of attention to child and family differences in studies of the relations between parenting and preschoolers' self-regulation. Individual differences, however, have been a primary focus in Kochanska's investigations of the development of one aspect of self-regulation—conscience—in the toddler and early childhood years.

Conscience has been construed as an "inner guiding system responsible for the gradual emergence and maintenance of self-regulation" (Kochanska & Aksan, 2006, p. 1587) and encompasses moral emotions (e.g., guilt upon transgression), moral conduct (e.g., helping another in distress), and moral cognitions (e.g., awareness of behavioral standards). Kochanska's program of research (e.g., Kochanska & Aksan, 2006) has revealed that the association between conscience-related aspects of self-regulation and parenting is moderated by child temperament. Links between successful conscience development and supportive, inductive, and warm parenting are strongest for children who are relatively fearful and anxious. For fearless children, however, conscience is best predicted by a "mutually responsive orientation" in both child and parent, which leads to the child's willingness to comply with parental directives and act in accordance with their standards and values.

In summary, self-regulation skills increase dramatically in the preschool years, as reflected in the child's growing abilities to inhibit inappropriate action, delay gratification, be guided by conscience, and comply with directives. These skills have important implications for the young child's ability to initiate and maintain positive relationships with peers and adults, as well as providing the child with a sense of control over self and environment.

Social Problem Solving

Social problem solving is the second foundational skill set in our model of social–emotional competence. Hannah's attempts to persuade her mother to allow her to wear the new shoes to school could be conceptualized within a social problem-solving model, in which a variety of strategies (e.g., crying, bargaining) might be used to achieve the goal, with the outcome conceptualized as a success or failure. Because thinking and emotion work together in such goal-directed situations, it is important to address even young children's skills in *thinking* about interpersonal interactions, going beyond their emotional experience, knowledge, regulation, and expression. Responsible decision making assumes importance as the everyday social interactions of preschoolers increase in frequency and complexity. Young children must learn to process social information—to encode and analyze social situations, set social goals, determine effective ways to solve peer conflict, and actually perform these behaviors (Crick & Dodge, 1994). In a meta-analysis of interventions focusing on such social problem solving, children's use of such decision-making skills were in fact found to be related to improved social behavior (Denham & Almeida, 1987). More recent reports (e.g., Greenberg, Kusche, & Riggs, 2001; Youngstrom et al., 2000) have shown comparable results, with added specifications of a link between social problem solving and academic success, as well as the advantages of learning specifically *prosocial* problem solutions.

Thus, each aspect of social information processing, the backbone of responsible decision making, may be related to preschoolers' competence. For example, *encoding* of social information is differentially related to social functioning; Coy, Speltz, DeKlyen, and Jones (2001) found that preschool boys diagnosed with oppositional defiant disorder generated more aggressive alternative solutions than did peers without this disorder. In tracing the reason for these aggressive solutions, Coy et al. found that the diagnosed boys demonstrated less accurate encoding of social information; however, they did *not* differ from nondiagnosed boys in interpreting the information once it was encoded. Similarly, diagnosed and nondiagnosed boys did not differ on response evaluation (see also Gouze, 1987). This pattern of findings is not, however, universal. Webster-Stratton and Lindsay (1999) reported that conduct problems in young children are indeed associated with deficits in awareness of social cues (encoding), but that these problems coexist with problematic interpretations (e.g., overestimating their own ability to perform competently and more often misattributing others' actions as hostile).

Regarding other aspects of social problem solving, Neel, Jenkins, and Meadows (1990) showed that aggressive and nonaggressive preschoolers differed not so much in the number or overall repertoire of their alternative problem-solving strategies but did differ in two dimensions: (1) their *favored type of strategy*, with aggressive children preferring intrusive strategies; and (2) their *goals* in interaction, with aggressive children tending to have goals of stopping or preventing others' behaviors, and nonaggressive children more often citing information gathering and relationship enhancement as social goals. With respect to *response access or construction*, and *response decision* processes, Musun-Miller (1993) has shown that preschoolers who could predict positive outcomes for social situations were liked better by same-sex peers than those who predicted less positive outcomes.

In summary, evidence suggests that during the preschool period, encoding, especially with reference to others' emotions, may be of central importance in social problem solving. Also, some investigators have found the *interpreting*, *goal*, and *response* aspects of social problem solving to be relevant as early as the preschool years.

In another new development, the social information-processing theory that forms a foundation for training in responsible decision making has been expanded to include emotional information and content at every step (Lemerise & Arsenio, 2000). This union of social information processing and emotions illustrates well our thinking about social–emotional competence during the preschool period: Children often attempt to understand their own and others' behavior, and emotions play a role in this understanding, conveying crucial interpersonal information that can guide interaction (Dodge, Laird, Lochman, Zelli, & Conduct Problems Prevention Research Group, 2002). For example, to decide what to do when trying to join a group of other preschoolers working on a puzzle, a young child would need to encode information from the setting; this might include the context, others' behavior, and others' affect, as well as one's own. Next, this information would need to be interpreted; these interpretations might differ depending on one's own emotional arousal. For example, a shy, socially inhibited child might perceive the facial expressions of peers as less than friendly. After interpretation, the child must consider various alternative means of joining the group, based on his or her goals— and here again, the shy, fearful child may have very different goals than would a bolder child. We consider that any measure of social problem solving should include assessment of emotions at each juncture in the process.

Not surprisingly, parental disciplinary strategies and beliefs are associated with their young children's social problem-solving skills. However, most research in this area has examined only associations of children's generation of alternative solutions, or response construction, to problematic social interchanges. Given this limitation, extant findings suggest that trained mothers can effectively instill social problem-solving thinking strategies in their children (Shure, 1983), with such teaching related to improvements in their children's social problem skills and behaviors. More generally, both earlier (e.g., Pettit, Dodge, & Brown, 1988) and current (Haskett & Willoughby, 2007) research indicate that parents' negative child-related beliefs (e.g., endorsement of aggression), emotional distress, and childrearing practices (e.g., restrictive discipline, harsh, insensitive parenting, or, conversely, preventive teaching) are related in expected directions to children's abilities to generate useful solutions to social problems (in the research of Haskett and Willoughby, intent attributions formed part of the social problem-solving latent variable as well).

Prosocial Behavior

A third skills set that we believe underlies social–emotional competence is the ability and motivation to act in ways that benefit others. Hannah's, albeit unsuccessful, attempt to alleviate Kate's separation distress is an example of such other-oriented concern. A large body of research links young children's prosocial behaviors (e.g., helping, cooperating, sharing, comforting) to relationship, peer group, and self-system indices of social–emotional competence (see reviews by Eisenberg, Fabes, & Spinrad, 2006; Penner, Dovidio, Piliavin, & Schroeder, 2005). For example, Clark and Ladd (2000) found that the tendency to

act empathically toward peers was positively related to number of friendships, friendship quality (greater harmony and less conflict), and peer acceptance. Sebanc (2003)
reported a link between observed prosocial behaviors and support from friends. Similarly,
preschoolers with friends have been found to display more frequent prosocial responses
(e.g., approaching, comforting) to peer distress than do those without friends (Farver &
Branstetter, 1994). Farver and Branstetter also found that prosocial responses were correlated with the frequency of successful play initiations and invitations. In addition, the use
of prosocial strategies (e.g., cooperation, alliance formation) in acquiring resources from
peers predicts parent-rated social competence (Hawley, 2002; Walker, 2005).

The developmental timing and origins of prosocial behavior have been a subject of
much theoretical consideration. From some theoretical perspectives, prosocial behavior
in young children would be relatively unexpected. In classical Freudian theory (Freud,
1933/1968), for example, prosocial behavior is rooted in the superego, which emerges
from identification with the same-sex parent—a process that does not occur until the
end of the preschool period. Similarly, from a Piagetian perspective (Piaget, 1967), the
hypothesized egocentrism of the preoperational stage would interfere with preschoolers'
capacity to act to benefit another until role-taking skills increase in later in childhood.

However, there is ample evidence that young children are capable of, and motivated
to, engage in spontaneous prosocial behaviors such as helping, cooperating, sharing,
comforting, and defending (e.g., Grusec, 1991; Hay, Payne, & Chadwick, 2004), although
sometimes at relatively low frequencies. In one of the earliest observational studies of
young children's responses to peer distress, for example, Murphy (1937) found evidence
of sympathy and comforting in 2-year-olds. Such prosocial acts not only increase over
early childhood but also appear to become more selective (for a review of age-related
changes, see Eisenberg et al., 2006).

This early emergence of prosocial behaviors is more consistent with ethological and
social learning theories than with psychoanalytic and cognitive-developmental approaches.
For example, ethologists have emphasized the existence and functional importance of
dominance hierarchies in reducing aggression and conflict in preschool groups (e.g.,
McGrew, 1972). Such hierarchies are established through the use of prosocial, as well as
aggressive, strategies. Indeed, ethologically oriented researchers have established connections between the frequency of prosocial acts and dominance status in preschool
classrooms (e.g., Pellegrini et al., 2007; Walker, 2005). Hawley (2002) put 3- to 6-year-old
children in a limited resource situation, in which they had to negotiate preferred access
to an attractive toy. Prosocial strategies (e.g., cooperation, reconciliation) were effective
in achieving such access and positively related to independent ratings of social competence. The use of such prosocial strategies following conflict would be likely to facilitate
positive relationships with peers, who may assist in future conflicts and minimize the
likelihood of subsequent victimization (Pellegrini et al., 2007; McGrew, 1972). Thus, in
this context, prosocial actions help to achieve simultaneously all three elements in our
competence model: improving group status, meeting individual needs, and maintaining
positive relationships.

From a behavioral–social learning theoretical perspective, we also might not be surprised to find young children acting in prosocial ways. Here, the focus is on how prosocial
behaviors and norms are acquired, shaped, and maintained through imitation, coaching,
and reinforcement, particularly within parent–child relationships. There is a long history
of research examining parental predictors of prosocial behaviors in young children. In

recent comprehensive literature reviews, Eisenberg et al. (2006) and Thompson (2006) concluded that parental warmth, responsiveness, connectedness, inductive discipline, and authoritative parenting often have been positively associated with children's prosocial behaviors, although results have been somewhat inconsistent and/or weak. Secure attachment also appears to promote prosocial behavior in children, perhaps through facilitating a "mutual responsive orientation" (Kochanska & Aksan, 2004), enhancing imitation of parental prosocial acts and internalization of parental values.

Although many researchers have shown that prosocial behaviors can be altered through reinforcement and modeling (e.g., Eisenberg et al., 1993; Grusec & Redler, 1980), they appear to be less responsive to such influences than are other social behaviors, such as aggression (Eisenberg et al., 2006; Grusec, 1991). For example, spontaneous helping occurs relatively frequently in 4-year-olds, in spite of low rates of parental reinforcement, infrequent empathy teaching, and mixed messages about their appropriateness and desirability (Grusec, 1991; Grusec, Davidov, & Lundell, 2002). This inconsistency between aspects of parenting and children's prosocial behavior may be explained by research indicating that young children's altruistic behavior is related to myriad nonparenting variables (see review by Eisenberg et al., 2006), including temperamental sociability (e.g., Eisenberg-Berg & Hand, 1979), moral reasoning (e.g., Eisenberg, Pasternack, Cameron, & Tyron, 1984), genetic predispositions (e.g., Knafo & Plomin, 2006), emotion regulation (e.g., Eisenberg et al., 2000), and positive emotionality (e.g., Eisenberg et al., 2000).

Other Foundational Skills

Our model of social–emotional competence (Figure 9.1) has a wide base, representing the large range of skills that are important in helping the child achieve social success at relationship, group, and self-efficacy levels. In the social awareness skills "box," for example, the abilities to identify and act upon one's awareness of the thoughts and feelings of others have long been recognized as central to social competence. Traditional social-cognitive developmental theory (e.g., Selman, 1980) suggests that preschoolers' ability to understand others' thoughts and feelings is substantially hampered by the dominance of their own thoughts and feelings. However, more recent research shows that preschoolers' awareness of others' thoughts and feelings is well developed during, and certainly by the end of, the preschool period (Denham & Kochanoff, 2002). Moreover, this knowledge of emotions during early childhood is often predictive of both teacher and peer ratings of overall social competence, both concurrently and longitudinally (e.g., Denham et al., 2002).

Alongside this specific knowledge of emotions, an increasing focus on young children's realization that others have minds, the contents of which may differ from one's own (Astington & Jenkins, 1995; Wellman & Woolley, 1990), has led to studies examining its relation to socially competent behavior (Capage & Watson, 2001; Cassidy, Werner, Rourke, Zubernis, & Balaraman, 2003; Walker, 2005). In general, these studies suggest that theory of mind skills are often, although not always and not necessarily strongly (and not necessarily in the same ways for girls and boys; see Walker, 2005), related to the demonstration of socially competent behavior.

We identify *communication abilities* and *sociodramatic play* as examples of additional foundational skills in our model. For example, McCabe (2005) found that preschoolers

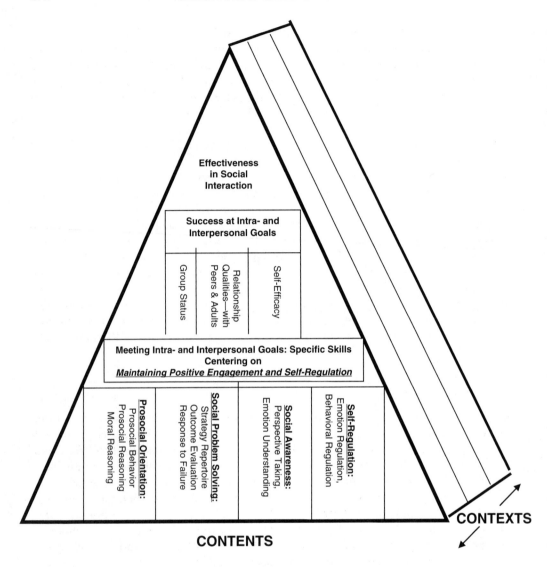

FIGURE 9.1. Adaptation and integration of Rose-Krasnor's (1997) model of social competence.

with specific language impairments were rated by both parents and teachers as having lower social competence than were peers without such communication difficulties. They were also more socially isolated. Furthermore, cooperative fantasy play provides a rich context for social development (see review by Rubin, Fein, & Vandenberg, 1983), including opportunities to learn communication skills, emotion regulation, symbolic thinking, and role taking. It may also provide an opportunity for the development of peer relationships and be especially important in successful friendship formation (Gottman, 1983). In addition, the benefits of social play may be lasting. Complex social play in toddlerhood and preschool, for example, predicts more prosocial activity and less aggression in midchildhood (Howes & Phillipsen, 1998).

Future Directions

Affective Processes

A pressing need in more fully fleshing out young children's social–emotional competence is to extend our focus to processes involved in competent responding. To this end, Halberstadt, Denham, and Dunsmore (2001) created a model of *affective social competence* (ASC), which comprises three integrated and dynamic components—sending emotional messages, receiving emotional messages, and experiencing emotion. Central and interconnected abilities within each component include the following skills: (1) awareness and identification of affect of self, peers, and adults (e.g., using prosocial display rules of emotion to be kind to others); (2) ability to work within a complex and constantly changing social environment; and (3) management/regulation. Thus, the ASC model highlights process; it also emphasizes moment-to-moment changes in social partners and allows for the differing cultural meanings inherent in social interaction, which impact social–emotional competencies. This model may be used in conjunction with the model put forward herein, especially to suggest ways in which to gain access to the social–emotional world of young children and to measure their behavior.

Cultural Considerations

Cultural differences in the foundational skills associated with competence have received increasing attention, much of which has focused on how the relation between these skills and social adjustment may vary as a function of the "collectivistic versus individualistic" nature (Triandis, 1993) of specific cultures. A common finding in this regard is that shyness is frequently associated with peer rejection and psychosocial maladjustment in more individualistic Western cultures, but it does not have the same negative associations in collectivist societies, such as China (e.g., Chen, Rubin, & Li, 1995; see Chen, Chung, & Hsiao, Chapter 24, this volume). Other research has shown culturally based differences in how parents socialize competence in young children, as reflected in parental values, goals, styles, and behaviors (Rubin & Chung, 2006). For example, Chinese mothers are more likely than European American mothers to rate individual traits (e.g., politeness, calmness) and to engage in socialization practices (e.g., authoritarian discipline) that are consistent with collectivistic values (e.g., Jose, Huntsinger, Huntsinger, & Liaw, 2000; Keller et al., 2007; Liu et al., 2005).

Although some aspects of competence (e.g., relationship quality) may be similar across cultures, the relative balance between autonomy and connectiveness may vary as a function of the culture's "collectivistic versus individualistic" orientation. However, even this perspective may be overly simplistic. The commonly held view of autonomy and connectedness as "opposing" human dimensions (e.g., Bakan, 1966) may itself be culturally bound. In an integrative literature review, Miller (2004) identified this tension between autonomy and connectedness as the "deep structure" common to theories of social development. She argued for the need to recognize cultural variations in which autonomy and connectedness coincide rather than "pull in opposite directions." In such situations, for example, fulfilling culturally defined relationship obligations is not seen as conflicting with autonomy, because individuals feel that they have freely chosen such duties. In addition, Harkness (2002) has articulated the limitations of categorizing cultures as either collectivist or individualistic—a dichotomy that, among other difficulties, fails to address within-culture variation and does not clarify the relations among values, socialization strategies, and children's social behavior.

Clearly, there is a need to understand more about the meaning and development of social competence across cultures, and how children from different cultures, and those who interact with them, view competence (Rubin, 2007; Rubin, Cheah, & Menzer, in press). Substantive cross-cultural collaborations are needed, in which researchers question implicit assumptions that may restrict how they measure and understand competence. More attention to within-culture variations in the meaning and expression of competence is also warranted, especially for situations in which children may be exposed to potentially incompatible competence models.

Measurement and Analysis

The conceptualization of competence put forward in this chapter presents considerable challenges for measurement and data analyses. First, social effectiveness, the essence of our competence definition, is a complex construct. Judgments of effectiveness may differ depending on who is doing the judging, the time frame involved (immediate vs. long term), and the situational or cultural context. In addition, interactions often involve multiple goals simultaneously (e.g., obtain a toy from a friend, maintain the friendship, not be noticed by the classroom bully), only some of which may successfully be met. Second, as described earlier, the process-oriented nature of social competence requires "online" measurement. Such an approach involves assessment of affective and motivational components, as well as skills level. Furthermore, the transactional character of competence means that it needs to be measured within relationship contexts. The SRM approach, although highly informative, has design requirements that are very difficult for researchers to meet. Other techniques that allow estimates of individual and partner effects (e.g., intraclass correlations) should be used more widely. Third, it is relatively surprising that researchers have not made more frequent use of latent variables in structural equation modeling to capture common variance among social competence indicators. Such procedures would increase our understanding of the nature of competence, as well as reduce problems due to unreliability of measurement.

Summary

In this chapter, we have described a transactional, multilevel model of social–emotional competence that proposes effectiveness as the highest level construct. Effectiveness is indexed by success in inter- and intrapersonal domains that are in turn supported by a range of skills and motivations. We focused on social problem solving, prosocial behavior, and self-regulation as three representative "skills boxes" to illustrate relevant developmental theory, processes, and advances. Cultural considerations, process orientation, and measurement/analysis issues were identified as important areas for future work.

We began this chapter with a brief glimpse of Hannah, our prototypical preschooler. The skills she brings to the social challenges of her everyday experiences help her meet her own developmental needs, as well as to build positive relationships with the peers and adults in her life. At the same time, with the assistance of supportive social partners, these experiences provide opportunities for her to improve and extend her skills. These emerging abilities will increase her competence to negotiate new social challenges. Understanding the complex ways that this process occurs is an important and exciting prospect for researchers and all those who interact with young children.

References

Astington, J. W., & Jenkins, J. M. (1995). Theory of mind development and social understanding. *Cognition and Emotion, 9*, 151–165.

Bakan, D. (1966). *The duality of human existence.* Chicago: Rand McNally.

Baltes, P., & Silverberg, S. (1994). The dynamics between dependency and autonomy: Illustrations across the life-span. In D. Featherman, R. Lerner, & M. Perlmutter (Eds.), *Life-span development of behavior* (Vol. 12, pp. 41–90). Hillsdale, NJ: Erlbaum.

Belsky, J., Garduque, L., & Hrncir, E. (1984). Assessing performance, competence, and executive capacity in infant play: Relations to home environment and security of attachment. *Developmental Psychology, 20*, 406–417.

Blair, K. A., Denham, S. A., Kochanoff, A., & Whipple, B. (2004). Playing it cool: Temperament, emotion regulation, and social behavior in preschoolers. *Journal of School Psychology, 42*, 419–443.

Block, J. H., & Block, J. (1980). The role of ego-control and ego-resiliency in the organization of behavior. In W. A. Collins (Ed.), *The Minnesota Symposia on Child Psychology: Vol. 13. Development of cognition, affect, and social relations* (pp. 39–101). Hillsdale, NJ: Erlbaum.

Calkins, S. D., & Fox, N. A. (2002). Self-regulatory processes in early personality development: A multilevel approach to the study of childhood social withdrawal and aggression. *Development and Psychopathology, 14*, 477–498.

Capage, L., & Watson, A. C. (2001). Individual differences in theory of mind, aggressive behavior, and social skills in young children. *Early Education and Development, 12*, 613–628.

Cassidy, K. W., Werner, R. S., Rourke, M., Zubernis, L. S., & Balaraman, G. (2003). The relationship between psychological understanding and positive social behaviors. *Social Development, 12*, 198–221.

Chen, X., Rubin, K. H., & Li, Z. (1995). Social functioning and adjustment in Chinese children: A longitudinal study. *Developmental Psychology, 31*, 531–539.

Clark, K. E., & Ladd, G. W. (2000). Connectedness and autonomy support in parent–child relationships: Links to children's socioemotional orientation and peer relationships. *Developmental Psychology, 36*, 485–498.

Coie, J. D., Cillessen, A. H., Dodge, K. A., Hubbard, J. A., Schwartz, D., Lemerise, E. A., et al. (1999). It takes two to fight: A test of relational factors and a method for assessing aggressive dyads. *Developmental Psychology, 35*, 1179–1188.

Cook, W. L. (2000). Understanding attachment security in family context. *Journal of Personality and Social Psychology, 78*, 285–294.

Coy, K., Speltz, M. L., DeKlyen, M., & Jones, K. (2001). Social cognitive processes in preschool boys with and without oppositional defiant disorder. *Journal of Abnormal Child Psychology, 29*, 107–119.

Crick, N., & Dodge, K. A. (1994). A review and reformulation of social-information-processing mechanisms in children's social adjustment. *Psychological Bulletin, 115*, 74–101.

Denham, S. A., & Almeida, M. C. (1987). Children's social problem-solving skills, behavioral adjustment, and interventions: A meta-analysis evaluating theory and practice. *Journal of Applied Developmental Psychology, 8*, 391–409.

Denham, S. A., Caverly, S., Schmidt, M., Blair, K., DeMulder, E., Caal, S., et al. (2002). Angry and aggressive children and emotional perspective taking ability. *Journal of Child Psychology and Psychiatry, and Allied Disciplines, 43*, 901–916.

Denham, S. A., & Holt, R. W. (1993). Preschoolers' likability as cause or consequence of their social behavior. *Developmental Psychology, 29*, 271–275.

Denham, S. A., & Kochanoff, A. (2002). "Why is she crying?": Children's understanding of emotion from preschool to preadolescence. In L. Feldman Barrett & P. Salovey (Eds.), *The wisdom in feelings: Psychological processes in emotional intelligence* (pp. 239–270). New York: Guilford Press.

Derryberry, D., & Rothbart, M. (1988). Arousal, affect, and attention as components of temperament. *Journal of Personality and Social Psychology, 55,* 958–966.

Dodge, K. A., Laird, R., Lochman, J. E., Zelli, A., & Conduct Problems Prevention Research Group. (2002). Multidimensional latent-construct analysis of children's social information processing patters: Correlations with aggressive behavior problems. *Psychological Assessment, 14,* 60–73.

Eisenberg, N., Fabes, R. A., Carlo, G., Speer, A. L., Switzer, G., Karbon, M., et al. (1993). The relations of empathy-related emotions and maternal practices to children's comforting behavior. *Journal of Experimental Child Psychology, 55,* 131–150.

Eisenberg, N., Fabes, R. A., Guthrie, I. K., & Reiser, M. (2000). Dispositional emotionality and regulation: Their role in predicting quality of social functioning. *Journal of Personality and Social Psychology, 78,* 136–157.

Eisenberg, N., Fabes, R. A., Nyman, M., Bernzweig, J., & Pinuelas, A. (1994). The relations of emotionality and regulation to children's anger-related reactions. *Child Development, 65,* 109–128.

Eisenberg, N., Fabes, R. A., & Spinrad, T. L. (2006). Prosocial development. In W. Damon & R. M. Lerner (Editors-in-Chief) & N. Eisenberg (Vol. Ed.), *Handbook of child psychology* (6th ed., Vol. 3, pp. 646–718). Hoboken, NJ: Wiley.

Eisenberg, N., Pasternack, J. F., Cameron, E., & Tyron, K. (1984). The relation of quantity and mode of prosocial behavior to moral cognition and social style. *Child Development, 55,* 1479–1485.

Eisenberg-Berg, N., & Hand, M. (1979). The relationship of preschoolers' reasoning about prosocial moral conflicts to prosocial behavior. *Child Development, 50,* 356–363.

Farver, J. M., & Branstetter, W. H. (1994). Preschoolers' prosocial responses to their peers' distress. *Developmental Psychology, 30,* 334–341.

Freud, S. (1968). *New introductory lectures on psychoanalysis.* London: Hogarth. (Original work published 1933)

Funder, D. C., Block, J. H., & Block, J. (1983). Delay of gratification: Some longitudinal personality correlates. *Journal of Personality and Social Psychology, 44,* 1198–1213.

Gjerde, P. F., Block, J., & Block, J. H. (1986). Egocentrism and ego resiliency: Personality characteristics associated with perspective-taking from early childhood to adolescence. *Journal of Personality and Social Psychology, 51,* 423–434.

Gottman, J. M. (1983). How children become friends. *Monographs of the Society for Research in Child Development. Vol. 48*(No. 201).

Gouze, K. R. (1987). Attention and social problem solving as correlates of aggression in preschool males. *Journal of Abnormal Child Psychology, 15,* 181–197.

Greenberg, M. T., Kusche, C. A., & Riggs, N. (2001). The P(romoting) A(lternative) TH(inking) S(trategies) Curriculum: Theory and research on neurocognitive and academic development. *CEIC Review, 10*(6), 22–23, 26.

Grusec, J. (1991). Socializing concern for others in the home. *Developmental Psychology, 27,* 338–342.

Grusec, J. E., Davidov, M., & Lundell, L. (2002). Prosocial and helping behavior. In P. K. Smith & C. H. Hart (Eds.), *Blackwell handbook of childhood social development* (pp. 457–474). Oxford, UK: Blackwell.

Grusec, J. E., & Goodnow, J. J. (1994). Impact of parental discipline methods on the child's internalization of values: A reconceptualization of current points of view. *Developmental Psychology, 30,* 4–19.

Grusec, J. E., & Redler, E. (1980). Attribution, reinforcement, and altruism: A developmental analysis. *Developmental Psychology, 16,* 525–534.

Halberstadt, A. G., Denham, S. A., & Dunsmore, J. (2001). Affective social competence. *Social Development, 10,* 79–119.

Harkness, S. (2002). Culture and social development: Explanations and evidence. In P. K. Smith & C. H. Hart (Eds.), *Blackwell handbook of childhood social development* (pp. 60–77). Oxford, UK: Blackwell.

Haskett, M. E., & Willoughby, M. (2007). Paths to child social adjustment: Parenting quality and children's processing of social information. *Child: Care, Health and Development, 33*, 67–77.

Hawley, P. H. (2002). Social dominance and prosocial and coercive strategies of resource control in preschoolers. *International Journal of Behavioral Development, 26*, 167–176.

Hay, D. F., Payne, A., & Chadwick, A. (2004). Peer relations in childhood. *Journal of Child Psychology and Psychiatry, 45*, 84–108.

Howes, C. (1987). Social competence with peers in young children: Developmental sequences. *Developmental Review, 2*, 252–272.

Howes, C., & Phillipsen, L. (1998). Continuity in children's relations with peers. *Social Development, 7*, 340–349.

Jose, P. E., Huntsinger, C. S., Huntsinger, P. R., & Liaw, F. R. (2000). Parental values and practices relevant to young children's social development in Taiwan and the United States. *Journal of Cross-Cultural Psychology, 31*, 677–702.

Karreman, A., van Tuijl, C., van Aken, M. A., & Dekovic, M. (2006). Parenting and self-regulation in preschoolers: A meta-analysis. *Infant and Child Development, 15*, 561–579.

Kashy, D., & Kenny, D. A. (2000). The analysis of data from dyads and groups. In H. T. Reis & C. M. Judd (Eds.), *Handbook of research methods in social and personality psychology* (pp. 451–477). New York: Cambridge University Press.

Keller, H., Abels, M., Lo, W., Su, Y., Wng, Y., Borke, J., et al. (2007). Socialization environments of Chinese and Euro-American middle-class babies: Parenting behaviors, verbal discourses and ethnotheories. *International Journal of Behavioral Development, 31*, 210–217.

Kieras, J. E., Tobin, R. M., Graziano, W. G., & Rothbart, M. K. (2005). You can't always get what you want: Effortful control and children's responses to undesirable gifts. *Psychological Science, 16*, 391–396.

Knafo, A., & Plomin, R. (2006). Prosocial behavior from early to middle childhood: Genetic and environmental influences on stability and change. *Developmental Psychology, 42*, 771–786.

Kochanska, G., & Aksan, N. (2004). Conscience in childhood: Past, present, and future. *Merrill–Palmer Quarterly, 50*, 299–310.

Kochanska, G., & Aksan, N. (2006). Children's conscience and self-regulation. *Journal of Personality, 74*, 1587–1617.

Kochanska, G., Murray, K. T., & Harlan, E. T. (2000). Effortful control in early childhood: Continuity and change, antecedents, and implications for social development. *Developmental Psychology, 36*, 220–232.

Kopp, C. B. (1982). Antecedents of self-regulation: A developmental perspective. *Developmental Psychology, 18*, 199–214.

Kopp, C. B., & Wyer, N. (1994). Self-regulation in normal and atypical development. In D. Cicchetti & S. Toth (Eds.), *Rochester Symposium on Developmental Psychopathology: Vol. 5. Disorders and dysfunctions of the self* (pp. 31–56). Rochester, NY: University of Rochester Press.

Lemerise, E. A., & Arsenio, W. F. (2000). An integrated model of emotion processes and cognition in social information processing. *Child Development, 71*, 107–118.

Liu, M., Chen, X., Rubin, K. H., Zheng, S., Cui, L., Li, D., et al. (2005). Autonomy- vs. connectedness-oriented parenting behaviors in Chinese and Canadian mothers. *International Journal of Behavioral Development, 29*, 489–495.

McCabe, P. C. (2005). Social and behavioral correlates of preschoolers with specific language impairment. *Psychology in the Schools, 42*, 373–387.

McGrew, W. C. (1972). *An ethological study of children's behaviors*. London: Metheun.

Miller, J. G. (2004). The cultural deep structure of psychological theories of social development. In R. J. Sternberg & E. L. Grigorenko (Eds.), *Culture and competence: Contexts of life success* (pp. 111–138). Washington, DC: American Psychological Association.

Mischel, W., Shoda, Y., & Rodriguez, M. L. (1989). Delay of gratification in children. *Science, 244*, 933–938.

Murphy, L. (1937). *Social behavior and child personality: An exploratory study of the roots of sympathy.* New York: Columbia University Press.

Musun-Miller, L. (1993). Social acceptance and social problem-solving in preschool children. *Journal of Applied Developmental Psychology, 14*, 59–70.

Neel, R. S., Jenkins, Z. N., & Meadows, N. (1990). Social problem-solving behaviors and aggression in young children: A descriptive observational study. *Behavioral Disorders, 16*, 39–51.

Parker, J. G., & Gottman, J. M. (1989). Social and emotional development in a relational context: Friendship interaction from early childhood to adolescence. In T. J. Berndt & G. W. Ladd (Eds.), *Peer relationships in child development* (pp. 95–131). New York: Wiley.

Pellegrini, A. D., Roseth, C. J., Mliner, S., Bohn, C. M., Van Ryzin, M., Vance, N., et al. (2007). Social dominance in preschool classrooms. *Journal of Comparative Psychology, 121*, 54–64.

Penner, L. A., Dovidio, J. F., Piliavin, J. A., & Schroeder, D. A. (2005). Prosocial behavior: Multilevel perspectives. *Annual Review of Psychology, 56*, 365–392.

Pettit, G. S., Dodge, K. A., & Brown, M. M. (1988). Early family experience, social problem solving patterns, and children's social competence. *Child Development, 59*, 107–120.

Piaget, J. (1967). *Six psychological studies.* New York: Vintage.

Rawn, C. D., & Vohs, K. D. (2006). The importance of self-regulation for interpersonal functioning. In K. D. Vohs & E. J. Finkel (Eds.), *Self and relationships: Connecting intrapersonal and interpersonal processes* (pp. 15–31). New York: Guilford Press.

Riggs, N. R., Jahromi, L. B., Razza, R. P., Dillworth-Bart, J. E., & Mueller, U. (2006). Executive function and the promotion of social–emotional competence. *Journal of Applied Developmental Psychology, 27*, 300–309.

Robins, L. N., & Rutter, M. (1990). *Straight and devious pathways from childhood to adulthood.* Cambridge, UK: Cambridge University Press.

Rose-Krasnor, L. (1997). The nature of social competence: A theoretical review. *Social Development, 6*, 111–135.

Rothbart, M. K., & Bates, J. E. (2006). Temperament. In N. Eisenberg (Vol. Ed.) & W. Damon & R. Lerner (Series Eds.), *Handbook of child psychology: Vol. 3. Social, emotional, and personality development* (6th ed., pp. 99–166). Hoboken, NJ: Wiley.

Rubin, K. H. (2007, April). *Peer interactions and relationships: Looking through the glass culturally.* Invited keynote address, Society for Research in Child Development, Boston, MA.

Rubin, K. H., Bukowski, W. M., & Parker, J. G. (2006). Peer interactions, relationships, and groups. In W. Damon & R. M. Lerner (Editors-in-Chief) and N. Eisenberg (Vol. Ed.), *Handbook of child psychology* (6th ed., Vol. 3, pp. 571–645). Hoboken, NJ: Wiley.

Rubin, K. H., Cheah, C. S. L., & Menzer, M. (in press). Peers. In M. Bornstein (Ed.), *Handbook of cross-cultural developmental science.* London: Psychology Press.

Rubin, K. H., & Chung, O. B. (Eds.). (2006). *Parental beliefs, parenting, and child development in cross-cultural perspective.* London: Psychology Press.

Rubin, K. H., Fein, G., & Vandenberg, B. (1983). Play. In P. H. Mussen (Series Ed.) & E. M. Hetherington (Vol. Ed.), *Handbook of child psychology: Vol. 4. Socialization, personality, and social development* (4th ed., pp. 693–744). New York: Wiley.

Rubin, K. H., & Rose-Krasnor, L. (1992). Interpersonal problem solving. In V. B. VanHassett & M. Hersen (Eds.), *Handbook of social and behavioral development* (pp. 1–18). Hillsdale, NJ: Erlbaum.

Ryan, R. M., & Deci, E. L. (2000). Self-determination theory and the facilitation of intrinsic motivation, social development, and well-being. *American Psychologist, 55*, 68–78.

Sebanc, A. M. (2003). The friendship features of preschool children: Links with prosocial behavior and aggression. *Social Development, 12*, 249–268.

Selman, R. L. (1980). *The growth of interpersonal understanding.* New York: Academic Press.

Selman, R. L., Watts, C. L., & Schultz, L. H. (1977). *Fostering friendship: Pair therapy for treatment and prevention*. Hawthorne, NY: Aldine de Gruyter.

Shure, M. (1983). Enhancing childrearing skills in lower income women. *Issues in Mental Health Nursing, 5*, 121–138.

Spinrad, T. L., Eisenberg, N., Cumberland, A., Fabes, R. A., Valiente, C., Shepard, S. A., et al. (2006). Relation of emotion-related regulation to children's social competence: A longitudinal study. *Emotion, 6*, 498–510.

Thompson, R. A. (1994). Emotion regulation: A theme in search of definition. *Monographs of the Society for Research in Child Development, 59*, 25–52, 250–283.

Thompson, R. A. (2006). The development of the person: Social understanding, relationships, conscience, self. In N. Eisenberg (Vol. Ed.) & W. Damon & R. Lerner (Series Eds.), *Handbook of child psychology: Vol. 3. Social, emotional, and personality development* (6th ed., pp. 24–98). Hoboken, NJ: Wiley.

Triandis, H. C. (1993). Collectivism and individualism as cultural syndromes. *Cross-Cultural Research, 27*, 155–180.

Vaughn, B. E., Kopp, C. B., & Krakow, J. B. (1984). The emergence and consolidation of self-control from eighteen to thirty months of age: Normative trends and individual differences. *Child Development, 55*, 990–1004.

Vygotsky, L. (1978). *Mind in society: The development of higher psychological processes*. Cambridge, MA: Harvard University Press.

Walker, S. (2005). Gender differences in the relationship between young children's peer-related social competence and individual differences in theory of mind. *Journal of Genetic Psychology, 166*, 297–312.

Waters, E., & Sroufe, L. A. (1983). Social competence as a developmental construct. *Developmental Review, 3*, 79–97.

Webster-Stratton, C., & Lindsay, D. W. (1999). Social competence and conduct problems in young children: Issues in assessment. *Journal of Clinical Child Psychology, 28*, 25–43.

Weir, R. C., & Gjerde, P. F. (2002). Preschool personality prototypes: Internal coherence, cross-study replicability, and developmental outcomes in adolescence. *Personality and Social Psychology Bulletin, 28*, 1229–1241.

Wellman, H. M., & Woolley, J. D. (1990). From simple desires to ordinary beliefs: The early development of everyday psychology. *Cognition, 35*, 245–275.

Yeates, K. O., Bigler, E. D., Dennis, M., Gerhardt, C. A., Rubin, K. H., Stancin, T., et al. (2007). Social outcomes in childhood brain disorder: A heuristic integration of social neuroscience and developmental psychology. *Psychological Bulletin, 133*, 535–556.

Yeates, K. O., & Selman, R. L. (1989). Social competence in the schools: Toward an integrative developmental model for intervention. *Developmental Review, 9*, 64–100.

Youngstrom, E., Wolpaw, J. M., Kogos, J. L., Schoff, K., Ackerman, B., & Izard, C. (2000). Interpersonal problem solving in preschool and first grade: Developmental change and ecological validity. *Journal of Clinical Child Psychology, 29*, 589–602.

CHAPTER 10

Friendship in Early Childhood

CAROLLEE HOWES

For a toddler or a young preschooler, a friend is someone to play with—when a mother's friend comes over to visit with her daughter; when neighbors meet at a park; when it is outside time in child care; at an older sister's birthday party; when a cousin stays overnight; when a best friend visits for a playdate.

Young children often join the words "play" and "friend" together: "You can't be my friend if you don't let me play. I'll be your friend if you will let me play." And adults often reinforce the confounding of "friend" and "play": "Play together nicely with your friends," "Play like friends," and "Go and play with your friends." Friends are exciting and fun to play with, but friendships involve more than playing together. Friends can make children sad—when they cannot play together; when a friend moves away; when a friend hurts their feelings. And friends can mend hurt feelings by comforting and sharing.

The everyday language of young children and of the adults who care for them demonstrates the importance of young children's friendships in regulating the course of their play. Young children's emergent play skills can make playing with more than one or two children difficult, because too many ideas and actions require coordination to make the play go smoothly. Corsaro's (1981) classic ethnographic study suggested that young children use the language of being a friend to include and exclude children from play.

Compared to the friendships of older children, early friendships appear to be based more on companionship and the compatibility of play style than on intimacy and affection (Brownell & Brown, 1992; Gifford-Smith & Brownell, 2003). Yet both theory and a rich empirical literature suggest that the early friendships of young children are more than fleeting relationship phenomena (Hinde, 1979; Hinde, Titmus, Easton, & Tamplin, 1985). Observational studies of toddlers and preschool-age children within stable peer groups indicate that young children do form reciprocated friendships (Howes, 1983; Vandell & Mueller, 1980) that are based on differentiated interactions (Ross, Conant, Cheyne, & Alevizos, 1992). Within these early friendships, children share feelings and ideas, mutual affection and attachment, and concern for each other (Dunn, 2004; Howes & Lee, 2006). And when circumstances allow, that is, when parents do not shift children out of the peer group, early friendships may persist over several years (Howes & Phillipsen, 1992; Walden, Lemerise, & Smith, 1999).

In this chapter, theories of friendship, particularly as they apply to early childhood, are briefly described. Methods used to examine the friendships of young children are introduced. Thereafter, empirical studies of friendship in early childhood are reviewed.

Relevant Theories

Much of the early research on young children's friendships is indebted to the writings of Hinde (1979) and other ethologists (i.e., Blurton-Jones, 1972). These scholars turned their attention from animals to children in social groups during the early human ethology movement in the 1970s. For example, Hinde provided a schema for categorizing relationships and emphasized the importance of relationships. According to Hinde, a relationship may best be understood by examining not only the interactions between dyadic partners but also the unique contributions of each partner (Hinde & Stevenson-Hinde, 1976).

The understanding of early friendship formation is also informed by attachment theory (Bowlby, 1969/1982). The processes of relationship formation embedded in Bowlby's attachment theory are applicable to friendship relationship (Howes, 1996). According to this interpretation, relationships (whether attachment or playmate relationships) develop through multiple and recursive interactive experiences. "Recursive interactions" are well-scripted social exchanges that are repeated many times with only slight variation (Bretherton, 1985). From these experiences, the child internalizes a set of fundamental social expectations about the behavioral dispositions of the partner (Bowlby, 1969/1982). These expectations form the basis for the development of an internal working model of relationships. Thus, through repeated experiences of social and social pretend play with a particular peer, a child forms an internal representation of a relationship with a playmate. Some playmate relationships evolve into friendships. It is important to note that the child's representation of the partner comprises cognitions and affect derived from both the structure and the content of social experiences with that partner. A child who engages in repeated and complex interactions with a given playmate is likely to represent the partner as a friend. Furthermore, the content of interactions is likely to influence the quality of the resulting relationship.

Making and keeping friends requires social and emotional regulation skills and social cognition. Thus, theories of social and emotional socialization and of social cognition are relevant to the understanding of early friendships. For example, Selman (1980) and Youniss (1980) proposed that children's understanding of friendship relationships is dependent on underlying cognitive-developmental changes. Perspective taking, affect recognition, and communicative skills; the understanding of intentions, desires, and belief in others; and social information-processing skills and social problem solving all underlie friendship formation in young children (Brownell & Brown, 1992; Dunn, 2004; Gifford-Smith & Brownell, 2003). To form friendships, children must recognize the potential friend as a social actor and be aware of the reciprocal nature of social behaviors in social interaction. Dunn (e.g., Dunn & Hughes, 2001) has argued that early friendships make an important contribution to the development of social-cognitive and social skills beyond experiences with adults. Unlike adult–child interaction, young friends create cooperative play and resolve conflicts in the context of shared, age-appropriate interests (e.g., building a tall block building; playing at being bus drivers). Gottman (1986) has provided a framework that attends to the affective quality of social conversations among young friends, thus contributing to understanding of the functions and quality of early friendships. As young friends share the enactment and development of fantasy themes in mutually created social pretend play, they create intimacy through emotional disclosure.

It is important to note that theories of early friendship have, by and large, been developed with little regard for notions of culture (see Chen, Chung, & Hsiao, Chapter 24, this volume). Rogoff's theory of the cultural nature of human development makes a useful contribution to theories of early friendships by placing early friendships within their cultural communities. In this framework, a cultural community is defined as a grouping of people who participate in a shared set of practices and traditions. In this regard, peer groups represent a form of cultural community (Howes & Ritchie 2002; Rogoff, 2003). As cultural communities, peer groups construct shared understandings and meanings in forms that include shared scripts for pretend play, games, conversations, knowledge of who hangs out with whom, who can and cannot be trusted to gossip without hurting other people's feelings, and ways to behave within the group. These shared understandings and meanings constitute the practices of the peer community. Peer communities have shared histories as well as practices. Children who participate over time in a given peer group can remind each other of events that have meaning only within the context of the peer group.

Placing the development of early friendships within cultural communities helps to resolve the question of whether early friendships are fleeting or more like the intimate friendship relationships of older children. For example, consider that children are simultaneously members of (1) *informal peer groups* formed by living within a neighborhood, by being part of a group of families that spends holidays or vacations together, or occasionally having a playdate; and (2) *formal peer groups*, such as those found within a child care center. The practices or ways of doing things within each of these peer communities are specific to the peer group. These peer-group-specific practices influence friendships formation. For example, cross-gender or cross-age friendships may flourish in informal neighborhood peer groups and be discouraged within classroom-based peer groups. Peer groups in child care may facilitate cross-ethnic, cross-religious, or cross-class friendships that are more difficult within peer groups in informal settings. Toddlers' friendships in a drop-in child care program may end when their mothers' schedules change.

Central Issues in the Study of Early Friendships

Issues in the study of early friendships mirror the levels of social organization initially introduced by Hinde (1979): the child, the dyad, and the peer group. Issues relevant to the child or individual level are developmental changes, changes that enable young friendships, and changes enhanced by friendships. Another central issue is the attachment theory–driven question of whether close relationships with adults are associated with the prevalence and quality of young children's friendships. Issues relevant to the dyadic level include identifying and assessing friendship, and friendship quality and identification of who becomes friends with whom. Finally, the influence of the wider culture and the context of the peer group are central issues that we describe below.

Developmental Changes

Individual changes in domains linked to relationship development make it possible for children to form friendships that comprise more than momentary play companionships. In part, social interactions with peers (and perhaps especially friends) enable the development of capacities that are important for the development of friendships. For example, within friendship dyads, toddlers and preschool-age children repeat, expand, and elaborate shared social pretend-play themes. These expanded pretend-play episodes are important in the development of perspective-taking skills that increase children's capacities to understand, support, and be concerned about the feelings of the other children (Dunn, 2004). In turn, these perspective-taking or mind-reading skills (Dunn, 2004) enable narrative capacities (Howes & Wishard, 2004; Kyratzis & Green, 1997).

Friendship dyads, perhaps as much or more than parent–child or sibling dyads (Dunn, 2004), are contexts within which children develop social understandings, particularly about emotions and relationships, interpersonal skills in resolving conflicts, and moral understanding and sensitivity. Talk within young friendship dyads includes a fair amount of gossip, sharing knowledge and opinions about their social world of peers (Dunn, 2004; Gottman, 1983). These exchanges provide practice in disclosure and in sharing feelings. Such talk also enhances children's social understandings of themselves, of others, and of social rules. For example, one recent ethnographic study of talk among preschoolers found that friends' talk indexed the social organization of the peer group and included discussions of emotions (Kyratzis, 2001; Kyratzis, Marx, & Wade, 2001). Interaction with peers also allows the formation of working models or internal representations of social relationships (Bretherton, Ridgeway, & Cassidy, 1990). All of these developments make it possible for children to develop affective-based relationships.

The friendships of toddlers and preschoolers can also be considered contexts for development in some of these same areas. Children who are friends have an easier time than children who are not friends in entering play groups and engaging in complex social and social pretend play (Gottman, 1983; Hinde et al., 1985; Howes, 1988). Young friends do engage in conflict—preschool friends engage in more conflicts than nonfriends; however, conflict within friend dyads is resolved differently than within nonfriend dyads (Hinde et al., 1985). Friends, compared to nonfriends, are more likely to negotiate, to compromise in reaching a solution, and to stay in proximity and continue playing after a dispute (Dunn, 2004; Hinde et al., 1985). Disputes between young friends also provide contexts for learning to resolve moral dilemmas (e.g., how to share the toys fairly; whether it is acceptable for a friend to tease the partner's younger sibling).

Assessing Friendship in Early Childhood: Identifying Friendship Dyads and the Quality of Their Friendship

The issues relevant to friendship measurement for toddlers and preschoolers are similar to those for older children. These central issues pertain to identifying reciprocal friendships and the behavioral characteristics of each partner, noting whether behavioral (or other) similarities exist; and examining the quality of the friendship. These issues are particularly problematic in studies of young children, who may not be reliable interviewees about their friendships.

Identifying Friendships

Toddlers' and preschool children's friendships are often identified behaviorally (Howes, 1983). Children are considered to be friends if they play in close proximity, engage in complex games, and express shared positive affect (Howes, 1996; Vandell & Mueller, 1980). Behavioral identification requires observation over relatively long time periods and on multiple occasions. This methodology precludes the possibility of discovering friendships beyond the contexts being observed.

A potentially more efficient way to identify early friendships may be to ask mothers to name their children's best friends (Howes, with Unger, & Matheson, 1992; Rubenstein & Howes, 1976). This method, however, may lead to the identification of a best friend as the child with whom the *mother* feels most comfortable.

By age 3, children in stable peer groups can reliably report reciprocated friendships using sociometric picture techniques (Howes, 1988). Teachers as well are able to identify friendships in their classrooms (Sebanc, 2003). Both of these methods are classroom-based, so neighborhood or family network friendships are not identified. Thus, it may be that some young children who appear to be friendless in school have friends elsewhere.

Describing Friendships

Preschool-age children, who are just beginning to be able to identify friends in a socio-metric format, are not yet able to describe features or qualitative dimensions of their friendships. Friendships, even first friendships, are not always positive. Aggression, bullying, and unresolved conflict between young friends can have the same negative consequences for children as they do in the negative friendships of older children (Sebanc, 2003). Early studies of the features and quality of the friendships of young children used naturalistic observations (Howes, 1988, 1996). Subsequently Park (now Kerns) developed a friendship quality Q-sort for videotaped dyadic interaction (Park, Keng-Ling, & Ramsay, 1993; Park & Waters, 1989). Other observational taxonomies were developed by Young-blade (Youngblade & Belsky, 1992; Youngblade & Dunn, 1995). Sebanc (2003) developed a teacher questionnaire that differentiates between friendships on the basis of support, intimacy, conflict, and asymmetry.

In general, friendship researchers find that children of all ages form friendships with others who are similar to themselves (Rubin, Bukowski, & Parker, 2006). Similarity can refer to demographic characteristics (gender, race, or home language), or to behaviors and interaction styles. Friendships of toddlers' and preschoolers' that are formed in diverse peer groups are less likely than the friendships of older children to be of the same sex and ethnicity (Howes & Phillipsen, 1992; Howes & Wu, 1990). By late preschool age, children tend to form same-sex friendships, but their friendships cross ethnic lines (Howes & Lee, 2007; Howes & Phillipsen, 1992).

Friendship Formation

Preschool children in well-established groups (Gottman, 1983) and somewhat older children in newly formed groups form friendships with children who are similar in play style (Rubin, Lynch, Coplan, Rose-Krasnor, & Booth, 1994; Serbin & Sprafkin, 1986). Researchers have speculated that these shared activity preferences draw young peers together. Recent work by Gleason, Gower, Hohmann, and Gleason (2005) suggests that similar temperament also moves children together, with boys more likely to select high-activity and high-impulsivity friends and girls more likely to select low-activity friends.

By the toddler period, some children are markedly aggressive or socially inhibited (Rubin, Burgess, Dwyer, & Hastings, 2003; Rubin, Burgess, & Hastings, 2002; Rubin, Hastings, Chen, Stewart, & McNichol, 1998). These aggressive or withdrawn young children may face challenges in forming positive friendships. For example, in a Head Start study, Snyder, Horsch, and Childs (1997) reported that preschool-age children tend to form friendships with children similar to themselves in aggression, and when aggressive children become friends with other aggressive agemates, their friendships appear to contribute to increases in individual levels of aggression over time.

Preschool children engage in both relational and physical aggression (Burr, Ostrov, Jansen, Cullerton-Sen, & Crick, 2005). Burr et al. found that relationally aggressive preschool-age girls used relational aggression to maintain their friendship status over a school year. For these children, the phrase "I'll be your friend if . . . " was a short-term, effective strategy for maintaining friendships, although relationally and physically aggressive children have difficulty in the long term establishing and maintaining positive friendships (Grotpeter & Crick, 1996).

Less is known about the early friendships of socially withdrawn toddlers and preschoolers (see Rubin, Bowker, & Kennedy, Chapter 17, this volume). Children who begin kindergarten withdrawing from peers appear to be initially dependent on their teachers but are indistinguishable from their peers in adjustment over time (Ladd & Burgess, 1999). However, studies of older children suggest that children who are friendless are also likely to be socially timid, socially sensitive, socially anxious, and lonely (Gazelle & Rudolph, 2004; Ladd & Troop-Gordon, 2003). And if these socially withdrawn older children do form best-friend friendships, then they tend to be with other socially withdrawn children, and the friendships are not always supportive or fun (Rubin, Wojslawowicz, Rose-Krasnor, Booth-LaForce, & Burgess 2006). We can speculate that younger, initially shy children may also be challenged in forming close and positive friendships in toddler and preschool peer groups, but remaining withdrawn may depend less on the child and more on the support provided for forming relationships.

Children's Close Relationships with Parents and Teachers

Based on a meta-analysis that included older children, as well as toddlers and preschoolers, it has been reported that children who have secure attachment relationships with their primary caregiver are more likely than insecure children to have friendships with peers (Schneider, Atkinson, & Tardiff, 2001). The influence of the child–mother attachment relationship on very young children's friendship formation may depend on the age at which the child is introduced to the peer group and on the context of the care setting. For example, when children enter stable peer groups (preschool, child care), the nature of the attachment relationship with their teacher predicts friendship formation and friendship quality (Howes, 1999). Indeed, even for children with difficult parent–child relationships, a secure relationship with a teacher can predict the formation of positive relationships with peers (Howes & Ritchie, 1999, 2002). Thus, the presence of an attachment figure within the peer context appears to provide a secure (or not) base for young children encountering their first peer group to explore social relationships with peers.

It bears noting that young children who have close ties with their parents tend to form friendships with children who also have secure child–parent attachments, and children with insecure child–parent attachment form friendships with children who have similar attachments (Denham & Holt, 2001). Relatedly, Sroufe (1983) has reported that in peer groups with an overrepresentation of preschoolers with insecure child–parent attachments, an overabundance of acrimonious peer relationships occurs.

Culture and Context for Early Friendships

Culture

Although friendships may be part of the social fabric in all cultures (Rubin, Bukowski, et al., 2006), cultural goals shape the activities and practices that parents provide for their young children. Hofstede (2007; Hofstede & McCrae, 2004) broadly classified cultures as collectivist or individualist in goals for interpersonal relationships. "Collectivist" cultures place value on cohesive groups, usually based on extended families. "Individualistic" cultures place less value on ties between individuals. These different cultural goals are expected to lead to different activities and practices. For example, in cultural groups categorized as having collectivist goals, parents might be expected to seek out opportunities for their young children to develop stable friendship relationships with either cousins and other family members or nonrelated peers. In contrast, in cultural groups categorized as having individualistic goals, parents would be expected to be more invested other goals (e.g., school readiness), and less likely to find opportunities for young children to have sustained contact with peers.

Current research on very young children's friendships has not been informed by systematic study of variations in cultural goals, although a comparative study of parental ethnotheories about close relationships outside the family reported differences between parents of preschoolers in Norway, the United States, Turkey, and Korea (Aukurst, Edwards, Kumru, Knoche, & Kim, 2003). Korean parents were more likely than the other parents to report that their child had a best friend in preschool and to value close relationships outside of the family.

Context

Both within and between cultural groups, parents' goals and values for social relationships outside the family, as well as constraints on their time and resources, determine the context within which young children may form friendships. Much of the classic research on friendship formation in young children was conducted in nursery schools, preschools, and child care centers (e.g., Issacs, 1937; Reed, 1950; Howes, 1988). Nursery schools and preschools for children of more affluent parents have traditionally been seen by parents as opportunities to promote social development in children. Child care programs for infants and toddlers are closely tied to working mothers and provide opportunities for relatively small and stable groups of children to have extended social contact. Extended family households may value interaction and close relationships among cousins and siblings more than friendships between children of unacquainted mothers (Howes, Guerra Wishard, & Zucker, 2008). But they, too, provide a small and stable group of agemates with extended social contacts and opportunities for close relationships.

The context of the peer group influences whether early friendships can be identified. In nursery school, child care, and Head Start programs, young children can choose their friends, without their parents preselecting them. Friendship formation is monitored by teachers. Susan Isaacs (1937), an early peer researcher, studied children in nursery schools and described their friendships as close, stable, and tied to the development of complex social pretend play. Howes (1983) described toddler friendships in a historical period when infants and toddlers of working mothers were first included in child care centers. In a manner similar to Isaacs, she described toddler friendships as stable, affective relationships. More recent research on friendships in young children has been conducted in Head Start centers serving primarily low-income African American families (Vaughn, Colvin, Azria, Caya, & Krzysik, 2001). Friendships developed in these Head Start programs were described as affectionate and as sources of social support beyond that provided by extended family members (Bost, 1995).

Based on the peer groups that were available for them to study (e.g., milk distribution centers in New York City's Central Park; Buhler, 1930; Maudry & Nekula, 1939), pioneer toddler peer researchers in the 1930s concluded that infants and toddlers engaged in games and other early forms of peer interaction, but not friendships. Milk distribution centers were unlikely to include stable peer groups, a necessary prerequisite for identifying friendships. In more contemporary times, mothers of young children who do not work may take their children to a neighborhood park, to a "Mommy and me" class, or arrange playdates (Haight & Miller, 1992; Ladd & Hart, 1992). These children have their friends preapproved by parents, and parents, not teachers, monitor the course of the friendship (Newson & Newson, 1970). These friendships tend to be described as playmate companions rather than affective intimate relationships (Haight & Miller, 1992).

In informal contexts in which both the mother and the child are involved in the friendship formation context, there are associations between the behaviors and features of parent- and child-formed friendships. Dunn's (2004) research suggests that mothers' styles of conflict and resolution with their children are tied to their children's style of conflict and resolution with their own friends. For example, the children of mothers who encourage cooperative problem solving have more positive conflict resolutions in their disputes with friends. Likewise, parents who are active in arranging opportunities for peer play, and who indirectly supervise play, have children with more friends (Kerns, 1998). Some work on the intergenerational continuity of peer relations further suggests that mothers' recollections of their own childhood peer relations may influence maternal activities, with mothers who recall themselves as anxious being more active in arranging their own children's peer experiences, including encouraging friendship with some peers and not others (Putallaz, Costanzo, Grimes, & Sherman, 1998; Putallaz, Costanzo, & Smith, 1991; Putallaz, Klein, Costanzo, & Hedges, 1994).

Some preschool-age children have little opportunity to form friendships. In poverty-stricken or dangerous neighborhoods, outside play with neighbor peers may rarely occur. Children whose families move frequently or who themselves move among relatives or are in and out of foster care are unlikely to form friendships (Cochran & Davila, 1992). Children with these difficult life circumstances often have parents with difficulties in social relationships, who may not value or encourage friendships in their children (Cochran & Davila, 1992). Also, these children are unlikely to be in studies of early friendships, unless they attend a center-based early childhood program.

The Influence of Social and Emotional Climate on Early Friendship

Researchers have suggested that children who live in highly conflicted families may be less successful at forming positive peer friendships. The mechanisms that may mediate the relation between family climate and the establishment and maintenance of early friendship may include children's behavioral inclinations (e.g., aggression) and their inability to regulate negative emotions (e.g., anger). For young children who form friendships within peer groups that are monitored and supervised by family members (e.g., playdates) or within expanded families, the social and emotional climate in these families is expected to be associated with the quality of children's friendships (Ladd & Pettit, 2002).

Most research on the social and emotional climate of the peer group has occurred in preschool or child care classrooms rather than in family settings. Based on aggregated observations of children's interactions or global assessments, classrooms can be rated as negative to positive in social and emotional climate (Hamre, 2008; Pianta, LaParo, & Hamre, 2004). In positive-climate classrooms, the affective tone of interaction is warm and positive, and children play together and engage in prosocial behaviors. Children who attend classrooms with more positive social and emotional climates are more likely to form close relationships with peers (Howes & Ritchie, 2002; Solomon, Watson, Delucchi, Schaps, & Battistich, 1988; Watson & Battistich, 2006).

Summary

Young friendships become possible because children develop working models of intimate relationships, the capacity to coordinate social interactions, and the capacity to coregulate emotions. And friendships reinforce children's abilities to coregulate interaction, play, and emotions. Furthermore, friendships appear to lead to the development of social understandings of relationships, conflict resolution, and shared emotion regulation.

Researchers have established valid and reliable measurements of friendship and friendship quality in young children. Because of verbal and cognitive limitations, young children's friendship quality has been measured with reference to adult perceptions rather than as seen through the eyes of the child.

The youngest children's friendships differ from those of older children in that toddlers and young preschoolers often become friends with children who are unlike themselves in terms of gender and ethnicity. Young child friendships are similar to older child friendships in that the partners tend to share common interests and behavioral styles. Furthermore, children with similar histories of adult attachment relationships tend to become friends. Children with more secure child–adult relationships are more likely than children with less secure child–adult attachments to form friendships and to experience more positive friendships.

Early friendships are embedded within cultures, and cultural goals shape the contexts of encounter between young peers. Within and across cultures, parents have different goals and values for close relationships outside of families. These goals and values may in part determine the kind of friendships available to young children. With reference to contexts, toddlers and preschoolers can only make friends within the peer group that their parents select. For many young children, early friendships occur within informal peer groups organized and monitored by parents. Only those toddlers and young children who attend center-based child care and preschool can select friendships from a larger peer group that does not include parental monitoring. Within these classroom contexts, the social and emotional climate influences the nature of the friendships that are formed. Within both classroom and family contexts, more positive social and emotional climates quantitatively predict more friendships and qualitatively predict more positive friendships among young children.

The broader question is whether it matters if very young children have friends. For concurrent development, children appear to benefit in terms of social and emotional development. Friends do seem to play a unique role in social and emotional development; young children, even children in supportive families, miss a friend who moves away (Dunn, 2004; Park et al., 1993). There is some evidence that having a friend can provide a preschooler emotional support in the absence of parents at child care (Howes et al., 1992), at the birth of a sibling (Vandell, 1987), and in the face of the everyday fears evoked by fantasy play (Gottman, 1986). Making a transition within preschool classrooms or between preschools (Howes, 1983), and from preschool to formal school (Ladd, Kochenderfer, & Coleman, 1996), is more successful when children move with their friends. And Kramer and Gottman (1992) found that children who played better and were better able to resolve conflicts with their friends had more positive sibling interaction after the birth of a sibling (Kramer & Gottman, 1992).

Relatively few longitudinal studies of friendship that begin in the toddler and preschool period exist. Dunn (2004) studied children with their siblings and their friends from toddlerhood to middle childhood. She found that the social understanding of both partners in the preschool friendship and their shared relationship experiences predicted the quality of later friendships. Both Kramer (Kramer & Kowal, 2005) and Howes (Howes & Aikins, 2002; Howes & Phillipsen, 1998; Howes & Tonyan, 2000) reported continuity in friendship quality of children from the toddler and preschool developmental period into adolescence. From these data, it would appear that friendships provide the young child with some developmental advantages; in the long term, good friendships seem to predict more good friendships. It remains for further research to ascertain what disadvantages, if any, accrue to a child without young friendships, or to children with a series of unfortunate friendships.

Future Directions

Theoretical formulations that explain and aid understanding of how friendships are formed, the qualitative nature of the relationship, and the consequences of development of friendships—not only for the individual children but also for the peer group that hosts the friendship—must be sufficiently complex to account for both individual development and contextual features. It is rare for developmental psychologists to consider simultaneously a theory of affective development in a dyadic relationship and a theory of how culture influences development. Current formulations of attachment theory (Cassidy & Shaver, 1999) provide a nuanced outline of what could be a theory of relationship formation, accounting for concurrent influences of social and emotional climate and intergenerational influences and continuity. Attachment theory also provides a framework for understanding the co-creation of relationship quality and the influence of working models of relationships on subsequent relationships. Yet attachment theory does not provide a framework for cultural influences on young friendships. Such a framework is necessary, because young friendships are embedded within goals, values, and practices specific to the cultural communities of the adults who ultimately have control over peer-group composition. To move beyond the study of young friendships formed within dominant-culture families, the field needs a theory of cultural influence on relationship development. Hofstede and McCrae (2004) provide a broad framework for considering cultural goals as collectivist or individualistic, and Rogoff (2003) provides a framework for explaining everyday practices that create opportunities for peer encounters.

Each of these theories is limiting; although they suggest the significance of intimate dyadic relationships, they do not provide an account of relationship formation. In ongoing research, Howes and colleagues (Howes, Sanders, & Lee, 2008) have moved toward an integration between theories of culture and theories of relationship formation. They have attempted to explain the formation of socially skilled, affective, and intimate relationships between young children who differ in race and home language. They are also examining the influence of adults on children who are constructing relationships with peers (Howes & Lee, 2007; Howes & Shivers, 2006). We know little about the short- and long-term developmental consequences of children from diverse backgrounds who have (or do not have) opportunities to form early friendships outside (and within) their families' cultural communities.

References

Aukurst, V. G., Edwards, C. P., Kumru, A., Knoche, L., & Kim, M. (2003). Young children's close relationships outside the family: Parental ethnotheories in four communities in Norway, United States, Turkey, and Korea. *International Journal of Behavioral Development, 27,* 481–494.

Blurton-Jones, N. (1972). *Ethological studies of child behavior.* New York: Cambridge University Press.

Bost, K. K. (1995). Mother and child reports of preschool children's social support networks network correlates of peer acceptances. *Social Development, 4,* 149–164.

Bowlby, J. (1982). *Attachment and loss: Vol. 1. Attachment.* London: Hogarth. (Original work published in 1969)

Bretherton, I. (1985). Attachment theory: Retrospect and prospect. *Monographs of the Society for Research in Child Development, 50,* 3–35.

Bretherton, I., Ridgeway, D., & Cassidy, J. (1990). The role of internal working models in the attachment relationship can it be studied in three year olds? In M. Greenberg, D. Cicchetti, & E. M. Cummings (Eds.), *Attachment during the preschool years* (pp. 273–308). Chicago: University of Chicago Press.

Brownell, C., & Brown, E. (1992). Peers and play in infants and toddlers. In J. VanHasselt & M. Herson (Eds.), *Handbook of social development* (pp. 183–200). New York: Plenum Press.

Buhler, C. (1930). *The first year of life.* New York: Day.

Burr, J. E., Ostrov, J. M., Jansen, E. A., Cullerton-Sen, C., & Crick, N. R. (2005). Relational aggression and friendship during early childhood: I won't be your friend. *Early Education and Development, 16,* 161–183.

Cassidy, J., & Shaver, P. R. (1999). *Handbook of attachment theory and research.* New York: Guilford Press.

Cochran, M., & Davila, V. (1992). Societal influences on children's peer relationships In R. D. Parke & G. W. Ladd (Eds.), *Family–peer relationships: Modes of linkage* (pp. 191–212). Hillsdale, NJ: Erlbaum.

Corsaro, W. A. (1981). Friendship in the nursery school: Social organization in a peer environment. In S. R. Asher & J. M. Gottman (Eds.), *The development of children's friendships* (pp. 207–241). Cambridge, UK: Cambridge University Press.

Denham, S., & Holt, R. W. (2001). Preschoolers at play: Co-socializers of emotional and social competence. *International Journal of Behavioral Development, 25*, 290–301.

Dunn, J. (2004). *Children's friendships*. Malden, MA: Blackwell.

Dunn, J., & Hughes, C. (2001). "I got some swords and you're dead!": Violent fantasy, antisocial behavior, friendship, and moral sensibility in young children. *Child Development, 72*, 491–505.

Gazelle, H., & Rudolph, K. D. (2004). Moving towards and moving away from the world: Social approach and avoidance in anxious youth. *Child Development, 75*, 829–849.

Gifford-Smith, M. E., & Brownell, C. (2003). Children's peer relationships: Social acceptance, friendship, and peer networks. *Journal of School Psychology, 41*, 235–284.

Gleason, T. R., Gower, A. L., Hohmann, L. M., & Gleason, T. C. (2005). Temperament and friendships in preschool age children. *International Journal of Behavioral Development, 29*, 336–344.

Gottman, J. (1983). How children become friends. *Monographs of the Society for Research in Child Development, 43*(3, Serial No. 201).

Gottman, J. M. (1986). The world of coordinated play: Same and cross-sex friendships in young children. In J. Gottman & J. Parker (Eds.), *Conversations of friends* (pp. 139–191). New York: Cambridge University Press.

Grotpeter, J. K., & Crick, N. R. (1996). Relational aggression, overt aggression, and friendship. *Child Development, 67*, 2328–2338.

Haight, W., & Miller, P. (1992). The development of everyday pretend play: A longitudinal study of mothers' participation. *Merrill–Palmer Quarterly, 38*, 331–349.

Hamre, B. (2008). Learning opportunities in preschool and elementary classrooms. In R. C. Pianta, M. J. Cox, & K. Snow (Eds.), *School readiness, early learning and the transition to kindergarten* (pp. 219–239). Baltimore: Brookes.

Hinde, R. A. (1979). *Towards understanding relationships* London: Academic Press.

Hinde, R., & Stevenson-Hinde, J. (1976). Towards better understanding relationships. In P. Bateson & R. Hinde (Eds.), *Growing points in ethology*. New York: Cambridge University Press.

Hinde, R., Titmus, G., Easton, D., & Tamplin, A. (1985). Incidence of friendships and behavior towards strong associates vs. nonassociates in preschoolers. *Child Development, 56*, 234–245.

Hofstede, G. (2007). A European in Asia. *Asian Journal of Social Psychology, 10*, 16–21.

Hofstede, G., & McCrae, R. R. (2004). Personality and culture revisited: Linking traits and dimensions of culture. *Cross-Cultural Research, 38*, 52–87.

Howes, C. (1983). Patterns of friendship. *Child Development, 54*, 1041–1053.

Howes, C. (1988). Peer interaction of young children. *Monographs of the Society for Research in Child Development, 53*(1, Serial No. 217).

Howes, C. (1996). The earliest friendships. In W. M. Bukowski, A. F. Newcomb, & W. W. Hartup (Eds.), *The company they keep: Friendships in childhood and adolescence* (pp. 66–86). New York: Cambridge University Press.

Howes, C. (1999). Attachment relationships in the context of multiple caregivers. In J. Cassidy & P. R. Shaver (Eds.), *Handbook of attachment theory and research* (pp. 671–687). New York: Guilford Press.

Howes, C., & Aikins, J. W. (2002). Peer relations in the transition to adolescence. In H. W. Reese & R. Kail (Eds.), *Advances in child development and behavior* (pp. 195–230). New York: Academic Press.

Howes, C., Guerra Wishard, A., & Zucker, E. (2008). Migrating from Mexico and sharing pretend with peers in the United States. *Merrill–Palmer Quarterly, 54*, 256–288.

Howes, C., & Lee, L. (2006). Peer relations in young children. In L. Balter & C. S. Tamis-Le Monda (Eds.), *Child psychology: A handbook of contemporary issues* (pp. 135–152). New York: Taylor & Francis.

Howes, C., & Lee, L. (2007). If you are not like me, can we play?: Peer groups in preschool. In B. Spodek & O. Saracho (Eds.), *Contemporary perspectives on research in social learning in early childhood education*. Durham, NC: Information Age.

Howes, C., & Phillipsen, L. (1992). Gender and friendship: Relationships within peer groups of young children. *Social Development, 1,* 230–242.

Howes, C., & Phillipsen, L. C. (1998). Continuity in children's relations with peers. *Social Development, 7,* 340–349.

Howes, C., & Ritchie, S. (1999). Attachment organizations in children with difficult life circumstances. *Developmental and Psychopathology, 11,* 254–268.

Howes, C., & Ritchie, S. (2002). *A matter of trust: Connecting teachers and learners in the early childhood classroom.* Teachers College Press.

Howes, C., Sanders, K., & Lee, L. (2008). Entering a new peer group in ethnically and linguistically diverse child care classrooms. *Social Development, 17,* 922–940.

Howes, C., & Shivers, E. M. (2006). New child–caregiver attachment relationships: Entering child care when the caregiver is and is not an ethnic match. *Social Development, 15,* 343–360.

Howes, C., & Tonyan, H. (2000). Links between adult and peer relationships across four developmental period. In K. A. Kerns, J. M. Contreras, & A. M. Neal-Barnett (Eds.), *Examining associations between parent–child and peer relationships* (pp. 85–113). New York: Greenwood.

Howes, C., with Unger, O. A., & Matheson, C. C. (1992). *The collaborative construction of pretend social pretend play functions.* Albany: State University of New York Press.

Howes, C., & Wishard, A. G. (2004). Revisiting sharing meaning: Looking through the lens of culture and linking shared pretend play through proto narrative development to emergent literacy. In E. Zigler, D. G. Singer, & S. J. Bishop-Josef (Eds.), *Children's play: The roots of literacy* (pp. 143–158). Washington, DC: Zero to Three.

Howes, C., & Wu, F. (1990). Peer interactions and friendships in an ethnically diverse school setting. *Child Development, 61,* 537–541.

Issacs, S. (1937). *Social development in children: A study of beginnings.* New York: Harcourt Brace.

Kerns, K. (1998). Attachment security, parent peer management practices and peer relationships in preschool. *Merrill–Palmer Quarterly, 44,* 504–522.

Kramer, L., & Gottman, J. (1992). Becoming a sibling: "With a little help from my friends." *Developmental Psychology, 28,* 685–699.

Kramer, L., & Kowal, A. K. (2005). Sibling relationship quality from birth to adolescence: The enduring contributions of friends *Journal of Family Psychology, 19,* 503–511.

Kyratzis, A. (2001). Emotion talk in preschool same-sex friendship groups: Fluidity over time and context. *Early Education and Development, 12,* 359–392.

Kyratzis, A., & Green, J. (1997). Jointly constructed narratives in classrooms: Co-construction of friendship and community through language. *Teaching and Teacher Education, 31,* 17–37.

Kyratzis, A., Marx, T., & Wade, E. R. (2001). Preschoolers communicative competence: Register shifts in the marking of power in different contexts friendship group talk. *First Language, 21,* 387–431.

Ladd, G. W., & Burgess, K. B. (1999). Charting the relationship trajectories of aggressive, withdrawn, and aggressive/withdrawn children during early grade school. *Child Development, 70,* 910–929.

Ladd, G. W., & Hart, C. H. (1992). Creating informal play opportunities are parents' and preschoolers' initiations related to children's competence with peers? *Developmental Psychology, 28,* 1179–1187.

Ladd, G. W., Kochenderfer, B. J., & Coleman, C. C. (1996). Friendship quality as a predictor of young children's early school adjustment. *Child Development, 67,* 1103–1118.

Ladd, G. W., & Pettit, G. (2002). Parenting and the development of children's peer relationships. In M. H. Bornstein (Ed.), *Handbook of parenting* (Vol. 5, pp. 377–409). Mahwah, NJ: Erlbaum.

Ladd, G. W., & Troop-Gordon, W. (2003). The role of chronic peer difficulties in the problems of children's psychological adjustment. *Child Development, 74,* 1344–1367.

Maudry, M., & Nekula, M. (1939). Social relations between children of the same age during the first two years of life. *Journal of Genetic Psychology, 54,* 193–215.

Newson, J., & Newson, E. (1970). *Four years old in an urban community*. Harmondsworth, UK: Penguin.

Park, K. A., Keng-Ling, L., & Ramsay, L. (1993). Individual differences and developmental changes in preschool friendships. *Developmental Psychology, 29*, 264–270.

Park, K. A., & Waters, E. (1989). Security of attachment and preschool friendships. *Child Development, 60*, 1076–1081.

Pianta, R. C., LaParo, K. M., & Hamre, B. (2004). *Classroom assessment scoring system*. Unpublished measure, University of Virginia, Charlottesville, VA.

Putallaz, M., Costanzo, P. R., Grimes, C. L., & Sherman, D. M. (1998). Intergenerational continuities and their influences on children's social development. *Social Development, 7*, 389–427.

Putallaz, M., Costanzo, P. R., & Smith, R. B. (1991). Maternal recollections of childhood peer relations: Implications for their children's social competence. *Journal of Social and Personal Relationships, 8*, 403–422.

Putallaz, M., Klein, T. P., Costanzo, P. R., & Hedges, L. A. (1994). Relating mothers' social framing to their children's entry competence with peers. *Social Development, 3*, 222–237.

Reed, K. H. (1950). *The nursery school: A human relationships laboratory*. Philadelphia: Saunders.

Rogoff, B. (2003). *The cultural nature of human development*. New York: Oxford University Press.

Ross, H. S., Conant, C. L., Cheyne, J. A., & Alevizos, E. (1992). Relationships and alliances in the social interactions of kibbutz toddlers. *Social Development, 1*, 1–17.

Rubenstein, J., & Howes, C. (1976). The effects of peers on toddler's interactions with mother and toys. *Child Development, 47*, 597–605.

Rubin, K. H., Bukowski, W., & Parker, J. (2006). Peer interactions, relationships, and groups. In N. Eisenberg, W. Damon, & R. Lerner (Eds.), *Handbook of child psychology: Vol. 3. Social, emotional, and personality development* (pp. 571–645). Hoboken, NJ: Wiley.

Rubin, K. H., Burgess, K. B., Dwyer, K. M., & Hastings, P. D. (2003). Predicting preschoolers' externalizing behaviors from toddler temperament, conflict, and maternal negativity. *Developmental Psychology, 39*, 164–176.

Rubin, K. H., Burgess, K. B., & Hastings, P. D. (2002). Stability and social-behavioral consequences of toddlers' inhibited temperament and parenting behaviors. *Child Development, 73*, 483–495.

Rubin, K. H., Hastings, P., Chen, X., Stewart, S., & McNichol, K. (1998). Interpersonal and maternal correlates of aggression, conflict, and externalizing problems in toddlers. *Child Development, 69*, 1614–1629.

Rubin, K. H., Lynch, D., Coplan, R., Rose-Krasnor, L., & Booth, C. L. (1994). "Birds of a feather . . . ": Behavioral concordances and preferential personal attraction in children. *Child Development, 65*, 1778–1785.

Rubin, K., Wojslawowicz, J. C., Rose-Krasnor, L., Booth-LaForce, C., & Burgess, K. B. (2006). The best friendships of shy/withdrawn children. *Journal of Abnormal Child Psychology, 34*, 143–157.

Schneider, B. H., Atkinson, L., & Tardiff, C. (2001). Child–parent attachment and children's peer relations: A quantitative review. *Developmental Psychology, 37*, 86–100.

Sebanc, A. M. (2003). The friendship features of preschool children: Links with prosocial behavior and aggression. *Social Development, 12*, 249–268.

Selman, R. (1980). *The growth of interpersonal understanding*. New York: Academic Press.

Serbin, L., & Sprafkin, C. (1986). The salience of gender and the process of sex typing in three to seven-year-old children. *Child Development, 57*, 1186–1199.

Snyder, J., Horsch, E., & Childs, J. (1997). Peer relationships of young children: Affiliative sources and the shaping of aggressive behavior. *Journal of Clinical Child Psychology, 26*, 145–156.

Solomon, D., Watson, M. S., Delucchi, K. L., Schaps, E., & Battistich, V. (1988). Enhancing children's prosocial behavior in the classroom. *American Educational Research Journal, 25*, 527–554.

Sroufe, L. A. (1983). Infant–caregiving attachment and patterns of maladaptation in preschool. In M. Permutter (Ed.), *Minnesota symposium on child psychology* (Vol. 16, pp. 41–81). Hillsdale, NJ: Erlbaum.

Vandell, D. (1987). Baby sister/baby brother: Reactions to the birth of a sibling and patterns of early sibling relations. In F. F. Schacter & R. K. Stone (Eds.), *Parental concerns about siblings: Bridging the research–practice gap* (pp. 13–37). New York: Haworth Press.

Vandell, D., & Mueller, E. (1980). Peer play and friendships during the first two years. In H. C. Foot, A. J. Chapman, & J. R. Smith (Eds.), *Friendships and social relationships in children* (pp. 181–208). New York: Wiley.

Vaughn, B. E., Colvin, T. N., Azria, M. R., Caya, L., & Krzysik, L. (2001). Dyadic analysis of friendship in a sample of preschool-age children attending head start: Correspondence between measures and implications for social competence. *Child Development, 72,* 862–878.

Walden, T., Lemerise, E., & Smith, M. C. (1999). Friendship and popularity in preschool classrooms. *Early Education and Development, 10,* 351–371.

Watson, M., & Battistich, V. (2006). Building and sustaining caring communities. In C. M. Evertson & C. S. Weinstein (Eds.), *Handbook of classroom management* (pp. 253–280). Mahwah, NJ: Erlbaum.

Youngblade, L. M., & Belsky, J. (1992). Parent–child antecedents of 5-year-olds' close friendships a longitudinal analysis. *Developmental Psychology, 28,* 700–713.

Youngblade, L. M., & Dunn, J. (1995). Individual differences in young children's pretend play with mother and siblings links to relationships and understanding of other people's feelings and beliefs. *Child Development, 66,* 1472–1492.

Youniss, J. (1980). *Parents and peers in social development.* Chicago: University of Chicago Press.

CHAPTER 11

Structural Descriptions of Social Transactions among Young Children

Affiliation and Dominance in Preschool Groups

BRIAN E. VAUGHN
ANTÓNIO JOSÉ SANTOS

Describing and explaining the benefits and costs of sociality have occupied the attention of political, social, and economic philosophers and social, behavioral, and developmental scientists for over 400 years (e.g., Hobbes, Locke, Rousseau, Smith, Marx, Darwin, G. S. Hall, Baldwin, Freud, Kropotkin, J. Moreno, Hinde, Kummer, McGrath, to name a few). The fundamental questions have been why and how it is that self-interest becomes subordinated (or not) to the interests of group comembers and why or how group norms, values, and structures change as a consequence of the actions of their constituent members and/or the embedding contexts of the group. Whereas philosophical treatments emphasized broad questions about "human nature" (e.g., egoist vs. communal) and the functional attributes of the groups (e.g., task-oriented or norm-enforcing), scientific approaches have tended to be pragmatic and problem focused (e.g., What sorts of structural features characterize different kinds of groups? Do groups have a "developmental" history? To what extent do group structures create affordances and/or impose constraints on the actions and developmental trajectories of members?). Wherever the emphasis was placed and whichever questions were asked, not until the last 80+ years have transactions within children's groups been considered relevant to those questions. In the first half of the 20th century, something of an intellectual sea change appears to have occurred in the behavioral sciences, and several researchers initiated studies of children's groups (e.g., Almack, 1922; Bott, 1928; Chevaleva-Janovskaja, 1927; Hagman, 1933; Hubbard, 1929; Wellman, 1926). For the most part, these studies were not directed at resolving arguments about human nature; rather, they were intended to provide information for educators, health care professionals, parents, and other adults who dealt with children on a routine basis.

With the introduction of sociometric theory by J. Moreno (e.g., 1932, 1933, 1934), the trickle of group studies with children became a torrent (e.g., Biehler, 1954; Dunnington, 1957a; Frankel, 1946; F. Moreno, 1942). J. Moreno's original formulation (1933, 1934) emphasized group structure as a function of the patterns of sympathy, antipathy, and indifferent feelings among group comembers. Studies with children emphasized notions of sociometric *status* based on aggregated sympathetic and antipathetic feelings of group comembers (e.g., F. Moreno, 1942; Dunnington, 1957a) and also raised questions about the uses of the technique for preschool-age children (e.g., Dunnington, 1957b; Marshall, 1957). These exchanges resulted in the picture sociometric task (McCandless & Marshall, 1957), which became the method of choice for obtaining positive and negative sociometric data from very young children. One effect of the emphasis on sociometric *status* and the introduction of the picture method was that assessments of acceptance and rejection replaced questions about affiliative structures and their affordances with questions about individual differences. Although children's affiliative structures remained salient to sociologists of childhood (e.g., Leinhardt, 1972) and to human ethologists (e.g., McGrew, 1972), developmental scientists did not return to the study of affiliative structures at the group level until the 1980s, and then from very different intellectual perspectives and with different methods (e.g., Cairns, 1983; Strayer, 1980a, 1980b; Strayer, Tessier, & Gariépy, 1985).

Of course, connection, cooperation, harmony, and friendship within the group always coexist with separation, competition, conflict, and enmity between comembers, and transactions within these latter relational categories give rise to structures that are in a dialectical relation with structures of affiliation. Whereas affiliative structures tend to reflect similarities among group members (the term "homophily" is used to describe such similarities; McPherson, Smith-Lovin, & Cook, 2001), the second set of structures reflects the coordination of power relations among group members that have their bases in comember asymmetries with regard to some physical–behavioral dimension and/or with regard to control of a desirable resource. Because size and directed aggression leading to submission ("agonistic" behavior) are often essential components of the asymmetries between group members, and because both concepts originated in ethology (a.k.a. behavioral biology and, recently, behavioral ecology), the term "social dominance" is used to characterize the structural properties of groups serving to regulate ingroup agonism (see Wilson [1975] for a discussion of the natural history of this concept, and Vermeij [2004] for an analysis of power as a control parameter driving evolutionary change at species, clade, and ecosystem levels).

Although agonism (both attack and submission components) contributes to dyadic dominance, it is a mistake to assume that the terms "dominance" and "aggressiveness" are synonymous. Whereas, "aggression" is a descriptor relevant to a specific category of acts initiated by an individual and "aggressiveness" is a trait descriptor referring the tendency of an individual to use aggressive acts, "dominance" is a relational term reflecting a pattern of exchanges within a dyad with respect to the initiation of an attack/threat *and* a submissive response and/or with respect to control of desired resources. These exchanges may be observed directly but are often inferred, such as when one child leaves a location or object at the approach of a peer, without a threat or implication of directed aggression from the other child. When one interactant initiates most frequently and the other responds by submitting to the initiator most frequently, the dyad is described as having established a dominance relationship. Initiations can be very subtle and may not reach the threshold of aggression, as such. Consequently, socially dominant children may not typically behave aggressively with subordinate children, and the most dominant children in a group may display aggressive behavior infrequently (e.g., Strayer, 1980b; Strayer & Strayer, 1976). Conversely, highly aggressive children would not achieve social dominance in their group if they lost most of the contests they initiated. At the group level, a dominance structure describes the ordering of established dominance relationships at the dyadic level. When these structures are transitive and rigid (i.e., when A is dominant to B, and B is dominant to C, then A also is dominant to C, and when there is an asymmetry with regard to initiations at the dyadic level with very few or no "reversals" at different positions in the structure), their organization is linear and hierarchical (Strayer, 1980a, 1981). It is important to keep in mind, however, that whereas the group dominance structure emerges from individual acts and reactions at the dyadic level, it is not reducible to rates or frequencies of individual actions.

The preceding remarks were intended to demarcate the scope and boundaries of the review to follow, but before embarking on our analysis and integration it will be helpful to offer a definition of "social structures" and to acknowledge the intellectual ecology that frames our interpretation of the research to be reviewed. There are at least three different ways that this concept has been used: (1) relative to the relations between entities or groups within larger social systems; (2) relative to the institutional and social norms, and the cognitive processes that influence individual behaviors within larger social systems; and (3) as a relatively enduring pattern of social arrangements or interrelations within a specific society, organization, or group (see Dornbusch, Glasgow, & Lin, 1996). The studies we review deal with small groups of preschool-age children, and the third approach to defining social structures is most relevant for our purposes, in part because enduring patterns of social arrangements can be observed at both macrostructural (e.g., whole group) and microstructural (e.g., dyad) levels. Because the embedding contexts (for a relevant discussion, see Arrow, McGrath, & Berdahl, 2000) and social ecologies (e.g., Strayer, 1989) can differ across groups, it is possible that affiliation and dominance structures will not always take the same forms in every group.

Regarding the intellectual ecology to which we adapted and have adopted, for various aesthetic and convenience reasons, we found the paradigms offered by evolutionary theory and behavioral biology (aka ethology, social ethology, behavioral ecology) to be attractive. Darwinian theory, especially as articulated in *The Expression of Emotion in Man and Animals* (Darwin, 1872), made the biological bases of human social behavior a legitimate target for scientific exploration (e.g., Hinde, 1974). Ethological theory and method, as summarized definitively by Tinbergen (1951), was deliberately oriented to the behavior of nonhuman animals and tended to emphasize causation and the ontogeny of behavior patterns through time (only two of Tinbergen's four "why" questions relevant to the causes of behavior; see Hinde, 1966). Special emphasis on Tinbergen's other two "why" questions (the adaptive function of behavior and the evolution of behavioral structure) characterized social ethology, which branched from the classical root in the 1960s and 1970s (e.g., Crook, 1970a, 1970b; Kummer, 1968, 1971). Crook (1970a) suggested that three interdependent features of social behavior should be the topics of social ethology: (1) comparative study of social structure and communicative behavior in relation to dynamics of the physical habitat; (2) analysis of relations between social organization in stable groups and general features of population dynamics; and (3) behavioral processes that maintain group structure, regulate social change, and determine differential reproductive success of group members. Importantly, social ethologists saw no a priori reason to exclude human social behavior from their scientific studies (but for a classical treatment of human behavior, see Eibl-Eibesfeldt, 1989). Although very little research with children addresses Crook's second topic, a number of ethological studies have addressed the first and third topics.

For both classic and social ethology, emphasis is placed on the observation and analysis of behavior in natural settings. Whereas in classical ethology, the primary objects studied and explained are the "fixed action patterns" characteristic of the species, in social ethology, social transactions and the structures emergent from those transactions constitute the primary entities for study. By definition, "social transactions" involve two or more actors, and the sequences are less "fixed" than may be true for patterns of individual acts. Even so, initial formulations from social ethology suggested that the structural features of groups were species-specific adaptations analogous to fixed action patterns. Longer observations in more groups and species revealed a wealth of diversity and complexity among primates, and early assumptions about the fixed quality of social structures were replaced by the notion that social groups were dynamic systems whose structural organization reflected an ongoing interaction of behavioral and ecological processes operating within the adaptive range tolerable for the species (Crook, 1970b).

This shift in assumptions about social organization raised the salience of adaptive function to a central focus for social ethology. Moreover, diversity of social adaptation could be documented for both individuals and groups as they respond to the interplay of behavioral and local ecological processes over ontogenetic and phylogenetic time. For individuals, diversity of function allows for the practice in multiple social roles with many partners, which may benefit both the self and social partners (i.e., why play is valued by the immature). At the group level, norms may evolve; for example, the punishment of noncooperative group comembers, even when interactants engage only in a single exchange (e.g., Boyd, Gintis, Bowles, & Richerson, 2003; Boyd & Richerson, 2002). In short, the discipline of social ecology opened possibilities for resolving questions regarding relations between developing individuals and the groups in which they are embedded. We found the reliance on naturalistic field observations, the intimate connection between method and theory, and the possibility that outsiders could remove disciplinary boundaries separating behavioral and social science domains to be aesthetically pleasing. For newly minted developmental scientists, social ethology offered novel questions to answer. As corollaries to the Tinbergen "why" questions, Kummer (1971) framed the research program for the new field with reference to five issues, adding emphases on dynamics (i.e., change as a fundamental feature of living systems) and time (development as both a process and a context, and phylogenetic processes linked to development). These are paraphrased below:

1. *Structural analysis*: a description of the organizational conditions of a living system, such as the anatomical underpinnings of a particular behavior pattern or the spatial arrangement of group members.
2. *Causal analysis*: the necessary and sufficient conditions, or the underlying processes that lead to the appearance of the behavioral structures under study.
3. *Functional analysis*: the immediate outcome, or emerging processes associated with the observed activity that increase the survival value or reproductive success of the living system.

4. *Ontogeny*: the study of organic, social, and ecological processes that shape changes during the course of individual development.
5. *Phylogeny*: the long-term processes that determine survivorship and directly shape the genetic heritage on which ontogeny depends.

Kummer (1971) identified two parameters for describing the grouping tendencies in a given species or population: (1) the distribution of individuals in space over time, and (2) the frequency and quality of interindividual communication. Frequently, temporal stability of a group structure is assessed by documenting the persistence of these parameters through time. However, because demonstrations of temporal stability serve primarily to validate initial descriptive analyses of group organization, Kummer stressed that descriptions must be complemented by causal and/or functional analysis of the derived social structures. That is to say, what transactions produce these structures and what are they good for?

Well before the formal promotion of social ethology/ecology to the status of a discipline, comparative psychologists and primatologists had argued that social organization involved a constant dialectic between cohesive and dispersive forces operating within the group. The necessity to optimize (or at least satisfice) the balance between these forces explained both affiliative and dominance structures and the temporal stability of primate groups. Social "cohesion" was thought to depend upon common interests in specific ecological contexts or with regard to control of resources; social "dispersion" derived from the inevitable conflicts of interest arising because some individuals attempted to maximize access to resources at the expense of group comembers (e.g., Carpenter, 1942; Yerkes, 1939). Applying these issues and insights to the study of children's groups seemed an obvious "next step."

Affiliation and Affiliative Structures in Preschool Children's Groups

Dictionary definitions of the term "affiliation" emphasize formal and/or informal connections, association, or bonds between entities (individuals, groups, or institutions), with stated or implied rules governing their affiliation. For preschool children, affiliations are usually inferred from assessments of social transactions, from child interviews, or from the reports of adults. When information about all (or most) children in a group is obtained, the multiple dyadic connections linking each individual to others in the group is referred to as an "affiliation network." For young children, the "rules" governing affiliation are informal and typically involve an obligation to play together (e.g., Corsaro, 1979; Howes, 1988). Repeated violation of the play rule usually results in the disruption or dissolution of the affiliative relationship (at least for a period of time).

Although developmental (e.g., Parten, 1932) and ethnographic studies (e.g., Corsaro, 1985), of affiliation and social participation have a long history in studies of preschoolers, these have tended to emphasize normative trends in the quality of social participation or the motives underlying participation rather than the properties of regularity and predictability giving rise to affiliative structures. Sociometric methods might have produced useful structural data for preschool children (e.g., Frankel, 1946), but the this approach was co-opted for the purposes of identifying individual differences with respect to the quality of social behavior in the 1940s and 1950s (e.g., McCandless & Marshall, 1957), and these possibilities were not realized. For adults, sociometry served as primary data for directed graphic theory and associated analytic strategies (e.g., Harary, Norman, & Cartwright, 1978; J. Moreno, 1955) and the analysis of social networks (e.g., Wasserman, Faust, & Iacobucci, 1994), both of which are mature fields of study in the social sciences today. More recently, social network concepts have crossed disciplinary boundaries and have enriched subdisciplines within the behavioral and developmental sciences.

A range of social network studies have been initiated with groups of preschool children; however, these come in two varieties (i.e., egocentric and sociocentric). "Egocentric" networks start from the perspective of the person and assess the connections between that person and the social world (e.g., Bost, 1995; Bost, Cielinski, Washington, & Vaughn, 1994; Reid, Landesman, Treder, & Jaccard, 1989). Egocentric network data often identify a range of individual differences related to a variety of physical, social, and mental health outcomes (e.g., Bost, Vaughn, Washington, Cielinski, & Bradbard, 1998); however, these data do not identify structural features of the peer group. Consequently, the usefulness of egocentric network data is uncertain regarding questions about affiliative structures, and we do not further discuss this body of research. In contrast, "sociocentric" network assessments assume a bounded group (e.g., classroom, grade level, work group, agency) and attempt to identify affiliations within the bounded group. Interview, survey, and observation formats have been used to collect network information with adults, adolescents, and older children (e.g., Almack, 1922; Cairns, Leung, Buchanan, & Cairns, 1995; Wasserman et al., 1994; Wellman, 1926); however, interview and survey methods have not been used successfully with preschool children. Cairns et al. (1995) referred to the older child's responses in terms of a "social-cognitive map" (SCM) of the group. Preschool-age children rarely report groups larger than dyads, and they tend to be more accurate about their own dyadic participation (e.g., Hagman, 1933) than about the partners of their classmates (Bost, personal communication, November 15, 2006; Martin, personal communication, March 28, 2007). For this reason, the SCM approach to data acquisition is not widely used with young children.

Observational studies of social preferences were pioneered in the 1920s (e.g., Bott, 1928; Hubbard, 1929), and Hagman (1933) was the first to compare children's reports of their play partners with observations of who played with whom. Chevaleva-Janovskaja (1927) studied a large number of preschool groups and documented the extent of homogeneity with respect to age and sex typical of these groups, anticipating Maccoby and Jacklin (1987) by 60 years. For several reasons, direct observations of naturally occurring behavior of preschool children fell from fashion in developmental research during the 1950s and 1960s, and such research was reported less and less often in journals such as *Child Development*. It was not until human ethologists started studying children (e.g., Blurton-Jones, 1972; McGrew, 1972; Strayer & Strayer, 1976) that developmental scientists returned to the preschool classroom in larger numbers.

We noted earlier that affiliative structures reflect within-group homophilies. It has been widely noted (e.g., LaFreniere, Strayer, & Gauthier, 1984; Maccoby & Jacklin, 1987; Martin, Ruble, & Szkrybalo, 2002; Serbin, Moller, Gulko, Powlishta, & Colburne, 1994; Vaughn et al., 2000) that sex structures affiliation from the early years of life forward (the first homophily). The tendency to interact with same-sex partners appears by the middle of the second year, at least in observational studies, and increases over the preschool years (e.g., LaFreniere et al., 1984). Fabes, Martin, and Hanish (2004) suggest that the tendency to seek out same-sex play partners both reinforces and shapes developmental patterns of gender-typed behavior in young children. Of course, preschool children do not choose playmates randomly from the roster of same-gender children in their groups; additional constraints apply.

McPherson et al. (2001) suggested that homophilies could be grouped into "status" and "behavioral" categories. With the exception of sex, most status variables identified by McPherson et al. as important for adults (e.g., race/ethnicity, age, socioeconomic status [SES], religious affiliation) have not been reported to be meaningful in specifying affiliative structures for preschoolers. It is possible that these status dimensions are not salient for preschool children. It is also the case that variability along dimensions of age, SES, and religious affiliation variables tends to be low in most preschool groups (e.g., most classes are age-graded, and most programs serve families who are roughly equivalent for SES indicators). Thus, potential effects of status are not observed. Behavioral homophilies have also received attention (e.g., Martin, Fabes, Hanish, & Hollenstein, 2005; Pellegrini, Long, Roseth, Bohn, & van Ryzin, 2007); however, as Fabes et al. (2004) note, behavioral homophilies are often gender-typed, and it is difficult to distinguish behavioral homophilies from status homophilies when interpreting preschooler's peer preferences. It is also true that similarity, however categorized, rarely links a child to specific group members in a manner allowing a depiction of the network of social affiliations in the group, above the level of dyadic friendships (but for a nuanced integration of local experience in a group with within-sex differences in activity preference, see Pellegrini, Long, et al., 2007).

This was the problem Strayer (e.g., 1980a, 1980b) attempted to resolve by introducing behavioral sociometry to child ethology. "Behavioral sociometry" is based on observations of directed affiliative behaviors, where "affiliative behaviors" are approaches, directed interactions (excluding attacks and threats), visual attention, and physical proximity. Affiliative links between any pair of group members may be unilateral (when one dyad member is the primary initiator of directed acts) or bilateral (when both dyad members direct acts to each other), and the significance of a link may be determined by comparing the relative frequency of initiated acts to a fixed value (the average of initiated acts directed to all groupmates). Following J. Moreno's (1934) method, Strayer prepared behavioral sociograms for his preschool groups to summarize their affiliation structures (e.g., Strayer et al., 1985).

Behavioral sociograms provide a range of insights into group organization and function including mutual/bilateral exchange of bids, identification of cohesively connected subgroups of children within the classroom group, and centers of behavioral exchange within the larger group that extend the utility of sociometric data beyond the individual-difference information contained in total acceptance or total rejection scores. Strayer's graphs (e.g., 1980b) revealed substantial symmetry between members of the network (at least at the dyadic level) with regard to the exchange of affiliative initiations. In contrast with idealized dominance structures (i.e., as transitive and hierarchical), affiliative networks were neither linear nor hierarchical. Even so, the information in the sociograms proved analytically intractable and did not easily lend itself to quantitative comparisons within or across groups, in part because each group could be described with a unique sociogram, and in part because slight alterations in the cut point could produce different sociograms for a given group. It was not until school-age children's social networks emerged as a topic of study (e.g., Cairns, Cairns, Neckerman, Gest, & Gariépy, 1988) that new approaches to the characterization of affiliative structures for preschool children were described.

As noted earlier, the SCM procedure is based on nominations of peers who "hang out together," and the demands of the task make it inappropriate for preschool-age children. Investigators studying young children have necessarily relied on *observations* of affiliative behavior within the group to identify subgroups within preschool classes (e.g., Martin & Fabes, 2001; Santos, Vaughn, & Bonnet, 2000; Strayer & Santos, 1996). Santos, Strayer, and associates (Santos et al., 2000; Santos & Strayer, 1997; Strayer & Santos, 1996) examined proximity matrices of children in preschool classrooms who had been observed over a period of several weeks (up to 2,000 observations in a given classroom). In the Strayer and Santos study, the analyses grouped together children with similar profiles of proximity to all other class members. Distinct subgroups of children were observed in all classrooms, and both average subgroup size and the degree of mutuality of affiliative exchanges tended to increase with age. Furthermore, the proportion of children identified as members of subgroups increased from about 50% for the youngest children to over 90% for the oldest children.

Santos et al. (2000) used these procedures for grouping children to describe the affiliation structure for a single classroom of 4- to 5-year-old children as it evolved over the school year. For the most part, the subgroup structure remained intact across three waves of data collection, and children who were ungrouped at the beginning of the year tended to become group members in subsequent waves of data collection. Santos et al. also reported the existence of a new subgroup category. These were children with similar profiles of proximity vis-à-vis other classmates but who did not show significant proximity to each other. They referred to these cases as "aggregates" or "low mutual proximity" (LMP) subgroups. Finally, Santos et al. showed that the subgroups could be ordered by sociometric rank (average of subgroup members) and that preferences for subgroup members were greater in subgroups with higher sociometric rank. Taken together, the results reported by Santos, Strayer, and associates indicate that preschool classes can be subdivided reliably into coherent subgroups that exchange affiliative behaviors and sociometric preferences; nevertheless, these data present static pictures of the group and do not describe the emergence or change of structures at the group level.

Martin et al. (2005) modeled changing affiliative structures by applying dynamic systems principles to subgroup formation and maintenance using state space grid methods (e.g., Lewis, Zimmerman, Hollenstein, & Lamey, 2004). Not surprisingly, over 70% of all social initiations were directed to a same-sex peer and children tended to return to same-sex play more rapidly than they returned to mixed-sex play. However, partner behavioral style was also a significant predictor of initiation preference and, for some children, was more influential than sex. The status homophily (i.e., sex) also influenced the affect expressed in interactive contexts. Positive affect was nearly three times more likely with same-sex than with other-sex partners and, for girls, negative affect was almost four times more likely when interacting with a boy. These findings suggest the possibility that whereas status homophilies may bring children together, it is the affect expressed in the subgroup that determines whether the subgroup becomes a high mutual proximity or LMP type. The exchange and the balance of positive versus negative affects may also contribute to subgroup changes over time (e.g., expelling members, incorporating new members, replacing members who leave the class; see Schmidt & Griffin, 2007).

The social ecology and dynamic systems approaches to studying affiliative structures are complementary in terms of enlarging our understanding of why and how children choose specific partners from available peers. The kinds of data used in both approaches are identical, but the clustering algorithms (e.g., Santos & Strayer, 1997) aggregate observations across time and link specific individuals together (but not what it is that linked individuals *do* together), whereas dynamical analyses preserve the temporal ordering of social transactions but do not easily preserve the identities of interactive partners (thus identifying what happens when, but not with whom). A challenge for future work with preschool groups will be to integrate these approaches in a single investigation to understand both how subgroups emerge in newly formed classrooms and how established subgroups are maintained over the school year. To the extent that specific partners provide unique opportunities to exercise motor, social, and academic skills, it seems likely that stable subgroups will influence behavior, affect experiences, and cognitions of subgroup members (e.g., Daniel, Santos, Vaughn, & Peceguina, 2007; Pellegrini, Long, et al., 2007). Thus, subgroups may provide specific affordances for comembers and may contribute to the construction of social roles, social norms, and social ecologies characteristic of preschool classrooms.

Dominance Structures in Preschool Children's Groups

Whereas affiliative structures reflect cohesive, interdependent features of group life that emerge from social exchanges underlying social preferences, dominance relationships and dominance structures reflect self-interest and dyadic asymmetries regarding social power. The concepts of dominance and hierarchy were imported by child ethologists from animal studies, especially studies on nonhuman primates (e.g., see reviews by Bernstein, 1980; Dewsbury, 1982). As with nonhuman primates, the early ethological studies of dominance in children used direct observations of dyadic conflicts to determine "winners" and "losers" (e.g., Abramovitch, 1976; McGrew, 1972; Sluckin & Smith, 1977; Strayer, Chapeskie, & Strayer, 1978; Strayer & Strayer, 1976; Vaughn & Waters, 1980). These studies showed that "attack–submit" and/or "win–loss" matrices for most, if not all, preschool groups could be arranged in a manner consistent with the presence of a dominance hierarchy, although the linearity and rigidity (i.e., proportion of dominance "reversals" in the matrix) of these hierarchies varied across studies and hierarchies based on conflicts over resources were not always strongly correlated with hierarchies based only on outcomes of attack–submit encounters (e.g., Vaughn & Waters, 1981).

Cross-sectional studies have shown that linear dominance hierarchies can be inferred from the directed agonism of toddlers as young as 15 to 18 months of age. Strayer and Trudel (1984) found that nearly 75% of peer dyads in toddler classrooms engaged in agonistic exchanges with distinct "attacker" versus "submission" roles. Hawley and Little (1999) reported a similar percentage for toddlers based on teacher's judgments of dominance. In Strayer's studies (e.g., 1989), the percentage of observed dominance dyads declined (to 55% for 3-year-olds and to 40% for 5-year-olds), but the rigidity and stability of hierarchies increased over this period. The reduced number of observed attacks leading to submission after 3 years of age is consistent with the often reported finding that physical aggression declines in frequency and as a proportion of overall social initiations after age 3 (e.g., Tremblay, 2002), but it raises questions about the structural features of dominance hierarchies. For example, how is it that groups of older children (in which the rates of aggressive exchanges are reduced and in which fewer dominance–subordinate relationships can be directly observed) have dominance structures that are more linear/ transitive and more rigid than for groups of younger children?

Drawing on the nonhuman primate data, Strayer (e.g., 1989) suggested that one consequence of an established dominance hierarchy in a given group should be the reduction of frequencies of within-group aggression, in part because members are aware of group dominance relations, and they behave so as to reduce the likelihood of conflicts with members whose rank is higher than their own. Strayer concluded that the relatively more advanced cognitive capacities of older (compared to younger) preschool children should make it more likely that they are consciously aware of the dominance status of peers. Findings relevant to this interpretation for preschool children are mixed, with some (e.g., Pellegrini, Roseth, et al., 2007) finding reduced rates of aggression after dominance hierarchies are established, and others (e.g., Vaughn & Waters, 1981) failing to find a decline in aggressive initiations. From another perspective, Hawley (1999) suggested that dominant children achieve and maintain rank in the group by using *both* prosocial and coercive behavioral strategies, and that the decline of aggression in young children's groups after age 3 may reflect increasing awareness of the utility of prosocial means for getting one's way.

Whether due to prowess as aggressors, to their success in securing access to resources, or to other factors, dominant individuals are central members of their groups. Chance (1967; Chance & Jolly, 1970) was one of the first to refer to dominant individuals in primate groups as "centers of attention." Observational studies of children verified that dominant children did command the visual attention of their peers (e.g., Abramovitch, 1976; Hold-Cavell & Borsutzky, 1986; LaFreniere & Charlesworth, 1983; Pellegrini, Roseth, et al., 2007; Vaughn & Waters, 1980, 1981), and Vaughn, Vollenweider, Bost, Azria-Evans, and Snider (2003) found similar results when the assessment of dominance was based on observer Q-sort ratings rather than on observed conflicts. Of course, there are several reasons why dominant children might be targets of peers' visual attention. On the one hand, to the extent that dominant children are leaders who control salient resources, paying attention to their behavior could be a means of obtaining information about the quality of the immediate social context and the direction of ongoing activities. On the other hand, if peers perceive dominant children as potentially dangerous, keeping an eye on them should be a useful strategy for avoiding potentially damaging interactions. To date, the relevant data are more consistent with the former interpretation than with the latter.

Both Chance (1967) and Seyfarth (1977) stressed that primate social activities are influenced by dominance status differences among group members. The underlying principle is attraction to high rank, with dominant individuals receiving more than their share of the total positive activity within the group. As a result, dominance status coordinates the distribution of affiliative investment (e.g., social grooming for monkeys) in the group. Strayer and associates (e.g., Strayer & Nöel, 1986) reported that dominant children tend to intervene in conflicts between other group members and these children also tend to be preferred targets for peers' positive affiliative bids. The results of these studies instantiate for preschool children the general truth that power is attractive (for a review and theoretical integration, see Keltner, Gruenfeld, & Anderson, 2003); however, Vaughn and Waters (1981) counterargued that it was not social power per se but rather *social competence* that attracted peer attention and affiliative bids. They suggested that social competence was an important antecedent to both dominance (e.g., by choosing which opponents to engage and at what intensity) and peer popularity (e.g., by choosing specific partners as playmates and as recipients of cooperative support in nonplay endeavors). These competing interpretations were not reconciled until the mid-1980s, when Charlesworth and associates (e.g., Charlesworth & Dzur, 1987; Charlesworth &

LaFreniere, 1983) showed that preschool children use both prosocial and coercive tactics in their attempts to maximize access to classroom resources; that is, dominant children seemed to know that they did not necessarily need to fight with or threaten their peers to get what they wanted.

Based on empirical and conceptual arguments, Charlesworth (1988) suggested that the criterion for dominance in humans should be shifted from directed agonism leading to submission to success in gaining and maintaining control over salient resources (see discussion by LaFreniere, 1996). This reorientation represented a break with ethological traditions insofar as most ethologists considered preferential access to resources to be a consequence of dominance rather than its criterion. Nevertheless, Charlesworth's conceptualization accounted for findings that frequency or intensity of aggressive behavior did not necessarily distinguish children at different positions in group dominance hierarchies (e.g., Pellegrini, Roseth, et al., 2007) and that high rates of initiating aggression did not necessarily translate into increased utilization of resources (e.g., LaFreniere, 1996; LaFreniere & Charlesworth, 1987). Furthermore, when dominance is conceptualized in terms of resource control, the relevance of prosocial behaviors, including cooperation, sharing, and providing assistance/support to peers, for achieving dominance becomes apparent. Likewise, psychological manipulation and deception (including self-deception) may also have a role in resource control. Recent discussions of social dominance in children's groups take Charlesworth's position on resource control as their starting point (e.g., Hawley, 1999; Roseth, Pellegrini, Bohn, van Ryzin, & Vance, 2007).

In her theory of social dominance, Hawley (1999) adopted a position that was even further from ethology than the view Charlesworth had articulated. Drawing on sociobiology and evolutionary psychology (e.g., Alexander, 1979; Cosmides & Tooby, 1987; MacDonald, 1988; Trivers, 1971), she suggested that social dominance was a result of "asymmetries among individuals in their ability to prevail in competition" (pp. 97–98) over salient resources, and that *any* strategy (e.g., coercion, cooperation, deception) could at different times or in different social contexts be used to acquire those resources. Of course, a range of parameters contributed to success in competitions over resources, including age, size, and motivation, as well as skills honed by practice. Perhaps more important than these were the attributes of group members. Hawley (1999) assumed that children assessed their position in the group and adjusted their control strategies according to the dominance status of their dyadic competitor. Finally, she argued that defining dominance as the strategic use of behavior and cognition to control resources supported a developmental perspective on social dominance that had not emerged from either ethological or sociobiological treatments of dominance. In her model, coercive strategies emerged first, between 1.5 and 3 years of age, followed by mixed coercive and prosocial strategies between 4 and 7 years of age, and finally by the separation of coercive and prosocial strategies around 8 years of age, with individuals specializing in prosocial resource control strategies being seen as "leaders" and individuals specializing in coercive strategies being seen as "bullies" (p. 110).

Although many hypotheses implied by Hawley's model lie beyond the scope of this review, her research in toddler and preschool groups has been largely consistent with her theoretical premises. For example, Hawley and Little (1999) determined the dominance ranks of toddler-age children in small groups, then examined dyadic play interactions in laboratory tasks designed to have a central attractive aspect presumed to interest both interactants. Consistent with predictions from Hawley's model, dominance rank was associated with individual-level characteristics (e.g., level of development, motivation), and interactions in the dyads were mediated by dominance rank. Dominant dyad members exploited the attractive component of the task more than did subordinate members. Dyadic dominance also predicted greater engagement and direction of mutual play in the dyad tasks, and lower levels of passive onlooking and imitation of partner. As predicted, children at the middle of the dominance ranking acted "dominant" when paired with lower ranking peers and "subordinate" when paired with higher ranking peers. Overall, these findings support Hawley's (1999) conceptual model, although the dyadic play data suggest that dominant children may use prosocial strategies for resource control at earlier ages than she originally suggested.

In subsequent studies with older preschoolers, Hawley (2002, 2003) suggested that children using both prosocial and coercive strategies for resource control succeeded in controlling resources more effectively than did children using only prosocial strategies (although these "bistrategic" children did not differ significantly from peers using only coercive strategies). Both prosocial and coercive resource control strategies were positively predicted by parent ratings of child social competence (Hawley, 2002), but bistrategic children were more preferred by peers in a sociometric task than were children using only coercive resource control strategies (bistrategic children also had higher preference scores than did average and noncontrolling children; Hawley, 2003). Hawley reported that bistrategic children evidenced more advanced moral reasoning than did either highly prosocial controllers or average and noncontrolling children, but were not different from highly coercive controlling children. Taken together, these results are broadly consistent with her conceptual framework and also with the notion that dominance may be an indicator of *social competence* (Vaughn, 1999). Consistent with this conclusion, Vaughn et al. (2003) reported that preschool children scoring higher on a *Q*-sort scale labeled "dominant–aggressive" had higher scores on a composite measure of social competence, even after controlling for coercive aggression.

The study of dominance in preschool groups has changed considerably over the past 30+ years, from ethologically grounded, descriptive studies demonstrating that hierarchically organized dominance structures based on dyadic agonism were present in most, if not all, groups to sociobiologically informed, quantitative, model-driven studies testing explicit hypotheses concerning the expression of dominance strategies at varying developmental time points. Most investigators studying dominance consider resource control rather than outcomes of directed agonism as the primary criterion of social dominance. One consequence of this shift has been the explicit connection between coercive and prosocial behavior in the service of competition, which hints at links between the dominance and affiliative group structures. At the same time, the shift in conceptual grounding (from social ethology to sociobiology) of research on dominance emphasizes its functional aspects for individuals at the expense of its structural aspects; that is, to the extent that dominance "hierarchies" are group-level structures with functional consequences for the group, these consequences are no longer central in dominance research. This loss of research diversity is regrettable, because it severs historical ties with concerns of primatologists and sociologists who have studied social influence at the group and subgroup levels. When dominance is treated as an individual-difference variable, the social negotiations maintaining group dominance structures are obscured, as well as the subtle interplay of affiliation preferences and dominance that characterize the day-to-day interactions of group members. Furthermore, taking an evolutionary–psychological perspective on dominance implies that prosocial behavior may function as a sophisticated competitive tactic rather than a distinct facet of human sociality (see Kropotkin, 1902).

Groups of Preschool Children: Integrating Affiliation and Dominance

At the outset of this chapter, we suggested that social and behavioral scientists recognize that most human activity takes place in groups, and that these groups both provide affordances for and impose constraints on actions of and interactions between members. Most group research addresses in one way or another questions concerning these affordances and/or constraints. For children, salient groups include families and peers, with peers being encountered most frequently in the context of child care and educational settings (at least in modern cultures with industry and/or service-based economies). Although it is historically true that formally organized peer groups were not normative until children reached primary school, for the last 25 years it has become normative that children are in formal group care with peers from 2–3 years of age forward. Thus, it is reasonable to study the structural features of their groups and to consider the results in light of findings with older children and adults (not to mention other group-living mammals and birds). Interestingly, when preschool children are aggregated into groups, they face the same challenges facing groups of older children, adolescents, and adults. What is perhaps more interesting is the degree of similarity in solutions to these problems across developmental periods and across taxa.

When children join a group (either at group formation or when entering an established group), they face two critical challenges with regard to their peer comembers: (1) determining the resource value (which may be denominated in terms of homophily along salient dimensions, such as sex, motivation for social engagement, play skills, availability, etc.) of comembers, and (2) assessing the relative differences between themselves and group comembers along dimensions of action and cognition relevant to power. Assuming no foreknowledge about peer resource value and power differences at the outset, the period of group formation will likely resemble a scramble competition (Packer, 2000; Pellegrini, 2008) in which children initiate interaction and change partners frequently to discover the best playmates available in the group and their social power relative to group comembers. From this scramble, which may take days or weeks to complete, affiliation preferences and social networks, as well as dominance orders, emerge. Although the data relevant to this assumption are sparse, findings suggest that both affiliative networks and dominance hierarchies are present in preschool groups within several weeks after group formation. From the perspective of this chapter, it is of interest that a given set of transactions at the dyadic level, immediately following group formation, may determine both resource value of group comembers *and* dyadic dominance status.

Vaughn and Waters (1981) reported significant rank stability for social dominance across adjacent terms of the preschool academic year for a class of 4- and 5-year-olds, suggesting early formation of the hierarchy in preschool classrooms. Strayer (1989) and Roseth et al. (2007) predicted and observed that aggressive contests declined over the course of the preschool academic year after the dominance hierarchy was established. In a comparable analysis of social network data, Santos et al. (2000) found that proximity-based affiliation structures identified in the first term of the preschool academic year were largely reproduced in data collected during the winter and spring terms for a classroom of 4- and 5-year-olds. What is not clear from these studies is whether the described emergent social structures required extensive sampling or testing of peer qualities on a one-to-one basis (as suggested by the "scramble" hypotheses discussed earlier) or whether children can acquire this information by watching the interactions of their peers, even those with whom they, themselves, do not interact.

If the primary structural features of groups emerge from a scramble-like competition shortly after the onset of group formation, how might these two structural aspects be related or integrated, and how should this integration be described and analyzed? Given the discussions of dominance highlighting the competence and prosocial behaviors of socially dominant preschool children (e.g., Hawley, 2002, 2003), it might seem that power and affiliation structures should overlap. Intuition in this instance proves a poor guide. First, a critical challenge for an integrative analysis of affiliative and dominance structures concerns relations of order. Whereas dominance hierarchies reflect asymmetries between group members and can be reduced to rank orders for analysis, affiliation networks reflect symmetries among subgroup members and do not reduce to a rational rank order. Practically speaking, this means that dominant children can be described in terms of individual-level trait or behavioral descriptors that correlate with dominance rank (e.g., Hawley, 2002; LaFreniere & Charlesworth, 1987; Pellegrini, Roseth, et al., 2007), but subgroups in an affiliative network must be described using group-level descriptors that explain within-subgroup similarity but are not necessarily useful for characterizing between-subgroup differences. A second challenge concerns the loss of information entailed by shifting from a directed graph representation to rank orders. For example, when dominance structures are reduced to ranks and associated with other individual difference variables, we may learn who does *what*, but we lose information about who does what *to whom*. Affiliation structures add information about who does what *with whom* and on *whose behalf* to the pool of information about group functioning.

In an attempt to resolve the ordering problem for affiliation structures, Santos and associates (Santos, 1993; Santos & Winegar, 1999) described subgroup distinctions in terms of peer acceptance (i.e., the tendency of social subgroups to be composed of children with relatively similar levels of peer acceptance, such that the subgroups can be rank-ordered) and showed that such orderings are related to indicators of in- versus out-group preferences on both interaction and sociometric measures (i.e., greater ingroup preference with higher sociometric status). In future studies, it will be useful to collect dominance and affiliation data together, to discover whether children with similar positions in the dominance hierarchy seek out each other as interaction partners, or whether the subgroups are mixed with respect to dominance status.

Summary and Conclusion

In retrospect, it is curious that studies linking dominance status and affiliative networks have not been reported, because most conceptualizations of dominance presume that dominant group members are highly salient to others. As such, dominant children might be expected to receive interactive bids from less dominant group members and to be members of preferred social subgroups. Strayer and Nöel (1986) reported that highly dominant children were sometimes prosocially aggressive (e.g., defending a lower-status peer from attack), and that other members of the group showed approval of aggressive behavior in these circumstances. Similarly, Hawley (2002) reported that socially dominant preschoolers engaged in more prosocial (*and* coercive) behavior in a dyadic play task than did subordinate children (i.e., low resource controllers from teacher ratings) and Pellegrini (2008) reported that children more successful in scramble competitions tended to display more cooperative behavior than did less successful children.

Strayer (1989) interpreted his data on third-party interventions in dyadic conflict to mean that social competence entails the co-adaptation of affiliative and dominance motivations. His position is more nuanced and appealing than the sociobiological argument, in that he suggests that affiliation and dominance have distinct motivational systems, with different evolutionary and ontogenetic histories, rather than being alternative pathways to resource control. Social integration and life success require skills supported by both motivational domains for members of mammalian social species, perhaps especially when the evolutionary history of those species suggests intense intergroup competition, as is the case for many primates, including *Homo sapiens* (e.g., Bloom, 1997; Manson & Wrangham, 1991). The extant empirical literature suggests that both integration and competition are salient features of children's groups, and that affiliative and dominance motivational systems are complexly interrelated at the level of the individual child. It seems plausible that the transactions between the group structures associated with these motivational systems should reflect this complexity as well. Discovering when, how, and to what end these structural interactions occur will no doubt become the central topic of this chapter in the next edition of this *Handbook*.

Acknowledgments

Preparation of this chapter was supported in part by National Science Foundation Grant Nos. BCS 99-05926, BCS 01-26163, and BCS 06-23019, and by Fundação para a Ciência e Tecnologia Grant No. POCTI/PSI/46739/2002. We wish to thank F. F. Strayer, Anthony Pellegrini, João R. Daniel, Inês Peceguina, and William Griffin for their insightful comments on an earlier version of this chapter. (All errors and misstatements remain the responsibility of the authors.)

References

Abramovitch, R. (1976). The relation of attention and proximity to rank in preschool children. In M. R. A. Chance & R. R. Larsen (Eds.), *The social structure of attention* (pp. 153–176). London: Wiley.

Alexander, R. D. (1979). *Darwinism and human affairs*. Seattle: University of Washington Press.

Almack, J. C. (1922). The influence of intelligence on the selection of associates. *School and Society, 16*, 529–530.

Arrow, H., McGrath, J. E., & Berdahl, J. L. (2000). *Small groups as complex systems: Formation, coordination, development, and adaptation*. Thousand Oaks, CA: Sage.

Bernstein, I. S. (1980). Dominance: A theoretical perspective for ethologists. In D. R. Omark, F. F. Strayer, & D. G. Freedman (Eds.), *Dominance relations: An ethological view of human conflict and social interaction* (pp. 71–84). New York: Garland Press.

Biehler, R. F. (1954). Companion choice behavior in kindergarten. *Child Development, 25*, 45–55.

Bloom, H. (1997). *The Lucifer principle: A scientific expedition into the forces of history*. New York: Atlantic Monthly Press.

Blurton-Jones, N. (1972). *Ethological studies of child behavior*. Cambridge, UK: Cambridge University Press.

Bost, K. K. (1995). Mother and child reports of preschool children's social support networks: Network correlates of peer acceptance. *Social Development, 4*, 149–164.

Bost, K. K., Cielinski, K. L., Washington, W., & Vaughn, B. E. (1994). Social networks of children attending Head Start from the perspective of the child. *Early Childhood Research Quarterly, 9,* 441–462.

Bost, K. K., Vaughn, B. E., Washington, W. N., Cielinski, K. L., & Bradbard, M. (1998). Social competence, social support, and attachment: Demarcation of construct domains, measurement, and paths of influence for preschool children attending Head Start. *Child Development, 69,* 192–218.

Bott, H. (1928). Observation of play activities in a nursery school. *Genetic Psychology Monographs, 4,* 44–88.

Boyd, R., Gintis, H., Bowles, S., & Richerson, P. J. (2003). The evolution of altruistic punishment. *Proceedings of the National Academy of Sciences USA, 100,* 3531–3535.

Boyd, R., & Richerson, P. J. (2002). Group beneficial norms can spread rapidly in a structured population. *Journal of Theoretical Biology, 215,* 287–296.

Cairns, R. B. (1983). Sociometry, psychometry, and social structure: A commentary on six recent studies of popular, rejected, and neglected children. *Merrill–Palmer Quarterly, 29,* 429–438.

Cairns, R. B., Cairns, B. D., Neckerman, H. J., Gest, S. D., & Gariépy, J.-L. (1988). Social networks and aggressive behavior: Peer support or peer rejection? *Developmental Psychology, 24,* 815–823.

Cairns, R. B., Leung, M.-C., Buchanan, L., & Cairns, B. D. (1995). Friendships and social networks in childhood and adolescence: Fluidity, reliability, and interrelations. *Child Development, 66,* 1330–1345.

Carpenter, C. R. (1942). Sexual behavior of free ranging rhesus monkeys: Periodicity of estrus, homo- and autoerotic and nonconformist behavior. *Journal of Comparative Psychology, 33,* 147–162.

Chance, M. R. A. (1967). Attention structure as a basis for primate rank order. *Man, 2,* 503–518.

Chance, M. R. A., & Jolly, C. J. (1970). *Social groups of monkeys, apes and men.* London: Jonathan Cape.

Charlesworth, W. R. (1988). Resources and resource acquisition during ontogeny. In K. B. M. Donald (Ed.), *Sociobiological perspectives on human development* (pp. 24–77). New York: Springer.

Charlesworth, W. R., & Dzur, C. (1987). Gender comparisons of preschoolers' behavior and resource utilization in group problem solving. *Child Development, 58,* 191–200.

Charlesworth, W. R., & LaFreniere, P. (1983). Dominance, friendship, and resource utilization in preschool children's groups. *Ethology and Sociobiology, 4,* 175–186.

Chevaleva-Janovskaja, E. (1927). Groupements spontanés d'enfants à l'age préscolaire [Spontaneous groupings of preschool-age children]. *Archives de Psychologie, 20,* 219–223.

Corsaro, W. A. (1979). "We're friends, right?": Children's use of access rituals in a nursery school. *Language in Society, 8,* 315–336.

Corsaro, W. A. (1985). *Friendship and peer culture in the early years.* Norwood, NJ: Ablex.

Cosmides, L., & Tooby, J. (1987). From evolution to behavior: Evolutionary psychology as the missing link. In J. Dupre (Ed.), *The latest on the best: Essays on evolution and optimality* (pp. 277–306). Cambridge, MA: MIT Press.

Crook, J. H. (1970a). Social organization and the environment: Aspects of contemporary social ethology. *Animal Behavior, 18,* 197–209.

Crook, J. H. (1970b). The socio-ecology of primates. In J. H. Crook (Ed.), *Social behaviour in birds and mammals: Essays on the social ethology of animals and man* (pp. 103–166). London and New York: Academic Press.

Daniel, J. R., Santos, A. J., Vaughn, B. E., & Peceguina, I. (2007, April). *Affiliative structures in Portuguese preschool groups: A social network analysis.* Poster presented at the Biennial Meeting of the Society for Research in Child Development, Boston.

Darwin, C. (1872). *The expression of emotions in man and animals.* New York: Appleton.

Dewsbury, D. A. (1982). Dominance rank, copulatory behavior, and differential reproduction. *Quarterly Review of Biology, 57,* 135–159.

Dornbusch, S. M., Glasgow, K. L., & Lin, I.-C. (1996). The social structure of schooling. *Annual Review of Psychology, 47,* 401–429.

Dunnington, M. J. (1957a). Behavioral differences of sociometric status groups in a nursery school. *Child Development, 28,* 139–114.

Dunnington, M. J. (1957b). Investigation of areas of disagreement in sociometric measurement of preschool children. *Child Development, 28,* 93–102.

Eibl-Eibesfeldt, I. (1989). *Human ethology: Foundations of human behavior.* New York: Aldine.

Fabes, R. A., Martin, C. L., & Hanish, L. D. (2004). The next 50 years: Considering gender as a context for understanding young children's peer relationships. *Merrill–Palmer Quarterly, 50,* 260–273.

Frankel, E. B. (1946). The social relationships of nursery school children. *Sociometry, 9,* 210–225.

Hagman, E. P. (1933). The companionships of preschool children. *University of Iowa Studies in Child Welfare, 7,* 10–69.

Harary, F., Norman, R. Z., & Cartwright, D. (1978). *Structural models: An introduction to the theory of directed graphs.* New York: Wiley.

Hawley, P. H. (1999). The ontogenesis of social dominance: A strategy-based evolutionary perspective. *Developmental Review, 19,* 97–132.

Hawley, P. H. (2002). Social dominance and prosocial and coercive strategies of resource control in preschoolers. *International Journal of Behavioral Development, 26,* 167–176.

Hawley, P. H. (2003). Strategies of control, aggression, and morality in preschoolers: An evolutionary perspective. *Journal of Experimental Child Psychology, 85,* 213–235.

Hawley, P. H., & Little, T. (1999). On winning some and losing some: A social relations approach to social dominance in toddlers. *Merrill–Palmer Quarterly, 45,* 185–214.

Hinde, R. A. (1966). *Animal behaviour: A synthesis of ethology and comparative psychology.* New York: McGraw-Hill.

Hinde, R. A. (1974). *Biological basis of human social behavior.* New York: McGraw-Hill.

Hold-Cavell, B. C., & Borsutzky, D. (1986). Strategies to obtain high regard: Longitudinal study of a group of preschool children. *Ethology and Sociobiology, 7,* 39–56.

Howes, C. (1988). Peer interaction of young children. *Monographs of the Society for Research in Child Development, 53*(Serial No. 217), 1–92.

Hubbard, R. M. (1929). A method of studying spontaneous group formation. In D. S. Thomas (Ed.), *Some new techniques for studying social behavior* (pp. 76–85). New York: Columbia University Press.

Keltner, D., Gruenfeld, D. H., & Anderson, C. (2003). Power, approach, and inhibition, *Psychological Review, 110,* 265–284.

Kropotkin, P. (1902). *Mutual aid: A factor of evolution.* London: Heinemann.

Kummer, H. (1968). *Social organization of Hamadryas baboons: A field study.* Chicago: University of Chicago Press.

Kummer, H. (1971). *Primate societies: Group techniques of ecological adaptations.* Chicago: Aldine.

LaFreniere, P. J. (1996). Co-operation as a conditional strategy among peers: Influence of social ecology and kin relations. *International Journal of Behavioral Development, 19,* 39–52.

LaFreniere, P. J., & Charlesworth, W. R. (1983). Dominance, affiliation and attention in a preschool group: A nine-month longitudinal study. *Ethology and Sociobiology, 4,* 1–14.

LaFreniere, P. J., & Charlesworth, W. R. (1987). Effects of friendship and dominance status on preschoolers resource utilization in a cooperative/competitive paradigm. *International Journal of Behavioral Development, 10,* 345–358.

LaFreniere, P., Strayer, F. F., & Gauthier, R. (1984). The emergence of same-sex affiliative preferences among preschool peers: A developmental/ethological perspective. *Child Development, 55,* 1958–1965.

Leinhardt, S. (1972). Developmental change in the sentiment structure of children's groups. *American Sociological Review, 37,* 202–212.

Lewis, M., Zimmerman, S., Hollenstein, T., & Lamey, A. V. (2004). Reorganization in coping behavior at 1½ years: Dynamic systems and normative change. *Developmental Science, 7,* 56–73.

Maccoby, E. E., & Jacklin, C. N. (1987). Gender segregation in childhood. In H. W. Reese (Ed.), *Advances in child development and behavior* (Vol. 20, pp. 239–287). Orlando, FL: Academic Press.

MacDonald, K. B. (1988). *Sociobiological perspectives on human development.* New York: Springer-Verlag.

Manson, J. H., & Wrangham, R. W. (1991). Intergroup aggression in chimpanzees and humans. *Current Anthropology, 32,* 369–390.

Marshall, H. R. (1957). An evaluation of sociometric–social behavior research with preschool children. *Child Development, 28,* 131–137.

Martin, C. L., & Fabes, R. A. (2001). The stability and consequences of young children's same sex peer interactions. *Developmental Psychology, 37,* 431–446.

Martin, C. L., Fabes, R. A., Hanish, L. D., & Hollenstein, T. (2005). Social dynamics in the preschool. *Developmental Review, 25,* 299–327.

Martin, C. L., Ruble, D. N., & Szkrybalo, J. (2002). Cognitive theories of early gender development. *Psychological Bulletin, 128,* 903–933.

McCandless, B. R., & Marshall, H. R. (1957). A picture sociometric technique for preschool children and its relation to teacher judgments of friendship. *Child Development, 28,* 139–149.

McGrew, W. C. (1972). *An ethological study of children's behavior.* New York: Academic Press.

McPherson, M., Smith-Lovin, L., & Cook, J. M. (2001). Birds of a feather: Homphily in social networks. *Annual Review of Sociology, 27,* 415–444.

Moreno, F. B. (1942). Sociometric status of children in a nursery school group. *Sociometry, 4,* 395–341.

Moreno, J. L. (1932). *Application of the group method to classification.* New York: National Committee on Prisons and Prison Labor.

Moreno, J. L. (1933). Psychological organization of groups in the community. In *Handbook of mental deficiency* (pp. 5–35). Boston: Association for Mental Deficiency.

Moreno, J. L. (1934). *Who shall survive?* Washington, DC: Nervous and Mental Disease Publishing Company.

Moreno, J. L. (1955). Contributions of sociometry to research methodology in sociology. In A. P. Hare, E. F. Borgatta, & R. F. Bales (Eds.), *Small groups: Studies in social interaction* (pp. 99–107). New York: Knopf.

Packer, G. A. (2000). Scramble in behaviour and ecology. *Philosophical Transactions of the Royal Society of London, 355,* 1637–1645.

Parten, M. B. (1932). Social participation among pre-school children. *Journal of Abnormal Psychology, 24,* 243–269.

Pellegrini, A. D. (2008). *The roles of aggressive and affiliative behaviors in resource control: A behavioral ecological perspective,* Unpublished manuscript, University of Minnesota, Minneapolis, MN.

Pellegrini, A. D., Long, J. D., Roseth, C. J., Bohn, C. M., & van Ryzin, M. (2007). A short-term longitudinal study of preschoolers' sex segregation: The role of physical activity, sex, and time. *Journal of Comparative Psychology, 121,* 282–289.

Pellegrini, A. D., Roseth, C. J., Mliner, S., Bohn, C. M., van Ryzin, M., Vance, N., et al. (2007). Social dominance in preschool classrooms. *Journal of Comparative Psychology, 121,* 54–64.

Reid, M., Landesman, S., Treder, R., & Jaccard, J. (1989). My family and friends: Six- to twelve-year-old children's perceptions of social support. *Child Development, 60,* 896–910.

Roseth, C. J., Pellegrini, A. D., Bohn, C. M., van Ryzin, M., & Vance, N. (2007). Follow the leader: An observational, longitudinal study of preschool dominance and social exchange, *Journal of School Psychology, 45,* 479–497.

Santos, A. J. (1993). *Preschool affiliative networks: A socio-structural analysis of the behavioral ecology of natural peer groups.* Unpublished doctoral thesis, Department of Psychology, University of Québec, Montréal, Canada.

Santos, A. J., & Strayer, F. F. (1997). A socio-structural analysis of preschool children's affiliative behavior. *Advances in Ethology: Contributions to the XXV International Etiology Conference, 32,* 115.

Santos, A. J., Vaughn, B. E., & Bonnet, J. (2000). L'influence du réseau affiliatif sur la répartition de l'attention sociale chez l'enfant en groupe préscolaire [The influence of the social network on the distribution of social attention in a preschool children's group]. *Revue des Sciences l'Education, 26,* 17–34.

Santos, A. J., & Winegar, L. T. (1999). Child social ethology and peer relations: A developmental review of methodology and findings. *Acta Ethologica, 2,* 1–11.

Schmidt, S. K., & Griffin, W. A. (2007). Signals of play: An ABM of affective signatures in children's playgroups. In T. Terano, S. Takahashi, D. Sallach, & J. Rouchier (Eds.), *Proceedings of the First World Congress on Social Simulation* (pp. 283–294). London: Springer-Verlag.

Serbin, L. A., Moller, L. C., Gulko, J., Powlishta, K. K., & Colburne, K. A. (1994). The emergence of gender segregation in toddler playgroups. In C. Leaper (Ed.), *Childhood sex segregation: Causes and consequences* (pp. 7–17). San Francisco: Jossey-Bass.

Seyfarth, R. M. (1977). A model of social grooming among adult female monkeys. *Journal of Theoretical Biology, 65,* 671–698.

Sluckin, A., & Smith, P. K. (1977). Two approaches to the concept of dominance in preschool children. *Child Development, 48,* 917–923.

Strayer, F. F. (1980a). Social ecology of the preschool peer group. In W. A. Collins (Ed.), *Development of cognition, affect and social relations: Minnesota Symposia on Child Psychology* (Vol. 13, pp. 165–196). Hillsdale, NJ: Erlbaum.

Strayer, F. F. (1980b). Child ethology and the study of preschool social relations. In H. Foot, T. Chapman, & J. Smith (Eds.), *Childhood friendships and peer relationships* (pp. 235–265). London: Wiley.

Strayer, F. F. (1981). The organization and coordination of asymmetrical social exchange among preschool children: A biological view of social power. In M. Watts (Ed.), *Research methods in bio-politics* (pp. 33–49). San Francisco: Jossey-Bass.

Strayer, F. F. (1989). Co-adaptation within the peer group: A psychobiological study of early competence. In B. Schneider, G. Attili, J. Nadel, & R. Weisman (Eds.), *Social competence in developmental perspective* (pp. 145–174). Dordrecht, the Netherlands: Kluwer.

Strayer, F. F., Chapeskie, T. R., & Strayer, J. (1978). The perception of preschool social dominance. *Aggressive Behavior, 4,* 183–192.

Strayer, F. F., & Nöel, J. M. (1986). The prosocial and antisocial functions of preschool aggression: An ethological study of triadic conflict among young children. In C. Zahn-Waxler, E. M. Cummings, & R. Iannotti (Eds.), *Altruism and aggression: Biological and social origins* (pp. 107–134). New York: Cambridge University Press.

Strayer, F. F., & Santos, A. J. (1996). Affiliative structures in preschool peer groups. *Social Development, 5,* 117–130.

Strayer, F. F., & Strayer, J. (1976). An ethological analysis of social agonism and dominance relations among preschool children. *Child Development, 47,* 980–989.

Strayer, F. F., Tessier, O., & Gariépy, J. L. (1985). L'activité et le réseau cohésif chez lex enfants d'´age préscolaire [Behavior and cohesive networks of preschool-age children]. In R. Tremblay, M. Provost, & F. F. Strayer (Eds.), *Éthologie et dévelopment de l'enfant* (pp. 291–308). Paris: Editions Stock/Laurence Pernoud.

Strayer, F. F., & Trudel, M. (1984). Developmental changes in the nature and functions of social dominance during the preschool years. *Ethology and Sociobiology, 5,* 279–295.

Tinbergen, N. (1951). *The study of instinct.* New York: Oxford University Press.

Tremblay, R. E. (2002). Prevention of injury by early socialization of aggressive behavior. *Injury Prevention, 8,* 17–21.

Trivers, R. L. (1971). The evolution of reciprocal altruism. *Quarterly Review of Biology, 46,* 35–57.

Vaughn, B. E. (1999). Power is knowledge (and *vice versa*): A commentary on "On winning some and losing some: A social relations approach to social dominance in toddlers." *Merrill–Palmer Quarterly, 45*, 215–225.

Vaughn, B. E., Azria, M. R., Krzysik, L., Caya, L. R., Bost, K. K., Newell, W., et al. (2000). Friendship and social competence in a sample of preschool children attending Head Start. *Developmental Psychology, 36*, 326–338.

Vaughn, B. E., Vollenweider, M., Bost, K. K., Azria-Evans, M. R., & Snider, J. B. (2003). Negative interactions and social competence for preschool children in two samples: Reconsidering the interpretation of aggressive behavior for young children. *Merrill–Palmer Quarterly, 49*, 245–278.

Vaughn, B. E., & Waters, E. (1980). Social organization among preschool peers: Dominance, attention, and sociometric correlates. In D. Omark, F. Strayer, & D. Freedman (Eds.), *Dominance relations: Ethological perspectives on human conflict* (pp. 359–379). New York: Garland Press.

Vaughn, B. E., & Waters, E. (1981). Attention structure, sociometric status, and dominance: Interrelations, behavioral correlates, and relationships to social competence. *Developmental Psychology, 17*, 275–288.

Vermeij, G. (2004). *Nature: An economic history*. Princeton, NJ: Princeton University Press.

Wasserman, S. S., Faust, K., & Iacobucci, D. (1994). *Social network analysis: Methods and applications*. New York: Cambridge University Press.

Wellman, B. (1926). The school child's choice of companions. *Journal of Educational Research, 14*, 126–132.

Wilson, E. O. (1975). *Sociobiology: The new synthesis*. Cambridge, MA: Harvard University Press.

Yerkes, R. M. (1939). Social dominance and sexual status in the chimpanzee. *Quarterly Review of Biology, 14*, 115–136.

PART IV

Middle Childhood and Early Adolescence

CHAPTER 12

Friendship as Process, Function, and Outcome

WILLIAM M. BUKOWSKI
CLAIRNEIGE MOTZOI
FELICIA MEYER

For children, adolescents, and adults, friendship is a sought after and ubiquitous experience. Nearly all children and adolescents want to be involved in friendships and most of them claim to have a friend or consider a subset of their peers to be their friends (Dunn, 1993; Lindsey, 2002). Children and adolescents ascribe multiple positive features to their friendship experiences and expect to derive multiple benefits from them (Youniss, 1980). Even at a young age, children see friendship as a form of interaction and relationship that has distinct features, processes, and benefits (Bigelow, 1977). Aside from interaction with their parents, children of all ages spend more time with friends than they do with other individuals, and they wish to share special events and adventures with them (Rubin, Bukowski, & Parker, 2006).

Friendship can be found at all times of life except perhaps in early infancy. In this way, friendship is the relationship that brings the lifespan together (Bukowski & Sippola, 2005). Nearly everyone has had friendship relations, often at every time of life (Hartup & Stevens, 1997). In this way, it is difficult not to recognize friendship as the quintessential form of peer relationship and as a basic feature of human life from early childhood to old age. For these reasons, it is not surprising that the first published study of peer relations was a comparison of children with and without friends (Monroe, 1898).

Friendship is not just of interest to developmental psychologists. It has also attracted the attention of philosophers, writers, moviemakers, song writers, and others. Both ancient and modern philosophers have tried to understand friendship as a social construct that is imbued with moral expectations and responsibilities, and as a basic form of human experience that gives meaning to life (Badhwar, 1993). Writers of fiction often depict the intricate fabric and texture of friendships especially as they serve as the basic ground or as turning points in the lives of their characters. For instance, J. K. Rowling's stories about Harry Potter, the most successful series of books ever written, are essentially descriptions

217

of what it is like to go through childhood and early adolescence in the company of one's friends (Bukowski, 2001).

The goal of this chapter is to ask several fundamental questions about friendship and its developmental significance. We review theory and empirical studies related to how friendship is defined and to the effects that it has on behavioral and affective development and well-being. Specifically, we first discuss three defining features of friendship: reciprocated liking, similarity, and coordination and responsivity. Then we examine certain functions of friendship, such as validation, protection from risk factors, and moral development, and their relation to adjustment.

The basic approach of our discussion is based on Hinde's (1995) model of relationships. According to Hinde, the functions, meanings, expectations, and emotions that comprise a friendship relation come from the reliable succession of interactions that occurs between friends. In turn, they account for many of the internalized benefits of friendship. For this reason, an account of friendship needs to describe the interactions that distinguish friendship from other kinds of interaction, and the relationship properties and function that are believed to result from these interactions. We have organized this chapter according to a set of statements that describe both friendship and the contribution that friendship makes to development.

Critical Issues: Features of Friendship

Friendship can be defined as the strong, positive affective bonds that exist between two persons and that are intended to facilitate the accomplishment of socioemotional goals (Hartup & Stevens, 1997; Hinde, 1987). At the center of a friendship are the egalitarian interactions in which a person is attracted to another who is attracted in return. Such interactions carry different types of expectations. For example, friends are expected to spend more time with each other, or to have a positive "cost–benefit" relationship. Additionally, friends are expected to be available to offer help, companionship, security, and emotional support.

Hartup and Stevens (1997) explained that these expectations vary across the lifespan. In young children, friendships are characterized by the presence of common activities and concrete reciprocities. In school-age children, the nature of the friendship relationship changes with the development of new cognitive and emotional skills that allow children to spend more time with their friends, to share their interests and beliefs, and also to engage in more intimate interactions characterized by self-disclosure. In older individuals, friendships are seen as relations in which one can receive support from a significant other; in other words, the friend is perceived as a dependable and understanding person (Hartup, 1996; Hartup & Stevens, 1997).

Friendship as Reciprocated Liking

In regard to the operational definitions that have been proposed for "friendship," there is nearly universal agreement that measures of friendship need to capture both the level of reciprocity and the level of closeness that occurs between two individuals. For this reason, the most basic measures of whether a child is part of a friendship involve an index of whether two children show a high level of liking for each other. Although these measures have typically involved the assessment of whether two children choose each other as their first or second best friends in a nomination-based sociometric questionnaire, other techniques have been used. A review by Erdley, Nangle, and Gold (1998) showed that at least five operational definitions have been proposed to index whether a child is engaged in a friendship. These techniques involve a nomination procedure in which a child chooses from a pool of peers the children whom he/she regards as his or her best friend, or a rating scale procedure in which each child rates every other child in the peer group according to how much he or she likes the child, or a combination of nomination and rating scale data. Typically the ratings are made with a 5-point scale in which a score of 1 indicates a high level of disliking and a 5 indicates a high level of liking.

As indicated earlier, the most commonly or widely used measure is the index of reciprocated best friend nominations from a sociometric questionnaire. This measure has been used extensively and is typically regarded as the most conservative definition of friendship. Alternatively, Bukowski and Hoza (1989) proposed a second definition that identifies dyads as friends if the two children give one another high ratings (4 or 5). This definition is less conservative than the first definition because children may be more inclined to give an unlimited number of high scores with a rating scale procedure than with a nomination technique. Nevertheless, even with these potentially less conservative criteria, it would still be clear that the two partners would have high levels of liking for each other.

The other three definitions use a combination of nomination-based and rating scale measures. A third technique, used by Howes (1990), defined "friendships" as dyads in which one child nominated the other child as a best friend, and the other child rated that peer with a 5 on the rating scale. With this definition there is a relatively high level of mutual liking, even though one of the dyad members does not specifically identify the other as a best friend. A fourth definition is more lenient. It conceptualizes friendships as dyads in which one child nominates the other as a best friend, and both children give the other a rating of at least 4 on the rating scale (see Jones, 1985). Finally, a fifth definition is even less restrictive. Specifically, Berndt (e.g., Berndt, Hawkins, & Hoyle, 1986; Berndt & Perry, 1986) defined as friends dyads in which either of the two peers nominated the other, and the two had an average mutual peer rating of 4 or greater on the rating scale measure.

Erdley et al. (1998) conducted a comparative analysis of these definitions using two criteria. One criterion was the average number of friendships that each of these five techniques identified. The other was the stability of the friendships identified with each technique. In regard to the first criterion, the second definition (mutual highest ratings) and the fifth definition (reciprocity on either the rating scale or the nomination measure and at least a score of 4 on the rating scale) identified the largest number of friendships, whereas the first definition (mutual nominations) produced the lowest number. They assessed the stability of the friendship dyads identified with each definition by examining whether they were observed at each of two times separated by an 8-week interval. The stability of the dyads varied little as a function of the operational definition that was used. The friendship dyads identified with the first definition (mutual nominations) appeared to be a bit less stable than those identified with the other techniques (57% vs. an average of 61%). This difference, however, may have been offset by the narrowness of this definition. In spite of the more conservative nature of this definition, it still identified friendship dyads that were as stable as those identified by much less restrictive measures. Accordingly, it may be the case that this definition (i.e., reciprocated nominations) deserves to be the most widely used measure of friendship.

Friendship as Responsivity, Cooperation, and Coordination

The definitions of friendship presented in the previous section refer only to the most basic criterion or feature of friendship (i.e., mutual liking). Certainly, there is more to friendship than this fundamental defining characteristic. In this section, we show that the interactions of friends differ substantially from the interactions of nonfriends. The centerpiece of this discussion is well known, specifically, that reciprocity is a fundamental characteristic of friendship. Beyond the simple reciprocity of liking discussed in the previous section, we show that reciprocity between friends can be seen in several domains, including affect and behavior. "Reciprocity" refers to the tendency of two persons to act in the same way, either simultaneously or in sequence (Hinde, 1979). Typically, reciprocity is directional in the sense that actions of friends are directed toward each other, such as when one friend does something and the other friend responds (Ross, Cheyne, & Lollis, 1988). The responsiveness between friends is often symmetrical, because each friend contributes equally to the interaction and neither of the two partners dominates the other.

Evidence of the presence of affective and behavioral reciprocity as a central feature is seen clearly in the findings of a meta-analysis of studies of friendship. Newcomb and Bagwell (1995) organized the rich set of interactions that had been studied in friendship research into four broadband categories: positive engagement, conflict management, task activity, and relationship properties. In each of these four areas substantial differences were found between the interactions of friends and nonfriends. The overall size of this difference for the category of positive engagement was nearly half of a standard deviation (Cohen's $d+ = 0.472$). Similar differences were found on each of the four types of interaction within this category: a difference of nearly two-thirds of a standard deviation on social contact, one-half a standard deviation on talking, and roughly one-third of a standard deviation on cooperation and positive affect. Smaller differences were seen on conflict management (Cohen's $d+ = 0.128$); however, consistent with comments we made earlier, there were large differences between the forms of interaction within this category. Although there were no differences on measures of conflict instigation, a difference of at least moderate size was found on measures of conflict resolution. For the category of task activities, an overall small effect was observed (Cohen's $d+ = 0.224$), but again, the size of the difference between the interactions of friendship varied across the particular measures in this category. A moderate difference (roughly two-fifths of a standard deviation) was found for measures of task performance, whereas a nonsignificant difference was found for measures of basic communication. With regard to indices of relationship properties, moderate to large differences were observed across several dimensions (overall Cohen's $d+ = 0.397$). These dimensions included similarity (roughly 0.4 of a standard deviation), equality (0.4), dominance (–0.2), mutual liking (0.75), closeness (0.61) and loyalty (0.54).

Although there were some age differences, Newcomb and Bagwell's (1995) findings can be generalized across the childhood and adolescent periods. For example, even during the preschool period, children's behavior with their friends differs from how they behave with children they know but who are not their friends. In addition to differences on features such as supportiveness and exclusivity (Sebanc, 2003), differences can be seen in the interactions of friends and of nonfriends as young as 3½ years on measures such as the directness and frequency of social overtures, the degree of engagement in social interactions, and complexity in play behavior (Dunn & Cutting, 1999; Dunn, Cutting, & Fisher, 2002). As well, preschool-age friends tend to cooperate and exhibit more positive social behaviors with each other than with nonfriends (e.g., Dunn et al., 2002). It is known also that friendship stability in the preschool years varies across friendships and is related to patterns of interaction. Ladd, Kochenderfer, and Coleman (1996), for example, have shown that, compared with unstable friendships in early childhood, stable friendships involve higher levels of positive friendship qualities (e.g., validation) and lower levels of negative friendship qualities (e.g., low conflict) are most likely to be stable.

Although preschool children have been shown to engage in more conflicts overall with friends than with other peers (Hartup, Laursen, Stewart, & Eastenson, 1988), the way that friends resolve conflicts has been shown to be more cooperative. Specifically, compared with nonfriends, preschool friends engage in more arguments, more assaults and threats, and more reactive hostility, such as refusals and oppositions (Dunn & Cutting, 1999; Laursen & Hartup, 1989). These differences are likely due to the larger amount of time that friends spend interacting with each other. It is the manner in which friends, relative to nonfriends, resolve conflicts that shows the higher level of responsivity that friends have for each other. For example, Hartup and his colleagues (1988) also reported qualitative differences in how preschool friends and nonfriends resolve conflicts, and in the likely outcomes of these conflicts. Friends, as compared with nonfriends, make more use of negotiation and disengagement, and they make relatively less use of winner-take-all strategies in their resolution of conflicts. In terms of conflict outcomes, friends are more likely than nonfriends to have equal resolutions. Also, following conflict resolution, friends are more likely than nonfriends to stay in physical proximity and continue to engage in interaction.

Two studies conducted with school-age children demonstrate quite clearly the differences shown in Newcomb and Bagwell's (1995) meta-analysis. In one study, pairs of 7- and 8-year-old children, equally divided between friends and nonfriends, were observed while watching a comedy film (Foot, Chapman, & Smith, 1977). The interactions of the two children in each pair were coded into five categories (laughing, smiling, looking, talking, and touching). In each of these categories, the observed frequencies and durations were higher for the pairs of friends than for the nonfriends. More importantly, a higher level of interdependence was observed between the children in the friend pairs than in the nonfriend pairs. Specifically, children in the friend pairs were more likely than the children in the nonfriend pairs to respond to the behavior of their partner. An example of a response would be when one child would laugh after the other child had laughed. These findings point to the much higher level of coordinated positive affect in friendship.

Similarly, Newcomb and Brady (1982) observed the interaction of pairs of school-age and early adolescent boys who were either friends or acquaintances as they worked with a "puzzle box," a brightly colored wooden case about the size of a small footlocker. It included 15 features. Five features could be manipulated by a single child (e.g., a combination lock hooked to a latch on the outside of the box), five needed the coordination of two people (e.g., a flashlight that could be illuminated only if each of the two children pushed buttons located at different places on the box), and five could be manipulated by one child or by two (e.g., playing with two cars kept in a drawer in the box). As in the Foot et al. (1977) study regarding matched affect (e.g., mutual laughter), differences were observed between the friend and acquaintance pairs on all measures of coordinated positive affect (e.g., mutual laughing). Differences were also observed on measures of coordinated activity. Friends were more likely than acquaintances to share activities and to participate in features that required the action of two people. Most importantly, the friend pairs were more likely to engage in exploration together. These findings point to the overall higher level of coordination and mutual responsivity for friends relative to nonfriends in both *affect* and *behavior*.

Friendship as Similarity

Insofar as mutual responsivity and coordinated action are central features of friendship, it follows that there would be greater similarity between friends than between nonfriends. Already several studies have provided support for the hypothesis that similarity underlies attraction (Byrne & Griffit, 1966) and is a key component of friendship. Beginning in the preschool years, children appear to be attracted to, and to become friends with, peers whose behavioral tendencies are similar to their own (Rubin et al., 2006). Similarity between friends has been shown on several dimensions, including prosocial and antisocial behaviors (Haselager, Hartup, van Lieshout, & Riksen-Walreaven, 1998; Liu & Chen, 2003; Poulin & Boivin, 2000; Poulin et al., 1997), shyness and internalized distress (e.g., Hogue & Steinberg, 1995; Rubin, Wojslawowicz, Burgess, Booth-LaForce, & Rose-Krasnor, 2004), sociability, peer popularity, and academic achievement and motivation (Altermatt & Pomerantz, 2003; Gest, Graham-Berman, & Hartup, 1991; Liu & Chen, 2003). The extent of similarity appears to vary across friendships. Hamm (2000), for example, showed that similarity to friends on a particular dimension varied across children largely due to the importance the child ascribed to it. For example, similarity to one's friend on academic performance was highest among children who saw academic performance as important.

The observation of similarity between friends on any particular dimension begs the question of whether this similarity existed before the friendship developed and served as the basis of attraction (i.e., similarity is a selection effect), or whether it was the result of the interactions between the friends (i.e., similarity is due to socialization). Currently there is evidence for both of these processes. In a recent longitudinal study of alcohol use, friends were shown to be similar to each other from the outset, indicating a selection effect, and to maintain or increase this similarity as their friendship continued, indicating a socialization effect (Popp, Laursen, Kerr, Stattin, & Burk, 2008). One important finding from this study was the decrease in similarity between peers after the friendship ended. Although these findings are limited to alcohol use, it is likely that they would generalize to other characteristics, especially those that are social in nature. Other similarities might be more difficult to "socialize" but could still lead to a selection effect (e.g., temperament—shyness, gregariousness, etc.).

Summary: Friendship Characteristics

In this section we have presented evidence that friendships differ from other peer dyads in several critical ways. Beyond the basic difference on mutual liking, interactions between friends differ from those of nonfriends in the coordination, responsivity, and similarity in their affect and behavior. Currently, the origins of these differences and their significance are not entirely clear. Through reciprocated liking, similarity, and responsivity and coordination, friendship provides children with dyadic experiences that are not available to children without friends. Thus, might the experience of having a friend affect not only children's adjustment but also their development of social competence?

Critical Issues: Friendship Functions and Outcomes

Friendship as Validation

The features of friendship we described in the previous section have provided the basis for theory regarding the effects of friendship. Consistent with the ideas of Hinde (1995), the implicit point of a large share of theory about friendship is that the interactions that define friendship create properties of relationships that in turn have direct or indirect effects on development. The best known theory of friendship can be found in the writing of the American psychiatrist Harry Stack Sullivan (1953). Sullivan proposed that the "chumships" or close, intimate mutual relationships that children have with their same-sex peers, are distinct from the hierarchical relationships that children experience with their parents and, as a result, are a child's first true interpersonal experience. According to Sullivan, the experience of reciprocity and exchange in friendship gives youngsters a sense of well-being and validation, which in turn would have a particularly strong effect on the development of the self-concept. This validation derives from children's recognition of the positive regard and care that the friend holds for them. Sullivan went so far as to argue that the positive experiences of having a "chum" in adolescence could be powerful enough to enable adolescents to overcome trauma that may have resulted from prior family experiences. In this way, Sullivan saw friendship as a security system that would protect children from sources of risk within the family.

An implied aspect of Sullivan's (1953) theory is that it is the features or provision of friendship that matter. "Relationship provisions" refer to the experiences, opportunities, and affordances of relationships (Furman & Buhrmester, 1985; Weiss, 1974). For example, companionship, intimacy, and even conflict have all been shown to be present in friendships and to offer direct benefits, as well as opportunities to develop social competencies (Furman & Robins, 1985; Hartup, 1996; Weiss, 1974). According to this view, children seek specific types of support in their relationships with others. Six basic social provisions—attachment (affection, security, and intimate disclosure), reliable alliance (a lasting, dependable bond), enhancement of worth, companionship, guidance, and nurturance—have been identified as critical features of friendship (Bukowski & Hoza, 1989).

Although very few, if any, studies have directly assessed how particular provisions or features of friendship affect well-being, there is some empirical evidence to support Sullivan's general claim that the experience of being friended affects adjustment. For example, children who have friends are known to be more self-confident than those who do not (Hartup, 1996; Newcomb & Bagwell, 1995). Friended children also tend to be less lonely and depressed than children who are friendless (Parker & Asher, 1993). In addition, children who have more friendships appear to be more involved in school and perform better academically (Berndt et al., 1986). Moreover, even when the effects of peer-group acceptance have been accounted for, researchers have found that children who have multiple friends are more academically proficient and less lonely (Ladd et al., 1997; Vandell & Hembree, 1994).

In two recent studies, friendship status was used as a mediator or as a moderator of other aspects of peer experience on developmental outcomes. Using a sample of older school-age children, Nangle, Erdley, Newman, Mason, and Carpenter (2003) used path analysis to examine whether friendship status mediates the association between being well-liked by peers (i.e., being accepted) and feeling lonely. Their model, supported by

their data, used acceptance as an antecedent to friendship, which in turn negatively predicted loneliness and depression. More recently, Laursen, Bukowski, Aunola, and Nurmi
(2007) showed that during the transition period of the entry into primary school, friendship protected at-risk children from both externalizing and internalizing problems. For
example, social isolation was observed to be a significant predictor of increases in internalizing and externalizing problems for friendless children but not for friended children.
Also, initial internalizing and externalizing problems were related to increases across time
in social isolation for friendless children but not for friended children.

In spite of these findings that show an association between friendship and multiple
measures of adjustment, clear evidence of a direct effect of friendship on measures of
the self-concept is still lacking. Creative longitudinal studies that provide direct assessment of how the self is related to friendship are needed; that is, there is a need for studies to assess whether having a friendship is associated with changes in children's beliefs
about themselves over time.

Friendship as Protection from Family-Related Risk Factors

One approach to understanding the effects of peer relationships on adjustment is to
examine whether they moderate the association between risk factors and adjustment
(Bukowksi & Adams, 2005). Indeed, protection figures among the numerous functions
that have been ascribed to friendship (Bukowski, 2001). As we noted earlier, a central
proposal of Sullivan's (1953) theory of interpersonal relationships was that positive experiences with peers, especially the experiences of a close friendship or "chumship" in early
adolescence, may be so powerful as to enable adolescents to overcome the "warps" that
may have resulted from social experiences within the family. Recently, researchers have
begun to investigate the possible protective functions of friendships and whether, as Sullivan believed, the experience of friendship may buffer children from stresses in their lives.
One such line of research examines whether the developmental significance of friendship is higher for children whose relationships with parents are less than optimal, in other
words, whether the link between parenting and child outcomes of a maladaptive nature
can be attenuated by a child's friendship quality or status in the peer group (Rubin et al.,
2006). However, only a limited number of studies have investigated friendships or peer
relationships more broadly in this way.

In a longitudinal study of 138 fourth and fifth graders, Gauze, Bukowski, Aquan-
Assee, and Sippola (1996) found that the association between family adaptability and
cohesion and children's perceived social competence and self-worth was stronger for
those without a friend or with lower quality friendships. In other words, low cohesion and
low adaptability in the family (as rated by parents) was significantly associated with lower
levels of perceived social competence and self-worth. However, this association was not
significant for early adolescents who had a high-quality or a reciprocated best friendship.
More specifically, Gauze and colleagues observed stronger moderating effects for the
friendship quality measure than for the friendship reciprocity measure. Thus, although
simply having a friend protected early adolescents from the effect of low family functioning, having a high-quality friendship was an even better protector. They concluded that
the significance of having a friend or of being in a high-quality friendship depends on
one's experiences within the family. Therefore, friendships may be critically important
for the adjustment of children from less optimal family environments.

In another study, Rubin and colleagues (2004) examined whether friendship quality would serve as a moderator to protect young adolescents with poor parent–child relationships from negative outcomes. They found that parental support (from the mother and father) and friendship quality made both independent and interactive contributions in the prediction of fifth graders' social and emotional adjustment. Interestingly, friendship quality moderated different parenting–outcome relations for boys compared to girls. Among the specific effects uncovered, the authors found that low maternal support was associated with lower perceived social competence among boys who also reported low-quality friendships. Furthermore, high friendship quality buffered the effects of low maternal support on girls' internalizing difficulties.

In a longitudinal study that followed early adolescents from the fifth until the seventh grade, Lansford, Criss, Pettit, Dodge, and Bates (2003) found that high levels of friendship quality and peer-group affiliation attenuated the association between unilateral parental decision making and adolescent externalizing behavior, especially when adolescents associated with peers low in antisocial behavior. Peer-group affiliation also served as a protective factor for adolescents exposed to low parental supervision and awareness. In contrast, having low-quality peer relationships and interacting with peers perceived to be highly antisocial amplified the association between unilateral parental decision making and adolescent externalizing behavior. Finally, this study found stronger support for the moderating role of peer groups than that of friendships.

A study by Criss, Pettit, Bates, Dodge, and Lapp (2002) using a younger sample yielded similar results. They examined family adversity, positive peer relationships, and children's externalizing behavior. Results indicated that peer acceptance moderated the relation between the three measures of family adversity, namely, ecological disadvantage, violent marital conflict and harsh discipline, and externalizing behavior. In contrast, friendship only moderated one of the measures of family adversity—harsh discipline. Specifically, at low levels of positive peer relations, the association between family adversity and child externalizing behavior was significant, whereas at high levels of positive peer relationships, this association was no longer significant.

In a 3-year longitudinal study of maltreated children and early adolescents, Bolger, Patterson, and Kupersmidt (1998) found that, as expected, greater severity and chronicity of maltreatment were associated with greater difficulties in self-esteem and peer relationships (i.e., lower peer acceptance). However, the association between child abuse and subsequent self-esteem was not significant among children with high-quality friendships or with a reciprocated best friendship. In fact, for some groups of maltreated children, namely, those who experienced chronic maltreatment or were physically abused, having a good friend was associated with an improvement in self-esteem over time. The authors concluded that both friendship quality and reciprocated friendship moderated the association between maltreatment and self-esteem.

Similarly, Schwartz, Dodge, Pettit, and Bates (2000) conducted two longitudinal studies investigating the moderating role of friendship in the pathway between early harsh home environment and later victimization in the peer group. In both studies, living in an early harsh, punitive, and hostile family environment was associated with higher levels of subsequent peer victimization for children who had a low number of friendships in elementary school. However, this association was not significant for children with an extensive friendship network (i.e., numerous friendships). In other words, the presence of an extensive friendship network moderated the association between harsh home environment and peer-group victimization both in younger and older elementary school-age children even when researchers controlled for the effect of peer-group acceptance.

Finally, Laible, Carlo, and Raffaelli (2000) investigated the impact of parent and peer attachment on levels of depression and anxiety in a sample of middle adolescents (mean age of 16 years). As expected, adolescents with high levels of parent and peer attachment were best adjusted, whereas those with low levels of parental and peer attachment were least well adjusted. The main finding of this study was that adolescents who reported high peer attachment but low parent attachment were better adjusted than those who reported high parent attachment but low peer attachment.

van Aken and Asendorpf (1997), who examined social support and compensation across various relationships in early adolescents' social networks, did not find support for the protective effects of peer relationships. As they expected, they found that children receiving low support from their mother, their father, or their classmates reported lower general self-worth. More importantly, they found that low support by one parent could only be compensated for by a supportive relationship with the other parent; in other words, it could not be compensated for by classmates. However, we should note that this study measured social support from classmates with whom the child interacted on a regular basis, but who were not necessarily friends; the authors did not identify whether the classmates were considered friends by the child in question.

The results by van Aken and Asendorpf (1997) contradict those obtained in an earlier study (Wehner & Furman, 1989) that investigated patterns of significant relationships in children's social networks and the impact of these relations on adjustment. In this study, adolescents were asked to rate their relationships with several individuals, including parents and friends. On the one hand, the authors found that the presence of two or more unsatisfying relationships, regardless of type (parent or best friend), was associated with poor self-reported adjustment. On the other hand, they found that children who benefited from two satisfying relationships showed relatively better self-reported adjustment, especially if one of the two relationships was with a best friend.

Overall, these studies provide evidence that friendships and the broader peer group can offset the risk implications of problematic family environments. To summarize, researchers have found that peer relationships moderate effects of family experiences on various aspects of children's adjustment, such as social competence (Gauze et al., 1996; Rubin et al., 2004), self-esteem (Bolger et al., 1998; Gauze et al., 1996; Rubin et al., 2004), internalizing difficulties (Rubin et al., 2004), externalizing difficulties (Criss et al., 2002; Lansford et al., 2003), peer victimization (Schwartz et al., 2000), and depression and anxiety (Laible et al., 2000).

Friendship as Protection from Victimization

Friendship has also been seen as a protective factor against victimization. Independent proposals by Davies (1982) and Rizzo (1989) ascribe a specifically protective function to friendship. Each claimed that a critical function of friendship was to protect at-risk children from victimization by peers. Consistent with the view that close relationships function as security systems (Sullivan, 1953), each of these theorists claimed that children who are at risk due to their own individual characteristics, such as being aggressive or withdrawn, will be spared from victimization by having a friend. These claims have been supported in one-time-only studies by Bukowski and Sippola (1995) and Hodges, Malone, and Perry (1997). These studies have shown that children who are at risk for victimization because of their own personal characteristics (e.g., aggression and withdrawal) are less likely to experience victimization within the peer group if they are friended rather than friendless. Further evidence of the protective effects of friendship with respect to victimization may be drawn from research by Hodges, Boivin, Vitaro, and Bukowski (1999), who found that peer victimization predicted increases in internalizing and externalizing difficulties across the school year for those children who lacked a mutual best friendship. The relation between peer victimization and internalizing and externalizing problems was nonsignificant for children who possessed a mutual best friendship, indicating that friendship may function protectively for children who are victimized by their peers. (Other studies of the interface between friendship and victimization can be found in the chapter by Salmivalli and Peets; Chapter 18, this volume).

Friendship as Morality

An important but often implied feature of theory and descriptions of friendship is that it can be a moral relationship. Inherent in the protective functions ascribed to friendship is the idea that friendship serves to minimize harm and maximize adaptation. In this way, friendship ensures that persons are treated fairly and are free from harm. Moreover the provisions associated with friendship (e.g., help, nurturance) possess a moral tone in the sense that they refer to the care and attention that friends devote to each other's needs and well-being. Certainly, children conceptualize friendships as having moral purposes. Even young school-age children see loyalty, help, and trust as essential features of friendships (Bigelow, 1977). These properties may be seen as not only properties of goodness but also a commitment to one's friend, his or her well-being, and the friendship itself; that is, insofar as care is a central feature of morality, and that care is a central feature of friendship, friendship and morality are inextricably interrelated (see Bukowski & Sippola [1996] for a longer discussion of these ideas).

In addition to conceptualizing friendship as serving moral functions, friendship has also been implicated in the processes underlying moral development. For Piaget (1932), moral development occurs as a function of co-construction between equals. Although Piaget may not have said so explicitly, the kind of cooperation and mutual sensitivity that he believed was fundamental to the process of moral development appears to be highly characteristic of friendship. Piaget recognized the importance of the interactive links between friends, and he believed that the interaction and mutual respect found in friendship would lead to processes of collaboration and cooperation that were necessary for the development of morality judgment. Kohlberg (1963) was more explicit than Piaget in his emphasis on friendship as part of the process of moral development. Kohlberg referred to the process of "moral attachment," which involves a child's basic imitation and perceived similarity to a friend. He believed that it was through this "attachment" that a child would develop a sense of a "shared self" with a friend that would in turn lead to a heightened sensitivity to the friend's perspective and needs. According to Kohlberg, this sensitivity would enhance one's sense of obligation or responsibility to the friend's welfare and promote the child's motivation to maintain the friendship itself.

The ideas expressed by Piaget and Kohlberg can also be seen in the writings of Sullivan (1953), who believed that the trust, intimacy, commitment, and affection that characterize friendship may make it a unique setting for moral development. He argued that the sense of collaboration that emerges between friends during preadolescence corresponds with an increased need for interpersonal intimacy. According to Sullivan, it is through collaboration with friends that young adolescents develop an increasing sensitivity to others' needs. Sullivan wrote that it is within the bounds of friendship that a young adolescent develops a sense of "what … I [should] do to contribute to the happiness or to support the prestige and feeling of worth-whileness of my chum" (Sullivan, 1953, p. 245). Clearly, Sullivan saw the affective ties of friendship as a precondition for the acquisition of particular moral sensitivities.

The recognition that friendship is imbued with moral concerns is not new. Instead it is truly an ancient premise of Western civilization. It is not surprising that the richest conceptualization of friendship are found not in modern texts or articles but instead in the writing of Aristotle 2,400 years ago. Aristole had a very differentiated view of friendship and recognized multiple forms of friendship. Like modern theorists, he believed that goodness is a central purpose of friendship, but he realized that it could serve other purposes also, specifically, pleasure or goodness (see Bukowski & Sippola, 1996). Although the relevance of much of Aristotle's thinking about friendship is not immediately clear, his idea that friendship can serve many purposes and his belief in the link between friendship and good are ideas that peer researchers may wish to consider seriously in either their hypotheses about friendship or their measurements of it.

Summary

In this chapter we have tried to make several points about friendship and development. Using the ideas of Hinde as the conceptual point of departure for this study we followed a trail from basic definitions of friendship to theory about the place of friendship in complex processes such as well-being and morality. Although it is often conceptualized in a very simple way (i.e., as mutual liking), friendship relies on a complex set of interactions that involve high rates of mutual responsivity in regard to both affect and behavior. We showed that interactions between friends are very different than the interactions between nonfriends. This level of mutual responsiveness is likely to be both a consequence and an antecedent of the similarity observed between friends; that is, the tendency of children to be like their friends makes it easier for friends to share affect and action, and their sharing of emotions and experience is in turn likely to increase interpersonal similarity. The sense of personal connection that friends derive from these opportunities for shared affect and behavior is purported to give friendship the capacity to enhance one's sense of well-being and to protect at-risk youth from problems within their families and the peer group. It also provide opportunities for the development of moral sensitivities. In spite of its constant presence in the literature on developmental psychology, friendship remains a ripe area for research on the features and effects of peer relations.

Acknowledgments

We are grateful for the grants or fellowships from the Social Science and Humanities Research Council of Canada that support our work.

References

Altermatt, E. R., & Pomerantz, E. M. (2003). The development of competence-related and motivational beliefs: An investigation of similarity and influence among friends. *Journal of Educational Psychology, 95,* 111–123.

Badhwar, N. K. (1993). The nature and significance of friendship. *Friendship: A philosophical reader.* Ithaca, NY: Cornell University Press.

Berndt, T. J., Hawkins, J. A., & Hoyle, S. G. (1986). Changes in friendship during a school year: Effects on children's and adolescents' impressions of friendship and sharing with friends. *Child Development, 57,* 1284–1297.

Berndt, T. J., & Perry, T. B. (1986). Children's perceptions of friendships as supportive relationships. *Developmental Psychology, 22,* 640–648.

Bigelow, B. J. (1977). Children's friendship expectations: A cognitive developmental study. *Child Development, 48,* 246–253.

Bolger, K. E., Patterson, C. J., & Kupersmidt, J. B. (1998). Peer relationships and self-esteem among children who have been maltreated. *Child Development, 69,* 1171–1197.

Bukowski, W. M. (2001). Friendship and the worlds of childhood. In D. Nangle & C. Erdley (Eds.), *The role of friendship in psychological adjustment: New directions for child and adolescent development* (No. 91, pp. 93–106). San Francisco: Jossey-Bass.

Bukowski, W. M., & Adams, R. (2005). Peer relations and psychopathology: Markers, mechanisms, mediators, moderators, and meanings. *Journal of Clinical Child and Adolescent Psychology, 34,* 3–10.

Bukowski, W. M., & Hoza, B. (1989). Popularity and friendship: Issues in theory, measurement, and outcome. In T. J. Berndt & G. W. Ladd (Eds.), *Peer relations in child development* (pp. 15–45). New York: Wiley.

Bukowski, W. M., & Sippola, L. K. (1995, April). *Friendship protects "at risk" children from victimization by peers.* Paper presented at the Biennial Meeting of the Society for Research in Child Development, Indianapolis, IN.

Bukowski, W. M., & Sippola, L. K. (1996). Friendship and morality: (How) are they related? In W. M. Bukowski, A. F. Newcomb, & W. W. Hartup (Eds.), *The company they keep: Friendship during childhood and adolescence* (pp. 238–261). New York: Cambridge University Press.

Bukowski, W. M., & Sippola, L. K. (2005). Friendship and development: Putting the most human relationship in its place. In R. Larson & L. Jensen (Eds.), *New directions for child and adolescent development* (pp. 91–98). San Francisco: Jossey-Bass.

Byrne, D., & Griffit, W. (1966). A developmental investigation of the law of attraction. *Journal of Personality and Social Psychology, 4*(6), 699–702.

Criss, M. M., Pettit, G. S., Bates, J. E., Dodge, K. A., & Lapp, A. L. (2002). Family adversity, positive peer relationships and children's externalizing behavior: A longitudinal perspective on risk and resilience. *Child Development, 73*(4), 1220–1237.

Davies, B. (1982). *Life in the classroom and playgrounds.* London: Routledge.

Dunn, J. (1993). *Young children's close relationships: Beyond attachment.* London: Sage.

Dunn, J., & Cutting, A. (1999). Understanding others and individual differences in friendship interactions in young children. *Social Development, 8,* 201–219.

Dunn, J., Cutting, A., & Fisher, N. (2002). Old friends, new friends: Predictors of children's perspective on their friends at school. *Child Development, 73,* 621–635.

Erdley, C. A., Nangle, D. W., & Gold, J. A. (1998). Operationalizing the construct of friendship among children: A psychometric comparison of sociometric-based definitional methodologies. *Social Development, 7,* 62–71.

Foot, H. C., Chapman, A. J., & Smith, J. R. (1977). Friendship and social responsiveness in boys and girls. *Journal of Personality and Social Psychology, 35,* 401–411.

Furman, W., & Buhrmester, D. (1985). Children's perceptions of the personal relationships in their social networks. *Developmental Psychology, 21,* 1016–1024.

Furman, W., & Robbins, P. (1985). What's the point: Selection of treatment objectives. In B. Schneider, K. H. Rubin, & J. E. Ledingham (Eds.), *Children's peer relations: Issues in assessment and intervention* (pp. 41–54). New York: Springer-Verlag.

Gauze, C., Bukowski, W. M., Aquan-Assee, J., & Sippola, L. K. (1996). Interactions between family environment and friendship and associations with self-perceived well-being during early adolescence. *Child Development, 67,* 2201–2216.

Gest, S. D., Graham-Bermann, S. A., & Hartup, W. W. (1991). Peer experience: Common and unique features of number of friendships, social network centrality, and sociometric status. *Social Development, 10,* 23–40.

Hamm, J. V. (2000). Do birds of a feather flock together?: The variable bases for African American, Asian American, and European American adolescents' selection of similar friends. *Developmental Psychology, 36*(2), 209–219.

Hartup, W. W. (1996). The company they keep: Friendships and their developmental significance. *Child Development, 67,* 1–13.

Hartup, W. W., Laursen, B., Stewart, M. A., & Eastenson, A. (1988). Conflicts and the friendship relations of young children. *Child Development, 59,* 1590–1600.

Hartup, W. W., & Stevens, N. (1997). Friendships and adaptation in the life course. *Psychological Bulletin, 121,* 355–370.

Haselager, G. J. T., Hartup, W. W., van Lieshout, C. F. M., & Riksen-Walraven, J. M. A. (1998). Similarities between friends and nonfriends in middle childhood. *Child Development, 69,* 1198–1208.

Hinde, R. A. (1979). *Towards understanding relationships.* London: Academic Press.

Hinde, R. A. (1987). *Individuals, relationships and culture.* Cambridge: Cambridge University Press.

Hinde, R. A. (1995). A suggested structure for a science of relationships. *Personal Relationships, 2,* 1–15.

Hodges, E., Boivin, M., Vitaro, F., & Bukowski, W. M. (1999). The power of friendship: Friendship as a factor in the cycle of victimization and maladjustment. *Developmental Psychology, 35,* 94–101.

Hodges, E. V. E., Malone, M. J., & Perry, D. G. (1997). Individual risk and social risk as interacting determinants of victimization in the peer group. *Developmental Psychology, 33,* 1032–1039.

Hogue, A., & Steinberg, L. (1995). Homophily of internalized distress in adolescent peer groups. *Developmental Psychology, 31,* 897–906.

Howes, C. (1990). Social status and friendship from kindergarten to third grade. *Journal of Applied Developmental Psychology, 11,* 321–330.

Jones, D. C. (1985). Persuasive appeals and responses to appeals among friends and acquaintances. *Child Development, 56,* 757–763.

Kohlberg, L. (1963). Moral development and identification. In H. W. Stevenson (Ed.), *Child psychology: 62nd yearbook of the National Society for the Study of Education.* Chicago: University of Chicago Press.

Ladd, G. W., Kochenderfer, B. J., & Coleman, C. C. (1996). Friendship quality as a predictor of young children's early school adjustment. *Child Development, 67,* 1103–1111, 1118.

Laible, D. J., Carlo, G., & Raffaelli, M. (2000). The differential relations of parent and peer attachment to adolescent adjustment. *Journal of Youth and Adolescence, 29*(1), 45–59.

Lansford, J. E., Criss, M. M., Pettit, G. S., Dodge, K. A., & Bates, J. (2003). Friendship quality, peer group affiliation, and peer antisocial behavior as moderators of the link between negative parenting and adolescent externalizing behavior. *Journal of Research on Adolescence, 13,* 161–184.

Laursen, B., Bukowski, W. M., Aunola, K., & Nurmi, J. E. (2007). Friendship moderates prospective associations between social isolation and adjustment problems in young children. *Child Development, 78,* 1395–1404.

Laursen, B., & Hartup, W. W. (1989). The dynamics of preschool children's conflicts. *Merrill–Palmer Quarterly, 35,* 281–297.

Lindsey, E. W. (2002). Preschool children's friendships and peer acceptance: Links to social competence. *Child Study Journal, 32*, 145–156.

Liu, M., & Chen, X. (2003). Friendship networks and social, school, and psychological adjustment in Chinese junior high school students. *Psychology in the Schools, 40*, 5–17.

Monroe, W. S. (1898). Social consciousness in children. *Psychological Review, 5*, 68–70.

Nangle, D., Erdley, C., Newman, J., Mason, C., & Carpenter, E. (2003). Popularity, friendship quality, and friendship quality: Interactive influences on children's loneliness and depression. *Journal of Clinical Child and Adolescent Psychology, 32*, 546–555.

Newcomb, A., & Bagwell, C. (1995). Children's friendship relations: A meta-analytic review. *Psychological Bulletin, 117*, 306–347.

Newcomb, A. F., & Brady, J. E. (1982). Mutuality in boys' friendship relations. *Child Development, 53*, 392–395.

Parker, J. G., & Asher, S. R. (1993). Friendship and friendship quality in middle childhood: Links with peer group acceptance and feelings of loneliness and social dissatisfaction. *Developmental Psychology, 29*, 611–621.

Piaget, J. (1932). *The moral judgment of the child*. Glencoe, IL: Free Press.

Popp, D., Laursen, B., Kerr, M., Stattin, H., & Burk, W. (2008). Modeling homophily over time with an actor–partner interdependence model. *Developmental Psychology, 44*, 1028–1039.

Poulin, F., & Boivin, M. (2000). The role of proactive and reactive aggression in the formation and development of boys' friendships. *Developmental Psychology, 36*, 233–240.

Poulin, F., Cillessen, A., Hubbard, J., Coie, J. D., Dodge, K. A., & Schwartz, D. (1997). Children's friends and behavioural similarity in two social contexts. *Social Development, 6*, 244–236.

Rizzo, T. A. (1989). *Friendship development among children in school*. Norwood, NJ: Ablex.

Ross, S. H., Cheyne, J. A., & Lollis, S. P. (1988). Defining and studying reciprocity in young children. In S. Duck (Series Ed.) & S. Duck, D. H. Hay, S. E. Hobfoll, W. Ickes, & B. M. Montgomery (Vol. Eds.), *Handbook of personal relationships: Theory, research and interventions* (pp. 143–160). London: Wiley.

Rubin, K. H., Bukowski, W. M., & Parker, J. G. (2006). Peer interactions, relationships and groups. In W. Damon (Series Ed.) & N. Eisenberg (Vol. Ed.), *The handbook of child psychology* (6th ed., pp. 571–645). New York: Wiley.

Rubin, K. H., Wojslawowicz, J. C., Burgess, K. B., Booth-LaForce, C., & Rose-Krasnor, L. (2004). *The best friendships of shy/withdrawn children*. Unpublished manuscript, University of Maryland.

Schwartz, D., Dodge, K. A., Pettit, G. S., & Bates, J. E. (2000). Friendship as a moderating factor in the pathway between early harsh home environment and later victimization in the peer group. *Developmental Psychology, 36*(5), 646–662.

Sebanc, A. M. (2003). The friendship features of preschool children: Links with prosocial behavior and aggression. *Social Development, 12*, 249–268.

Sullivan, H. S. (1953). *The interpersonal theory of psychiatry*. New York: Norton.

van Aken, M. A. G., & Asendorpf, J. (1997). Support by parents, classmates, friends and siblings in preadolescence: Covariation and compensation across relationships. *Journal of Social and Personal Relationships, 14*, 79–93.

Vandell, D. L., & Hembree, S. (1994). Peer social status and friendship: Independent contributors to children's social and academic adjustment. *Merrill–Palmer Quarterly, 40*, 461–477.

Wehner, E. A., & Furman, W. (1989, July). *A typology of social networks and its relation to adjustment*. Paper presented at the biennial meeting of the International Society for the Study of Behavioral Development, Jyvaskula, Finland.

Weiss, R. S. (1974). The provisions of social relationships. In Z. Ruibin (Ed.), *Doing unto others* (pp. 17–26). Englewood Cliffs, NJ: Prentice-Hall.

Youniss, J. (1980). *Parents and peers in social development: A Sullivan–Piaget perspective*. Chicago: University of Chicago Press.

CHAPTER 13

The Behavioral Basis of Acceptance, Rejection, and Perceived Popularity

STEVEN R. ASHER
KRISTINA L. McDONALD

Scholars have long been interested in learning about the kinds of behavioral characteristics that lead children and adolescents to be accepted versus rejected by their peers. Indeed, every decade since the 1930s has brought forward major studies of this topic (e.g., Bukowski, Gauze, Hoza, & Newcomb, 1993; Chen, Rubin, & Sun, 1992; Cillessen & Mayeux, 2004; Coie, Dodge, & Coppotelli, 1982; Coie & Kupersmidt, 1983; Crick & Grotpeter, 1995; Dodge, Coie, Pettit, & Price, 1990; French, 1988; Gottman, Gonso, & Rasmussen, 1975; Hartup, Glazer, & Charlesworth, 1967; Koch, 1933; Ladd & Oden, 1979; Marshall & McCandless, 1957; Northway, 1944; Parkhurst & Asher, 1992; Putallaz & Gottman, 1981; Rubin & Mills, 1988; Wright, Giammarino, & Parad, 1986). This is not to say that there was a steady stream of research in every decade. As Hartup (1970) noted, there was a significant lull in research on this topic in the 1960s. Indeed, although there were classic studies from the 1930s through the early 1970s, a critical mass of research on this topic only began to emerge in the late 1970s, hitting full stride in the 1980s and 1990s, with continuing progress being made in the past ten years.

Research on the behavioral correlates of acceptance–rejection has been reviewed regularly and thoroughly by scholars such as Coie, Dodge, and Kupersmidt (1990), Hartup (1970, 1983), Ladd (2005), Newcomb, Bukowski, and Pattee (1993), Bierman (2004), and Rubin, Bukowski, and Parker (2006). We build on this foundation by summarizing what has been learned about general and social task-specific forms of behavior associated with acceptance and rejection. In this context, we briefly describe the research settings and methods used to examine the behavioral basis of acceptance and rejection. We then describe the primary behavioral characteristics that have been found to be associated with being liked versus disliked by peers, and we highlight important social tasks, only some of which have been studied. Following this, we discuss a newer, but related, line of inquiry in peer relations research, namely, studies of the behavioral correlates of *perceived popularity*. This topic draws a contrast between sociometric popularity (being highly accepted or liked by peers) and being "popular" in the everyday sense that other children view the child as a highly visible, central, and/or a prestigious and influential member of the peer group. The chapter then concludes with recommendations for future research.

The Behavioral Basis
of Acceptance and Rejection

Research Settings and Methods

Research on the behavioral basis of acceptance and rejection has typically been conducted in naturalistic settings, primarily schools, or in laboratory settings specifically designed to elicit or amplify behaviors of interest. Some researchers productively combine these settings in a sequential way by doing sociometric and peer or teacher behavioral assessments in schools, then bringing selected children into the laboratory for more intensive behavioral observations or individual interviews. Occasionally, summer camps have been used as a research setting (e.g., Parker & Seal, 1996; Wright et al., 1986), although for various pragmatic reasons, including sample size and representativeness, this setting, as well as other nonschool settings (e.g., afterschool programs, youth sports programs, religiously affiliated youth groups, scouting groups), have been underutilized.

One advantage of schools as a research setting is that the behavioral correlates of acceptance can be studied in large, intact groups where children have a long-term shared history of interaction and know each other well. Because school attendance is typically mandated, most children can be found in public or private schools, with the exception of a small percentage of children who are home-schooled. As a result, samples are likely to be reasonably representative of the community, especially when schools from different neighborhoods within a school district are included. Furthermore, the school context ensures a large number of peer respondents when students are sociometrically surveyed about their feelings toward class- or grademates. This large pool of sociometric raters means that the sociometric scores children receive from others have the potential to be highly reliable (see Cillessen, Chapter 5, this volume), even during the preschool years (Asher, Singleton, Tinsley, & Hymel, 1979). Likewise, a large peer group gives researchers a pool of raters for assessing behavioral style. This means that the reliability and validity of children's behavior scores (averaged across raters) are likely to be satisfactory even if certain children in a class or grade level are not perceptive observers. Additionally, the school context enables researchers to observe children with different types of interaction partners and in different school settings (classroom, playground, lunchroom, etc.), important factors yet to be fully explored in this literature.

Measuring Acceptance and Rejection

For the most part, researchers use one of two sociometric measurement approaches to assess whether children are accepted or rejected by peers. Rating scale measures of peer acceptance involve asking children to rate on a Likert scale how much they like each class- or grademate. For example, children have been asked to indicate on a 3-, 5-, or 7-point scale (the number of points on the scale varies based on the age of the children) how much they like to play with each of the other members of their class. Children's received ratings are then averaged and standardized within gender and class or grade (for an early example, see Oden & Asher, 1977). Researchers either treat this score as a continuous measure or group children into low-, average-, or high-acceptance groups.

A second method is to gather "positive" and "negative" nominations from each child of most and least liked peers. Typically, children have been asked to nominate three classmates for each category, although unlimited nominations may have psychometric advantages. The positive and negative nomination approach dates back to the early years of sociometric research (e.g., Northway, 1944) and was revised years later by Peery (1979), Coie et al. (1982), and Newcomb and Bukowski (1983). Most and least liked nominations can be used to calculate a continuous social preference score, as well as to categorize children as sociometrically popular, average, rejected, or neglected. Again, for more information on the topic of sociometric assessment, please refer to Cillessen, Chapter 5, this volume.

Measuring Behavior

A traditional strength of research on the behavioral correlates of peer acceptance and rejection has been the creative use of direct observation measures of behavior in naturalistic and laboratory settings. Whereas naturalistic observations have the potential for greater external validity by observing children in their everyday environments, laboratory or analogue methods allow for greater experimental control and are helpful for evoking and studying behaviors that occur less frequently in natural settings. Many of the classic studies in the field have had an observational component. In her pioneering study, Koch (1933) used a thorough time-sampling procedure in which she observed children in various preschool settings for 400 thirty-second intervals. In the 1970s, Gottman et al. (1975) used a very extensive coding system, studying children in both working-class and middle-class schools, and observing them in the classroom, in gym, at recess, and in other play periods. Moving to the 1980s, a set of studies by Coie and Kupersmidt (1983), Dodge (1983), Putallaz and Gottman (1981), and Putallaz (1983) pioneered the technique of observing children in new groups of previously unfamiliar peers to eliminate the effects of prior reputation on behavior, thereby demonstrating that behavior contributes to sociometric status rather than simply being the consequence of a prior reputation. This tradition of assessing children in newly formed groups continues to the present (e.g., Gazelle et al., 2005).

Within the literature on the behavioral correlates of sociometric status, researchers have also assessed behavior by asking peers to describe one another through peer nomination inventories, by having teachers complete behavior ratings about their students, and by presenting children with hypothetical situations (i.e., scenarios or vignettes) and asking them to act out (role play) or describe what they would do. These latter descriptions may be open-ended or children may be asked to indicate, through ratings, the likelihood that they would carry out various behavioral strategies.

All of these assessment methods have a long history, with evidence of validity. Still, it is important to acknowledge that each approach has strengths and weaknesses (see Bierman, 2004). For example, direct behavioral observations have no equal for capturing detailed descriptions of interaction processes. By contrast, peer assessments are useful when large samples are involved and the goal is to assess a wide variety of general behavioral characteristics, capitalizing on children's knowledge of one another over time and across contexts.

Broad Research Strategies and the Need for Theory

Evidence for the behavioral correlates of acceptance and rejection comes from two types of studies. One type is designed to characterize children's behavioral style in general, and without regard to specific situations. A second type of study assesses children's responses to specific social situations (also referred to as "social tasks") and attempts to provide a picture of how children who are accepted and rejected differ in their approach to particular situations that arise in everyday life.

Regardless of the research approach, rarely have studies of the behavioral dynamics associated with acceptance and rejection been presented in the context of explicitly stated theory. However researchers appear to have adopted a general social learning perspective that assumes that behaviors will lead to liking by peers if the behaviors are "rewarding" to the other person (for early influential studies that implicitly adopted this perspective, see Hartup et al., 1967; Gottman et al., 1975). Accordingly, researchers appear to have chosen behaviors to study based on intuitions about what kinds of behaviors would be appreciated or be rewarding to other children. However, this begs the question of what it is that children find "rewarding." Everyday observations suggest that children cannot bribe their way into being liked simply by giving goodies to their peers. So what is it that makes certain behaviors attractive or unattractive, rewarding or not rewarding?

In an attempt to address this kind of issue, Asher and Williams (1987) proposed that children approach their interactions with others with an implicit set of "core questions," and that these questions serve as guides for implicitly evaluating another person's behavior (for a more recent discussion, see Troop & Asher, 1999). The core questions Asher and Williams postulated were as follows:

1. Is this child fun to be with?
2. Is this child trustworthy?
3. Do we influence each other in ways that I like?
4. Does this child facilitate and not undermine my goals?
5. Is this child similar to me?
6. Does this child make me feel good about myself?

Asher and Williams then proposed that various behavioral characteristics gain their power because they speak to certain core questions. For example, the power of aggression lies in its relevance to several questions. A child interacting with an aggressive peer is likely to conclude that the other child is neither fun to be with nor trustworthy, and that the child seeks to have influence in ways that are not acceptable. What Asher and Williams did not indicate is that these core questions do not arise out of nowhere. Instead the six core questions are likely rooted in children's (and adults') basic needs for: (1) companionship; (2) trust in their surroundings; (3) autonomy and some measure of control over their environment; (4) agency, mastery, and efficacy; (5) a sense of connection and of belonging with kindred spirits; and (6) a sense of worthiness and value about oneself. Over the decades, many scholars have written about the primacy of such needs (e.g., Baumeister & Leary, 1995; Bowlby, 1969; Deci & Ryan, 1985; Erikson, 1950; Shrauger, 1975). However, scholars who study the behavioral correlates of acceptance and rejection rarely discuss the ways that the behaviors they study are powerful because they speak to peoples' fundamental needs and perhaps, therefore, to some connected core questions that guide peoples' evaluations of others. One potential benefit of incorporating this perspective is that it might suggest other behavioral characteristics that are relevant to acceptance and rejection but have not yet been studied.

Type I Studies: Characterizing Children's General Behavioral Style

Fortunately, although efforts to ground research in this topic area to theory have been few, scholars in this field have had excellent intuitions about what behavioral characteristics to study. A large body of research indicates that certain broad categories of behavior and certain task-specific behaviors are consistently linked with acceptance and rejection. Indeed, the pattern of evidence emerging from the 75-year history of behavioral correlates research has been consistent and clear. Well-liked children tend to be prosocial in the sense that they are cooperative, friendly, helpful, and kind. These children also tend to be leaders and to be (nonaggressively) assertive. They also tend not to be highly disruptive nor to exhibit high levels of verbal, physical, or social/relational aggression. Highly accepted children tend not to be withdrawn or submissive with peers, and they tend to be more competent academically. Finally, although these characteristics have been studied far less frequently, these children tend to have better senses of humor and are more likely to be physically well-coordinated and better athletes.

By contrast, rejected children tend to show heightened levels of aggression and disruptive behavior, and higher levels of withdrawn/submissive forms of behavior. Regardless of whether rejected children exhibit an externalizing versus an internalizing pattern, they tend to exhibit lower levels of prosocial behavior (e.g., Parkhurst & Asher, 1992). The prosocial skills deficits of rejected children have provided a large part of the rationale for teaching positive relationship skills to various subtypes of peer-rejected children (for reviews, see Asher, Parker, & Walker, 1996; Bierman & Powers, Chapter 33, this volume).

Although there is wide agreement that far more research is needed on developmental changes in the behavioral correlates of status (for a discussion of the limited work in this area, see Rubin et al., 2006), there is some evidence to suggest that physical aggression may become a weaker correlate of status as children grow older (e.g., Cillessen & Mayeux, 2004). Partly this could result from children moving into the different organizational structures provided by middle schools versus elementary schools. The larger number of children with whom aggressive children come into contact during a given day increases the opportunity to find and befriend similar peers who are also aggressive. This process could result in a greater number of children providing "like most" nominations to an aggressive child, thereby weakening the negative correlation between peer acceptance scores and aggression. Of course, this would not explain changes in the correlation over age/grade level that occur within the elementary school context (see Sandstrom & Coie, 1999). However, it does imply that using a rating scale sociometric measure would be instructive for learning how aggressive children are viewed by *all* of their classmates or grademates, not just those who name them as their three "like most" peers. It would also be instructive to learn how the behavioral characteristics of aggressive children's "like most" *nominators* change over age. This would address the hypothesis that the negative correlation between aggression and acceptance becomes weaker over age/grade level, because aggressive children increasingly befriend one another.

Until fairly recently, most of what was known about the behavioral correlates of acceptance and rejection was based on North American samples. This was a significant limitation given that the meaning of interpersonal behavior is interpreted through a cultural lens, and what is socially appropriate in one culture may or may not be so in another.

It seems plausible that cultural frames of reference would affect how children evaluate peers' behavior and whether they like or dislike another child (Chen, French, & Schneider, 2006). This recognition makes it important to compare the behavioral correlates of acceptance and rejection among people of varying cultures or cultural subgroups.

Cross-cultural comparisons to date have revealed considerable similarities in the behaviors associated with acceptance and rejection in various cultures. For example, among Chinese students, similar to children in Canada and the United States, being prosocial and sociable is positively associated with acceptance (e.g., Chang, 2004; Chen, Li, Li, Li, & Liu, 2000). Being sociable and a leader has been linked with higher acceptance in Italy as well (Casiglia, Lo Coco, & Zappulla, 1998). Furthermore, aggression has been linked to peer rejection in Italian children (e.g., Casiglia et al., 1998; Tomada & Schneider, 1997), Cuban children (e.g., Valdivia, Schneider, Chavez, & Chen, 2005), and Chinese children (e.g., Chen et al., 1992).

There has been research on the extent to which forms of withdrawn behavior are linked with rejection cross-culturally. Withdrawn behavior has been found to be associated with peer rejection in the United States (e.g., Rubin, Burgess, & Coplan, 2002), Canada (e.g., Hymel, Rubin, Rowden, & LeMare, 1990), Cuba (Valdivia et al., 2005), Russia (e.g., Hart et al., 2000), and Italy (e.g., Casiglia et al., 1998). However, preliminary evidence indicates that in Eastern cultures, a pattern of shyness/sensitivity may be positively associated with acceptance. Chen et al. (1992) found that Chinese children who were shy-sensitive (i.e., feelings get hurt easily, very shy, usually sad) were better liked by peers. They suggested that in China, compliance, reservedness, and obedience were valued, and inhibition was considered a sign of maturity.

However, the positive association between certain forms of withdrawal and acceptance has not been replicated in all studies with Chinese children (Chang, 2004; Hart et al., 2000; Schwartz, Chang, & Farver, 2001). These discrepancies may be due to different ways of operationalizing withdrawal, the examination of different subtypes of withdrawn behavior (see Coplan, Rubin, Fox, Calkins, & Stewart, 1994), or the historical period when the research was conducted. For example, Hart et al. (2000) found that preschoolers who were more reticent, as rated by teachers (i.e., wandered aimlessly, appeared to be doing nothing, stared at other children without interacting with them, watched others play), were more likely to be rejected by peers in the United States, Russia, and China. Furthermore, Chen, Cen, Li, and He (2005) found that the association between shyness-sensitivity and acceptance varied by the cohort being studied, such that an association that was positive in the 1990 cohort was negative by 2002. This suggests that the meaning of shy-sensitive behavior may have changed in China over time, perhaps as the country moved in a more Western-style economic direction.

Variation in the behaviors associated with acceptance and rejection has also been studied in different contexts or subgroups of a population. For example, in a classic study, Wright et al. (1986) found that in groups in which a majority of boys were aggressive, children who were more withdrawn were the most rejected, and aggression was not predictive of liking. On the other hand, in groups with boys that were predominately low in aggression, boys who were aggressive were more likely to be rejected, whereas withdrawn behavior was not significantly associated with acceptance. The importance of context is further illustrated through more recent examinations of variation in behavior–acceptance associations by classroom or group composition (Boivin, Dodge, & Coie, 1995; Chang, 2004; Stormshak et al., 1999). These studies have replicated the finding that the relation between negative social behaviors and status is attenuated when negative behaviors are normative.

Wright et al. (1986) suggested that prosocial behaviors may be universally associated with peer acceptance and their data were supportive of this possibility. Likewise, Stormshak et al. (1999) found that prosocial behavior was positively linked to acceptance, regardless of the group composition. However, Boivin et al. (1995) did not find a positive association between acceptance and positive social behavior in groups that were low on these behaviors, and Chang (2004) found that higher classroom levels of assertive prosocial behavior strengthened the positive association between this form of behavior and peer acceptance, although this context effect was smaller than those for aggression and withdrawal. Chang suggested that the contextual effect for prosocial behavior may be smaller than for aggression and withdrawal because prosocial behavior is a more dominant norm; thus, there is less variation in prosocial behavior across contexts. Clearly, more work is needed on context effects on the behavior–acceptance connection, but it is good to have studies like these emerging in this literature and setting the stage for further inquiry.

Type II Studies: Characterizing Behavior in Response to Specific Social Tasks

Within the literature on the behavioral correlates of status is a set of studies that takes a social tasks approach. This research has its roots in conceptual and empirical work by investigators such as Goldfried and D'Zurilla (1969), McFall (1982), and Dodge, McClaskey, and Feldman (1985). A major assumption underlying social tasks–based research is that people's social relationship problems are not necessarily pervasive across all situations, but may instead be highly specific to certain situations that are especially problematic for them.

Research focused on children's behavior in response to specific social tasks, from its beginning in the early 1980s, has typically made use of either observations in specially structured laboratory (analogue) situations (e.g., Putallaz & Gottman, 1981) or vignette measures that present hypothetical situations to children and ask them what they would do (e.g., Dodge, 1980; Renshaw & Asher, 1983). Rarely do investigators ask teachers or peers to make their behavioral ratings or nominations with respect to specific situations, although this could be done if informants, especially teachers, were trained to observe situations carefully (Coie et al., 1990). An example of more situated teacher assessments is Dodge and Coie's (1987) work asking teachers and peers to distinguish between proactive and reactive aggression (e.g., "uses physical force to dominate" vs. "when teased strikes back").

Table 13.1 presents a list of everyday social tasks faced by children, adolescents, and adults. The list is illustrative rather than complete, and we present it in the hope of stimulating research on the many very interesting tasks that have been insufficiently studied to date. Inherent in a social tasks perspective is the assumption that the various tasks on this list have their own distinct challenges and call upon skills and knowledge that are task specific. The value of a social tasks approach for studying the behavioral correlates of liking and disliking lies in its potential for uncovering very specific behavioral processes within particular social situations. The social tasks approach is valuable because it moves our analysis beyond generalizations about "macro" levels of behavioral description (e.g., highly accepted children are prosocial) to a more textured and nuanced description of what well-accepted children or rejected children do in specific situations. A social tasks approach also contributes by informing the design of interventions; that is, learning about what well-accepted children do in specific situations can inform the content that is taught to children who are having peer relationship problems. Finally, a social tasks

TABLE 13.1. An Incomplete List of Social Tasks

Entering a Group	Helping
Responding to Ambiguous Provocation	Asking for Help
Managing Conflict	Responding to Cheating/Unfairness
Coping with False Accusations	Resisting Distraction by Others
Listening	Persuading
Negotiating Rules	Achieving Equity/Fairness
Retrieving Belongings	Complimenting
Generating "Fun" Ideas	Coping with Frustrating Situations
Sharing Resources/Belongings	Getting Picked for Teams/Activities
Maintaining Interaction	Expressing Affection
Making Requests	Coping with Teasing
Eliciting Disclosure	Avoiding Dangerous Peer Contexts
Self-Disclosure	Comforting
Responding to Requests	Defending Self
Expressing Appreciation	Communicating Contingently
Coping with Public Failure	Sticking Up for a Friend
Coping with Rejection	Refusing a Dare
Dealing with Losing	Responding to Winning/Success
Apologizing	Keeping Secrets
Forgiving	Terminating Interaction

approach provides a potentially productive way of thinking about individual differences in the sense that children differ greatly in their profiles of social tasks proficiency. For example, some children who may know how to enter a group may not manage conflicts competently. Other children may be relatively competent at sharing resources but have trouble coping when teased.

Of all the social tasks listed in Table 13.1 (and, again, this list is likely far from complete), fewer than 10 have been given research attention in the literature on the behavioral correlates of peer acceptance. However, the research that does exist on children's responses to these situations indicates the considerable promise of a social tasks perspective for identifying specific behavioral strategies that well-accepted and poorly accepted children employ. The early work on peer group entry indicated that well-accepted children enter groups by taking the frame of reference of the children who are already interacting, then saying something relevant to the group activity (Putallaz & Gottman, 1981; Putallaz, 1983). Research on ambiguous provocation by Dodge (1980) and others led to evidence that not only do aggressive–rejected children aggress more in response to being harmed when the intent of the actor is not perfectly clear but they also fail to ask for clarification of the other person's intent before responding with hostility (Erdley & Asher, 1996). There is also a small body of work on children's responses to help-seeking and help-giving tasks (Gottman et al., 1975; Ladd & Oden, 1979; Rose & Asher, 2004), and a growing body of research on how children respond to various types of conflicts of interest with a peer (e.g., Chung & Asher, 1996; Hopmeyer & Asher, 1997; Rabiner & Gordon, 1992; Rose & Asher, 1999; Troop-Gordon & Asher, 2005). In these studies, too, poorly accepted children prove to be not only aggressive but also lacking in a sophisticated understanding of how to meet the specific challenges of the social tasks they are confronting. For example, whereas highly accepted children propose nonaggressive but verbally assertive ways of handling conflict, children low in peer acceptance are more likely to propose seeking out help from adults (Hopmeyer & Asher, 1997).

Game situations are potentially rich contexts, because a wide variety of social tasks arise and children can pursue a wide variety of goals (Taylor & Asher, 1984). In a laboratory/analogue observational study by Hubbard (2001), confederate actors interacted with participants in two game-playing contexts, one in which a confederate played fairly and the other in which a confederate cheated. Hubbard found that rejected children expressed more anger during the game in which the confederate cheated than did children with average sociometric status, but differences were not significant in the fair play condition. Rejected children also expressed more happiness during turns when they were winning the game than did average children. These findings have relevance to two of the social tasks in Table 13.1, namely, responding to cheating/unfairness and responding to one's own winning or public success. Overall, the Hubbard findings suggest that rejected children would not be perceived by peers to be "good sports" in game situations. This inference is also consistent with a follow-up analogue observational study by R. M. Rubin and Hubbard (2002), who found that rejected children were more likely both to cheat and to brag in a game situation.

In contrast to the growing number of cross-cultural studies on the "broad category" correlates of status (prosocial behavior, aggression, withdrawal, etc.), very little cross-cultural research examines the behavioral correlates of status at the social tasks level. Our hypothesis is that there will be cultural differences at the social tasks level (e.g., the particular ways that children deal with conflict), such that the specific behavioral strategies that correlate with acceptance will vary by culture even though generalizations about macro-level categories (e.g., prosocial behavior) will still generally apply across cultures.

The Distinction between Sociometric Popularity (Acceptance) and Perceived Popularity

In the sociology of education field, there is a long tradition of studying what leads children and adolescents to be "popular" in the peer group. Sociologists in this tradition use the term "popular" in a way that is much closer to the meaning of "popularity" in colloquial language. For them, "popularity" refers to dimensions such as status, visibility, and being socially central or prominent. Coleman's (1961) *The Adolescent Society* provides an early example of this sort of work. Coleman surveyed students to learn about the characteristics (good looks, personality, athletic ability, good grades, etc.) students thought led to popularity in their high schools. Although there was similarity in the factors that led to popularity among students from different schools, there was also sufficient variability to suggest school-based differences. This tradition in the sociology of education continues (e.g., Adler & Adler, 1998; Eder, 1985; Merten, 1997) and adds a great deal of information to what we know about peer groups.

In the last 10 years, research on the behavioral correlates of acceptance and rejection has given rise to an independent but related line of inquiry, conducted primarily by psychologists, that examines the behaviors associated with being perceived as popular. This work highlights the point that researchers who have studied sociometric popularity (meaning "popular" in the sense of being well-liked) are not studying the same construct of popularity as that used by the layperson or studied by sociologists. Most researchers within this new line of inquiry (e.g., Cillessen & Mayeux, 2004; Hawley, 2003; LaFontana & Cillessen, 2002; Parkhurst & Hopmeyer, 1998; Rose, Swenson, & Waller, 2004) measure "perceived popularity." The measurement of perceived popularity is based on the peer group's perceptions of who is popular. Researchers typically ask children to nominate who in their class or grade is "popular." Then they divide the number of nominations a child receives by the number of possible nominations he or she could have received and standardize this proportion by class or grade. The resulting score is an index of perceived popularity.

Perceived popularity, according to this methodology, overlaps to some extent not only with the characteristics associated with being sociometrically popular but also to some extent with characteristics associated with controversial sociometric status and even with rejected status (e.g., see Coie et al., 1982). Indeed, Parkhurst and Hopmeyer's (1998) study was motivated partly by conversations with students who expressed dislike for students they considered to be popular. Overall, the correlation between perceived popularity and sociometric popularity ranges from moderate to strong (Hawley, 2003; Cillessen & Mayeux, 2004; LaFontana & Cillessen, 2002; Parkhurst & Hopmeyer, 1998; Vaillancourt & Hymel, 2006), but as children get older and enter high school this association may weaken, especially so for girls (Cillessen & Mayeux, 2004). Consistent with the finding that perceived popularity overlaps to some degree with controversial status, students high in perceived popularity are also high in social impact (Parkhurst & Hopmeyer, 1998), meaning that they receive many "liked most" and "liked least" nominations.

Moving to a discussion of the specific correlates of perceived popularity, research indicates that being perceived as popular is highly associated with dominance and power (Hawley, 2003; Vaillancourt & Hymel, 2006), prosocial behavior (LaFontana & Cillessen, 2002), having a good sense of humor (Vaillancourt & Hymel, 2006), and other peer-valued characteristics, such as academic competence, athletic ability, being attractive, and being stylish and wealthy (LaFontana & Cillessen, 2002; Vaillancourt & Hymel, 2006). Perceived popularity is also negatively associated with withdrawal (LaFontana & Cillessen, 2002) and being easy to push around (Parkhurst & Hopmeyer, 1998). Additionally, perceived popularity has been positively linked with both physical and relational aggression (Cillessen & Mayeux, 2004; LaFontana & Cillessen, 2002; Parkhurst & Hopmeyer, 1998; Rose et al., 2004).

Consistent with this diverse and seemingly contradictory set of correlates, Rodkin, Farmer, Pearl, and Van Acker (2000, 2006) have identified two different subsets of popular children. Rodkin et al. (2000, 2006) measure the construct of popularity by asking teachers to rate children on three items: "popular with boys," "popular with girls," and "has lots of friends." In a study of boys, the children the researchers labeled as "model" boys were high on popularity, high on academic and physical competence, high on affiliative behaviors, and low on teacher-rated aggression. The children labeled as "tough" boys were found to be high on popularity, aggression, and physical competence. Both "model" and "tough" children were also found (using a social network measure) to be socially central (Rodkin et al., 2000, 2006) and perceived by peers as "cool" (Rodkin et al., 2006).

The association between perceived popularity and different forms of aggression has been further explored to piece apart the mechanisms of influence. Longitudinal research suggests that aggression, especially relational aggression, and perceived popularity are intertwined and may serve to reinforce each other over time. Cillessen and Mayeux (2004) found that perceived popularity predicted increases in relational aggression over time, and that relational aggression in middle school also predicted subsequent increases in perceived popularity. They suggest that children who attain social prominence increase their use of relational aggression as a means to maintain their status. Additionally, the link between overt aggression and perceived popularity could be explained by the link between relational aggression and perceived popularity. Overt and relational aggression are positively associated, and Rose et al. (2004) found that when controlling for relational aggression, the association between overt aggression and perceived popularity was no longer significant. This important finding substantially qualifies the picture regarding the linkage between physical aggression and perceived popularity.

An understanding of perceived popularity and associated behavioral character- istics is further complicated by gender, age, and contextual differences. For example, perceived popularity may not be significantly associated with aggression in elementary school, but as children transition into middle and high school this association increases (Cillessen & Mayeux, 2004; Rose et al., 2004). It has been suggested that the skills needed to use aggression to maintain status are complex and develop with age (Cillessen & Rose, 2005). Additionally, the link between relational aggression and perceived popularity may be stronger for girls than for boys (Cillessen & Mayeux, 2004; Rose et al., 2004). There is also evidence that there may be differences across ethnic groups that deserve further exploration (e.g., LaFontana & Cillessen, 2002; Rodkin et al., 2006). For example, the association between sociometric popularity and perceived popularity is greater for Euro- pean American than for African American or Latino children (LaFontana & Cillessen, 2002).

The association between perceived popularity and aggression, especially relational aggression, may be of relevance to understanding how aggressive behaviors come to be maintained by the peer group even though these same behaviors are generally corre- lated with peer dislike. The focus on perceived popularity and its behavioral correlates is relatively new in peer relations research. As exploration continues in this area, including observational and experimental studies, we will learn much more about the mechanisms underlying how behavior and perceived popularity are associated and how one's reputa- tion for being popular emerges in the peer group.

Future Directions

Despite the 75-year history of research on the behavioral dynamics that give rise to accep- tance and rejection, some surprising gaps in our knowledge need attention. Two of these are research on developmental changes and on gender differences in the correlates of acceptance versus rejection. Surprisingly, despite repeated calls for inquiry into these areas, relatively little work has addressed how the correlates of status change with age or differ as a function of gender. With regard to developmental change, for various reasons, it seems likely that certain behavioral characteristics become more or less prominent as children's criteria for evaluating their relationships evolve or as their skills for attending to and interpreting the behavior of others increases. These kinds of developmental changes would make it possible for children and adolescents to notice certain forms of behavior that might earlier have escaped their notice. Consider, for example, the way behavior that is particularly self-focused/narcissistic (a more difficult pattern of behavior to detect than physical aggression) might affect the peers of a 5-year-old versus a 17-year-old.

Likewise, there has been relatively little work on whether the behavioral processes that lead to acceptance and rejection differ by gender. Is this because researchers have examined their data on the behavioral correlates of status separately by gender, found little of interest, and then pooled their data across gender (for a discussion of how this may happen in the broader gender differences literature, see Maccoby & Jacklin, 1974)? Or has there been a failure to examine some of the behavioral characteristics that might show differential associations to status for boys versus girls? For example, the processes that lead to girls versus boys being viewed as a "fun partner" might differ. McDonald, Putallaz, Grimes, Kupersmidt, and Coie (2007) found that sociometrically popular girls gossiped more with their friends than did rejected girls. Would this be equally true for boys?

It may be that there are not many significant developmental or gender differences in the correlates of status at the macro level of prosocial, aggressive, or disruptive behavior. For example, prosocial behavior is likely to be a very powerful influence on acceptance for boys and for girls and at every age level. However, more subtle behavioral processes (e.g., communicating contingently with an interaction partner who is confiding) may show differential associations with status at different ages or for boys versus girls. These processes cannot easily be detected by asking children to make peer nominations or even by asking adults to complete behavioral rating forms. Most people do not mentally code the behavior of others at the same fine-grained level of analysis as a researcher who creates elaborate and highly differentiated coding systems to understand interpersonal processes. It took videotaping of interaction and a relatively sophisticated coding system to identify the processes involved in successful peer-group entry (Putallaz & Gottman, 1981) and it will take comparable work to study the diverse social tasks of everyday life that heretofore have been given very little attention.

This brings us to another major suggestion, namely, that scholars in the field continue to do intensive behavioral observation research rather than coming to rely increasingly on peer assessments or teacher ratings. The peer relations literature, broadly, continues to make creative use of behavioral observation methodology (e.g., Hubbard, 2001; McDonald et al., 2007; Underwood, Scott, Galperin, Bjornstad, & Sexton, 2004), but within the specific field of the behavioral correlates of sociometric status in the past decade, far more research has used peer assessments than has used direct observations of behavior. On the one hand this is surprising because, historically, naturalistic and laboratory/analogue observational studies were among those classic studies that captured scholars' interests in this topic area and helped to significantly advance our knowledge. However, the increasing reliance on peer and teacher assessments is also understandable given the kinds of research questions of recent interest. It requires very large sample sizes to compare subgroups of children who only can be identified in sufficient numbers by starting with a large pool of research participants. Behavior observation is an expensive methodology, and it is difficult to do this work with large sample sizes. Likewise, as our interest in context and culture has grown, so too have the challenges of doing work in multiple schools or multiple countries. This, too, makes behavior observations more difficult to realize when hundreds of children in each context or country are included. Likewise, exciting longitudinal research, which is inherently more time consuming and expensive, can lead researchers to forgo direct observation, especially when a large sample of children is followed over time. Cost and time considerations work against direct observations as other aspects of the research design become more ambitious.

The relative neglect of direct observational assessments in this area of research is a lost opportunity, especially given new wireless transmission technologies for recording behavior and conversations at an unobtrusive distance (e.g., Asher, Rose, & Gabriel, 2001; Pepler & Craig, 1995). The ability to study conversation can be especially productive. For example, Asher et al. (2001) used wireless audio and video recording at school to identify 32 different kinds of interpersonal rejection, some of which were rather subtle and unexpected, that would have been very difficult to identify without the recording and analysis of conversation. Research using this technology is important for another reason. Without recording conversation, we may be misled by interactions that from a distance look neutral but would be coded as prosocial or aggressive if the content of the children's speech could be recorded.

Our next suggestion concerning future directions is also methodological and involves the increased use of experimental designs. A potentially powerful way to study the behaviors that lead to liking versus disliking is to systematically vary child characteristics to learn how much children like a child who displays certain characteristics. The power of this methodology is that one can test very specific hypotheses about the effects of a particular behavioral characteristic, without the presence of confounding behavioral characteristics or reputational factors.

Surprisingly, there has been a relative dearth of experimental studies in recent years aimed at learning about the characteristics that lead children to be liked versus disliked by their peers. Three studies from the 1980s illustrate the potential of this kind of work. DiLorenzo and Foster (1984) presented children with a video of two boys in several different interaction scenarios. After each scenario, children were asked to rate how much they liked each boy in the video. They found that children liked boys more when they initiated interaction cooperatively rather than uncooperatively, and that they liked the responder more when he was compliant rather than noncompliant. Darby and Schlenker (1982) used written scenarios to depict a child who, in certain conditions, hurt another child. Children liked the target more when he or she gave more elaborate apologies rather than when apologies were brief and could be thought of as perfunctory. Parker (1986) used another variation of this methodology that may be particularly appropriate for young children. A child interacted with a partner who either did or did not engage in very specific communicative behaviors. In this case, the partner was a large, toy-like character (described to children as an extraterrestrial) whose voice was that of a human observing through a one-way mirror and communicating through a speaker located inside the toy. Parker was interested in learning about the conversational processes that led to friendship between the child and the "playmate," but a similar methodology could be used to study liking versus disliking outcomes. Still another variation would be to bring together a child with a confederate child whose behavior is systematically varied across experimentally designed conditions. The previously discussed work by Hubbard (2001) illustrates this possibility.

A logical extension of these experimental studies would be to identify children who are low on certain behaviors, teach children specific relevant skills, and learn whether the increase in those behaviors (compared to a control condition) leads to corresponding changes in how well a child is liked. Something akin to this approach was taken in early social skills training studies (e.g., Oden & Asher, 1977; Ladd, 1981; Bierman, 1986). Indeed, Bierman found that the more children exhibited the behavioral processes they were taught, the more their liking by peers increased. The field needs more experiments like this to test hypotheses derived from the correlational studies. Such work would also be consistent with the humanistic values and goals underlying research on the behavioral characteristics associated with peer acceptance.

References

Adler, P. A., & Adler, P. (1998). *Peer power: Preadolescent culture and identity*. New Brunswick, NJ: Rutgers University Press.

Asher, S. R., Parker, J. G., & Walker, D. L. (1996). Distinguishing friendship from acceptance: Implications for intervention and assessment. In W. M. Bukowski, A. F. Newcomb, & W. W. Hartup

(Eds.), *The company they keep: Friendship during childhood and adolescence* (pp. 366–405). New York: Cambridge University Press.

Asher, S. R., Rose, A. J., & Gabriel, S. W. (2001). Peer rejection in everyday life. In M. R. Leary (Ed.), *Interpersonal rejection* (pp. 105–142). New York: Oxford University Press.

Asher, S. R., Singleton, L. C., Tinsley, B. R., & Hymel, S. (1979). A reliable sociometric measure for preschool children. *Developmental Psychology, 15,* 443–444.

Asher, S. R., & Williams, G. A. (1987). Helping children without friends in home and school contexts. In *Children's social development: Information for teachers and parents.* Urbana, IL: University of Illinois (ERIC Document Reproduction Service No. ED 283 625).

Baumeister, R. F., & Leary, M. R. (1995). The need to belong: Desire for interpersonal attachments as a fundamental human motivation. *Psychological Bulletin, 117,* 497–529.

Bierman, K. L. (1986). Process of change during social skills training with preadolescents and its relation to treatment outcome. *Child Development, 57,* 230–240.

Bierman, K. L. (2004). *Peer rejection: Developmental processes and intervention strategies.* New York: Guilford Press.

Boivin, M., Dodge, K. A., & Coie, J. D. (1995). Individual–group behavioral similarity and peer status in experimental play groups of boys: The social misfit revisited. *Journal of Personality and Social Psychology, 69,* 269–279.

Bowlby, J. (1969). *Attachment and loss: Vol. 1. Attachment* (2nd ed.). New York: Basic Books.

Bukowski, W. M., Gauze, C., Hoza, B., & Newcomb, A. F. (1993). Differences and consistency between same-sex and other-sex peer relationships during early adolescence. *Developmental Psychology, 29,* 255–263.

Casiglia, A. C., Lo Coco, A., & Zappulla, C. (1998). Aspects of social reputation and peer relationships in Italian children: A cross-cultural perspective. *Developmental Psychology, 34,* 723–730.

Chang, L. (2004). The role of classroom norms in contextualizing the relations of children's social behaviors to peer acceptance. *Developmental Psychology, 40,* 691–702.

Chen, X., Cen, G., Li, D., & He, Y. (2005). Social functioning and adjustment in Chinese children: The imprint of historical time. *Child Development, 76,* 182–195.

Chen, X., French, D. C., & Schneider, B. H. (2006). Culture and peer relationships. In X. Chen, D. C. French, & B. H. Schneider (Eds.), *Peer relationships in a cultural context* (pp. 3–22). New York: Cambridge University Press.

Chen, X., Li, D., Li, Z., Li, B., & Liu, M. (2000). Sociable and prosocial dimensions of social competence in Chinese children: Common and unique contributions to social, academic and psychological adjustment. *Developmental Psychology, 36,* 302–314.

Chen, X., Rubin, K. H., & Sun, Y. (1992). Social reputation and peer relationships in Chinese and Canadian children: A cross-cultural study. *Child Development, 63,* 1336–1343.

Chung, T., & Asher, S. R. (1996). Children's goals and strategies in peer conflict situations. *Merrill–Palmer Quarterly, 42,* 125–147.

Cillessen, A. H. N., & Mayeux, L. (2004). From censure to reinforcement: Developmental changes in the association between aggression and social status. *Child Development, 75,* 147–163.

Cillessen, A. H. N., & Rose, A. J. (2005). Understanding popularity in the peer system. *Current Directions in Psychological Science, 14,* 102–105.

Coie, J. D., Dodge, K. A., & Coppotelli, H. (1982). Dimensions and types of status: A cross-age perspective. *Developmental Psychology, 57,* 557–570.

Coie, J. D., Dodge, K. A., & Kupersmidt, J. B. (1990). Peer group behavior and social status. In S. R. Asher & J. D. Coie (Eds.), *Peer rejection in childhood* (pp. 17–59). New York: Cambridge University Press.

Coie, J. D., & Kupersmidt, J. B. (1983). A behavioral analysis of emerging social status in boys' groups. *Child Development, 54,* 1400–1416.

Coleman, J. S. (1961). *The adolescent society: The social life of the teenager and its impact on education.* Westport, CT: Greenwood Press.

Coplan, R. J., Rubin, K. H., Fox, N. A., Calkins, S. D., & Stewart, S. (1994). Being alone, playing alone, and acting alone: Distinguishing among reticence and passive and active solitude in young children. *Child Development, 65,* 129–137.

Crick, N. R., & Grotpeter, J. K. (1995). Relational aggression, gender, and social-psychological adjustment. *Child Development, 66,* 710–722.

Darby, B. W., & Schlenker, B. R. (1982). Children's reactions to apologies. *Journal of Personality and Social Psychology, 43,* 742–753.

Deci, E. L., & Ryan, R. M. (1985). *Intrinsic motivation and self-determination in human behavior.* New York: Plenum Press.

DiLorenzo, T. M., & Foster, S. L. (1984). A functional assessment of children's ratings of interaction patterns. *Behavioral Assessment, 6,* 291–302.

Dodge, K. A. (1980). Social cognition and children's aggressive behavior. *Child Development, 51,* 162–170.

Dodge, K. A. (1983). Behavioral antecedents of peer social status. *Child Development, 54,* 1386–1399.

Dodge, K. A., & Coie, J. D. (1987). Social-information processing factors in reactive and proactive aggression in children's peer groups. *Journal of Personality and Social Psychology, 53,* 1146–1158.

Dodge, K. A., Coie, J. D., Pettit, G. S., & Price, J. M. (1990). Peer status and aggression in boys' groups: Developmental and contextual analyses. *Child Development, 61,* 1289–1309.

Dodge, K. A., McClaskey, C. L., & Feldman, E. (1985). A situational approach to the assessment of social competence in children. *Journal of Consulting and Clinical Psychology, 53,* 345–353.

Eder, D. (1985). The cycle of popularity: Interpersonal relations among female adolescents. *Sociology of Education, 58,* 154–165.

Erdley, C. A., & Asher, S. R. (1996). Children's social goals and self-efficacy perceptions as influences on their responses to ambiguous provocation. *Child Development, 67,* 1329–1344.

Erickson, E. H. (1950). *Childhood and society.* New York: Norton.

French, D. C. (1988). Heterogeneity of peer-rejected boys: Aggressive and non-aggressive subtypes. *Child Development, 59,* 976–985.

Gazelle, H., Putallaz, M., Li, Y., Grimes, C., Kupersmidt, J. B., & Coie, J. D. (2005). Anxious solitude across contexts: Girls' interactions with familiar and unfamiliar peers. *Child Development, 76,* 227–246.

Goldfried, M. R., & D'Zurilla, T. J. (1969). A behavioral–analytic model for assessing competence. In C. D. Speilberger (Ed.), *Current topics in clinical and community psychology* (pp. 151–198). New York: Academic Press.

Gottman, J., Gonso, J., & Rasmussen, B. (1975). Social interaction, social competence, and friendship in children. *Child Development, 46,* 709–718.

Hart, C. H., Yang, C., Nelson, L. J., Robinson, C. C., Olsen, J. A., Nelson, D. A., et al. (2000). Peer acceptance in early childhood and subtypes of socially withdrawn behavior in China, Russia, and the United States. *International Journal of Behavioral Development, 24,* 73–81.

Hartup, W. W. (1970). Peer interaction and social organization. In P. H. Mussen (Ed.), *Carmichael's manual of child psychology* (Vol. 2, 3rd ed., pp. 360–456). New York: Wiley.

Hartup, W. W. (1983). Peer relations. In P. H. Mussen (Series Ed.) & E. M. Hetherington (Vol. Ed.), *Handbook of child psychology, Vol. 4: Socialization, personality and social development* (4th ed., pp. 103–196). New York: Wiley.

Hartup, W. W., Glazer, J. A., & Charlesworth, R. (1967). Peer reinforcement and sociometric status. *Child Development, 38,* 1017–1024.

Hawley, P. H. (2003). Prosocial and coercive configurations of resource control in early adolescence: A case for the well-adapted Machiavellian. *Merrill–Palmer Quarterly, 49,* 279–309.

Hopmeyer, A., & Asher, S. R. (1997). Children's responses to peer conflicts involving a rights infraction. *Merrill–Palmer Quarterly, 43,* 235–254.

Hubbard, J. A. (2001). Emotion expression processes in children's peer interaction: The role of peer rejection, aggression, and gender. *Child Development, 72,* 1426–1438.

Hymel, S., Rubin, K. H., Rowden, L., & LeMare, L. (1990). Children's peer relationships: Longitudinal prediction of internalizing and externalizing problems from middle to late childhood. *Child Development, 61,* 2004–2021.

Koch, H. L. (1933). Popularity in preschool children: Some related factors and a technique for its measurement. *Child Development, 4,* 164–175.

Ladd, G. W. (1981). Effectiveness of a social learning method for enhancing children's social interaction and peer acceptance. *Child Development, 52,* 171–178.

Ladd, G. W. (2005). *Children's peer relations and social competence: A century of progress.* New Haven, CT: Yale University Press.

Ladd, G. W., & Oden, S. (1979). The relationship between peer acceptance and children's ideas about helpfulness. *Child Development, 50,* 402–408.

LaFontana, K. M., & Cillessen, A. H. N. (2002). Children's perceptions of popular and unpopular peers: A multi-method assessment. *Developmental Psychology, 38,* 635–647.

Maccoby, E. E., & Jacklin, C. N. (1974). *The psychology of sex differences.* Stanford, CA: Stanford University Press.

Marshall, H. R., & McCandless, B. R. (1957). A study in prediction of social behavior of preschool children. *Child Development, 28,* 149–159.

McDonald, K. L., Putallaz, M., Grimes, C. L., Kupersmidt, J. B., & Coie, J. D. (2007). Girl talk: Gossip, friendship, and sociometric status. *Merrill–Palmer Quarterly, 53,* 381–411.

McFall, R. M. (1982). A review and reformulation of the concept of social skills. *Behavioral Assessment, 4,* 1–33.

Merten, D. E. (1997). The meaning of meanness: Popularity, competition, and conflict among junior high school girls. *Sociology of Education, 70,* 175–191.

Newcomb, A. F., & Bukowski, W. M. (1983). Social impact and social preference as determinants of children's peer group status. *Developmental Psychology, 19,* 856–867.

Newcomb, A. F., Bukowski, W. M., & Pattee, L. (1993). Children's peer relations: A meta-analytic review of popular, rejected, neglected, controversial, and average sociometric status. *Psychological Bulletin, 113,* 99–128.

Northway, M. L. (1944). Outsiders: A study of the personality patterns of children least acceptable to their age mates. *Sociometry, 7,* 10–25.

Oden, S., & Asher, S. R. (1977). Coaching children in social skills for friendship making. *Child Development, 48,* 495–506.

Parker, J. G. (1986). Becoming friends: Conversational skills for friendship formation in young children. In J. M. Gottman & J. G. Parker (Eds.), *Conversations of friends: Speculations on affective development* (pp. 103–138). New York: Cambridge University Press.

Parker, J. G., & Seal, J. (1996). Forming, losing, renewing, and replacing: Applying temporal parameters to the assessment of children's friendship experiences. *Child Development, 67,* 2248–2268.

Parkhurst, J. T., & Asher, S. R. (1992). Peer rejection in childhood: Subgroup differences in behavior, loneliness, and interpersonal concerns. *Developmental Psychology, 28,* 231–241.

Parkhurst, J. T., & Hopmeyer, A. (1998). Sociometric popularity and peer perceived popularity: Two distinct dimensions of peer status. *Journal of Early Adolescence, 18,* 125–144.

Peery, J. C. (1979). Popular, amiable, isolated, rejected: A reconceptualization of sociometric status in preschool children. *Child Development, 50,* 1231–1234.

Pepler, D. J., & Craig, W. (1995). A peek behind the fence: Naturalistic observations of aggressive children with remote audiovisual recording. *Developmental Psychology, 31,* 548–553.

Putallaz, M. (1983). Predicting children's sociometric status from their behavior. *Child Development, 54,* 1417–1426.

Putallaz, M., & Gottman, J. M. (1981). An interactional model of children's peer group entry. *Child Development, 52,* 986–994.

Rabiner, D. L., & Gordon, L. V. (1992). The coordination of conflicting social goals: Differences between rejected and nonrejected boys. *Child Development, 63,* 1344–1350.

Renshaw, P. D., & Asher, S. R. (1983). Children's goals and strategies for social interaction. *Merrill–Palmer Quarterly, 29,* 353–374.

Rodkin, P. C., Farmer, T. W., Pearl, R., & Van Acker, R. (2000). Heterogeneity of popular boys: Antisocial and prosocial configurations. *Developmental Psychology, 36*, 14–24.

Rodkin, P. C., Farmer, T. W., Pearl, R., & Van Acker, R. (2006). They're cool: Social status and peer group supports for aggressive boys and girls. *Social Development, 15*, 175–204.

Rose, A. J., & Asher, S. R. (1999). Children's goals and strategies in response to conflicts within a friendship. *Developmental Psychology, 35*, 69–79.

Rose, A. J., & Asher, S. R. (2004). Children's strategies and goals in response to help-seeking and help-giving tasks within a friendship. *Child Development, 75*, 749–763.

Rose, A. J., Swenson, L. P., & Waller, E. M. (2004). Overt and relational aggression and perceived popularity: Developmental differences in concurrent and prospective relations. *Developmental Psychology, 40*, 378–387.

Rubin, K. H., Bukowski, W. M., & Parker, J. G. (2006). Peer interactions, relationships, and groups. In W. Damon (Series Ed.) & N. Eisenberg (Vol. Ed.), *Handbook of child psychology: Vol. 3. Social, emotional, and personality development* (6th ed., pp. 571–645). New York: Wiley.

Rubin, K. H., Burgess, K. B., & Coplan, R. J. (2002). Social withdrawal and shyness. In P. K. Smith & C. H. Hart (Eds.), *Blackwell's handbook of childhood social development* (pp. 329–352). London: Blackwell.

Rubin, K. H., & Mills, R. S. L. (1988). The many faces of social isolation. *Journal of Consulting and Clinical Psychology, 56*, 916–924.

Rubin, R. M., & Hubbard, J. A. (2002). Children's verbalizations and cheating behavior during game playing: The role of sociometric status, aggression, and gender. *Journal of Abnormal Child Psychology, 31*, 65–78.

Sandstrom, M. J., & Coie, J. D. (1999). A developmental perspective on peer rejection: Mechanisms of stability and change. *Child Development, 70*, 955–966.

Schwartz, D., Chang, L., & Farver, J. M. (2001). Correlates of victimization in Chinese children's play groups. *Developmental Psychology, 37*, 520–532.

Shrauger, J. S. (1975). Responses to evaluation as a function of initial self-perceptions. *Psychological Bulletin, 82*, 581–596.

Stormshak, E. A., Bierman, K. L., Bruschi, C. J., Dodge, K. A., Coie, J. D., & the Conduct Problems Prevention Research Group. (1999). The relation between behavior problems and peer preference in different classroom contexts. *Child Development, 70*, 169–182.

Taylor, A. R., & Asher, S. R. (1984). Children's goals and social competence: Individual differences in a game-playing context. In T. Field, J. L. Roopnarine, & M. Segal (Eds.), *Friendship in normal and handicapped children* (pp. 53–78). Norwood, NJ: Ablex.

Tomada, G., & Schneider, B. H. (1997). Relational aggression, gender, and peer acceptance: Invariance across culture, stability over time, and concordance among informants. *Developmental Psychology, 33*, 601–609.

Troop, W. P., & Asher, S. R. (1999). Teaching peer relationship competence in schools. In R. J. Stevens (Ed.), *Teaching in American schools* (pp. 141–171). Columbus, OH: Merrill.

Troop-Gordon, W. P., & Asher, S. R. (2005). Modifications in children's goals when encountering obstacles to conflict resolution. *Child Development, 76*, 568–582.

Underwood, M. K., Scott, B. L., Galperin, M., Bjornstad, G. J., & Sexton, A. M. (2004). An observational study of social exclusion under varying conditions: Gender and developmental differences. *Child Development, 75*, 1538–1555.

Vaillancourt, T., & Hymel, S. (2006). Aggression and social status: The moderating roles of sex and peer-valued characteristics. *Aggressive Behavior, 32*, 396–408.

Valdivia, I. A., Schneider, B. H., Chavez, K. L., & Chen, X. (2005). Social withdrawal and maladjustment in a very group-oriented society. *International Journal of Behavioral Development, 29*, 219–228.

Wright, J. C., Giammarino, M., & Parad, H. W. (1986). Social status in small groups: Individual–group similarity and the social misfit. *Journal of Personality and Social Psychology, 50*, 523–536.

CHAPTER 14

Social Exclusion
in Childhood and Adolescence

MELANIE KILLEN
ADAM RUTLAND
NOAH SIMON JAMPOL

Exclusion is a pervasive aspect of social life. As soon as groups form in early childhood, decisions are made about whom to include and whom to exclude. In fact, being excluded from social groups is endemic to peer interactions, relationships, and social groups from early childhood through adulthood. Moreover, exclusion may be a basic feature of group dynamics that derives from the basic processes underlying the evolution and maintenance of groups (Bukowski & Sippola, 2001). Although much research has been conducted on peer rejection from groups, most of this research is focused principally on the individual social deficits that lead individuals to reject and be rejected (Rubin, Bukowski, & Parker, 2006). Typically, research has focused on *individual* children who have been identified as victims (e.g., fearful, socially anxious, and shy) and/or bullies (e.g., aggressive and lacking sensitivity to social cues). The theoretical approach in this chapter focuses on the role of group membership and intergroup attitudes, providing a different, and complementary, way both to investigate and to explain exclusion.

An intergroup approach involves examining how identification with the ingroup or the outgroup bears on judgments and evaluations of exclusion (Abrams & Rutland, 2008; Killen, Margie, & Sinno, 2006). This approach investigates when and how variables such as gender, race, ethnicity, and culture are related to how children evaluate exclusion, identify with the group, and make judgments about intergroup and intragroup exclusion. We propose that there are times when children are rejected for reasons other than social deficits, as defined by personality characteristics. Instead, children are rejected on the basis of their group membership, such as gender, race, ethnicity, and culture, which may have little to do with their social competence skills (e.g., a girl may be rejected from an all-boys group for reasons other than her personality traits, solely because she is a girl). A burgeoning area of research provides empirical validation for this proposal, which reflects the central thrust of this chapter.

In this chapter, we review theory and research on exclusion from two developmental approaches: social-cognitive domain theory (Smetana, 2006; Turiel, 1998), which provides an intergroup framework for analyzing children's social reasoning about exclusion (Killen, 2007; Killen et al., 2006); and developmental subjective group dynamics (Abrams & Rutland, 2008; Abrams, Rutland, Cameron, & Ferrell, 2007), which provides a model for examining the within- and between-group dynamics regarding children's attitudes about exclusion. These two models are complementary theories that have generated research studies on exclusion in peer relationships, interactions, and groups.

Research stemming from the social-cognitive domain theory has shown that children use moral, social-conventional, and psychological reasons to exclude others (described in more detail later). Children often rely on social-conventional reasons, such as "group functioning," to justify their decisions to exclude. Research generated from the developmental subjective group dynamics model has provided detailed information about what contributes to group functioning; that is, what it is about groups that children focus on when identifying with the groups, and when rejecting someone who does not fit the norms of the groups. Thus, we begin with an overview of the central issues embedded in the topic of intergroup and intragroup exclusion, followed by a brief explanation of the theories, then a short review of the empirical research, concluding with a discussion of future directions.

Central Issues

Exclusion from groups, based on group membership, is multifaceted. On the one hand, decisions to exclude others can reflect prejudicial judgments, stereotyping, conventions, traditions, norms, and status quo. On the other hand, decisions to include others can reflect moral judgments about fairness, justice, and equality. The norms, beliefs, and attitudes about decisions to exclude others reveal much about how groups work, as well as the function of groups in everyday social life. For the most part, understanding exclusion in childhood has been conducted from a *developmental intergroup approach*, which draws on social-psychological constructs about groups (Abrams, Hogg, & Marques, 2005), as well as developmental theories about change, emergence, and social cognition (Killen et al., 2006; Rutland, 2004).

Developmental intergroup social cognition examines the origins of prejudice and stereotyping, as well as moral cognition about fair treatment of others. This research focuses on normative samples and how the majority, rather than the minority, may hold biases that are not optimal from a social competence viewpoint (Rutland, 2004). Importantly, research on exclusion in childhood provides a basis for understanding the developmental origins and emergence of attitudes that provide the seeds, in part, of societal conflict, such as intergroup antagonism, that unfortunately have generated societal strife and conflict around the globe.

Research on exclusion in childhood has been conducted on group categories that have (1) generated extreme societal conflict (e.g., gender, race, ethnicity, and nationality); (2) created stigma (e.g., obesity and handicapped status); and (3) enabled close examination of the components of exclusion, without the societal histories associated with the categories (e.g., minimal group paradigm). In this chapter, we discuss research findings on these various forms of exclusion.

What are the consequences of exclusion? Studies in the area of peer rejection have shown that extensive experiences of being rejected by peers result in depression, loneliness, and anxiety (Bierman, 2004). Interventions are designed to focus on improving rejected children's social skills and social competence. Exclusion based on group membership, such as gender, race, and ethnicity, contributes to prejudice, bias, and discrimination, which can have detrimental effects on children's academic performance, create a general environment that perpetuates hierarchies and inequalities, and lead to negative long-term outcomes, such as injustice in the workforce and societal setting. In the world of elementary and secondary schooling, students who experience bias are at risk for distress due to discrimination, particularly in adolescence (Fisher, Wallace, & Fenton, 2000), as well as stereotype threat (Good, Aronson, & Inzlicht, 2003).

At the same time, there exist some positive outcomes for experiences with exclusion, such as increased sensitivity to the wrongfulness of exclusion that results from reflecting on the experience of exclusion (Killen, Lee-Kim, McGlothlin, & Stangor, 2002). Empathy and perspective-taking skills can enable individuals who have experienced exclusion to judge that it is wrong to exclude others. This does not mean that the experience of exclusion is justified, but that the experience of it may lead one to be empathic toward others.

Another central issue is to identify how judgments about exclusion vary depending on the context, the target, and the reason for exclusion. The context involves multiple aspects of the group, including one's identity with the group and an understanding of the group dynamics (Nesdale & Brown, 2004). "Group dynamics" refers to the intragroup considerations that reflect relationships between ingroup and outgroup members, such as when children identify with an outgroup member who may provide instability to the ingroup, which may or may not disrupt the functioning of the group. The target of exclusion varies depending on the context, and research has shown that children's views about the legitimacy of exclusion vary depending on the target. Moreover the reasons to justify exclusion vary depending on the type of exclusion. In the next section, we outline theories from social cognition that have provided models to study social reasoning about exclusion, as well as social identity and group dynamics.

Relevant Theories

Social-Cognitive Domain Theory and Peer Relationships

Social-cognitive domain theory provides a theoretical framework to examine social reasoning about exclusion. This model proposes that three domains of knowledge—the moral (fairness, justice, equality, rights), social-conventional (traditions, customs, etiquette, rituals), and the psychological (personal, individual discretion, autonomy, theory of mind)—coexist within individual evaluations of social issues and are reflected in social reasoning about exclusion (Killen, 2007; Smetana, 2006). For example, one could view a decision to exclude as "unfair" (moral) or as legitimate to make the group work well (conventional) or as a personal choice (psychological). This model differs from the Kolhberg (1971) moral development model in that these forms of reasons exist in parallel in development, emerging at a very early age, and change in terms of the breadth, criteria, and nature of the justifications. In contrast, Kohlberg's theory was hierarchical in that young children were oriented to the self (personal), then to the group (conventions), finally arriving at an understanding of justice late in adolescence (morality). A domain approach provides a theory for examining the coexistence of children's moral, conventional, and personal reasoning in early development, and is consistent with many domain-specific views in cognitive development (Keil, 1981).

What makes the application of a social-cognitive domain model to the topic novel is that exclusion, from this view, is conceptualized as multifaceted rather than strictly moral or nonmoral. In social psychology, exclusion is often viewed as a "moral transgression," an act that has created societal discord and strife through ethnic cleansing and genocide (Opotow, 1990). Yet there are times when exclusion serves a purpose, that is, to make groups function well (Abrams et al., 2005). For example, a slow runner is excluded from the track team, and a weak violin player is excluded from the orchestra. In these cases, the reasons for exclusion are not group membership per se but competence and ability, which creates a strong and competitive track team or a beautiful sounding orchestra. Yet research in social psychology has shown that stereotypical expectations often involve confusion between competence and group membership (e.g., girls are slow at running; Latinos are bad at classical music); moreover, societal conventions and expectations are often used to justify inequities and allocation of resources in an unfair manner (Levy, Chiu, & Hong, 2006). Thus, understanding when and how children differentiate between competence and group membership is a key part of determining how children evaluate exclusion.

Developmental research in the area of peer relationships has shown the important connections between attitudes and behavior, a central issue for social-cognitive domain theory. Understanding individuals' intentions and motivations is necessary for interpreting the "moral" status of any action. Whether a person pushes someone to hurt that individual or to prevent him or her from being hit by a car is performing an act for very different motivations. Most peer research utilizes behavioral situations to assess the quality and type of peer relationships, complemented by children's nominations of peer behavior. Yet children's reports of their peers' social status are filtered through their social-cognitive interpretations of situations, which include motivations, intentions, and moral judgments.

What to one child may appear to be negative behavior may to another child be positive behavior, depending on the attributions of intention, as well as evaluations of the behavior under consideration (Lemerise & Arsenio, 2000). Moreover, attributions of intention are often related to intergroup variables, such as group membership. Who becomes liked or not liked as children get older is heavily influenced by variables such as social stigma, stereotyping, and bias. Thus, it is essential to measure children's social-cognitive perspectives to provide a full account of the role played by peer relationship, interactions, and groups in the healthy development of children's social lives. In fact, developmental research on social cognition has provided key information for interpreting children's and adolescents' social interpretation of peer exchanges and interactions.

The social-cognitive domain model is based on the notion that peer interactions provide an important foundation for the construction of social knowledge, as theorized by Piaget in his groundbreaking book about children's moral judgment (Piaget, 1932). Piaget theorized that peer interactions enable children to acquire an understanding of the "other," and that through exchanges involving conflict, as well as reciprocity, children develop concepts about equality and fairness. Although Piaget's work provided the basis for understanding when children view the fair treatment of all as obligatory, there has remained a gap in the social-cognitive domain research regarding when children rely on *stereotypical expectations* to treat others differently, as with exclusion (Killen, Richardson, & Kelly, in press). Social-psychological research with adults has provided extensive data on how adults hold stereotypes, biases, and prejudicial judgments about others based on group membership (Dovidio & Gaertner, 1998).

What are the developmental origins of these types of attitudes, and how do these types of judgments manifest in peer interactions, relationships, and groups? Drawing on both social-cognitive domain theory and social-psychological research on intergroup attitudes, such as developmental subjective group dynamics (DSGD), researchers in the area of moral judgment, along with those from areas such as social identity and group dynamics, have contributed to knowledge about developmental intergroup judgments, attitudes, and relationships, as evidenced in recent special issues of journals on developmental intergroup attitudes (Killen & McKown, 2005; Rutland, Abrams, & Levy, 2007).

Developmental Subjective Group Dynamics

What remains to be better understood in the peer relations literature is the role of identity and group membership in the process of social exclusion. Children at an early age develop a better understanding of the different groups that constitute their social world and begin to identity with these groups (Bennett & Sani, 2004; Ruble et al., 2004; Ruble & Martin, 1998). These groups range from broad social categories, such as ethnicity or gender, to unique groups, such as family, and temporary but significant groups, such as the school class. Social-developmental psychologists have long shown that children are excluded because of their group memberships (Aboud, 1988; Bigler, Jones, & Lobliner, 1997). This form of exclusion between children from different social groups (i.e., intergroup bias) develops because group memberships become an integral part of children's self-concepts. According to social identity theory (SIT; Tajfel & Turner, 1979), by excluding others from their social group, children are able to bolster their sense of social identity (Verkuyten, 2001; Nesdale & Brown, 2004) and present positive public selves to their peer group (Rutland, 2004).

Recently social-developmental psychologists have also begun to focus on how social identity can result in exclusion *within* groups. This should be of particular interest to those concerned with social exclusion *within* peer groups when group memberships are salient (e.g., ethnically heterogeneous schools). Here the issue is how children make sense of a situation in which identities are salient but particular peers differ from their fellow group members (Abrams et al., 2005).

The DSGD model (Abrams & Rutland, 2008; Abrams, Rutland, & Cameron, 2003) holds that children develop a *dynamic* relationship between their judgments about peers *within* groups and about groups as a whole (i.e., intergroup attitudes). As their social-cognitive development changes and children experience belonging to social groups, they are more likely to integrate their preferences for different groups, with their evaluations of peers within groups based on particular characteristics or behaviors. Specifically, the DSGD model proposes that children shift from evaluations of ingroup and outgroup members based solely on preference for members of their ingroup category (Aboud, Mendelson, & Purdy, 2003; Nesdale, 2008; Tajfel & Turner, 1979) to judgments that also differentiate among peers within groups. For example, children in a group identifying with a sports team may begin to change their attitudes about a member of the ingroup "team" who acts like or prefers members of a rival team (the outgroup). This change in social cognition means that children may often exclude a peer because he or she is from a different social group (i.e., intergroup bias) or exclude a peer from *within* their group who deviates from the group's social-conventional norms (i.e., intragroup bias), such as increased liking of an outgroup member.

This model contends that during middle childhood, deviant peers within the ingroup are judged negatively compared to similarly deviant outgroup peers (i.e., the "black sheep effect"; Marques, Yzerbyt, & Leyens, 1988). This *subjective* phenomenon is akin what occurs during the dynamics of real-life, face-to-face small groups, with efforts to exclude and differentiate between peers serving to constrain deviants to reinforce the boundaries of group norms (e.g., Schachter, 1961; Levine, 1989). However, if these dynamics occur when social identities are salient, exclusion between peers within groups (i.e., "differential evaluation") occurs simultaneously with the motivation to sustain a positive social identity and ingroup distinctiveness (SIT; Tajfel & Turner, 1979). The former process involves attention to individual peer group members to identify and devalue deviant peers (i.e., intragroup exclusion), thus upholding ingroup norms, and the latter process implies general exclusion of those from other groups. These two processes combined are considered subjective group dynamics.

During middle childhood and early adolescence children begin to recognize that deviant peer-group members constitutes a departure from norms that other group members would want to preserve (i.e., deviance is a variation among individuals that is relevant to their group membership). This recognition is compatible with the developmental literature on social perspective taking (Quintana, 1999; Selman, 1980), which shows that children develop the ability to take the perspective of others in social situations. Children in middle childhood sustain their social identity and intergroup differences by excluding deviant peers within their groups in favor of those who provide stronger support for ingroup norms (Abrams & Rutland, 2008). Therefore, children's developing social-cognitive capacity to focus on differences within groups sustains rather than diminishes intergroup bias, because the exclusion targets particular deviant peers within their group. How children evaluate exclusion based on various group memberships has been the focus of much recent research.

Thus, this review of recent theories indicates that several models are in place for investigating how children reason about exclusion, what happens when members of the group are deviant, and how that bears on their group identity. We now turn to the empirical literature to provide a brief review of recent studies on exclusion in childhood and adolescence.

Research Findings:
Social-Cognitive Domain Views of Exclusion

As described earlier, social-cognitive domain theory provides a means to analyze social reasoning about exclusion. To understand individual reasoning about exclusion, it is necessary to assess the context, target, and prior and current experiences of the potential excluder (Killen et al., 2006). Developmental intergroup approaches informed by social-cognitive domain theory have led to several lines of research examining both explicit judgments and implicit attitudes. In the area of explicit judgments, empirical studies have provided evidence regarding children's social reasoning and evaluations of exclusion incorporating moral, conventional, and psychological reasoning. Implicit attitudes have been measured by researchers using ambiguous pictures to measure children's attributions of intentions, in a manner similar to peer relations studies on the hostile attribution bias (with the difference being a focus on intergroup relationships).

Social categorization, stereotyping, and implicit attitudes can contribute to the development of prejudicial attitudes, and these attitudes can translate into exclusionary practices that may well have longlasting detrimental effects on the excluded individual (Dovidio, Glick, & Rudman, 2005; Killen, 2007). A review of explicit judgments includes the role of friendship, social cliques, and romantic relationships, each of which is a central aspect of peer relationships in social development, as well as social experience. Then, a review of research from the DSGD model is described, followed by a discussion of research on implicit attitudes in the area of intergroup peer relationships.

Friendship and Exclusion

As noted in the peer relationships literature, friendships may result from considerations of similarities, often based on the shared interests of a dyad or peer group (Rubin et al., 2006). Noting the significant role that shared interests can play, Killen and Stangor (2001) investigated the forms of reasoning used by children and adolescents when evaluating exclusion from activity-based peer groups who share interests (e.g., ballet, baseball). They introduced the role of group membership (gender and race) by asking children about exclusion of an individual who did not fit the stereotypical expectations of the group (e.g., gender: excluding a boy from ballet, a girl from baseball; race: excluding a white student from basketball or a black student from a math club). In this way, the assessment involved asking children whether it is legitimate to exclude someone from joining a group who shares an interest (e.g., likes ballet) but does not fit the stereotypical expectations for those who participate in the shared interests (e.g., boys in ballet). For straightforward exclusion decisions (e.g., "Is it all right or not all right to exclude a boy from a ballet club?"), the vast majority of first, fourth, and seventh graders evaluated such exclusionary acts as unfair and morally wrong. Shared interests were viewed as more important than stereotypical issues.

When asked to make complex judgments, however, such as who the group should pick when only one space was available and two children wanted to join, one who matched the stereotype and one who did not (e.g., "A boy and girl both want to join the ballet club. Who should the group pick?"), with age, participants focused on group functioning considerations and picked the child who fit the stereotype (e.g., "It will be weird to have a boy wearing leotards, so they should choose the girl"). Despite using moral reasoning to evaluate the straightforward exclusion vignette, the older sample used more social-conventional reasoning than did their younger counterparts when picking a new group member in the inclusion–exclusion scenario. Research with young children has also found similar findings with shared play activities, such as dolls and trucks (Theimer, Killen, & Stangor, 2001). Thus, with age, adolescents' awareness of group functioning considerations overwhelms their focus on fairness or equal opportunity in some contexts. This is important information for understanding adolescents' intentions about exclusion and inclusion.

Social Cliques and Exclusion

Social cliques in early adolescence reflect the emergence of overt and concrete attention to group functioning within peer relationships. Brown and colleagues (Brown & Lohr,

1987; Brown, Mounts, Lamborn, & Steinberg, 1993) identified the extensive and pervasive nature of social cliques for adolescents. Furthermore, the salience of these social groups in the context of exclusion judgments has been investigated by Horn (2003, 2006), who has documented the hierarchies and social status of social clique membership and how adolescents reason about exclusionary choices based on group membership.

Horn (2003) surveyed 9th- and 11th-grade adolescents, assessing attitudes and judgments regarding the choice to exclude someone from a social group (e.g., cheerleaders) on the basis of their peer-group membership (e.g., gothic); thus, participants were asked questions, such as "Is it all right or not all right for the cheerleaders to exclude a gothic from the team?" Whereas the vast majority of younger and older adolescents considered it wrong to consider group membership when deciding about the distribution of resources, only a simple majority viewed as wrong excluding someone from a social group on the basis of peer-group membership. Moreover, age-related differences were found regarding the use of stereotypes and conventional reasoning to justify the exclusion of a peer, with younger adolescents using these reasons more often than did older adolescents. Furthermore, 9th graders judged exclusion as less wrong overall than did 11th graders.

With age, the salience of social cliques diminishes, and with this knowledge comes reasoning that rejects the maintenance of group functioning and status quo in the context of exclusion. Horn's (2003) study supported Turiel's (1983) hypothesis regarding age-related decreases in the use of conventional reasoning. Horn identified what has been referred to as the "peak" for the dominance of social cliques in peer relationships with a demonstration of reliance on stereotyped reasoning in her 9th-grade sample. As adolescents get older, cliques diminish and romantic relationships become more dominant (Horn, 2003, 2006).

Romantic Relationships and Exclusion

Research has identified adolescent romantic relationships as highly influential and significant, providing adolescents with distinct and dynamic social experiences (Laursen & Bukowski, 1997). Furthermore, it has been theorized that the intimate component of peer relationships provides additional salience to the romantic aspect of adolescent life (Shulman, Laursen, Kalman, & Karpovsky, 1997). As these relationships emerge in early adolescence, balancing individuality with this newfound closeness becomes a challenge (Selman, 1990).

Moving beyond the demands of common interests and cliques, researchers have investigated social reasoning about exclusion within a romantic dating context (Killen, Stangor, Price, Horn, & Sechrist, 2004). Although Nucci (2001) has demonstrated that choice of friendships is categorized by children and adolescents as within the personal domain, and is differentiated from moral and social-conventional issues, which are regulated by principles and rules, little research has examined the role of group membership, such as race and ethnicity, in romantic relationships. Killen et al. (2002) demonstrated that children view it as wrong to refrain from being friends with someone because of their race, but what about dating? Dating is viewed as a highly personal decision; thus, one might expect that even in the context of race and ethnicity this type of decision remains a personal choice (Nucci, 1996). Participants were asked to evaluate three different decisions by a European American student regarding an African American student: (1) not to vote for someone for student council president because of race; (2) not to attend a baseball game with someone because of race; and (3) not to enter into a romantic relationship with someone because of race. Although individuals consider it wrong not to vote for a candidate based on race and fairly unreasonable not to attend a baseball game with someone of a different race, they viewed not dating someone on the basis of race as permissible and as a matter of personal choice. When social reasoning includes considerations of romantic relationships, not only are moral and social conventional forms of reasoning employed, but also personal reasons and appeals to autonomy enter into the decision to include or exclude a peer in this type of relationship.

Social Experience

Research findings support the viewpoint that individuals' daily experiences with exclusion are related to their attributions and judgments about exclusion, which has also been shown with aggression: Children who are aggressive attribute hostile bias in ambiguous situations (Crick & Dodge, 1994; Lemerise & Arsenio, 2000). For example, Horn (2006) found that adolescents who identified with low-status peer-group members (e.g., druggies) were more inclusive than their high-status group peers (e.g., jocks). Furthermore, high-status peer-group members used more conventional reasoning than their lower-ranking peers when making such exclusionary decisions (Horn, 2006). Horn (2003) also demonstrated that adolescent females rated exclusion as more wrong and provided more moral reasons for condemning exclusion than did males when evaluating exclusion decisions by members of social cliques. Killen and colleagues (2002) also found that European American females and minority participants evaluated exclusion as more wrong than their European American male counterparts, and used more moral reasoning than conventional reasoning in their evaluations. This diversity of evaluation is perhaps evidence of increased empathy on behalf of individuals who have had more personal experience with exclusion, be they racial minorities, females, or low-status peer-group members. Yet only recently has the experience of identifying with the ingroup or with members of the outgroup, as it pertains to exclusion, been investigated.

Developmental Social Group Dynamics View of Exclusion

The DSGD model, as described earlier, focuses extensively on how the motivation to sustain a positive social identity results in exclusion both between and within groups. Research following this developmental intergroup approach (Abrams & Rutland, 2008; Abrams et al., 2003) has investigated intergroup exclusion alongside construction of an experimental paradigm to examine how children would evaluate ingroup and outgroup peers who showed either "normative" (loyal) or "deviant" (disloyal) behavior. In experiments using nationality as the group membership (e.g., English, German), children were first asked to rate how they felt toward the ingroup as a whole and the outgroup as a whole (i.e., intergroup exclusion). Then the children heard descriptions of normative and deviant peers who were either in the same or in different groups. Normative peers made two positive statements about the ingroup, whereas deviant peers made one positive statement about the ingroup, but also one positive statement about the outgroup.

Initially, children were asked to evaluate the normative and deviant peers (i.e., intragroup exclusion). This should indicate whether the children were excluding peers *within* each social group. Importantly, then the children were asked to judge whether other peers from the ingroup and the outgroup would exclude or include the normative and deviant peers. This taps children's expectations about the way others exclude or include the peers. Subjective group dynamics should be evident in children who have correct expectations and, therefore, provide positive evaluations of peers who are acceptable to the *ingroup* rather than peers who are more acceptable to the outgroup.

Studies in intergroup contexts that used national groups (Abrams et al., 2003), summer school groups (Abrams et al., 2007) and minimal or "arbitrary" groups (Abrams, Rutland, Ferrell, & Pelletier, 2008) have shown that the relationship between exclusion among group members and exclusion within peer groups tends to be reliable after around age 7 years, when children can simultaneously exclude persons from other social groups and those within their own peer group that threaten the social-conventional norms central to their group. In addition, studies (e.g., Abrams et al., 2003, 2008) have shown that these different forms of social exclusion are more strongly linked when older children are more motivated to support their ingroup (i.e., show high intergroup bias or identify more strongly). This finding indicates that both types of social exclusion are related to the children's sense of social identity and their desire to maintain intergroup differences.

Peer Accountability and Exclusion

The DSGD model contends that peer-group accountability affects children's social exclusion judgments in intergroup contexts. Peer-group accountability involves children believing that their actions are visible and may be criticized or may have to be defended among their peer group. Much of middle childhood and early adolescence is spent among peers, either in education or play, so it is not surprising that social exclusion judgments are likely to be influenced by the degree to which children's words and actions are visible to their peer group. Research suggests that the development of exclusion judgments between peers within groups and between different social groups is sensitive to the normative aspects (i.e., what is acceptable behavior for the peer ingroup or outgroup) of the intergroup context (Abrams et al., 2007; Rutland, Cameron, Milne, & McGeorge, 2005). Thus, increasing children's *accountability* makes the norms of the peer group more salient. This should encourage self-presentational concerns among children and variations in their exclusion judgments. The result should either increase or decrease peer exclusion within groups and intergroup bias between groups depending on the prevailing norm within the peer group (e.g., racial exclusion is either unacceptable or legitimate).

Among both children and adults, accountability is known to affect exclusion judgments (Blanchard, Crandall, Brigham, & Vaughn, 1994; Jetten, Spears, & Manstead, 1997; Monteith, Deneen, & Tooman, 1996). Research also has shown that during middle childhood and adolescence, individuals begin to control their expressions of intergroup and intragroup bias to reflect self-presentational concerns and social norms (Abrams et al., 2007). During middle childhood, children, like adults, begin to show a tendency toward more or less social exclusion between and within groups depending on the dominant social norms in the specific intergroup context (Nesdale, Griffith, Durkin, & Maass, 2005). Thus, for example, heightening peer accountability in a competitive school or national intergroup context in which exclusion is tolerated or even encouraged may increase children's desire to exclude socially. In contrast, accountability may have the opposite effect in a racial intergroup context in which norms against explicit exclusion are typically prominent.

Bullying and Exclusion

Researchers are beginning to recognize the influence of social groups on children's bullying behavior and peer rejection generally (Jackson, Barth, Powell, & Lochman, 2006; Juvonen, Nishina, & Graham, 2006). On this basis, there is evidence that in some intergroups contexts and among certain groups, bullying and peer exclusion may simply become normative. In such situations, research from the DSGD model suggests a quite different view of the bully. As mentioned earlier, bullies are generally and consistently portrayed as having poor social understanding and deficient social-cognitive skills (Crick & Dodge, 1994). In contrast, in settings where bullying is normative and social identities are a central motivating factor, bullies often may have a good understanding of others' emotions and their social perspectives (Dunn, 2004; Sutton, Smith, & Swettenham, 1999). Arguably, good social understanding is especially important for indirect bullying that involves social exclusion of nontypical (here termed "deviant") members within a group (Bjorkqvist, Lagerspetz, & Kaukainen, 1992), because a bully is likely to require some understanding of group dynamics. We suggest that, in such contexts, bullies in the preadolescent years are likely to show a good understanding of subjective group dynamics and generally demonstrate social competence.

Group Dynamics, Morality, and Group-Based Exclusion

As described earlier, children's evaluations of peer behavior in any context may reflect a multitude of factors (Bukowski & Sippola, 2001; Killen, 2007; Turiel, 1998) relating to considerations of the self (e.g., individual autonomy), the group (e.g., norms or social conventions) and morality (e.g., fairness or justice). Abrams et al. (2008) examined how children employ both moral and social-conventional (i.e., group-based) criteria, such as loyalty, when deciding whether to exclude ingroup and outgroup peer members that deviate according to moral principles. They found that children excluded peers on the basis of both group membership *and* individual morality. Significantly, children favored not only ingroup peers over outgroup peers but also peers from either group who behaved according to moral principles over morally deviant peers from each group. Moreover, because these types of exclusion judgments involve different domains of reasoning (Turiel, 1998), group- and morality-based judgments occurred in parallel and were independent of each other.

These findings provide insight into how children approach morality in intergroup situations. Children do not seem to trade off between favoring people because of their group membership and favoring people because of their morality when they evaluate ingroup and outgroup peers. Rather, Abrams and colleagues showed that when moral violations are objectively uncorrelated with group membership, children use both morality *and* group memberships as independent bases to determine whom to exclude. This supports social-cognitive domain theory (Killen et al., 2002; Smetana, 2006) by showing that morality- and group-based judgments are not opposites. Instead, children employ both when engaging in social exclusion and peer rejection.

Although analyses of explicit judgments about exclusion and the group dynamics of ingroup and outgroup identification are informative regarding exclusion, social-psychological research has indicated that implicit attitudes are also related to decisions to include and exclude others (Dovidio, Kawakami, & Beach, 2001). Recent research with children has also revealed the ways that implicit attitudes are involved when children make judgments about peer relationships and interactions.

Implicit Attitudes about Peer Exchanges

Implicit attitudes provide an important complement to the investigation of individuals' explicit judgments, particularly when determining social cognition about attributions of intentions and bias. Developmental intergroup researchers have investigated children's implicit attitudes using a number of different techniques (Killen, McGlothlin, & Henning, 2008). These methods range from variants of the adult Implicit Association Test (IAT), which involves measuring latency responses on a computer screen to associations of good and bad words with black and white faces (Baron & Banaji, 2006), to forms of attributions about bias based on group membership in which the participant is unaware of the manipulation. The latter technique has been used to analyze how children and adolescents attribute intentions based on group membership in ambiguous situations (McGlothlin & Killen, 2006). Using ambiguous situations, modeled on earlier studies by Schofield (Sagar & Schofield, 1980) and Lawrence (1991). McGlothlin and Killen (2006) investigated the roles that race and intergroup contact played in children's perceptions of similarity between interracial peer dyads and judgments of cross-race friendships (Margie, Killen, Sinno, & McGlothlin, 2005; McGlothlin & Killen, 2005, 2006). Working within the context of children's everyday peer exchanges, researchers designed these studies to help them understand when children's biases based on group membership influence their interpretations of intentions in interracial dyadic exchanges.

Peer relationship researchers who used the ambiguous situations picture to determine when children overattribute hostile intentions found that aggressive children often attribute negative intentions in situations in which nonaggressive children do not (e.g., spilling milk is viewed as an intentional act by aggressive children, but as an accident by nonaggressive children; Crick & Dodge, 1994; Lemerise & Arsenio, 2000). McGlothlin and Killen (2006) created a twist on the methodology by introducing the race of the potential perpetrator as a variable, such that the perpetrator is black in one version of the ambiguous situation and white in another. This manipulation enables researchers to determine when children use race to attribution negative intentions unbeknownst to the participant, along with measuring other aspects of peer relationships, such as the potential for cross-race friendship and other aspects of intentional behavior. Using another measurement, the Perceptions of Similarity Task, children are asked to evaluate the similarity of children across a variety of factors, including both physical characteristics (e.g., skin color) and activity interests (e.g., playing basketball). This assessment provides a measure of how such evaluations affect the perception of similarity and potential for friendship.

Over three studies, first and fourth graders from a range of ethnic backgrounds, and in both low and high diversity schools, were asked to make judgments about intentions in ambiguous pictures, as well as the similarity of same-race and cross-race dyads, to determine how early implicit attitudes about race and ethnicity emerge. The ethnicity of participants in the three studies varied such that McGlothlin, Killen, and Edmonds (2005) examined European American children who attended ethnically diverse schools (heterogeneous); Margie et al. (2005) interviewed African American, Latino, and Asian American children who also attended ethnically diverse schools; and McGlothlin and

Killen (2006) interviewed European American children who attended ethnically homogeneous (predominantly European American demography) schools. Sampling from different racial and ethnic backgrounds, as well as from schools varying in ethnic student population, added the dimension of intergroup contact to children's perceptions of similarity.

The results indicated that children who attended heterogeneous schools were less likely than children who attended homogeneous schools to use race as a variable when attributing intentions in ambiguous situations. Yet for all children, expectations about cross-race potential declined with age. Fortunately, however, children at this age (early elementary school) focused primarily on shared or unshared activity interests, and not on differences in skin color (Margie et al., 2005; McGlothlin et al., 2005). This is important, because it indicates that given another salient variable, such as shared interests (Aboud et al., 2003), children focus on that more than on race or skin color. However, race was not completely ignored by the white children, who rated the same-race peer dyads (both black and white pairs) that shared the same activity interests as more similar than the cross-race peer dyads that also shared the same interests. In the unshared activity interest condition, the same-race black peer dyad was judged to be more similar than the same-race white peer dyad. White children attributed greater variability to the same-race white dyad (the ingroup) than to the same-race black dyad (the outgroup), referred to as the "outgroup homogeneity effect," because participants were attributing more homogeneity to the outgroup than to the ingroup.

Thus, whereas children from ethnic minority backgrounds did not use skin color as a basis for judgments of similarity, white children attending ethnically heterogeneous schools differentiated between some dyads based on race. Yet when assessing friendship potential, the majority of children judged that all dyads, same-race or cross-race, could be friends. Surprisingly, children from all backgrounds attending ethnically diverse schools, no matter how they viewed variability within and between groups, focused on the similarity of activity interests and not on race when determining the possibility of friendship.

Similarly, McGlothlin and Killen (2005) found that white children attending homogeneous schools also focused more often on shared (or unshared) sports interests than on race. Yet the racial makeup of the dyad was a factor in the similarity ratings. These white children rated the same-race black dyads as more similar than the same-race white dyads, again demonstrating an outgroup homogeneity effect. Similar to the participants in the heterogeneous schools, judgments of friendship potential of children in homogenous schools focused on activity interests to a greater extent than on skin color. When activity interests were shared, children were highly positive about the likelihood of friendship. When the dyad did not share activity interests, however, these white children evaluated friendship potential differently based on the racial makeup of the dyad. In particular, whereas two black characters were judged to have the greatest potential for friendship despite not sharing a sports interest, members of the cross-race dyad were judged as least likely to be friends.

Differences based on the ethnic composition of the schools (heterogeneous or homogenous) were also found with regard to judgments of friendship potential. Children in heterogeneous schools were more inclusive, overall, than were the white children in homogeneous schools; that is, children who attended ethnically diverse schools evaluated friendship as possible between children who did not share activity interests and/or skin color, whereas white children who attended ethnically homogeneous schools were less optimistic about friendship potential, especially when activity interest and race were not shared. Thus, the amount of contact children experienced with racial and ethnic groups other than their own at school influenced their decisions about friendship.

Extending the attribution of intention studies into adolescence, Killen, Kelly, Richardson, and Jampol (2007) examined the implicit racial biases and intergroup contact of middle school (8th grade) and high school (11th grade) students. In this study, a picture card–based assessment depicted interracial peer exchanges in school settings marked by ambiguity in intent. For example, one picture depicted a student who fell down in the hallway, with an onlooker who may have pushed him or her or is about to help him or her up. The results indicated that African American participants rated ambiguous interracial dyadic exchanges more positively than did European American participants (Killen et al., 2007); moreover, girls rated the interactions as more positive than did boys, and older adolescents rated the exchanges as more positive than did younger adolescents.

With age, and by gender and ethnicity, differences were found in the attributions of intentions regarding interracial interactions depicted in ambiguous picture cards. Furthermore, ethnic minority students were more likely to view as unfair a teacher or a peer accusing the protagonist of wrongdoing given that the intentions were ambiguously depicted; more information was warranted before making an accusation. These findings provide a window into the social competence of minority students about peer interactions, students who, themselves, may often experience unfair accusations based on race and ethnicity.

Future Directions

There are many promising integrative lines of research that might contribute to an understanding of how intergroup relationships bear on peer relationships in childhood and adolescence. Given the importance of peer relationships in social development and the pervasiveness of ingroup and outgroup dynamics, it is essential to understand how group membership plays a role in social development. Moral judgments, social identity, social competence, perspective taking, friendship, social cliques, and values all involve intergroup relationships and attitudes in various contexts throughout children's everyday lives.

For example, peer interactions contribute to the acquisition of moral principles about equality due to the reciprocity and perspective taking involved when children resolve conflicts with "equals" (peers). Yet when peers are different from the self on the basis of many variables, including group membership (e.g., gender and race), the acquisition process may look somewhat different. In a positive social environment with few stereotypical messages, children may readily identify with a range of other children, forming a strong sense of group identity when the group surpasses categories such as race, ethnicity, or gender (e.g., age: "We're all 4-year-olds"). In an environment in which categories such as race, ethnicity, and gender are made particularly salient and are justified as a basis for exclusion ("They are different from us" or "Girls are different from boys"), the outcome may be somewhat less social. Fortunately, children often find ways to interact and to exchange with peers in ways not expected or predicted by adults, and in these contexts, the salient group identity may continue to be one that "unites" rather than "divides," or one in which the ingroup is identified as greater than that defined by cultural or gender membership.

Conclusions

Our world is increasingly heterogeneous, multicultural, and mobile. On the one hand, heterogeneity offers a wealth of new experiences from which children can benefit by understanding new ways of living and being. On the other hand, heterogeneity can lead to stereotyping, bias, and prejudice. What makes a difference are the ways adults create positive learning environments, allowing children to interact with others from different ethnic, racial, and cultural backgrounds. Yet little is known about how group membership, such as gender, race, ethnicity, and culture, is related to decisions by peers to socialize with others, become friends, join groups, date, and ultimately decide to embark on new unions in the form of marriage. We propose that an integrative approach drawing on both social psychology and developmental psychology in the areas of peer interactions, group dynamics, moral cognition, and social reasoning, will provide essential information for the ontogenesis of exclusion and inclusion, that is, how it emerges, changes, and manifests in peer relationships throughout development.

References

Aboud, F. E. (1988). *Children and prejudice.* New York: Blackwell.

Aboud, F. E., Mendelson, M. J., & Purdy, P. (2003). Cross-race peer relations and friendship quality. *International Journal of Behavioral Development, 27,* 165–173.

Abrams, D., Hogg, M. A., & Marques, J. M. (2005). A social psychological framework for understanding social inclusion and exclusion. In D. Abrams, M. A. Hogg, & J. M. Marques (Eds.), *The social psychology of inclusion and exclusion* (pp. 1–24). New York: Psychology Press.

Abrams, D., & Rutland, A. (2008). The development of subjective group dynamics. In S. R. Levy & M. Killen (Eds.), *Intergroup relations: An integrative developmental and social psychological perspective* (pp. 47–65). Oxford, UK: Oxford University Press.

Abrams, D., Rutland, A., & Cameron, L. (2003). The development of subjective group dynamics: Children's judgments of normative and deviant in-group and out-group individuals. *Child Development, 74,* 1840–1856.

Abrams, D., Rutland, A., Cameron, L., & Ferrell, J. (2007). Older but wilier: In-group accountability and the development of subjective group dynamics. *Developmental Psychology, 43,* 134–148.

Abrams, D., Rutland, A., Ferrell, J. M., & Pelletier, J. (2008). Children's judgments of disloyal and immoral peers: Subjective group dynamics in minimal intergroup contexts. *Child Development, 79,* 444–461.

Baron, A. S., & Banaji, M. R. (2006). The development of implicit attitudes: Evidence of race evaluations from ages 6 and 10 and adulthood. *Psychological Science, 17,* 53–58.

Bennett, M., & Sani, F. (Eds.). (2004). *The development of the social self.* New York: Psychology Press.

Bierman, K. L. (2004). *Peer rejection: Developmental processes and intervention strategies.* New York: Guilford Press.

Bigler, R. S., Jones, L. C., & Lobliner, D. B. (1997). Social categorization and the formation of intergroup attitudes in children. *Child Development, 68,* 530–543.

Bjorkqvist, K., Lagerspetz, K. M. J., & Kaukainen, A. (1992). Do girls manipulate and boys fight?: Developmental trends in regard to direct and indirect aggression. *Aggressive Behavior, 18,* 117–127.

Blanchard, F. A., Crandall, C. S., Brigham, J. C., & Vaughn, L. A. (1994). Condemning and condoning racism: A social context approach to interracial settings. *Journal of Applied Psychology, 79,* 993–997.

Brown, B. B., & Lohr, M. J. (1987). Peer-group affiliation and adolescent self-esteem: An integration of ego-identity and symbolic interaction theories. *Journal of Personality and Social Psychology,* *52*, 47–55.

Brown, B. B., Mounts, N., Lamborn, S. D., & Steinberg, L. (1993). Parenting practices and peer groups affiliation in adolescence. *Child Development, 64*, 467–482.

Bukowski, W., & Sippola, L. (2001). Groups, individuals, and victimization: A view of the peer system. In J. Juvonen & S. Graham (Eds.), *Peer harassment in school: The plight of the vulnerable and victimized* (pp. 355–377). New York: Guilford Press.

Crick, N., & Dodge, K. A. (1994). A review and reformulation of social information-processing mechanisms in children's social adjustment. *Psychological Bulletin, 115*, 74–101.

Dovidio, J. F., & Gaertner, S. L. (1998). On the nature of contemporary prejudice: The causes, consequences, and challenges of aversive racism. In J. Eberhardt & S. T. Fiske (Eds.), *Confronting racism: The problem and the response* (pp. 3–32). Newbury Park, CA: Sage.

Dovidio, J. F., Glick, P., & Rudman, L. (2005). *On the nature of prejudice: Fifty years after Allport.* Oxford, UK: Blackwell.

Dovidio, J. F., Kawakami, K., & Beach, K. (2001). Implicit and explicit attitudes: Examination of the relationship between measures of intergroup bias. In R. Brown & S. L. Gaertner (Eds.), *Blackwell handbook of social psychology* (Vol. 4, pp. 175–197). Oxford, UK: Blackwell.

Dunn, J. (2004). *Children's friendships: The beginning of intimacy.* Oxford: Blackwell.

Fisher, C. B., Wallace, S. A., & Fenton, R. E. (2000). Discrimination distress during adolescence. *Journal of Youth and Adolescence, 29*(6), 679–695.

Good, C., Aronson, J., & Inzlicht, M. (2003). Improving adolescents' standardized test performance: An intervention to reduce the effects of stereotype threat. *Journal of Applied Developmental Psychology, 24*(6), 645–662.

Horn, S. (2003). Adolescents' reasoning about exclusion from social groups. *Developmental Psychology, 39*, 11–84.

Horn, S. (2006). Group status, group bias, and adolescents' reasoning about the treatment of others in school contexts. *International Journal of Behavioral Development, 30*, 208–218.

Jackson, M. F., Barth, J. M., Powell, N., & Lochman, J. E. (2006). Classroom contextual effects of race on children's peer nominations. *Child Development, 77*, 1325–1337.

Jetten, J., Spears, R., & Manstead, A. S. R. (1997). Strength of identification and intergroup differentiation: The influence of group norms. *European Journal of Social Psychology, 27*, 603–609.

Juvonen, J., Nishina, A., & Graham, S. (2006). Ethnic diversity and perceptions of safety in urban middle schools. *Psychological Science, 17*, 394–401.

Keil, F. C. (1981). Constraints on knowledge and cognitive development. *Psychological Review, 88*, 197–227.

Killen, M. (2007). Children's social and moral reasoning about exclusion. *Current Directions in Psychological Science, 16*, 32–36.

Killen, M., Kelly, M. C., Richardson, C., & Jampol, N. S. (2007). Adolescents' attributions of bias in interracial peer exchanges. Unpublished manuscript, University of Maryland.

Killen, M., Lee-Kim, J., McGlothlin, H., & Stangor, C. (2002). How children and adolescents evaluate gender and racial exclusion. *Monographs of the Society for Research in Child Development, 67*(4, Serial No. 271), 1–180.

Killen, M., Margie, N. G., & Sinno, S. (2006). Morality in the context of intergroup relationships. In M. Killen & J. G. Smetana (Eds.), *Handbook of moral development* (pp. 155–183). Mahwah, NJ: Erlbaum.

Killen, M., McGlothlin, H., & Henning, A. (2008). Explicit judgments and implicit attitudes: A developmental perspective. In S. Levy & M. Killen (Eds.), *Intergroup relations: An integrative developmental and social psychological perspective* (pp. 126–145). New York: Oxford University Press.

Killen, M., & McKown, C. (2005). How integrative approaches to intergroup attitudes advance the field. *Applied Developmental Psychology, 26*, 616–622.

Killen, M., Richardson, C., & Kelly, M. C. (in press). Developmental intergroup attitudes: Stereotyping, exclusion, fairness, and justice In J. F. Dovidio, M. Hewstone, P. Glick, & V. M. Esses (Eds.), *Handbook of prejudice and discrimination*. Thousand Oaks, CA: Sage.

Killen, M., & Stangor, C. (2001). Children's social reasoning about inclusion and exclusion in gender and race peer group contexts. *Child Development, 72,* 174–186.

Killen, M., Stangor, C., Price, B. S., Horn, S., & Sechrist, G. (2004). Social reasoning about racial exclusion in intimate and nonintimate relationships. *Youth and Society, 35,* 293–322.

Kohlberg, L. (1971). From is to ought: How to commit the naturalistic fallacy and get away with it in the study of moral development. In T. Mischel (Ed.), *Psychology and genetic epistemology* (pp. 151–235). New York: Academic Press.

Laursen, B., & Bukowski, W. M. (1997). A developmental guide to the organisation of close relationships. *International Journal of Behavioral Development, 21*(4), 747–770.

Lawrence, V. W. (1991). Effect of socially ambiguous information on white and black children's behavioral and trait perceptions. *Merrill–Palmer Quarterly, 37,* 619–630.

Lemerise, E., & Arsenio, W. F. (2000). An integrated model of emotion processes and cognition in social information processing. *Child Development, 71,* 107–118.

Levine, J. M. (1989). Reaction to opinion deviance in small groups. In P. B. Paulus (Ed.), *Psychology of group influence* (2nd ed., pp. 197–231). Hillsdale, NJ: Erlbaum.

Levy, S. R., Chiu, C. Y., & Hong, Y. Y. (2006). Lay theories and intergroup relations. *Group Processes and Intergroup Relations, 9,* 5–24.

Margie, N. G., Killen, M., Sinno, S., & McGlothlin, H. (2005). Minority children's intergroup attitudes about peer relationships. *British Journal of Developmental Psychology, 23*(2), 251–269.

Marques, J. M., Yzerbyt, V. Y., & Leyens, J. P. (1988). The black sheep effect: Judgmental extremity towards in-group members as a function of group identification. *European Journal of Social Psychology, 18,* 287–292.

McGlothlin, H., & Killen, M. (2005). Children's perceptions of intergroup and intragroup similarity and the role of social experience. *Applied Developmental Psychology, 26,* 680–698.

McGlothlin, H., & Killen, M. (2006). Intergroup attitudes of European American children attending ethnically homogeneous schools. *Child Development, 77,* 1375–1386.

McGlothlin, H., Killen, M., & Edmonds, C. (2005). European-American children's intergroup attitudes about peer relationships. *British Journal of Developmental Psychology, 23,* 227–249.

Monteith, M. J., Deneen, N. E., & Tooman, G. D. (1996). The effect of social norm activation on the expression of opinions concerning gay men and blacks. *Basic and Applied Social Psychology, 18,* 267–288.

Nesdale, D. (2008). Peer group rejection and children's intergroup prejudice. In S. R. Levy & M. Killen (Eds.), *Intergroup attitudes and relations in childhood through adulthood* (pp. 32–46). New York: Oxford University Press.

Nesdale, D., & Brown, K. (2004). Children's attitudes towards an atypical member of an ethnic ingroup. *International Journal of Behavioral Development, 28,* 328–335.

Nesdale, D., Griffith, J., Durkin, K., & Maass, A. (2005). Empathy, group norms and children's ethnic attitudes. *Journal of Applied Developmental Psychology, 26,* 623–637.

Nucci, L. P. (1996). Morality and the personal sphere of actions. In E. S. Reed, E. Turiel, & T. Brown (Eds.), *Values and knowledge* (pp. 41–60). Mahwah, NJ: Erlbaum.

Nucci, L. P. (2001). *Education in the moral domain.* Cambridge, UK: Cambridge University Press.

Opotow, S. (1990). Moral exclusion and injustice: An introduction. *Journal of Social Issues, 46,* 1–20.

Piaget, J. (1932). *The moral judgment of the child.* New York: Free Press.

Quintana, S. M. (1999). Role of perspective-taking abilities and ethnic socialization in development of adolescent ethnic identity. *Journal of Research on Adolescence, 19,* 161–184.

Rubin, K., Bukowski, W., & Parker, J. (2006). Peers, relationships, and interactions. In W. Damon & R. Lerner (Eds.), *Handbook of child psychology* (pp. 571–645). New York: Wiley.

Ruble, D. N., Alvarez, J., Bachman, M., Cameron, J., Fuligni, A., & Coll, C. G. (2004). The development of a sense of "we": The emergence and implications of children's collective identity.

In M. Bennett & F. Sani (Eds.), *The development of the social self* (pp. 29–76). East Sussex, UK: Psychology Press.

Ruble, D. N., & Martin, C. L. (1998). Gender development. In W. Damon & N. Eisenberg (Eds.), *Handbook of child psychology* (5th ed., Vol. 3, pp. 933–1016). New York: Wiley.

Rutland, A. (2004). The development and self-regulation of intergroup attitudes in children. In M. Bennett & F. Sani (Eds.), *The development of the social self* (pp. 247–265). East Sussex, UK: Psychology Press.

Rutland, A., Abrams, D., & Levy, S. R. (Eds.). (2007). Social identity and intergroup attitudes in children and adolescents [Special issue]. *International Journal of Behavioral Development, 31,* 417–418.

Rutland, A., Cameron, L., Milne, A., & McGeorge, P. (2005). Social norms and self-presentation: Children's implicit and explicit intergroup attitudes. *Child Development, 76,* 451–466.

Sagar, H. A., & Schofield, J. W. (1980). Racial and behavioral cues in black and white children's perceptions of ambiguously aggressive acts. *Journal of Personality and Social Psychology, 39,* 590–598.

Schachter, S. (1961). Deviation, rejection and communication. *Journal of Abnormal and Social Psychology, 46,* 190–207.

Selman, R. L. (1980). *The growth of interpersonal understanding: Development and clinical analyses.* San Diego: Academic Press.

Selman, R. L. (1990). Fostering intimacy and autonomy. In W. Damon (Ed.), *Child development today and tomorrow* (pp. 409–436). San Francisco: Jossey-Bass.

Shulman, S., Laursen, B., Kalman, Z., & Karpovsky, S. (1997). Adolescent intimacy: Revisited. *Journal of Youth and Adolescence, 26,* 597–617.

Smetana, J. G. (2006). Social domain theory: Consistencies and variations in children's moral and social judgments. In M. Killen & J. G. Smetana (Eds.), *Handbook of moral development* (pp. 119–154). Mahwah, NJ: Erlbaum.

Sutton, J., Smith, P. K., & Swettenham, J. (1999). Bullying and "theory of mind": A critique of the "social skills deficit" view of anti-social behaviour. *Social Development, 8,* 117–127.

Tajfel, H., & Turner, J. C. (1979). An integrative theory of intergroup conflict. In W. G. Austin & S. Worchel (Eds.), *The social psychology of intergroup relations* (pp. 33–47). Monterey, CA: Brooks/Cole.

Theimer, C. E., Killen, M., & Stangor, C. (2001). Preschool children's evaluations of exclusion in gender-stereotypic contexts. *Developmental Psychology, 37,* 1–10.

Turiel, E. (1983). *The development of social knowledge: Morality and convention.* Cambridge, UK: Cambridge University Press.

Turiel, E. (1998). The development of morality. In W. Damon (Ed.), *Handbook of child psychology: Vol. 3. Social, emotional, and personality development* (5th ed., pp. 863–932). New York: Wiley.

Verkuyten, M. (2001). "Abnormalization" of ethnic minorities in conversation. *British Journal of Social Psychology, 40,* 257–278.

CHAPTER 15

Conflict in Peer Relationships

BRETT LAURSEN
GWEN PURSELL

Interdependence fosters conflict. When lives are entwined, disagreement is inevitable. Most conflicts arise within a handful of close relationships. Family members and friends account for the majority of conflicts during early and middle childhood; romantic relationships are responsible for an added share during adolescence (Laursen & Collins, 1994). Differences in relationship properties give rise to differences in conflict behaviors. Close peer relationships are voluntary in contrast to family relationships, which are compulsory. Coercive conflict tactics, notably, anger and power assertion, are far more common with parents and siblings than with friends and romantic partners (Adams & Laursen, 2001). The implications and consequences of conflict also vary according to these relationship distinctions, perhaps because conflict is more a threat to the stability of peer relationships than to family relationships.

Friends and romantic partners hold special significance in the lives of children and adolescents, a significance that stems from the very nature of the relationship. The earliest friendships entail mutual expressions of affection and companionship (Dunn, 2004). Friends spend time together and share positive feelings toward one another. Young friends also demonstrate psychological and emotional intimacy, although this is more common during middle childhood. Across early and middle childhood, friends become important sources of support, both emotional and instrumental (Furman, 1989). Commitment and loyalty emerge during late childhood and early adolescence. The first romantic relationships appear about this time. These have most of the same properties as friendships, with the obvious addition of physical intimacy (Laursen, 1996). Greater closeness and interdependence mean that friends and romantic partners are increasingly important interpersonal resources.

Conflict threatens peer relationships and the resources they provide. Early in life, young children recognize and are able to articulate the potentially disruptive consequences that conflict poses to friendships (Dunn & Herrera, 1997). Children and adolescents seek to avoid conflict with their friends (and, later, with their romantic partners); when disagreements do arise, they often strive to resolve them in a mutually satisfactory manner. It is not so much that peer relationships dissolve in response to a single conflict episode; few friendships end with a big blowup (Hartup, 1992). Instead, chronic conflict appears to have a debilitative effect on the perceived quality of the relationship. Friendships and romantic relationships are predicated on mutually beneficial social exchanges. When exchanges cease to be favorable, relationship bonds deteriorate (Laursen & Hartup, 2002). Thus, conflict is an important factor that contributes to the overall climate of peer relationships.

Our chapter is divided into four sections. In the first section we describe some of the central issues that confront scholars of peer conflict. Definitions of conflict are reviewed, with an eye toward distinguishing conflict from related constructs. Measurement issues are discussed, with particular attention to biases inherent in assessment techniques. Developmental changes in characteristics of peer conflict are detailed, and distinctions between peer relationships in the management of conflict are explicated. In the second section we address relevant theory concerning the characteristics and consequences of peer conflict. Special attention is given to exchange theory as a framework for understanding normative conflict behavior in voluntary, close relationships. Competing conceptual claims are reviewed concerning the costs and benefits of conflict. Models that describe individual differences in conflict behavior are also considered. In the third section we describe select classical and contemporary research studies of conflict with friends and romantic partners. After a brief review of studies that describe normative features of peer conflict, we turn our attention to issues that have proven particularly vexing. The first of these research challenges concerns individual differences in peer conflict. The second challenge concerns dyadic differences in peer conflict. The third challenge concerns competing claims that peer conflict is both beneficial and detrimental to individual adjustment. In the fourth section we discuss future directions in theory and research on conflict with friends and romantic partners. Our focus is on the role of conflict in the maintenance and dissolution of friendships and romantic relationships.

Central Issues

Defining Conflict

What Conflict Is

Interpersonal conflict describes a state of disagreement that may be manifest in terms of incompatible or opposing behaviors and views. Subjective states of disagreement abound, but most scholars prefer objective indices that define conflict in terms of *overt behavioral opposition*. "Overt" means that behaviors signifying disagreement are directed toward the individual with whom one is disagreeing, in a manner that is understood by both participants to signify disagreement. Divergent opinions or actions expressed in the absence of the party with whom one is disagreeing do not qualify as interpersonal conflict, because they do not involve an exchange between two individuals. The same can be said of indirect conflicts, conflict through proxies, and most "he said, she said" disputes. "Behavioral" implies verbal or physical actions that convey disagreement. Put simply, conflict must be observable. Privately held opinions may contain the basic elements of disagreement, but they do not rise to the level of conflict unless they are expressed. "Opposition" connotes a contrary position or action. During a conflict, one party resists or contests the behaviors or views advanced by another party. Disagreement cannot occur in a vacuum; it must always be expressed in response to something someone else said or did.

What Conflict Is Not

To improve definitional clarity, interpersonal conflict is distinguished from the related constructs of aggression, dominance, competition, and anger. Interpersonal conflict should not be equated with aggression. Instances of verbal and physical aggression often take place in the context of conflict, but most conflicts between agemates do not contain aggression (Hartup & Laursen, 1993). Interpersonal conflict is also distinct from dominance. Although conflict is a prominent vehicle for the establishment and maintenance of dominance in peer relationships (LaFreniere & Charlesworth, 1987), disagreements are only one of the many ways that dominance is demonstrated. Furthermore, dominance does not appear to be a factor in most disputes between friends. Competition is not generally regarded as conflict, but we mention it here because early scholars considered scarce resource paradigms, such as the Prisoner's Dilemma, to be prototypical examples of conflict interchanges (e.g., Deutsch, 1973). It is true that competition often provokes conflict, but most forms of peer competition take place in artificial circumstances that replace the constraints that govern social exchanges between peers with norms that sanction oppositional behavior (Hartup, French, Laursen, Johnston, & Ogawa, 1993). Furthermore, most conflicts do not involve competition for resources. Finally, conflict and anger are distinct but overlapping constructs. Anger usually arises during conflict episodes; most conflicts, however, involve little or no negative affect. The closer the relationship, the less anger friends display during conflicts (Murphy & Eisenberg, 2002).

What Constitutes a Conflict

There is debate about the amount of opposition necessary for a conflict. Some scholars define conflict in terms of a single instance of opposition (Garvey, 1984). This unilateral definition of conflict requires oppositional behavior from one individual only. Consider two children who are playing a game together. After Child A moves a game piece, Child B protests that the move was out of turn. Regardless of Child A's response, Child B's opposition qualifies the episode as an example of unilateral conflict. Other scholars hold that a single opposition is a necessary but not sufficient condition for conflict (Maynard, 1985). This mutual definition of conflict requires oppositional behavior from both participants in a disagreement. Continuing with the previous example, the initial protest by Child B must be met with some form of objection or resistance by Child A, if the interaction is to qualify as a mutual conflict. The relative frequency of these two forms of conflict is not well documented. In one observational study, approximately one out of three disputes between preschool children was discontinued after the initial opposition (Laursen & Hartup, 1989).

The debate between one-turn and two-turn definitions is particularly relevant to observational studies in which the investigator can track behavioral exchanges. It is not clear that participants in self-report studies appreciate the distinction between unilateral and mutual disagreements and, when they do, there is little evidence that events are encoded in memory with sufficient precision that these different definitions can be applied accurately and reliably.

Measuring Conflict

Components of Conflict

Shantz (1987) characterized conflict as a "time-distributed social episode" that contains several distinct features, including initiation and opposition (behaviors that start the conflict), tactics and strategies (behaviors that perpetuate the conflict), resolution (behaviors that conclude the conflict), and outcome (consequences of the conflict). In addition to these sequential features, a conflict may additionally be described in terms of its frequency, affective tenor, and topic.

Dynamics of Conflict

Conflicts have been likened to a play or a novel, in that they tend to follow an organized sequence (Laursen & Collins, 1994). There are a protagonist and an antagonist (conflict participants), a theme (conflict topic), a complication (initial oppositional sequence), rising action (tactics and strategy), climax or crisis (resolution), and denouement (outcome). Plots unfold according to a prescribed sequence, and so do conflicts. Each comprises discrete units that combine to form a coherent whole. Three general patterns of conflict between friends have been identified (Laursen, Hartup, & Koplas, 1996): (1) coercion, which includes negative affect, aggression or power assertion, and unequal or unfavorable outcomes; (2) mitigation, which includes neutral or positive affect, negotiation, and equal or constructive outcomes; and (3) disengagement, which describes conflicts that have no resolution and no outcome. These patterns apply primarily to mutual conflicts; unilateral conflicts are best described as simple, affectively neutral compliance episodes (Laursen & Hartup, 1989).

There are other parallels between plots and conflicts. Both may be scripted and formulaic. Conflicts with similar distinguishing features fall into groups akin to genres, in which much of the action logically flows from participant roles and disagreement topics. Many conflicts proceed according to a script, in which participants assume well-rehearsed roles and interactions proceed in a familiar manner. Some scripts are driven by topics (e.g., object disputes). Other scripts are driven by relationship roles (e.g., behavior expected of friends). There is good evidence that a substantial proportion of marital conflicts are scripted (Gottman, 1993), but it is not clear whether the same can be said of conflicts between friends and romantic partners. We know that some conflict topics tend to elicit certain behaviors (Adams & Laursen, 2001). For instance, when adolescents describe disagreements that concern a violation of friendship norms, they report considerable anger and minimal negotiation.

Observing Conflict

Observations of conflict, either in the laboratory or *in vivo*, have the apparent advantage of objectivity. This advantage may be illusory. Laboratory interactions between parents and children reveal low agreement between insiders and outsiders as to whether an exchange involved conflict; participants were even less likely to agree with each other than to agree with an observer (Gonzales, Cauce, & Mason, 1996; Welsh, Galliher, & Powers, 1998). When friends do agree on the presence of conflict, their reports of affective intensity and outcomes have greater interrater reliability than their reports of resolutions (Burk &

Laursen, 2005; Simpkins, Parke, Flyr, & Wild, 2006). The fact that insiders do not agree with each other or with outsiders on key aspects of conflict has important implications, because it raises the possibility that subjective experiences of conflict may be the most important factor determining the consequences of conflict on individual adjustment.

Self-Reports of Conflict

Interview and questionnaire assessments of conflict have their own special challenges. The frequency and type of conflict reported by participants tends to vary as a function of the way conflict is defined and the time period for recollection. More conflict is reported when the term is defined as disagreeing than when it is defined as quarreling, fighting, or arguing. This is not surprising given that high-intensity disputes occur less frequently than low-intensity disputes. When asked to identify their most important disagreement, adolescents tend to select conflicts with high levels of anger (Laursen & Koplas, 1995), which suggests that angry conflicts are overrepresented in assessments limited to significant or salient conflicts.

Other factors influence self-reports of conflict. Questionnaires in which participants review a list of conflict topics and identify the number of disagreements arising during the previous day elicit more conflicts than daily records in which participants describe social interactions and note whether each contained a disagreement (Burk, Denissen, van Doorn, Branje, & Laursen, in press). Whether interaction-based assessments underestimate rates of conflict or topic-based assessments overestimate rates of conflict is not clear. Nor is it clear whether these different assessment tools elicit conflicts with specific characteristics.

Self-reports of conflict frequencies also vary according to the time interval for recall. Lower rates of conflict are reported by participants who are asked to recall conflict during the past week or month than by participants asked to report conflict during the previous day. Such response biases have origins in pragmatic inferences made by participants (Winkielman, Kanuper, & Schwarz, 1998). Long reference periods suggest that the investigator is looking for unusual, infrequent events, whereas short reference periods suggest that the investigator is looking for common, mundane events. It follows that longer reference periods probably underestimate the true incidence of disagreement. Note also that longer reference periods are subject to bias arising from relationship views (Feeney & Cassidy, 2003) and personality traits (Barrett, 1997; Schwarz & Bienias, 1990).

Responses to Hypothetical Conflict Scenarios

Children's conflict goals and strategies are often examined with hypothetical scenarios, in which participants are asked to imagine their response to a conflict vignette. Children report that their goals are typically related to their resolution strategies: Revenge and instrumental control goals predict assertive and hostile strategies, whereas relationship maintenance goals predict compromise strategies (Chung & Asher, 1996). Meta-analytic results indicate that hypothetical vignettes tend to overestimate the use of compromise and underestimate the use of coercion relative to rates obtained from self-reports and observations of actual conflicts (Laursen, Finkelstein, & Betts, 2001). One study directly comparing hypothetical vignettes to observed conflict behavior indicated that young children's responses to conflict vignettes have little relation to their behavior during real disagreements (Hay, Zahn-Waxler, Cummings, & Iannotti, 1992). Still, even if they are less than accurate representations of true conflict behavior, responses to hypothetical conflicts provide important insight into individual differences in responses to conflict.

Developmental Changes in Peer Conflict

Longitudinal studies that track the incidence and dynamics of peer conflict across childhood and adolescence are not available. Trends must be extrapolated from a series of cross-sectional and short-term longitudinal studies. This is particularly challenging when it comes to rates of conflict, because these are quite sensitive to the vagaries of measurement and definition.

Peer conflict initially emerges toward the end of the first year of life; violations of property rights or personal space that do not elicit protest at 6 months of age meet with resistance at 12 months of age, and by 21 months of age most children in peer settings are involved in disputes with playmates (Hay & Ross, 1982). Groups of preschool children average five to eight conflicts per hour during free play (Hay, 1984); preschool friends average almost three conflicts per hour (Hartup, Laursen, Stewart, & Eastenson, 1988). There appears to be little change in rates of conflict during the early primary school years (Howes & Wu, 1990), the last period for which comparable observational data are available. There are modest correlations between the frequency of conflict and the amount of daily social interaction with friends during adolescence (Laursen, 1995), but little is known about whether there are developmental changes in the rate of conflict per unit of social interaction. If this rate is stable, then the number of conflicts with peers should increase with age in a manner that roughly parallels increases in the amount of time spent with peers. There is reason to suspect, however, that the rate of conflict per unit of social interaction decreases with age, because global ratings of conflict with friends decline across middle childhood and adolescence (Clark-Lempers, Lempers, & Ho, 1991; Simpkins et al., 2006). The finding that youth engage in a significant number of disputes with their friends but perceive these relationships to be less quarrelsome than do others suggests that subjective perceptions are guided by features other than frequency counts.

Disputes between toddlers and preschool children are overwhelmingly focused on objects (Hay & Ross, 1982). Disagreements over the control of objects decline across middle childhood, whereas disagreements over the control of social behavior increase (Hartup & Laursen, 1993). By adolescence, most disputes with peers involve interpersonal concerns. Physical aggression declines across early childhood and is all but absent from conflicts during middle childhood (Shantz, 1987). Aggression does not disappear altogether; rather, physical aggression appears to be supplanted by verbal and relational aggression.

Conflict resolutions also change with age. Results from a meta-analysis examining the resolution of peer conflict during childhood, adolescence, and young adulthood indicate that coercion declines with age, accompanied first by increases in disengagement, then by increases in negotiation (Laursen et al., 2001). Reports of actual conflicts (exclusive of responses to hypothetical vignettes) indicate that most disputes between children are resolved with coercion, followed by equal levels of disengagement and negotiation. Disengagement becomes the primary means for settling disputes between adolescents, followed by coercion, then negotiation. By young adulthood, most disagreements with peers are resolved through negotiation, followed by disengagement and coercion. Given that angry, coercive disagreements are more apt than amicable disagreements to result in unequal outcomes and discontinued social interactions, conflict is likely to have more adverse consequences for the peer relations of young children than for those of older children and adolescents.

Relationship Differences in Peer Conflict

Children spend much of their free time interacting with friends; adolescents tend to divide their time between friends and romantic partners. Given that social interaction is a necessary prerequisite for conflict, it is perhaps not surprising to learn that children have more conflicts with friends than with nonfriends, and that adolescents have more conflicts with friends and romantic partners than with nonfriends. Controlling for social interaction closes the gap to the point that close peers have comparable rates of conflict to those of other peers (Hartup, 1992). This helps explain the meta-analytic finding that friends and nonfriends have a comparable incidence of conflict (Newcomb & Bagwell, 1995). Often (but not always), boys are found to have more conflicts with friends than girls.

Relationship differences in conflict topics become more differentiated with age. Young children engage in object disputes, regardless of their conflict partner (Hartup et al., 1988). As children get older, relationship concerns increasingly dominate disagreements between friends and nonfriends alike; nonfriends, however, also engage in a good deal of petty bickering over topics such as criticizing, teasing, and annoying behavior (Laursen, 1995). The concerns of romantic partners are similar to those of friends in many ways, although they also include disagreements over affection and sexual behavior.

There are important differences between friends and nonfriends in the management of conflict. Aggression and negative affect are rarer among friends than among nonfriends. This is not to say that friends never get angry; rather, friends tend to settle disputes in a manner that avoids lingering animosity. Conflict management tactics are the key to amicable solutions. Relative to acquaintances, friends and romantic partners are more apt to negotiate or to disengage from a dispute and less apt to pursue power assertive strategies, a trend that accelerates with age (Laursen et al., 2001). Peacemaking helps to explain why friends are more likely than nonfriends to resume social interactions (Verbeek & de Waal, 2001). Friends tend to make amends quickly, then return to play. Romantic partners report than conflict is as likely to improve their relationship as to have no impact; friends report that most conflicts have no bearing on their relationships, one way or another (Laursen, 1993). The latter findings suggest that when conflict arises, friends are content to close off the dispute and leave well enough along. Romantic partners, in contrast, engage in special efforts at constructive peacemaking.

Relevant Theory

Relationship Properties That Determine Conflict Behavior

Humans have a strong, innate need to belong that is manifest in a drive to form and maintain lasting, positive, and significant interpersonal relationships (Baumeister & Leary, 1995). We achieve this goal through interactions with individuals with whom we have formed stable and enduring bonds. This affiliative need probably has origins in the survival and reproductive benefits that accrue from membership in a group. It is not focused on a particular relationship, but it may have provided the impetus for additional evolved mechanisms that aid in the establishment and maintenance of different types of social relationships (Bugental, 2000). Although relationship categories are not hardwired, we believe that humans are predisposed to understand relationships in certain ways. Our interests lie in the reciprocity domain, because it is here that children learn to implement principles of social exchange, to manage reciprocal obligations, and to negotiate equivalent benefits.

Exchange theory starts from the premise that individuals strive to maximize their interpersonal outcomes. When individuals are free to select their interaction partners, they prefer those most likely to provide rewards (Homans, 1961). Interdependence describes conditions in which interaction outcomes are favorable for both participants. If mutually rewarding outcomes continue, short-term interdependencies may lead to long-term relationships (Kelley et al., 1983). Under these circumstances, participants come to depend on one another to provide essential resources in a variety of domains. It is important to note that strict equity is not the norm in most close relationships. Instead, friendships and romantic relationships are guided by communal norms, which include expectations of reciprocal exchanges that promote the well-being of the relationship and the individuals within it (Clark & Jordan, 2002). In communal relationships, benefits are distributed according to need, with the assumption that temporary inequalities will balance out over time.

Friendships and romantic relationships are, by definition, voluntary affiliations. Participation is not compulsory, and either member may dissolve the relationship at any time. Power in these relationships tends to be distributed evenly. Friendships and romantic relationships are horizontal or symmetrical in the sense that participants share equally in rights, privileges, and obligations. One party cannot dictate terms to the other, and both parties must agree on the distribution of outcomes for the relationship to remain close. Most voluntary relationships are transitory; they survive only as long as they serve the interests of both parties. Of course, in the absence of a suitable replacement, participants are loath to terminate a close relationship because of the emotional costs and the loss of benefits (Laursen & Hartup, 2002). The closer the relationship, the more difficult it is to discontinue it.

Conflict signals inequality, implying a perceived imbalance in rewards and costs. As such, it poses a critical challenge to friendships and romantic relationships, because failure to address the source of discord satisfactorily can undermine the foundation of voluntary, symmetrical relationships (Laursen, 1996). Conflict does more than just convey relationship threats; the mere act of disagreeing can be hazardous to relationships. Disagreement often evokes intense negative affect. For this reason, it is inherently unpleasant. It follows that frequent, angry conflicts change the calculus of a relationship by increasing the costs associated with social exchanges. Poorly managed conflicts also reduce the benefits of affiliation by disrupting ongoing interactions. When disputes are resolved in a manner that benefits one party but not the other, participants may be inclined to revisit communal assumptions.

The special properties of close peer relationships give rise to special patterns of conflict behavior. We have argued that friends and romantic partners are more apt than family members and other peers to use constructive forms of conflict management because of the greater potential of conflict to disrupt beneficial exchanges in voluntary, close relationships (Laursen et al., 1996). Some disagreement is necessary to settle differences, communicate expectations, and eliminate annoyances, so there is no reason to expect fewer conflicts among close peers than among others. Instead, differences should arise in the manner in which conflicts are managed. Friends and romantic partners should strive to minimize negative affect, coercive behavior, and win–lose outcomes, fostering continued social interaction between participants and mitigating perceptions of relationship damage. The threat that conflict poses to relationships is more distal than immediate; friendships and romantic relationships are less likely to end after a single dispute than they are to weaken in response to repeated disagreements that undermine closeness and alter perceptions about the commitment of participants to a communal orientation.

Developmental Shifts in Relationship Properties That Determine Conflict Behavior

As children grow older, they develop more mature views of peer relationships. Conceptions of friendship are hypothesized to progress from an ephemeral relationship designed to maximize personal benefits, to a short-term relationship dedicated to equality, and finally to a committed relationship designed to satisfy psychological needs (Selman, 1980). Young children are initially motivated by strictly selfish directives, but they soon realize that friendships differ in important ways from other relationships. An equal distribution of power forces children to embrace reciprocity (Piaget, 1932). Peer relations are initially premised on the principal of equal sharing. Symmetrical, reciprocal interactions foster cooperation and collaboration. This provides a foundation for the development of mutual respect and affection, which leads to practices that promote equality and mutual benefits (Youniss, 1980). Cognitive advances in role taking eventually foster another shift, from relationship algorithms based on equality to a more complex system based on participant contributions and needs. As appreciation for the importance of friendship develops, the overarching needs of the relationship are eventually elevated above the parochial needs of participants.

Commensurate changes in conflict management are anticipated. The emphasis that young friends place on equality suggests that conflict tactics will be dictated by anticipated outcomes; in some instances, fairness demands compromise, but in other instances, it requires coercion and concession. As children come to appreciate the impact their behavior has on others, their conflict tactics should gradually soften. Improved social skills also make it easier to get along with agemates. Friends learn to shun coercive, angry behaviors that inflict physical or psychological harm. Increasingly, friends agree to disagree, on the premise that an unresolved dispute is preferable to one that is settled by insistence. In this way, children learn to identify trivial disagreements that might derail ongoing exchanges. Not all disagreements can be ignored, however, and most youth eventually determine that it is incumbent on good friends to work through their disagreements, resolving them in a manner satisfactory to both parties. Compromise and negotiation gain prominence, with outcomes reflecting concern for long-term relationship consequences. One final point is worth noting. There must inevitably be a lag between relationship cognitions and relationship behavior, because it takes time to develop and hone social skills that are consistent with interpersonal aims (Hartup & Laursen, 1993). It follows that constructive conflict management tactics will be somewhat slower to emerge than constructive conflict management goals.

Individual and Dyadic Differences in Conflict Behavior

Diverse theoretical models have been invoked to account for individual differences in the rate and management of conflict. Most emphasize the importance of dispositions and social cognitions. In terms of dispositions, aggressive children are expected to be involved in more frequent disagreements and to have more difficulty managing disagreements constructively (Moffitt, Caspi, Rutter, & Silva, 2001). Children who have difficulties with emotional regulation and impulsivity should have similar difficulties avoiding and managing conflict (Eisenberg & Fabes, 2006). Temperamental and personality traits may also forecast contentiousness because irritable, disagreeable individuals tend to provoke discord and practice coercive conflict tactics (Graziano & Eisenberg, 1997). In terms of social cognitions, considerable attention has been given to social information-processing skills deficits and their links to hostile attribution biases (Crick & Dodge, 1994). Individuals who have difficulties encoding and interpreting information from the social world, and who fail to consider constructive alternatives to problems, may adopt provocative interaction styles and coercive conflict tactics. Dispositional and social-cognitive difficulties hinder social competence and damage peer reputations. For these and other reasons, peer conflict is expected to be a problem for rejected, socially maladept children.

Relationship characteristics should also have a bearing on conflict behaviors. Interpersonal conflict should reflect larger patterns of interacting within a relationship. Presumably, high-quality relationships have fewer sources of discontent than do low-quality relationships. Children in good quality relationships may also be more apt to practice constructive conflict management practices than those in poor-quality relationships (Laursen, 1996). Various dimensions have been proposed to account for these differences, including perceived support, felt security, anticipated relationship duration, and emotional distance.

The Correlates of Conflict

Conventional wisdom holds that conflict is bad for relationships and bad for individuals. We have already discussed how conflict is thought to undermine the benefits of affiliation and to erode the communal basis for exchanges. We have also alluded to assumptions that conflict has an adverse impact on individuals. Conflict can be stressful, particularly when it involves a lot of unresolved anger (Uchino, Cacioppo, & Kiecolt-Glaser, 1996). Too much conflict of this sort elevates the risk for stress-induced maladies. Conflict may also threaten individual adjustment by interfering with the provision of social support. Because social support helps to buffer against the deleterious mental and physical health consequences otherwise associated with stress (Cohen & Wills, 1985), conflict can exacerbate the consequences of stress if it dilutes support from the relationship in which it arises.

Beneficial outcomes have been hypothesized, too. Conflict is the primary vehicle whereby individuals work through interpersonal difficulties (Kelley et al., 1983). It follows that constructively managed conflict holds the potential to improve relationships. Of course, individuals also profit from relationship repair, but there may be other reasons to expect personal gain from conflict. First, conflict may help to right an injury or injustice. Second, conflict may promote individual growth. Dunn (2004) asserts that conflict with peers helps young children learn how to express and to defend their views. Piaget (1932) argues that children come to understand morality through disputes with peers over issues of justice. These conflicts may also promote cognitive-developmental advances by forcing children to abandon ineffective reasoning strategies. Cooper (1988) suggests that conflict helps youth establish an independent identity and a sense of autonomy. These and other benefits may be limited to instances in which conflict arises in the context of a supportive, nonthreatening relationship.

Classical and Contemporary Research

Normative Conflict Behavior

One of the earliest studies of peer conflict involved free-play observations of 40 children attending a laboratory nursery school (Green, 1933). Each dyad received a quarrelsomeness index representing the number of its quarrels divided by the number of opportunities for dyad members to play together. Each dyad also received a friendship index, representing the number of times the children played together divided by the number of opportunities to play together. The main findings bear repeating. "The ratio of quarreling to friendship decreases regularly with age. Boys are more quarrelsome than girls. ... Mutual friends are more quarrelsome, and mutual quarrelers are more friendly than the average, therefore, quarreling is a part of friendly social intercourse at these ages" (p. 251). Elaborating on these findings more than 50 years later, Hartup and colleagues (1988) demonstrated that the main difference between the conflicts of friends and those of nonfriends is not their rate of occurrence; rather, it is the manner in which the disagreements are managed. Compared to nonfriends, conflicts between friends involve less anger, less insistence, more equitable outcomes, and more postconflict social interaction.

There is an important exception to this rule. Social exchanges between friends are sensitive to environmental demands (Hartup & Laursen, 1993). Circumstances can make friends behave in a manner that would not otherwise be typical of their relationship. Closed-field settings describe circumstances in which sustained interaction is required; neither party is free to leave, and no alternative interaction partners are available. This contrasts with open-field settings, in which individuals come and go as they please. Competitive closed-field settings alter normal patterns of social exchange evinced in open-field settings. In competitive closed-field settings, friends share less and are more assertive than nonfriends (Fonzi, Schneider, Tani, & Tomada, 1997), and the conflicts of friends and nonfriends are as apt to be aggressive as they are to be conciliatory (Hartup et al., 1993). Experimental evidence on conflict behavior is lacking, but studies of resource distribution suggest that when competitive constraints are removed, friends behave in closed-field settings much as they do in open-field settings (Staub & Noerenberg, 1981).

Individual Differences in Conflict Behavior

Differences with Origins in Social Cognitions

The child's understanding of the social world has important implications for the way he or she manages disagreement. Social perspective-taking skills help the child appreciate that conflict behaviors have an impact on others (Selman, Beardslee, Schultz, Krupa, & Podorefsky, 1986). Developmental advances fostered by perspective taking promote a greater sensitivity to the risks that conflict poses to friendship. It follows that children with more sophisticated perceptions of friendships should adopt more constructive conflict management strategies. There is some evidence to support this claim: Levels of social understanding assessed at 3 and 4 years of age forecast observed rates of constructive and destructive conflict tactics with friends at 6 and 7 years of age (Dunn, 1999).

Social information-processing abilities have also been identified as a salient feature in responses to potentially provocative situations. Because social goals provide a framework for the processing of information about interpersonal behavior, they help to determine the behavioral response selected and implemented (Crick & Dodge, 1994). Reports of actual conflicts indicate that friendship conflict goals predict constructive conflict management tactics (Murphy & Eisenberg, 2002). Responses to hypothetical conflicts indicate that children who perceive the behavior of others as hostile report self-interested goals and confrontational or aggressive strategies for achieving these goals, whereas children who perceive the behavior of others as benign report constructive goals and accommodating strategies (Chung & Asher, 1996). Children who ascribe to self-interested goals and hostile strategies report the greatest conflict with their friends; children with constructive goals and accommodating strategies report the least conflict with their friends (Rose & Asher, 1999).

Differences with Origins in Social Competence

Children who are socially maladept have difficulties anticipating and avoiding conflict, and they lack the ability to manage conflict constructively. Considerable evidence links individual differences in social skills and emotional regulation to individual differences in conflict behavior. In one study, socially competent preschool children were less likely to be involved in angry conflicts and more likely to deal with angry conflicts directly and nonaggressively compared to children rated by teachers as less socially competent (Fabes & Eisenberg, 1992). Maternal and teacher ratings of emotional regulation were uniquely linked to displays of anger and the tendency to respond constructively (Eisenberg, Fabes, Nyman, Bernzweig, & Pinuelas, 1994). Similarly, among older children and adolescents, social functioning composites (derived from camp counselor ratings of social competence, self-regulation, and emotional regulation) uniquely predicted self-reports of constructive conflict strategies and conflict affective intensity (Murphy & Eisenberg, 1996). These and other studies suggest that the ability to manage conflict in a constructive manner, with minimal negative affect, is a hallmark of social competence.

Differences as a Function of Peer Social Status

Strong evidence ties social status to peer conflict behavior, which is perhaps not surprising given the links between social status and social competence. High-accepted preschool children have fewer and shorter disputes, with less negative affect and more positive affect, than low-accepted children (Putallaz, Hellstern, Sheppard, Grimes, & Glodis, 1995). Aggressive conflicts appear to account for most of the differences in conflict rates; high- and low-accepted children are involved in a similar number of nonaggressive conflicts (Arsenio & Cooperman, 1996). High- and low-status children also manage conflict differently. Teacher ratings of social preference are correlated with self-reports of nondestructive conflict tactics among U.S. and Indonesian school children (French, Pidada, Denoma, McDonald, & Lawton, 2005). Responses to hypothetical conflicts indicate that rejected children adopt aggressive tactics when encountering obstacles to conflict reso-lution, suggesting that low-accepted children focus on the instrumental rather than the relationship consequences of disagreements (Troop-Gordon & Asher, 2005). To date, no studies have examined conflict with friends or romantic partners, so it is not known whether social status differences are tied to the type and quality of the relationship in which disagreements arise.

Differences with Origins in Personality

There is good reason to assume that personality traits contribute to individual differences in conflict behavior. We have already discussed conflict in relation to emotional regula-tion, a disposition that has been implicated in different facets of personality, most nota-bly, agreeableness. Agency and communion, the core features of agreeableness, promote prosocial behavior and positive social relations, which in turn foster conciliatory conflict behavior. Among young children, prosociability is inversely associated with concurrent and prospective rates of conflict with friends (Dunn, Cutting, & Fisher, 2002). Among adolescents, agreeableness correlates positively with self-reports of constructive conflict resolutions and outcomes, and negatively with conflict anger and aggression (Jensen-Campbell & Graziano, 2001). It remains to be seen whether agreeableness is an indepen-dent predictor of conflict behavior, or whether its effects are mediated by social status and relationship quality.

Dyadic Differences in Peer Conflict Behavior

In general, participants in higher-quality friendships manage conflicts better than partici-pants in lower-quality friendships. Responses to hypothetical vignettes suggest that chil-dren who perceive higher levels of support from friends are less likely to endorse revenge as a conflict goal (Rose & Asher, 1999). We mentioned earlier the fact that friends hold disparate views of conflict events. One recent study attempted to disentangle these dif-fering viewpoints with techniques designed for interdependent data (Burk & Laursen, 2005). Both friends rated the quality of their relationship and described conflicts from the previous day. After parceling out the effects of negative relationship characteristics, friendship social support uniquely predicted the perceived impact of conflict on the relationship, such that disagreements tended to improve better-quality relationships and harm poorer-quality relationships. One friend's perceptions of relationship negativity independently predicted the other friend's reports of the impact that conflict had on the relationship, the anger expressed during the conflict, and the extent to which social interactions resumed after the conflict.

Peer relationships differ on a variety of attributes, and some of these differences are related to conflict behavior. Friendships characterized by high levels of controlling behavior also have frequent and intense conflicts (Updegraff et al., 2004). Friends who work collaboratively on a card-sorting task report less conflict anger and more compro-mise resolutions than friends who work independently on the task (Shulman & Laursen, 2002). The former are also more likely than the latter to report that conflict does not affect their relationship. Finally, observations indicate that adolescents in preoccupied romantic relationships have more frequent and more angry conflicts than adolescents in secure romantic relationships (Furman & Simon, 2006). Taken together, these studies suggest that interpersonal conflict is sensitive to a variety of peer relationship dimensions.

The Adjustment Correlates of Peer Conflict

Paradoxical Effects of Conflict

Peer conflict has been linked to both positive and negative outcomes. Chronic conflict and poorly managed conflict are characteristic of children and adolescents with adjustment difficulties. For instance, hostility and fighting with friends are associated with maternal reports of externalizing problems (Dunn, 2004). Antisocial friends perceive greater conflict in their relationship than do nonantisocial friends (Poulin, Dishion, & Haas, 1999). Similarly, school performance is negatively associated with the frequency of conflicts with friends (Adams & Laursen, 2007), and with the use of power assertive resolutions in conflicts with friends (Jensen-Campbell, Graziano, & Hair, 1996). But conflict is not uniformly detrimental. Consistent with Piaget's (1932) assertion that disagreement with agemates promotes cognitive development, there is evidence that peer conflict improves scientific reasoning (Azmitia & Montgomery, 1993). Observations of adolescents engaged in a problem-solving task revealed that conflicts containing transactive dialogue (i.e., elaborations or requests for elaboration) forecast subsequent increases in reasoning abilities. Cognitive performance was unrelated to participation in conflicts that lacked transactive dialogue, suggesting that the benefits of conflict may be limited to exchanges that require participants to articulate and defend a reasoned position. Taken together, these findings suggest a paradox: Is conflict beneficial and detrimental?

Addressing the Paradox

Two studies address the paradoxical effects of conflict. The first concerns associations between conflict with friends and adolescent emotional adjustment, as mediated by the perceived quality of the relationship (Demir & Urberg, 2004). Perceptions of conflict were positively associated with self-reported depressive symptoms, but this association was fully mediated by perceptions of friendship quality. Higher levels of conflict were associated with poorer-quality friendships, which in turn were linked to higher levels of depression. These findings raise the possibility that the consequences of conflict vary as a function of the quality of the relationship. To test this possibility, moderator analyses were applied to adolescent reports of conflict, friendship quality, and individual adjustment (Adams & Laursen, 2007). The results revealed nonlinear associations between the frequency of conflict and both delinquency and withdrawal that were moderated by perceived negativity. For adolescents in better-quality friendships, there was no change in withdrawal and delinquency as conflict increased from low to medium levels, but withdrawal and delinquency worsened as conflict increased from medium to high levels. In these relationships, conflict did not have an adverse impact on adjustment except among those reporting multiple daily disagreements. For adolescents in poorer-quality friendships, there was a positive linear association between the frequency of conflict and both delinquency and withdrawal. In these relationships, adjustment declined with each successive increase in conflict. The findings are consistent with the proposition that chronic conflict is debilitative, but moderate conflict may be benign or even beneficial for those who experience it in the context of a supportive relationship.

Future Directions

There is a critical need for theory and research describing the role of interpersonal conflict in the establishment, maintenance, and dissolution of friendships and romantic relationships (Hartup, 1992). Most of the work that addresses relationship trajectories concerns conflict in adult marital relationships. There are many reasons to suspect that these models do not easily generalize to child and adolescent friendships and romantic relationships. Chief among these reasons are their failure to account for developmental changes in individuals, the divergent nature of the resources exchanged at different age periods, and the unique constraints that accompany obligatory marital relationships.

Gottman and Parkhurst (1980) hypothesized that conflict is important to the development of friendship, because when unacquainted children get together and seek to establish common ground, efforts by one child to control the direction of play inevitably give rise to disagreements. Because disagreement is a natural by-product of play, friends must learn to defuse a dispute so they can continue playing. Available data indicate that disagreements do arise more frequently as children get acquainted. A study at a weeklong summer camp indicated that the incidence of quarreling among previously unacquainted youth increases over time (Furman, 1987), although this can be explained, at least in part, by increases in social interaction among preferred affiliates. Observations of previously unacquainted young children in closed-field dyadic play settings indicated that children who engage in more frequent disagreements are less likely to develop a friendship (Gottman, 1983). One of the characteristics that distinguish between children who hit it off and those who do not is their ability to return to play successfully after a conflict. Unfortunately, specific conflict tactics anticipating the resumption of play were not identified. Thus, we cannot say with any certainty whether or how conflict may promote or impede the development of friendship. We know only that intense and prolonged quarreling undermines interactions that are a necessary precondition for the establishment of friendship.

There is some evidence to suggest that rates of conflict are unrelated to the stability of established friendships (Berndt & Keefe, 1992; Bowker, 2004). Children rarely mention disagreements as a reason for terminating a friendship, and ethnographic observations of free play corroborate their claims (Rizzo, 1989). Dunn (2004) argues that rates of conflict are less important in distinguishing long-lived from short-lived friendships than is the successful management of conflict. In findings from a competitive closed-field task, dyads that used negotiation to resolve a resource-sharing dispute were more likely to remain friends over the course of the school year than were dyads that did not (Fonzi et al., 1997). As noted earlier, the unique nature of closed-field interchanges suggests that caution may be warranted in generalizing from this type of inquiry. The fact that longstanding friends fail to resolve a large proportion of their disputes may be seen as evidence that successful friendships do not require disagreements to be amicably resolved (Rizzo, 1992).

Speculation has far outpaced research on this topic. On the one hand, we think it unlikely that conflict has no bearing whatsoever on the longevity of a friendship or romantic relationship; marital relationships, which are far more difficult to dissolve, are clearly sensitive to the rate and management of conflict (Gottman, 1993). On the other hand, we know that relationship trajectories are more complicated and varied than our current models reflect; the prediction of stability must necessarily involve identifying relationship typologies and ascertaining the unique risks that conflict poses to each. We must do a better job accounting for the conflict's contribution to perceptions of relationship quality, because common sense tells us that unsatisfactory relationships tend to be jettisoned when more attractive alternatives are available.

Conclusion

Children know that friends are important, and that if they want to make and keep friends, they need to get along with them. From an early age, children hold nuanced views of their friendships and of the disagreements that arise within them. Erik, age 7, summed up the matter: "Kids who aren't your friends just try to get what they want or else tell the teacher. With your friends, things are different. You try to go half and half—like divide the stuff or do some of what you want to do and some of what your friend wants to do. You get along better that way." This deceptively simple formula explains how friends are supposed to behave. Unfortunately, when it comes to disagreements, things can get out of hand. These exceptions are what make the phenomenon and its consequences something more than what it is supposed to be.

Acknowledgment

Support for the preparation of this chapter was provided to Brett Laursen by the National Institute of Mental Health (Grant No. MH058116).

References

Adams, R., & Laursen, B. (2001). The organization and dynamics of adolescent conflict with parents and friends. *Journal of Marriage and Family, 63*, 97–110.

Adams, R. E., & Laursen, B. (2007). The correlates of conflict: Disagreement is not necessarily detrimental. *Journal of Family Psychology, 21*, 445–458.

Arsenio, W., & Cooperman, S. (1996). Children's conflict-related emotions: Implications for morality and autonomy. In M. Killen (Ed.), *Children's autonomy, social competence, and interactions with adults and other children: Exploring connections and consequences. New Directions for Child Development* (No. 73, pp. 25–39). San Francisco: Jossey-Bass.

Azmitia, M., & Montgomery, R. (1993). Friendship, transactive dialogues, and the development of scientific reasoning. *Social Development, 2*, 202–221.

Barrett, L. F. (1997). The relationships among momentary emotion experiences, personality descriptions, and retrospective ratings of emotion. *Personality and Social Psychology Bulletin, 23*, 1100–1110.

Baumeister, R. F., & Leary, M. R. (1995). The need to belong: Desire for interpersonal attachments as a fundamental human motivation. *Psychological Bulletin, 117*, 497–529.

Berndt, T. J., & Keefe, K. (1992). Friends' influence on adolescents' perceptions of themselves in school. In D. H. Schunk & J. L. Meece (Eds.), *Student perceptions in the classroom* (pp. 51–73). Hillsdale, NJ: Erlbaum.

Bowker, A. (2004). Predicting friendship stability during early adolescence. *Journal of Early Adolescence, 24*, 85–112.

Bugental, D. B. (2000). Acquisition of the algorithms of social life: A domain-based approach. *Psychological Bulletin, 126*, 187–219.

Burk, W. J., Denissen, J., van Doorn, M., Branje, S. J. T., & Laursen, B. (in press). The vicissitudes of conflict measurement: Stability and reliability in the frequency of disagreements. *European Psychologist.*

Burk, W. J., & Laursen, B. (2005). Adolescent perceptions of friendship and their associations with individual adjustment. *International Journal of Behavioral Development, 29,* 156–164.

Chung, T., & Asher, S. R. (1996). Children's goals and strategies in peer conflict situations. *Merrill–Palmer Quarterly, 42,* 125–147.

Clark, M. S., & Jordan, S. D. (2002). Adherence to communal norms: What it means, when it occurs, and some thoughts on how it develops. In B. Laursen & W. G. Graziano (Eds.), *Social exchange in development. New Directions for Child and Adolescent Development* (No. 95, pp. 3–25). San Francisco: Jossey-Bass.

Clark-Lempers, D. S., Lempers, J. D., & Ho, C. (1991). Early, middle, and late adolescents' perceptions of their relationships with significant others. *Journal of Adolescent Research, 6,* 296–315.

Cohen, S., & Wills, T. A. (1985). Stress, social support, and the buffering hypothesis. *Psychological Bulletin, 98,* 310–357.

Cooper, C. R. (1988). The role of conflict in adolescent–parent relationships. In M. R. Gunnar & W. A. Collins (Eds.), *The Minnesota Symposia on Child Psychology: Vol. 21. Development during the transition to adolescence* (pp. 181–187). Hillsdale, NJ: Erlbaum.

Crick, N. R., & Dodge, K. A. (1994). A review and reformulation of social information-processing mechanisms in children's social adjustment. *Psychological Bulletin, 115,* 74–101.

Demir, M., & Urberg, K. A. (2004). Friendship and adjustment among adolescents. *Journal of Experimental Child Psychology, 88,* 68–82.

Deutsch, M. (1973). *The resolution of conflict.* New Haven, CT: Yale University Press.

Dunn, J. (1999). Siblings, friends, and the development of social understanding. In W. A. Collins & B. Laursen (Eds.), *The Minnesota Symposia on Child Psychology: Vol. 30. Relationships as developmental contexts* (pp. 263–279). Mahwah, NJ: Erlbaum.

Dunn, J. (2004). *Children's friendships: The beginnings of intimacy.* Malden, MA: Blackwell.

Dunn, J., Cutting, A. L., & Fisher, N. (2002). Old friends, new friends: Predictors of children's perspective on their friends at school. *Child Development, 73,* 621–635.

Dunn, J., & Herrera, C. (1997). Conflict resolution with friends, siblings, and mothers: A developmental perspective. *Aggressive Behavior, 23,* 343–357.

Eisenberg, N., & Fabes, R. A. (2006). Emotion regulation and children's socioemotional competence. In L. Balter & C. S. Tamis-LeMonda (Eds.), *Child psychology: A handbook of contemporary issues* (2nd ed., pp. 357–381). New York: Psychology Press.

Eisenberg, N., Fabes, R. A., Nyman, M., Bernzweig, J., & Pinuelas, A. (1994). The relations of emotionality and regulation to children's anger-related reactions. *Child Development, 65,* 109–128.

Fabes, R. A., & Eisenberg, N. (1992). Young children's coping with interpersonal anger. *Child Development, 63,* 116–128.

Feeney, B. C., & Cassidy, J. (2003). Reconstructive memory related to adolescent–parent conflict interactions: The influence of attachment-related representations on immediate perceptions and changes in perceptions over time. *Journal of Personality and Social Psychology, 85,* 945–955.

Fonzi, A., Schneider, B. H., Tani, F., & Tomada, G. (1997). Predicting children's friendship status from their dyadic interaction in structured situations of potential conflict. *Child Development, 68,* 496–506.

French, D. C., Pidada, S., Denoma, J., McDonald, K., & Lawton, A. (2005). Reported peer conflicts of children in the United States and Indonesia. *Social Development, 14,* 458–472.

Furman, W. (1987). Acquaintanceship in middle childhood. *Developmental Psychology, 23,* 563–570.

Furman, W. (1989). Developmental changes in children's social networks. In D. Belle (Ed.), *Children's social networks and social supports* (pp. 151–172). New York: Wiley.

Furman, W., & Simon, V. A. (2006). Actor and partner effects of adolescents' romantic working models and styles on interactions with romantic partners. *Child Development, 77,* 588–604.

Garvey, C. (1984). *Children's talk.* Cambridge, MA: Harvard University Press.

Gonzales, N. A., Cauce, A. M., & Mason, C. A. (1996). Interobserver agreement in the assessment of parental behavior and parent–adolescent conflict: African American mothers, daughters, and independent observers. *Child Development, 67,* 1483–1498.

Gottman, J. M. (1983). How children become friends. *Monographs of the Society for Research in Child Development, 48*(3, Serial No. 201).

Gottman, J. M. (1993). The roles of conflict engagement, escalation, and avoidance in marital interaction: A longitudinal view of five types of couples. *Journal of Consulting and Clinical Psychology, 61,* 6–15.

Gottman, J. M., & Parkhurst, J. T. (1980). A developmental theory of friendship and acquaintanceship processes. In W. A. Collins (Ed.), *The Minnesota Symposia on Child Psychology: Vol. 13. Development of cognitions, affect, and social relations* (pp. 197–253). Hillsdale, NJ: Erlbaum.

Graziano, W. G., & Eisenberg, N. H. (1997). Agreeableness: A dimension of personality. In R. Hogan, J. Johnson, & S. Briggs (Eds.), *Handbook of personality psychology* (pp. 795–824). San Diego: Academic Press.

Green, E. H. (1933). Friendships and quarrels among preschool children. *Child Development, 4,* 237–252.

Hartup, W. W. (1992). Conflict and friendship relations. In C. U. Shantz & W. W. Hartup (Eds.), *Conflict in child and adolescent development* (pp. 186–215). New York: Cambridge University Press.

Hartup, W. W., French, D. C., Laursen, B., Johnston, M. K., & Ogawa, J. R. (1993). Conflict and friendship relations in middle childhood: Behavior in a closed-field situation. *Child Development, 64,* 445–454.

Hartup, W. W., & Laursen, B. (1993). Conflict and context in peer relations. In C. H. Hart (Ed.), *Children on playgrounds: Research perspectives and application* (pp. 44–84). Albany: State University of New York Press.

Hartup, W. W., Laursen, B., Stewart, M. I., & Eastenson, A. (1988). Conflict and the friendship relations of young children. *Child Development, 59,* 1590–1600.

Hay, D. F. (1984). Social conflict in early childhood. In G. Whitehurst (Ed.), *Annals of child development* (Vol. 1, pp. 1–44). Greenwich, CT: JAI.

Hay, D. F., & Ross, H. S. (1982). The social nature of early conflict. *Child Development, 53,* 105–113.

Hay, D. F., Zahn-Waxler, C., Cummings, E. M., & Iannotti, R. J. (1992). Young children's views about conflict with peers: A comparison of the daughters and sons of depressed and well women. *Journal of Child Psychology and Psychiatry, 33,* 669–683.

Homans, G. C. (1961). *Social behavior: Its elementary forms.* New York: Harcourt.

Howes, C., & Wu, F. (1990). Peer interactions and friendships in an ethnically diverse school setting. *Child Development, 61,* 537–541.

Jensen-Campbell, L. A., & Graziano, W. G. (2001). Agreeableness as a moderator of interpersonal conflict. *Journal of Personality, 69,* 323–362.

Jensen-Campbell, L. A., Graziano, W. G., & Hair, E. C. (1996). Personality and relationships as moderators of interpersonal conflict in adolescence. *Merrill–Palmer Quarterly, 42,* 148–164.

Kelley, H. H., Berscheid, E., Christensen, A., Harvey, J. H., Huston, T. L., Levinger, G., et al. (Eds.). (1983). *Close relationships.* New York: Freeman.

LaFreniere, P. J., & Charlesworth, W. R. (1987). Effects of friendship and dominance status on preschoolers' resource utilization in a cooperative/competitive situation. *International Journal of Behavioral Development, 10,* 345–358.

Laursen, B. (1993). The perceived impact of conflict on adolescent relationships. *Merrill–Palmer Quarterly, 39,* 535–550.

Laursen, B. (1995). Conflict and social interaction in adolescent relationships. *Journal of Research on Adolescence, 5*, 55–70.

Laursen, B. (1996). Closeness and conflict in adolescent peer relationships: Interdependence with friends and romantic partners. In W. M. Bukowski, A. F. Newcomb, & W. W. Hartup (Eds.), *The company they keep: Friendship in childhood and adolescence* (pp. 186–210). New York: Cambridge University Press.

Laursen, B., & Collins, W. A. (1994). Interpersonal conflict during adolescence. *Psychological Bulletin, 115*, 197–209.

Laursen, B., Finkelstein, B. D., & Betts, N. T. (2001). A developmental meta-analysis of peer conflict resolution. *Developmental Review, 21*, 423–449.

Laursen, B., & Hartup, W. W. (1989). The dynamics of preschool children's conflicts. *Merrill–Palmer Quarterly, 35*, 281–297.

Laursen, B., & Hartup, W. W. (2002). The origins of reciprocity and social exchange in friendships. In B. Laursen & W. G. Graziano (Eds.), *Social exchange in development. New Directions for Child and Adolescent Development* (No. 95, pp. 27–40). San Francisco: Jossey-Bass.

Laursen, B., Hartup, W. W., & Koplas, A. L. (1996). Towards understanding peer conflict. *Merrill–Palmer Quarterly, 42*, 76–102.

Laursen, B., & Koplas, A. L. (1995). What's important about important conflicts? Adolescents perceptions of daily disagreements. *Merrill–Palmer Quarterly, 41*, 536–553.

Maynard, D. W. (1985). How children start arguments. *Language in Society, 14*, 1–29.

Moffitt, T. E., Caspi, A., Rutter, M., & Silva, P. A. (2001). *Sex differences in antisocial behavior: Conduct disorder, delinquency, and violence in the Dunedin Longitudinal Study.* New York: Cambridge University Press.

Murphy, B. C., & Eisenberg, N. (1996). Provoked by a peer: Children's anger-related responses and their relations to social functioning. *Merrill–Palmer Quarterly, 42*, 103–124.

Murphy, B. C., & Eisenberg, N. (2002). An integrative examination of peer conflict: Children's reported goals, emotions, and behaviors. *Social Development, 11*, 534–557.

Newcomb, A. F., & Bagwell, C. L. (1995). Children's friendship relations: A meta-analytic review. *Psychological Bulletin, 117*, 306–347.

Piaget, J. (1932). *The moral judgment of the child.* London: Kegan Paul.

Poulin, F., Dishion, T. J., & Haas, E. (1999). The peer influence paradox: Friendship quality and deviancy training within male adolescent friendships. *Merrill–Palmer Quarterly, 45*, 42–61.

Putallaz, M., Hellstern, L., Sheppard, B. H., Grimes, C. L., & Glodis, K. A. (1995). Conflict, social competence, and gender: Maternal and peer conflicts. *Early Education and Development, 6*, 433–447.

Rizzo, T. A. (1989). *Friendship development among children in school.* Norwood, NJ: Ablex.

Rizzo, T. A. (1992). The role of conflict in children's friendship development. In W. A. Corsaro & P. J. Miller (Eds.), *Interpretive approaches to children's socialization. New Directions for Child Development* (No. 58, pp. 93–111). San Francisco: Jossey-Bass.

Rose, A. J., & Asher, S. R. (1999). Children's goals and strategies in response to conflicts within a friendship. *Developmental Psychology, 35*, 69–79.

Schwarz, N., & Bienias, J. (1990). What mediates the impact of response alternatives on frequency reports of mundane behaviors? *Applied Cognitive Psychology, 4*, 61–72.

Selman, R. L. (1980). *The growth of interpersonal understanding: Developmental and clinical analyses.* Orlando, FL: Academic Press.

Selman, R. L., Beardslee, W., Schultz, L. H., Krupa, M., & Podorefsky, D. (1986). Assessing adolescent interpersonal negotiation strategies: Toward the integration of structural and functional models. *Developmental Psychology, 22*, 450–459.

Shantz, C. U. (1987). Conflict between children. *Child Development, 58*, 283–305.

Shulman, S., & Laursen, B. (2002). Adolescent perceptions of conflict in interdependent and disengaged friendships. *Journal of Research on Adolescence, 12*, 353–372.

Simpkins, S. D., Parke, R. D., Flyr, M. L., & Wild, M. N. (2006). Similarities in children's and early adolescents' perceptions of friendship qualities across development, gender, and friendship qualities. *Journal of Early Adolescence, 26,* 491–508.

Staub, E., & Noerenberg, H. (1981). Property rights, deservingness, reciprocity, friendship: The transactional character of children's sharing behavior. *Journal of Personality and Social Psychology, 40,* 271–289.

Troop-Gordon, W., & Asher, S. R. (2005). Modifications in children's goals when encountering obstacles to conflict resolution. *Child Development, 76,* 568–582.

Uchino, B. N., Cacioppo, J. T., & Kiecolt-Glaser, J. K. (1996). The relationship between social support and physiological processes: A review with emphasis on underlying mechanisms and implications for health. *Psychological Bulletin, 119,* 488–531.

Updegraff, K. A., Helms, H. M., McHale, S. M., Crouter, A. C., Thayer, S. M., & Sales, L. H. (2004). Who's the boss? Patterns of perceived control in adolescents' friendships. *Journal of Youth and Adolescence, 33,* 403–420.

Verbeek, P., & de Waal, F. B. M. (2001). Peacemaking among preschool children. *Peace and Conflict: Journal of Peace Psychology, 7,* 5–28.

Welsh, D. P., Galliher, R. V., & Powers, S. I. (1998). Divergent realities and perceived inequalities: Adolescents', mothers', and observers' perceptions of family interactions and adolescent psychological functioning. *Journal of Adolescent Research, 13,* 377–402.

Winkielman, P., Kanuper, B., & Schwarz, N. (1998). Looking back at anger: Reference periods change the interpretation of emotion frequency questions. *Journal of Personality and Social Psychology, 75,* 719–728.

Youniss, J. (1980). *Parents and peers in social development: A Sullivan–Piaget perspective.* Chicago: University of Chicago Press.

CHAPTER 16

Aggression and Peer Relationships in School-Age Children
Relational and Physical Aggression in Group and Dyadic Contexts

NICKI R. CRICK
DIANNA MURRAY-CLOSE
PETER E. L. MARKS
NAZANIN MOHAJERI-NELSON

The study of the peer relationships of aggressive children has a long and rich history. Early on, studies tended to focus on the degree to which physically aggressive children were liked or disliked by their agemates, particularly their classmates at school. Since those groundbreaking investigations, many important advances have been made, including expansion of the types of aggression studied (e.g., relational aggression in addition to physical/verbal aggression,[1] proactive and reactive aggression), inclusion of aggressive girls rather than a primary focus on aggressive boys, and greater attention to the variety of peer relationships in which children engage (e.g., friendships, cliques). Our goal for this chapter is to provide a conceptual and empirical overview of our current understanding of the peer relationships of school-age, aggressive boys and girls, with an emphasis on physical and relational forms of aggression. Peer relationships discussed in this chapter include group metrics, such as peer status, perceived popularity, cliques, and crowds, as well as dyadic relations, specifically, friendships. Empirical studies of aggression and peer relationships are of two distinct types: studies that analyze the relationships of aggressive versus nonaggressive youth, and those that analyze the correlation between aggression and varying qualities of relationships (stability, closeness, etc.). As much as possible, we have identified which type of study is being presented, so that the reader can draw appropriate conclusions.

Theories Relevant to the Study of Peer Relations of Aggressive Children

A number of theoretical frameworks have been posited regarding the nature of aggressive children's peer relations, including social dominance theory, gender normativity theory, relational orientations, and homophily. *Social dominance theory* focuses on the evolutionary adaptiveness of certain behaviors that allow an individual to attain or control resources, and views aggression primarily as a means of achieving and maintaining dominance (Blanchard & Blanchard, 2003; Buss & Shackelford, 1997). From this perspective, social dominance is associated with popularity, because peers are attracted to dominant children's resources (e.g., Babad, 2001). This theory may also explain why differences in gender normative forms of aggression developed, positing that males (for whom reproductive fitness is often determined by short-term success) are more likely to use physical methods of aggressive dominance (i.e., physical aggression), whereas females (whose reproductive fitness is determined more by ability to survive) are more likely to use forms of aggression that are less likely to result in physical injury (e.g., relational aggression; Campbell, 1999). The fact that many children and adolescents employ gender normative methods of aggression to achieve popularity, often at the cost of being socially rejected, suggests that these evolved tendencies are being translated into specific, gender-differentiated behaviors.

Whereas some researchers focus on the use of aggression in attaining social dominance among humans, others stress the importance of both aggressive *and* prosocial actions in achieving dominance and status (Hawley, 2003; Parkhurst & Hopmeyer, 1998; Pellegrini, 2002). In this view, acts of leadership and cooperation, paired with deliberate acts of aggression, may be the most effective means for children and adolescents to gain status within the social hierarchy. In contrast, the *gender normativity theory* of aggression (Crick & Dodge, 1994; Crick & Rose, 2000) identifies how acts of aggression, particularly when they violate gender roles, lead to peer rejection. From this perspective, gender non-normative aggression (i.e., physical aggression for girls and relational aggression for boys) is actively discouraged by same-gender peers during middle childhood and adolescence, and is therefore expected to result in severe social sanctions. Gender normative aggression, on the other hand, is viewed by peers as inevitable (if undesirable) behavior. Thus, although both gender normative and non-normative aggression should predict social maladjustment (as well as having a substantial negative impact on victims), problems should be especially evident among users of gender non-normative forms.

A third theoretical perspective regarding the association between aggression and peer relationships involves gender differences in *relational orientations*. A number of researchers have identified the relative importance of interpersonal relationships for girls and agency for boys (Crick & Zahn-Waxler, 2003; Cross & Madsen, 1997; Rose & Rudolph, 2006) which have important implications for the development of aggression in the peer context. First, risk factors for aggressive conduct (e.g., peer rejection) may be more likely to result in relational aggression for girls and physical aggression for boys, because at-risk children employ aggressive behaviors that reflect the goals and values of their gender-segregated peer groups (Crick & Grotpeter, 1995; Crick & Zahn-Waxler, 2003). Second, maladaptive peer relationships (e.g., poor friendship quality) may be more likely to result from gender normative forms of aggression. For example, relational aggression may be especially disruptive and harmful to girls' friendships given their relative sensitivity to interpersonal stress (Rose & Rudolph, 2006).

A fourth theoretical perspective relevant to this body of work suggests that aggressive children tend to be in friendships and cliques with aggressive peers (Espelage, Holt, & Henkel, 2003; Xie, Cairns, & Cairns, 1999). This process, termed "homophily," may reflect the effects of selection or socialization (Espelage et al., 2003). From a selection perspective, children choose to affiliate with peers who are similar to themselves on a number of dimensions, including the tendency to behave aggressively. Aggressive children may choose aggressive friends and cliques, because such relationships provide support for existing behaviors, or because these children are rejected from the larger peer group and are therefore excluded from alternative peer relationships (Cairns, Cairns, Neckerman, Gest, & Gariepy, 1988; Xie et al., 1999). Moreover, once involved with aggressive peers, children often exhibit increases in their aggressive conduct. From a socialization perspective, aggressive friends and cliques provide support for aggression, leading to the development of such conduct over time (Cairns et al., 1988; Werner & Crick, 2004). The processes underlying such socialization include exposure to deviant models and reinforcement of aggressive behaviors (Bagwell & Coie, 2004; Dishion, McCord, & Poulin, 1999).

Review of Relevant Empirical Studies

Social Status

Social Preference[2]

A number of sociometric studies of both children and adolescents have shown that physical/verbal aggression is associated with low social preference (e.g., LaFontana & Cillessen, 2002; Rubin, Chen, & Hymel, 1993). However, it is important to consider acceptance and rejection separately, given that correlations between physical/verbal aggression and acceptance tend to be nonsignificant, whereas correlations between physical/verbal aggression and rejection tend to be moderately positive (Graham & Juvonen, 2002; see Rubin et al., 1993; Olweus, 1977). Studies looking categorically at acceptance- and rejection-based social status groupings (Coie, Dodge, & Coppotelli, 1982; see Cillessen, Chapter 5, this volume) seem to confirm that rejection, but not acceptance, is related to physical/verbal aggression. In a meta-analysis, Newcomb, Bukowski, and Pattee (1993) found that controversial and rejected elementary school children were significantly more physically/verbally aggressive than average children, who were themselves more aggressive than sociometrically popular and neglected children (see also Crick & Grotpeter, 1995; Tomada & Schneider, 1997). Similar results have been shown for adolescents (e.g., Coie et al., 1982). Whereas some researchers indicate that physical aggression may precede peer rejection in playgroup situations (Dodge, 1983), others have found that low social preference may predict increases in physical/verbal aggression over time for girls only (Prinstein & Cillessen, 2003). Longitudinal work considering associations between physical/verbal aggression and peer preference has, unfortunately, provided inconsistent support for relations in either direction (Cillessen & Mayeux, 2004).

It may seem surprising that physical/verbal aggression is related to rejection but not to acceptance given the theoretical link between these constructs.[3] Such a pattern of findings suggests that physically/verbally aggressive behavior does not affect how much a child or adolescent is liked by peers. What physically/verbally aggressive behavior *does* appear to do, however, is to cause the child to be *disliked* by peers. In fact, children who had good social skills received an equal number of acceptance nominations regardless of level of physical/verbal aggression (see Asher & McDonald, Chapter 13, this volume, for a discussion of relations between prosocial behavior and acceptance). Presumably, an aggressive child with high social skills will be liked by a portion of the peer group (perhaps a similarly deviant portion, as suggested by homophily theory) but disliked by victims of the aggression (see Campbell & Yarrow, 1961; Rose, Swenson, & Waller, 2004).

Similarly, evidence supports a significant association between both relational aggression and concurrently assessed peer rejection for middle childhood, adolescent, and young adult samples regardless of whether relational aggression was assessed as a continuous or categorical variable (e.g., Crick & Grotpeter, 1995; Henington, Hughes, Cavell, & Thompson, 1998; Storch, Werner, & Storch, 2003; Werner & Crick, 1999, 2004; Zalecki & Hinshaw, 2004) and between relational aggression and *future* peer rejection (e.g., Crick, 1996; Tomada & Schneider, 1997). In some studies, the latter association was found for girls only (Werner & Crick, 2004). Longitudinal studies have also shown that relational aggression predicts increases in peer rejection over time, particularly for girls (Crick, 1996). Studies employing peer acceptance or social preference as the index of peer status have found that relational aggression is negatively associated with concurrent and future peer acceptance/social preference (Henington et al., 1998; Tomada & Schneider, 1997), particularly for girls (Andreou, 2006; Crick, 1996; Roach & Gross, 2003). In addition, engaging in relational aggression is associated with reductions in peer acceptance over time (Tomada & Schneider, 1997). Evidence demonstrates that relational aggression is significantly associated with relatively high levels of concurrent and future peer rejection and low levels of social preference even after physical/verbal aggression has been statistically controlled (Crick, 1996; Henington et al., 1998; Rys & Bear, 1997; Zimmer-Gembeck, Geiger, & Crick, 2005). With the exception of one study (Henington et al., 1998), these associations were apparent for girls only. As with physically/verbally aggressive children, research with sociometric status groups has demonstrated that rejected and controversial status children are significantly more relationally aggressive than their peers (Crick & Grotpeter, 1995; Henington et al., 1998; Tomada & Schneider, 1997).

Taken together, these findings provide convincing evidence of an association between aggression and peer rejection for both physical/verbal and relational forms of aggression. However, only relational aggression appears to be related to relatively low peer acceptance. Furthermore, this association may be stronger for girls, a finding that supports the relational orientations theoretical perspective. Interestingly, though, both relational and physical/verbal aggression have been shown to be associated with controversial peer status, which, by definition, includes being both highly liked and disliked, a finding that may seem at odds with the results for relational aggression and peer acceptance. Further research is needed to clarify this issue.

Perceived Popularity

Recently, researchers have focused on the social status construct of perceived popularity. A number of studies have demonstrated that the relation between popularity and physical/verbal aggression may vary with age; at least two cross-sectional studies (LaFontana & Cillessen, 2002; Rose et al., 2004) have found that physical/verbal aggression is associated with lower popularity during middle childhood (see also Rodkin, Farmer, Pearl, & Van Acker, 2006) but higher levels of popularity by early adolescence (see also Parkhurst & Hopmeyer, 1998). At all grade levels, however, some aggressive children are also popular. For example, in a group of fourth- through sixth-grade students, Rodkin and his colleagues (2006) found that nearly one-fourth of children categorized as aggressive were also popular.

Relational aggression also appears to predict heightened perceived popularity among children in middle school but, with one exception (Andreou, 2006), not among children in elementary school (LaFontana & Cillessen, 2002; Rose et al., 2004; Lease, Kennedy, & Axelrod, 2002). Longitudinal results explicate these effects; across different lengths of time and among different age groups (fifth grade and older), higher levels of popularity have been related to increases in relational aggression (Cillessen & Mayeux, 2004; Prinstein & Cillessen, 2003; Rose et al., 2004). In general, higher relational aggression predicted increases in popularity during early adolescence, but not during middle childhood or middle adolescence. As Sandstrom and Cillessen (2006) noted, this pattern of relationships may be interpreted as indicating that either popular individuals must use increasing levels of coercion and social manipulation to retain their status and power, or that popularity itself is "corrosive" and inevitably leads powerful individuals to hurt others. In addition, the fact that relational aggression predicted popularity in middle school may help to explain the prevalence of relationally aggressive behaviors during this period.

One important question that has surfaced in recent years is whether the relation between physical/verbal aggression and perceived popularity during adolescence is a consequence of the association between physical/verbal aggression and relational aggression. Three studies of adolescents (Cillessen & Mayeux, 2004; Prinstein & Cillessen, 2003; Rose et al., 2004) have shown that, with relational aggression factored out, physical/verbal aggression has a nonsignificant (or, in a few cases, a low negative) relation to perceived popularity. Certainly, moderate correlations between physical/verbal and relational aggression (e.g., Crick & Grotpeter, 1995; Rose et al., 2004) suggest that a significant portion of individuals who are physically/verbally aggressive are also relationally aggressive, and that it may be this co-occurring relational aggression that allows these individuals to gain and maintain status within the social hierarchy (Sandstrom & Cillessen, 2006).

In summary, whereas all forms of aggression are negatively related to both peer preference and popularity during childhood, a shift seems to occur around the beginning of middle school. By early adolescence, physical/verbal and relational aggressive behaviors appear to be associated with increased popularity (i.e., social status and power), supporting social dominance theory but not gender normativity theory. Contrary to gender normativity predictions, relational aggression has been found more reliably to relate to rejection for girls than for boys. Furthermore, gender differences tend not to emerge in associations between peer preference and physical/verbal aggression (with some exceptions; e.g., Crick, 1996) or in associations between perceived popularity and either physical/verbal or relational aggression. Indeed, the implication that relational aggression may be more damaging to girls' peer relationships is more in line with the predictions of relational orientations theory than gender normativity theory.

Cliques

"Peer cliques," defined as voluntary, friendship-based peer networks, emerge in middle childhood and tend to include 3 to 10 members (Brown & Klute, 2003; Cairns et al., 1988). Research assessing the association between aggression and peer cliques has focused on (1) comparing clique involvement between aggressive and nonaggressive children and (2) assessing the similarity of aggressiveness in clique members.

Clique Involvement

Physically/verbally aggressive children and adolescents are as likely to be involved in social cliques as their nonaggressive peers (Bagwell, Coie, Terry, & Lochman, 2000; Cairns et al., 1988). In addition, children and adolescents may establish and maintain their prominence in cliques through aggressive behaviors (Adler & Adler, 1995; Xie, Farmer, & Cairns, 2003), leading them to be central members of prominent cliques in their classroom (i.e., high in "network centrality"; Rodkin, Farmer, Pearl, & Van Acker, 2000). Although some studies have found no relation between physical/verbal aggression and network centrality (Bagwell et al., 2000; Cairns et al., 1988; Xie, Cairns, & Cairns, 2002), other research suggests that physically/verbally aggressive children are more likely than their peers to be central clique members (Rodkin et al., 2000; Xie et al., 1999). These mixed findings may reflect the moderating role of culture and gender in this association. Aggression may only afford higher social positions when it is relatively normative in the larger peer group (Estell, Cairns, Farmer, & Cairns, 2002). In fact, in China (where aggression is highly discouraged), higher levels of general aggression (including both physical and relational aggression items) were associated with a lower likelihood of having ties to classroom cliques (Xu, Farver, Schwartz, & Chang, 2004). The association between physical/verbal aggression and clique membership appears to differ for males and females. In one study, higher levels of physical/verbal aggression predicted lower involvement in cliques for girls but were not related to clique membership for boys (Xie et al., 1999). Although physically/verbally aggressive boys tend to be nuclear clique members, such aggression is either not associated with clique centrality for girls (Xie et al., 1999, 2003) or it is actually related to *lower* centrality for girls (Farmer & Rodkin, 1996). These gender differences may reflect the greater social sanctions for girls who engage in physical aggression (Crick, 1997).

To date, few researchers have examined the association between clique membership and relational aggression. Clique members, particularly those high in network centrality, may be in a good position to employ relationally aggressive behaviors, because they have the power to threaten victims' social relationships effectively (Adler & Adler, 1995; Xie et al., 2002). Some research suggests that higher relational aggression is associated with heightened network centrality (Xie et al., 2002), particularly for girls (Xie et al., 2003). Overall, then, aggressive children are as likely to be clique members and are more likely to be central members of cliques than their peers. Initial work suggests that nuclear clique membership is positively associated with relational aggression for girls and physical/verbal aggression for boys.

Cliques with Aggressive Members

Physically/verbally aggressive children tend to be members of cliques with aggressive peers (Bagwell et al., 2000; Cairns et al., 1988; Xie et al., 1999), and longitudinal work supports the involvement of both selection and socialization processes (Espelage et al., 2003). Gender and age are also important factors involved in homophily. For boys, the similarity among clique members in physically/verbally aggressive behavior is evident during elementary school (Cairns et al., 1988; Xie et al., 1999; Xu et al., 2004). However, for girls, homophily in physical/verbal aggression does not emerge until middle school (Cairns et al., 1988; Xie et al., 1999).

Few researchers have assessed whether relationally aggressive children tend to belong to cliques with relationally aggressive peers. In one study, Espelage and colleagues (2003) found that both male and female adolescents exhibited similar levels of bullying behavior (including gossip and social exclusion) as members of their clique; in addition, involvement in bullying cliques predicted increases in adolescents' bullying over time. Overall, then, selection and socialization within cliques are evident for physical/verbal aggression, and preliminary work suggests that these processes may occur for relational forms of aggression as well. However, additional research is necessary to examine this hypothesis and to assess whether there are gender or cultural differences in homophily of relationally aggressive cliques.

Crowds

In contrast to cliques, "crowds" are defined as reputation-based social networks in which members do not necessarily spend time with one another, and often include groups such as "jocks," "brains," "loners," "druggies," "nerds," and "populars" (Brown, 1990). Crowds are larger than cliques (often greater than 10 members), and crowd membership is assigned by the consensus of the peer group (Brown, 1990). Crowds may be related to aggressive behavior, because certain behaviors may help peers assign individuals to particular crowds (e.g., substance use and "druggies"; Brown, Lohr, & Trujillo, 1990), and crowds may channel adolescents into certain activities and social relationships (Brown et al., 1990; Brown & Klute, 2003). The association between crowd membership and aggression has been understudied. However, research from related areas suggests that crowd membership is related to adolescent behavior and adjustment (e.g., alcohol consumption, sexual activity, and internalizing symptoms; Dolcini & Adler, 1994; LaGreca, Prinstein, & Fetter, 2001; Prinstein & LaGreca, 2002; Urberg, 1992).

It is plausible that certain crowds may be more aggressive (e.g., "burnouts") or nonaggressive (e.g., "nerds"); however, very little research has been conducted on crowd membership and aggression. Researchers have posited that some crowds (e.g., "populars") may be especially likely to employ relationally aggressive behaviors, because their prominent status in the peer group may make such conduct especially effective (Adler & Adler, 1995). In fact, adolescents sometimes consider exclusion, a relationally aggressive behavior, to be a legitimate response to threats to group functioning (Killen & Stangor, 2001), and adolescents are less likely to rate exclusion based on crowd membership as wrong relative to other transgressions (Horn, 2003). Furthermore, members of low-status crowds may be especially likely to be excluded, particularly by members of high-status crowds (Horn, 2006). Further research is sorely needed to determine whether crowd membership is associated with either physical or relational aggression.

Friendships

Children's friendships have been studied in a variety of ways; however, most investigators currently define a "friendship" in terms of its reciprocal nature; that is, each member of the dyad must consider the partner to be one of his or her best liked peers for the relationship to be identified as a friendship (Hartup & Stevens, 1997). Three indices have been shown to be particularly important for understanding children's friendships (Hartup & Stevens, 1997): (1) the degree to which children engage in friendships (having friends), (2) the characteristics of the friendships (friendship quality), and (3) the attributes of the friend (friend characteristics).

Having Friends

When researchers compared aggressive and nonaggressive children, physically/verbally aggressive children were reported to have the same number of mutual friendships as nonaggressive children (Brendgen, Vitaro, Turgeon, & Poulin, 2002; Ray, Cohen, Secrist, & Duncan, 1997). In fact, physically/verbally aggressive children were still selected as best friends by peers, even though, overall, they were rated to be less popular and more disliked (Cairns et al., 1988). Highly physically/verbally aggressive children were more likely to lose friends over the course of a summer school program, whereas moderately physically/verbally aggressive children displayed an increase in the number of friends (Hektner, August, & Realmuto, 2000). Relationally aggressive grade-schoolers have been found to be just as likely as nonaggressive peers to have at least one reciprocal friendship (Rys & Bear, 1997).

Friendship Quality

In more recent years, researchers have become interested in the quality of children's friendships, including the friendships of physically/verbally aggressive children. Compared to nonaggresive children, physically/verbally aggressive children tend to be involved in friendships with relatively high levels of conflict (Coie et al., 1999), coercion, and, among boys, reactive anger (Dodge, Price, Coie, & Christopoulos, 1990). Aggression is also correlated with low levels of positive qualities, such as closeness, security, and intimacy (Cillessen, Jiang, West, & Laszkowski, 2005; Grotpeter & Crick, 1996). In fact, Grotpeter and Crick (1996) concluded that physically/verbally aggressive children value the time they spend with friends but place little value on the emotional bonds, a finding verified by Bagwell and Coie (2004). Even when aggressive children did not self-report any differences in their friendship qualities, observers found that physically/verbally aggressive boys had fewer positive and reciprocal interactions than their peers (Bagwell & Coie, 2004). Furthermore, the friends of physically/verbally aggressive children reported more negative feelings toward the friendship (Brendgen et al., 2002).

When comparing the quality of friendship of children rated as aggressive, the relation between physical/verbal aggression and poor friendship quality was moderated by the function of the physically/verbally aggressive act. Specifically, proactively physically/verbally aggressive youth (i.e., youth who initiate aggression to achieve their own ends) reported satisfaction with their friendships and the support that they received from friends at the beginning of the year but had increasing levels of conflict over time (Poulin & Boivin, 1999). Conversely, reactively physically/verbally aggressive children (i.e., children who aggress in response to perceived provocation) reported less satisfaction with their friendships but higher levels of conflict. Finally, the best friends of proactively physically/verbally aggressive boys reported relatively high levels of conflict and dissatisfaction with the friendship; nonetheless, they were still selected as best friends more often than were reactively aggressive boys.

A number of studies have shown that the quality of the friendships of relationally aggressive children differ from those of nonaggressive children in important ways. Grotpeter and Crick (1996) found that, compared with peers, relationally aggressive children reported significantly higher levels of exclusivity (e.g., feeling jealous if a friend wants close ties with another peer), intimacy (e.g., sharing secrets), and relational aggression within their friendships. The authors hypothesized that relationally aggressive children may use the secrets shared by their friends to manipulate them into exclusive relationships (e.g., threatening to divulge a secret if the friend considers befriending someone else). Further evidence for a lack of harmony in the friendships of relationally aggressive children is that their friendships were characterized by high levels of conflict and low levels of positive friendship qualities (e.g., companionship; Cillessen et al., 2005).

Preliminary evidence has indicated that the quality of relationally aggressive children's friendships may vary for boys and girls. Relational aggression is particularly common in girls' friendships (Crick & Nelson, 2002); among adolescent girls, closeness to the friend has been positively associated with the degree of hurt felt when targeted by a friend's relational aggression (Remillard & Lamb, 2005). Recent findings indicate that the association between intimate disclosure by a friend and relational aggression may be stronger for girls than for boys; specifically, Murray-Close, Ostrov, and Crick (2007) found that increases in intimate disclosure over time by a close friend were associated with increases in relational aggression for girls only.

Friend Characteristics

Supporting the homophily theory of friendships (Kandel, 1978), Cairns et al. (1988) found that physically/verbally aggressive children and adolescents were more likely to befriend and associate with physically/verbally aggressive peers. Friendship with physically/verbally aggressive peers likely results in more aggressive behavior, because friends reinforce each others' behaviors (Dishion, Patterson, & Griesler, 1994). It is difficult to determine whether this similarity in physical/verbal aggression level among friends can be attributed to aggressive youths' selection of aggressive friends or to the socialization that occurs among friends (Kandel, 1978). In support of the selection perspective, boys with the same level of proactive physical/verbal aggression were more likely to initiate and maintain friendships over time, whereas boys who had discordant levels of proactive physical/verbal aggression were more likely to terminate their friendships (Poulin & Boivin, 2000). Some evidence suggests that aggressive children become friends *after* being rejected by nonaggressive children, rather than selecting each other based on behavioral similarities (Hektner et al., 2000).

In support of the socialization perspective, research suggests that physically/verbally aggressive children who befriend each other are at heightened risk for maintaining a stable level of aggressiveness over time, because they exert social pressure on each other to continue involvement in such conduct (Brendgen, Vitaro, & Bukowski, 2000). For example, in one study, adolescents transitioning into middle school were found to have stable levels of physical/verbal aggression, particularly if they had high rates of aggression at Time 1 *and* maintained their friendship with a physically/verbally aggressive peer (Adams, Bukowski, & Bagwell, 2005). In a longitudinal study, Warman and Cohen (2000) found that chronically physically/verbally aggressive children befriended other physically/verbally aggressive children, but children who discontinued their physically/verbally aggressive behaviors were more likely to have had nonaggressive friends. It is plausible that having nonaggressive friends could serve as a buffer against continued involvement in aggression; however, the evidence of such trends is limited and periodically contradicted. In fact, in a follow-up assessment, youth involved in the intervention did select less aggressive peers as friends, but the intervention did not impact the peer ratings of their physical/verbal aggressiveness (August, Egan, Realmuto, & Hektner, 2003).

With respect to relational aggression, levels of relational aggression of youth and their friends were significantly correlated for children (Werner & Crick, 2004) and adolescents (Cillessen et al., 2005). Friends' socialization effects were found for girls; that is, friends' levels of relational aggression predicted girls' own levels of relational aggression 1 year later. Some support for selection effects were also apparent for both genders; specifically, children's levels of relational aggression predicted friends' relational aggression 1 year later, suggesting that their friends may have selected them based on their aggressive conduct.

General Conclusions and Future Directions

This chapter focuses on a number of theoretical perspectives (e.g., social dominance theory; Blanchard & Blanchard, 2003; Buss & Shackelford, 1997), each of which makes a number of unique and at times competing predictions regarding how aggression develops in the peer context. For example, social dominance theory identifies how aggression may be used to attain short-term goals (e.g., gaining access to resources, high levels of perceived popularity, and central membership to cliques; LaFontana & Cillessen, 2002; Rose et al., 2004; Xie et al., 1999, 2003). However, behaving aggressively is also related to a host of negative outcomes (e.g., peer rejection). Thus, although aggression may yield some social benefits, it is also related to a number of indices of poor peer functioning.

Consistent with gender normativity theory (Crick, 1997), under some conditions, physical aggression appears to be more harmful to peer functioning for girls, whereas relational aggression is more harmful for boys. For example, physically/verbally aggressive girls do not enjoy the high network centrality that is typical of their male counterparts, and these girls may experience particularly high levels of peer rejection (Crick, 1997; Farmer & Rodkin, 1996). Parallel findings have been reported for relationally aggressive boys (Crick, 1997; Xie et al., 2003).

However, from the perspective that males and females differ in their relational orientations, peer relationship processes should be more strongly associated with relational aggression *for girls* and physical aggression *for boys*. In fact, a number of researchers have found that peer rejection, intimate exchange in friendships, and social network centrality are more strongly related to relational aggression for girls (Murray-Close et al., 2007; Werner & Crick, 2004), whereas high network centrality is more strongly related to physical aggression for boys (Xie et al., 2003). Therefore, the assessment of both relational and physical aggression is necessary to gain a gender-balanced understanding of the development of aggression in the peer group. Future work should examine the contexts in which gender normative aggression is associated with heightened peer problems (as predicted by relational orientation perspective) versus lower levels of peer problems (as predicted by gender normativity theory).

Finally, consistent with the homophily hypothesis, a number of studies have found that both physically/verbally and relationally aggressive children are more likely to have aggressive friends (e.g., Werner & Crick, 2004) and to be involved in aggressive cliques (e.g., Xie et al., 1999), and both selection and socialization processes appear to be involved (Espelage et al., 2003). Future research should examine the role of selection and socialization in additional peer networks, including crowds. Poulin and Boivin (2000) concluded that it is more plausible that aggressive children select each other as friends rather than socially influence each other into becoming aggressive, which might be due to lack of options when their efforts to befriend nonaggressive children are rejected (Hektner et al., 2000). Aggressive behaviors are also encouraged and reinforced by aggressive friends (Dishion et al., 1994). Disentangling the cyclical effects of selection and socialization of physically/verbally aggressive children and adolescents requires further longitudinal and intervention studies.

Beyond these important theoretical issues, a number of other facets of work on peer relations and aggression are worth consideration in future investigative efforts. First, it is important to note that the effects of peers on aggressive behaviors may differ depending on the level of analysis under consideration. Specifically, more proximal relationships may be especially influential, because children and adolescents spend more time with close friends, are more invested in these relationships (Brown, Dolcini, & Leventhal, 1997), and experience greater pressure to conform to their close friends than to their crowds (Urberg, 1992). In fact, although best friendships, clique involvement, and crowd membership are each uniquely associated with substance abuse, best friendships are an especially strong predictor (Hussong, 2002). Thus, although crowd membership may be related to aggressive conduct, it is likely that best friendships and clique involvement will be stronger predictors of such behavior. Research that systematically evaluates the relative strength and uniqueness of the influence of proximal and distal peer relationships on children's aggressive behavior seems warranted.

Second, some researchers have speculated that modest levels of aggression may not be harmful and may in some cases even be adaptive (Hawley, 1999; Little, Brauner, Jones, Nock, & Hawley, 2003), suggesting a potential curvilinear relation between aggression and adjustment. To date, little empirical work has examined whether the association between aggression and adjustment is curvilinear, and findings from the few studies that do exist are mixed. For example, in one study, moderately aggressive children exhibited increases in the number of friendships, whereas highly aggressive children lost friendships over time (Hektner et al., 2000). However, in another study, perceived popularity was more strongly related to high, rather than to moderate, levels of aggression (Prinstein & Cillessen, 2003). Despite the limited work available in this area, researchers appear to make different assumptions regarding this important question. For example, in some research studies (e.g., Bagwell et al., 2000), extreme groups of aggressive children are created, then aggressive children's adjustment is compared to that of their nonaggressive peers. This design is consistent with the assumption that only very high levels of aggression will be harmful. In contrast, other studies (e.g., Espelage et al., 2003) adopt dimensional models that assume a linear relationship between aggression and adjustment. Nevertheless, the question of whether aggression has a curvilinear association with adjustment outcomes is an important one, and research that empirically tests this possibility is warranted.

Clearly, we have made significant progress during the past couple of decades in our understanding of the peer relationships of aggressive, school-age children and adolescents. Future research may benefit from investigating a number of relatively understudied issues, including (1) the degree to which, and under what conditions, school-age, relationally aggressive children have friends; (2) the association between crowd membership and aggression; (3) the role of aggression in the maintenance and/or termination of friendships; and (4) the unique roles of specific forms of aggression within peer relationships. Of most benefit in future studies would be research with prospective and/

or experimental designs that can best uncover the processes by which peers influence engagement in aggressive behavior and vice versa.

Notes

1. A note on nomenclature: Traditionally, the term "overt aggression" has been used to describe measures of aggression that included both physical (e.g., hits, pushes) and verbal (e.g., teases, says mean things) components, or were less specific in terms of the avenue of harm (e.g., starts fights, disrupts). The term "overt aggression," however, is misleading, because some verbally aggressive behaviors can be indirect (e.g., sarcasm, backhanded complements), and some relationally aggressive behaviors can be overt (e.g., direct exclusion from the peer group). To allow for greater precision, we use the term "physical/verbal aggression" in this chapter when we refer to findings from studies that measured both physical and verbal aggression in their instruments. In a similar vein, studies of relational aggression described in this chapter have been limited to those in which the majority of the items used to measure relational aggression clearly described acts in which the vehicle of harm was damage to relationships. Given our use of this common definition across studies reviewed, we chose to use the term "relational aggression" consistently throughout, regardless of the term used by the authors (e.g., "social aggression") of each study.

2. In discussing relations between aggression and social status, a brief clarification of social status terminology is necessary. Whereas researchers have historically collected peer nomination-based measures of the affective variable "social preference" (as well as the constituent constructs of "acceptance" and "rejection"), research during the past decade has additionally looked at "perceived popularity," a reputational measure of an individual's place within the social status hierarchy (Parkhurst & Hopmeyer, 1998; Rose, Swenson, & Waller, 2004). Though a full discussion of the differences between these social status variables is beyond the scope of this chapter, Asher and McDonald (Chapter 13, this volume) provide a description of these constructs and their interrelations. Furthermore, it is worth noting that the majority of studies we cite did use standard social preference and perceived popularity nominations, and that results from the few studies that used peer "ratings" (e.g., Olweus, 1977) or variations in nomination wording (i.e., "Who do you like *to hang out with*"; Graham & Juvonen, 2002) did not vary appreciably from results of those using standard nominations. Except where otherwise noted, studies relating aggression to social preference or popularity used continuous measures of these variables.

3. Indeed, studies linking rejection, but not acceptance, to physical/verbal aggression have contributed to a call by researchers to differentiate between the constructs of acceptance and rejection (see Graham & Juvonen, 2002; Pakaslahti & Keltikangas-Järvinen, 2001; Parkhurst & Asher, 1992).

References

Adams, R. E., Bukowski, W. M., & Bagwell, C. (2005). Stability of aggression during early adolescence as moderated by reciprocated friendship status and friend's aggression. *International Journal of Behavioral Development, 29*, 139–145.

Adler, P. A., & Adler, P. (1995). Dynamics of inclusion and exclusion in preadolescent cliques. *Social Psychology Quarterly, 58*, 145–162.

Andreou, E. (2006). Social preference, perceived popularity, and social intelligence. *School Psychology International, 27*, 339–351.

August, G. J., Egan, E. A., Realmuto, G. M., & Hektner, J. M. (2003). Four years of the Early Risers Early-Age-Targeted Preventive Intervention: Effects on aggressive children's peer relations. *Behavior Therapy, 34*, 453–470.

Babad, E. (2001). On the conception and measurement of popularity: More facts and some straight conclusions. *Social Psychology of Education, 5*, 3–29.

Bagwell, C. L., & Coie, J. D. (2004). The best friendships of aggressive boys: Relationships quality, conflict management, and rule-breaking behavior. *Journal of Experimental Child Psychology, 88*, 5–24.

Bagwell, C. L., Coie, J. D., Terry, R. A., & Lochman, J. E. (2000). Peer clique participation and social status in preadolescence. *Merrill–Palmer Quarterly, 46*, 280–305.

Blanchard, D. C., & Blanchard, R. J. (2003). What can animal aggression research tell us about human aggression? *Hormones and Behavior, 44*, 171–177.

Brendgen, M., Vitaro, F., & Bukowski, W. M. (2000). Deviant friends and early adolescents' emotional and behavioral adjustment. *Journal of Research on Adolescence, 10*, 173–189.

Brendgen, M., Vitaro, F., Turgeon, L., & Poulin, F. (2002). Assessing aggressive and depressed children's social relations with classmates and friends: A matter of perspective. *Journal of Abnormal Child Psychology, 30*, 609–624.

Brown, B. B. (1990). Peer groups and peer culture. In S. S. Feldman & G. R. Elliott (Eds.), *At the threshold: The developing adolescent* (pp. 171–196). Cambridge, MA: Harvard University Press.

Brown, B. B., Dolcini, M. M., & Leventhal, A. (1997). Transformations in peer relationships at adolescence: Implications for health-related behavior. In J. Schulenberg, J. L. Maggs, & K. Hurrelmann (Eds.), *Health risks and developmental transitions during adolescence* (pp. 161–189). New York: Cambridge University Press.

Brown, B. B., & Klute, C. (2003). Friends, cliques, and crowds. In G. R. Adams & M. D. Berzonsky (Eds.), *Blackwell handbook of adolescence* (pp. 330–348). Malden, MA: Blackwell.

Brown, B. B., Lohr, M. J., & Trujillo, C. M. (1990). Multiple crowds and multiple lifestyles: Adolescents' perceptions of peer group stereotypes. In R. E. Muuss (Ed.), *Adolescent behavior and society* (4th ed., pp. 30–36). New York: McGraw-Hill.

Buss, D. M., & Shackelford, T. K. (1997). Human aggression in evolutionary psychological perspective. *Clinical Psychology Review, 17*, 605–619.

Cairns, R. B., Cairns, B. D., Neckerman, H. J., Gest, S. D., & Gariepy, J. L. (1988). Social networks and aggressive behavior: Peer support or peer rejection? *Developmental Psychology, 24*, 815–823.

Campbell, A. (1999). Staying alive: Evolution, culture, and women's intrasexual aggression. *Behavioral and Brain Sciences, 22*, 203–252.

Campbell, J. D., & Yarrow, M. R. (1961). Perceptual and behavioral correlates of social effectiveness. *Sociometry, 24*, 1–20.

Cillessen, A. H. N., Jiang, X. L., West, T. V., & Laszkowski, D. K. (2005). Predictors of dyadic friendship quality in adolescence. *International Journal of Behavioral Development, 29*, 165–172.

Cillessen, A. H. N., & Mayeux, L. (2004). From censure to reinforcement: Developmental changes in the association between aggression and social status. *Child Development, 75*, 147–163.

Coie, J. D., Cillessen, A. H., Dodge, K. A., Hubbard, J. A., Schwartz, D., Lemerise, E. A., et al. (1999). It takes two to fight: A test of relational factors and a method for assessing aggressive dyads. *Developmental Psychology, 35*, 1179–1188.

Coie, J. D., Dodge, K. A., & Coppotelli, H. (1982). Dimensions and types of status: A cross-age perspective. *Developmental Psychology, 18*, 557–570.

Crick, N. R. (1996). The role of overt aggression, relational aggression, and prosocial behavior in the prediction of children's future social adjustment. *Child Development, 67*, 2317–2327.

Crick, N. R. (1997). Engagement in gender normative versus nonnormative forms of aggression: Links to social-psychological adjustment. *Developmental Psychology, 33*, 610–617.

Crick, N. R., & Dodge, K. A. (1994). A review and reformulation of social information-processing mechanisms in children's social adjustment. *Psychological Bulletin, 115*, 74–101.

Crick, N. R., & Grotpeter, J. K. (1995). Relational aggression, gender, and social-psychological adjustment. *Child Development, 66*, 710–722.

Crick, N. R., & Nelson, D. A. (2002). Relational and physical victimization within friendships: Nobody told me there'd be friends like these. *Journal of Abnormal Child Psychology, 30*, 599–607.

Crick, N. R., & Rose, A. J. (2000). Toward a gender-balanced approach to the study of social–emotional development: A look at relational aggression. In P. H. Miller, E. Kofsky, & E. Scholnick (Eds.), *Toward a feminist developmental psychology* (pp. 153–168). New York: Routledge.

Crick, N. R., & Zahn-Waxler, C. (2003). The development of psychopathology in females and males: Current progress and future challenges. *Development and Psychopathology, 15*, 719–742.

Cross, S. E., & Madsen, L. (1997). Models of the self: Self-construals and gender. *Psychological Bulletin, 122*, 5–37.

Dishion, T. J., McCord, J., & Poulin, F. (1999). When interventions harm: Peer groups and problem behavior. *American Psychologist, 54*, 755–764.

Dishion, T. J., Patterson, G. R., & Griesler, P. C. (1994). Peer adaptations in the development of antisocial behavior: A confluence model. In L. R. Huesmann (Ed.), *Aggressive behavior: Current perspectives* (pp. 61–95). New York: Plenum Press.

Dodge, K. A. (1983). Behavioral antecedents of peer social status. *Child Development, 54*, 1386–1399.

Dodge, K. A., Price, J. M., Coie, J. D., & Christopoulos, C. (1990). On the development of aggressive dyadic relationships in boys' peer groups. *Human Development, 33*, 260–270.

Dolcini, M. M., & Adler, N. E. (1994). Perceived competencies, peer group affiliation, and risk behavior among early adolescents. *Health Psychology, 13*, 496–506.

Espelage, D. L., Holt, M. K., & Henkel, R. R. (2003). Examination of peer-group contextual effects on aggression during early adolescence. *Child Development, 74*, 205–220.

Estell, D. B., Cairns, R. B., Farmer, T. W., & Cairns, B. D. (2002). Aggression in inner-city early elementary classrooms: Individual and peer-group configurations. *Merrill–Palmer Quarterly, 48*, 52–76.

Farmer, T. W., & Rodkin, P. C. (1996). Antisocial and prosocial correlates of classroom social positions: The social network centrality perspective. *Social Development, 5*, 174–188.

Graham, S., & Juvonen, J. (2002). Ethnicity, peer harassment, and adjustment in middle school: An exploratory study. *Journal of Early Adolescence, 22*, 173–199.

Grotpeter, J. K., & Crick, N. R. (1996). Relational aggression, overt aggression, and friendship. *Child Development, 67*, 2328–2338.

Hartup, W. W., & Stevens, N. (1997). Friendships and adaptation in the life course. *Psychological Bulletin, 121*, 355–370.

Hawley, P. H. (1999). The ontogenesis of social dominance: A strategy-based evolutionary perspective. *Developmental Review, 19*, 97–132.

Hawley, P. H. (2003). Prosocial and coercive configurations of resource control in early adolescence: A case from the well-adapted Machivellian. *Merrill–Palmer Quarterly, 49*, 279–309.

Hektner, J. M., August, G. J., & Realmuto, G. M. (2000). Patterns and temporal changes in peer affiliation among aggressive and nonaggressive children participating in a summer school program. *Journal of Clinical Child Psychology, 29*, 603–614.

Henington, D., Hughes, J. N., Cavell, T. A., & Thompson, B. (1998). The role of relational aggression in identifying aggressive boys and girls. *Journal of School Psychology, 36*, 457–477.

Horn, S. S. (2003). Adolescents' reasoning about exclusion from social groups. *Developmental Psychology, 39*, 71–84.

Horn, S. S. (2006). Group status, group bias, and adolescents' reasoning about the treatment of others in school contexts. *International Journal of Behavioral Development, 30*, 208–218.

Hussong, A. M. (2002). Differentiating peer contexts and risk for adolescent substance use. *Journal of Youth and Adolescence, 31*, 207–220.

Kandel, D. B. (1978). Homophily, selection, and socialization in adolescent friendships. *American Journal of Sociology, 84*, 427–436.

Killen, M., & Stangor, C. (2001). Children's social reasoning about inclusion and exclusion in gender and race peer group contexts. *Child Development, 72*, 174–186.

LaFontana, K. M., & Cillessen, A. H. N. (2002). Children's perceptions of popular and unpopular peers: A multimethod assessment. *Developmental Psychology, 38*, 635–647.

LaGreca, A. M., Prinstein, M. J., & Fetter, M. D. (2001). Adolescent peer crowd affiliation: Linkages with health-risk behaviors and close friendships. *Journal of Pediatric Psychology, 26,* 131–143.

Lease, A. M., Kennedy, C. A., & Axelrod, J. L. (2002). Children's social constructions of popularity. *Social Development, 11,* 87–109.

Little, T. D., Brauner, J., Jones, S. M., Nock, M. K., & Hawley, P. H. (2003). Rethinking aggression: A typological examination of the functions of aggression. *Merrill–Palmer Quarterly, 49,* 343–369.

Murray-Close, D., Ostrov, J. M., & Crick, N. R. (2007). A short-term study of growth of relational aggression during middle childhood: Associations with gender, friendship intimacy, and internalizing problems. *Development and Psychopathology, 19,* 187–203.

Newcomb, A. F., Bukowski, W. M., & Pattee, L. (1993). Children's peer relations: A meta-analytic review of popular, rejected, neglected, controversial, and average sociometric status. *Psychological Bulletin, 113,* 99–128.

Olweus, D. (1977). Aggression and peer acceptance in adolescent boys: Two short-term longitudinal studies of ratings. *Child Development, 48,* 1301–1313.

Pakaslahti, L., & Keltikangas-Järvinen, L. (2001). Peer-attributed prosocial behavior among aggressive/preferred, aggressive/non-preferred, non-aggressive/preferred, and non-aggressive/non-preferred adolescents. *Personality and Individual Differences, 30,* 903–916.

Parkhurst, J. T., & Asher, S. R. (1992). Peer rejection in middle school: Subgroup differences in behavior, loneliness, and interpersonal concerns. *Developmental Psychology, 28,* 231–241.

Parkhurst, J., & Hopmeyer, A. (1998). Sociometric popularity and peer-perceived popularity: Two distinct dimensions of peer status. *Journal of Early Adolescence, 18*(2), 135–144.

Pellegrini, A. D. (2002). Affiliative and aggressive dimensions of dominance and possible functions during early adolescence. *Aggression and Violent Behavior, 7,* 21–31.

Poulin, F., & Boivin, M. (1999). Proactive and reactive aggression and boys' friendship quality in mainstream classrooms. *Journal of Emotional and Behavioral Disorders, 7,* 168–177.

Poulin, F., & Boivin, M. (2000). The role of proactive and reactive aggression in the formation and development of boys' friendships. *Developmental Psychology, 36*(2), 233–240.

Prinstein, M. J., & Cillessen, A. H. N. (2003). Forms and functions of adolescent peer aggression associated with high levels of peer status. *Merrill–Palmer Quarterly, 49*(3), 310–342.

Prinstein, M. J., & LaGreca, A. M. (2002). Peer crowd affiliation and internalizing distress in childhood and adolescence: A longitudinal follow-back study. *Journal of Research on Adolescence, 12,* 325–351.

Ray, G. E., Cohen, R., Secrist, M. E., & Duncan, M. K. (1997). Relating aggressive and victimization behaviors to children's sociometric status and friendships. *Journal of Social and Personal Relationships, 14*(1), 95–108.

Remillard, A. M., & Lamb, S. (2005). Adolescent girls' coping with relational aggression. *Sex Roles, 53,* 221–229.

Roach, C. N., & Gross, A. M. (2003). Assessing child aggression: A tale of two measures. *Child and Behavior Therapy, 25,* 19–38.

Rodkin, P. C., Farmer, T. W., Pearl, R., & Van Acker, R. (2000). Heterogeneity of popular boys: Antisocial and prosocial configurations. *Developmental Psychology, 36,* 14–24.

Rodkin, P. C., Farmer, T. W., Pearl, R., & Van Acker, R. (2006). They're cool: Social status and peer group supports for aggressive boys and girls. *Social Development, 15*(2), 175–204.

Rose, A. J., & Rudolph, K. D. (2006). A review of sex differences in peer relationship processes: Potential trade-offs for the emotional and behavioral development of girls and boys. *Psychological Bulletin, 132,* 98–131.

Rose, A. J., Swenson, L. P., & Waller, E. M. (2004). Overt and relational aggression and perceived popularity: Developmental differences in concurrent and prospective relations. *Developmental Psychology, 40*(3), 378–387.

Rubin, K. H., Chen, X., & Hymel, S. (1993). Socioemotional characteristics of withdrawn and aggressive children. *Merrill–Palmer Quarterly, 39*(4), 518–534.

Rys, G. S., & Bear, G. G. (1997). Relational aggression and peer relations: Gender and developmental issues. *Merrill–Palmer Quarterly, 43*, 87–106.

Sandstrom, M. J., & Cillessen, A. H. N. (2006). Likeable versus popular: Distinct implications for adolescent adjustment. *International Journal of Behavioral Development, 30*, 305–314.

Storch, E. A., Werner, N. E., & Storch, J. B. (2003). Relational aggression and psychosocial adjustment in intercollegiate athletics. *Journal of Sport Behavior, 26*, 155–168.

Tomada, G., & Schneider, B. H. (1997). Relational aggression, gender, and peer acceptance: Invariance across culture, stability over time, and concordance among informants. *Developmental Psychology, 33*, 601–609.

Urberg, K. A. (1992). Locus of peer influence: Social crowd and best friend. *Journal of Youth and Adolescence, 21*, 439–450.

Warman, D. M., & Cohen, R. (2000). Stability of aggressive behaviors and children's peer relationships. *Aggressive Behavior, 26*, 277–290.

Werner, N. E., & Crick, N. R. (1999). Relational aggression and social-psychological adjustment in a college sample. *Journal of Abnormal Psychology, 108*, 615–623.

Werner, N. E., & Crick, N. R. (2004). Maladaptive peer relationships and the development of relational and physical aggression during middle childhood. *Social Development, 13*, 495–514.

Xie, H., Cairns, R. B., & Cairns, B. D. (1999). Social networks and configurations in inner-city schools: Aggression, popularity, and implications for students with EBD. *Journal of Emotional and Behavioral Disorders, 7*, 147–156.

Xie, H., Cairns, R. B., & Cairns, B. D. (2002). The development of social aggression and physical aggression: A narrative analysis of interpersonal conflicts. *Aggressive Behavior, 28*, 341–355.

Xie, H., Farmer, T. W., & Cairns, B. D. (2003). Different forms of aggression among inner-city African-American children: Gender, configurations, and school social networks. *Journal of School Psychology, 41*, 355–375.

Xu, Y., Farver, J. M., Schwartz, D., & Chang, L. (2004). Social networks and aggressive behavior in Chinese children. *International Journal of Behavioral Development, 28*, 401–410.

Zalecki, C. A., & Hinshaw, S. P. (2004). Overt and relational aggression in girls with attention deficit hyperactivity disorder. *Journal of Clinical Child and Adolescent Psychology, 33*, 125–137.

Zimmer-Gembeck, M. J., Geiger, T. C., & Crick, N. (2005). Relational and physical aggression, prosocial behavior, and peer relations: Gender moderation and bidirectional associations. *Journal of Early Adolescence, 25*, 421–452.

CHAPTER 17

Avoiding and Withdrawing from the Peer Group

KENNETH H. RUBIN
JULIE C. BOWKER
AMY E. KENNEDY

In many ways this chapter concerns a topic unlike most that appear in this *Handbook*. Rather than focusing on the ways in which children and adolescents may interact with their peers, this chapter is centered on those children who, for whatever reason, engage rarely in peer interaction. As noted throughout this *Handbook*, children who are socially engaging and competent interact with peers in ways that allow the establishment and maintenance of positive relationships. Such children fare well in their social and academic lives. Alternatively, their socially unskilled counterparts often suffer from peer rejection, friendlessness, and loneliness; furthermore, they are thought to be at risk for a wide range of social–emotional and academic difficulties. In this chapter, we focus on children who avoid and rarely interact with their peers, and who suffer deeply for their withdrawal.

Historical Background

For at least two decades, researchers have argued that children who do not have adequate or "typical" peer interactions and peer relationship experiences may be at risk for later maladjustment. Such a conclusion has been reinforced by studies demonstrating that peer rejection in childhood predicts psychopathology and school dropout, among other negative consequences in adolescence and adulthood (for a relevant review, see Rubin, Bukowski, & Parker, 2006). From a purely clinical perspective, available evidence suggests that poor peer relationships are common reasons for children's referrals to child specialists. For example, Achenbach and Edelbrock (1981) reported that 30–75% of children (depending on age) referred to guidance clinics were reported by their mothers to experience peer difficulties (e.g., poor social skills, aggression). And peer difficulties are roughly twice as common among clinic children as among nonreferred children.

The group of children generally considered at highest risk for later psychiatric difficulty comprises mainly those whose interactions may best be described as hostile and aggressive. Aggressive children are often portrayed as emotionally dysregulated, atypical in the ways they think about social interactions and events, inaccurate in the ways they think about themselves and their social relationships, disruptive at home and school, and behaviorally agonistic in an often bullying manner (for a recent review, see Dodge, Coie, & Lynam, 2006). As it happens, one of the strongest correlates and predictors of peer rejection is aggressive behavior. Moreover, the emotional, cognitive, and self-system "baggage" that accompanies aggressive behaviors also predicts peer rejection. Thus, there appears to be a clear link between the frequency with which children display agonistic behavior and the establishment and maintenance of a negative peer reputation (Rubin, Bukowski, et al., 2006). Despite their agonistic inclinations, however, aggressive children have friends and are often members of cliques and peer networks. Their friends tend to resemble them behaviorally, and the networks they are involved in likewise comprise angry, aggressive peers (see Dishion & Piehler, Chapter 32, this volume). In these latter regards, aggressive behavior may be maintained and reinforced through the process of active deviancy training (Dishion, McCord, & Poulin, 1999).

For many years, it was posited that the straightest route to peer rejection and other, related peer difficulties began with aggressive behavior (e.g., refer to special issues/sections of *Child Development* and the *Merrill–Palmer Quarterly* in 1983!). More recently, however, a strong case has been made for the significance of social withdrawal in predicting negative peer concomitants and outcomes. This literature is reviewed herein.

Central Issues: Construct Definition

The construct of social withdrawal has many "faces" or forms and subtypes (Rubin & Mills, 1988) and, over the years, terms of reference such as "social withdrawal," "social isolation," "shyness" (fearful and self-conscious), and "behavioral inhibition" have been used interchangeably. Whereas these constructs may be related conceptually and statistically, they are not equivalent. As we have indicated elsewhere (e.g., Rubin & Asendorpf, 1993; Rubin & Coplan, 2007; Rubin, Burgess, & Coplan, 2002) "inhibition" may be defined as the disposition to display fearful, anxious behaviors in unfamiliar contexts. "Fearful shyness" represents inhibited behavior in the face of *social* novelty. "Self-conscious" shyness, which is thought to emerge between ages 4 and 5, refers to the display of socially wary behavior evoked by intrapersonal concerns of being negatively evaluated by others. Finally, "social withdrawal" refers to the consistent (across situations and over time) display of solitary behavior when encountering familiar and/or unfamiliar peers. The common thread binding each of these constructs is that the thought or presence of social company evokes reactions of fear or anxiety that result in attempts to cope or to self-regulate through socially restrained or avoidant behavior. Indeed, "anxious-solitude" is a recent term that denotes social withdrawal resulting from fear or anxiety (e.g., Gazelle & Ladd, 2003).

Importantly, not all forms of solitary behavior are elicited by fear or anxiety. For example, the experience of social rejection can result in being *isolated* by and removed from the group. In this regard, aggressive children may evidence solitude in groups that reject them (e.g., Hymel, Rubin, Rowden, & LeMare, 1990). Other children appear to prefer solitude and lack the desire to engage others in social interaction. These children have been described as "unsociable" (Asendorpf, 1993) or "socially disinterested" (Coplan, Prakash, O'Neil, & Armer, 2004). They appear to possess not only a low motivation to approach others, but also a low motivation to avoid social interaction (Asendorpf, 1993). In early childhood, these children tend to engage in solitary play marked by the quiescent, often sedentary exploration and construction of objects; at the same time, for many young children, this type of quiet, constructive solitude is not associated with either peer rejection or psychological maladaptation (Rubin, Coplan, Fox, & Calkins, 1995). Beyond the preschool years, however, unsociable children may experience increased peer and psychological difficulties when developmental norms move in the direction of increased socially interactive behavior, and their behavior comes to be viewed as socially inappropriate (Asendorpf, 1993; Rubin & Coplan, 2007).

Solitude that results from *social disinterest* has been contrasted with the display of anxious, *reticent* behavior, which appears to reflect an approach–avoidance conflict; reticent children watch others from afar and at the same time appear to desire the companionship of others (e.g., Asendorpf, 1993; Coplan et al., 2004). Unlike solitary exploration and construction (indicators of social disinterest), reticence both reflects and predicts peer rejection and psychosocial maladjustment (e.g., Rubin, Chen, McDougall, Bowker, & McKinnon, 1995). Significantly, little attention has been paid to different forms of social withdrawal *beyond the early childhood years*, an issue to which we return in the final section of this chapter.

In light of findings documenting significant, negative psychosocial correlates and consequences of social withdrawal (for a review, see Rubin, Burgess, Kennedy, & Stewart, 2003), it seems particularly important to understand not only its concomitants and consequences but also its origins. Thus, in this chapter, we begin with a brief review of relevant theory, followed by a description of factors that predict solitary behavior in the peer group. We follow with descriptions of the peer relationships and friendships of socially withdrawn children and young adolescents, and the social and emotional consequences of withdrawal. We conclude with a discussion of future research directions.

Relevant Theory

Theoretically derived statements about the etiology and psychological significance of social withdrawal were practically nonexistent until the 1980s (e.g., Rubin, 1982a). Those searching for relevant theory had to rely on classical writings pertaining to the significance of peer interaction for normal social, emotional, and cognitive growth. For example, in his early writings, Piaget (1932) posited that children's relationships with peers, unlike their relationships with adults, were relatively balanced, egalitarian, and fell along a more or less horizontal plane of power assertion and dominance. It was within this egalitarian context that Piaget believed peer interaction provided a unique cognitive and social-cognitive growth context for children. Piaget focused specifically on the relevance of disagreements with agemates and the opportunities for negotiation arising from disagreements. These naturally occurring differences of opinion were assumed to engender cognitive conflict that required both intra- and interpersonal resolution for positive peer exchanges and experiences to occur. The resolution of interpersonal disputes was thought to result in an enhanced understanding of others' thoughts and emotions, the broadening of one's social repertoire with which to solve interpersonal disputes and misunderstandings, and the comprehension of cause–effect relations in social interaction.

Empirical support for these notions derived from demonstrations that peer exchange, conversations, and interactions produced growth in social-cognitive development and social competence (e.g., Damon & Killen, 1982). Also in keeping with these theoretically driven findings, researchers found that perspective-taking skills could be improved through peer interactions, particularly those experiences that involved role play. In turn, such improvements predicted improvements in social competence (e.g., Selman & Schultz, 1990).

Peer interaction also allows children to understand the rules and norms of their peer subcultures (e.g., Fine, 1987). It is this understanding of norms and normative performance levels that engenders in the child an ability to evaluate his or her own competency levels against the perceived standards of the peer group. This latter view concerning self-definition and identity was addressed over 70 years ago in the writings of George Herbert Mead (1934). In his theory of symbolic interactionism, Mead suggested that exchanges among peers, whether experienced during cooperative or competitive activity, *or* during conflict or friendly discussion, enabled children to understand the self as both a subject and an object. Understanding that the self could be an object of others' perspectives gradually evolved into the conceptualization of a "generalized other" or an organized and coordinated perspective of the "social" group. In turn, recognition of the "generalized other" led to the emergence of an organized sense of self.

The classic *personality theory* of Sullivan (1953) has served as a guide for much research concerning children's peer relationships and social skills. Like Piaget, Sullivan believed that the concepts of mutual respect, equality, and reciprocity developed from peer relationships. Sullivan, however, emphasized the significance of "special" relationships—"chumships" or best-friendships—for the emergence of these concepts. Sullivan thought that in the early school years, whether friends or not, children were basically insensitive to their peers. During the juvenile years (late elementary school), however, children were thought to be able to recognize and value each other's personal qualities; as a consequence, peers gained power as personality-shaping agents. Sullivan's theory has proved influential in terms of the contemporary study of children's friendships (e.g., Furman, Simon, Shaffer, & Bouchey, 2002), as well as in the understanding of loneliness as a significant motivational force in development and adjustment (e.g., Asher & Paquette, 2003).

Learning and *social learning theory* have also stimulated current research on children's peer relationships and social skills. It was originally suggested, and it is now known, that children learn about their social worlds, and how to behave within them, through direct peer tutelage, as well as by observing each other. In this regard, children punish or ignore non-normative social behavior and reward or reinforce positively those behaviors viewed as culturally appropriate and competent (e.g., Dishion et al., 1999).

Taken together, these theories and data supportive of them have led psychologists to conclude that peer interactions and relationships are essential for normal social-cognitive and social–emotional development. But these theories are focused on the putative *benefits* of peer interactions and relationships. They "speak to" the development of competent behavioral styles and adaptive extrafamilial relationships. The theories offer little with regard to establishing how *insufficient* or *deficient* interactions and relationships can lead to maladaptive behavioral styles or to nonexistent or dysfunctional extrafamilial relationships. Yet if peer interaction does lead to the development of social competencies and the understanding of the self in relation to others, it seems reasonable to ponder the developmental consequences for those children who refrain from social interaction and avoid the company of their peers. It is this reasonable thought that drives much of the current research on social withdrawal.

Last and perhaps most important, current research on social withdrawal is also guided by *Hinde's model of relationships*, in which social withdrawal can be considered an *individual* characteristic that influences the presence or absence and quality of social exchanges ("interactions") and relationships (e.g., friendship). This characteristic is also likely to influence the individual's reputation and standing in the peer *group* (e.g., peer rejection). Thus, Hinde's (1987) conceptual model serves as a useful heuristic to present central lines of inquiry and major research findings regarding children who avoid and withdraw from the peer group. A more detailed description of the research on the developmental course of social withdrawal, as it is influenced by Hinde's model, is presented below.

Key Classical and Modern Research Studies

Biological and Parenting Factors

The Contribution of Biology to the Development of Social Withdrawal

To begin with a focus on the *individual* in Hinde's model, there is ample evidence to suggest that different forms of social withdrawal have varying biological and genetic roots. For example, to Kagan, Snidman, and Arcus (1993), some infants are genetically hardwired with a physiology that biases them to be cautious, timid, and wary in unfamiliar social and nonsocial situations. It is contended that "inhibited" children differ from their uninhibited counterparts in ways that imply variability in the threshold of excitability of the amygdala and its projections to the cortex, hypothalamus, sympathetic nervous system, corpus striatum, and central gray matter. In support of the argument that inhibition has a genetic basis, Hariri and colleagues (2002) reported that the presence of the short 5-hydroxytryptamine (5-HT) allele was associated with greater functioning of the amygdala in response to fearful stimuli in some individuals, but the same was not true for those individuals possessing the long 5-HT allele (Hariri et al., 2002). The functioning of the amygdala has long been associated with the display of inhibited behavior across species (e.g., Schwartz, Wright, Shin, Kagan, & Rauch, 2003).

Consistent with the argument that there is a *biological* basis to social wariness and inhibition is research that indicates a pattern of greater relative right frontal electroencephalographic (EEG) asymmetry associated with the display of behavioral inhibition in infancy (Calkins, Fox, & Marshall, 1996) and social reticence during the preschool years (Fox et al., 1995). Relatedly, Fox, Henderson, Rubin, Calkins, & Schmidt (2001) found that *continuously inhibited* children (high on behavioral inhibition at 14 or 24 months, and high on social reticence at 4 years) exhibited a pattern of greater relative right frontal EEG asymmetry at 9 months, 14 months, and 4 years compared to those children who did not remain continuously inhibited (high on behavioral inhibition at 14 or 24 months and low on social reticence at 4 years). These links between EEG asymmetry and shy/reticent behavior have been documented in middle childhood as well (e.g., Schmidt, Fox, Schulkin, & Gold, 1999).

Variations in the functioning of the autonomic nervous system have also been correlated with the display of shy/wary behavior in early childhood. For instance, *lower* cardiac vagal tone (an index of emotion dysregulation) is contemporaneously and predictively associated with the display of behavioral inhibition and socially reticent behavior in early childhood (Rubin, Hastings, Stewart, Henderson, & Chen, 1997). More recently, Henderson, Marshall, Fox, and Rubin (2004) found that two types of solitude (reticence and solitary–passive behavior) were associated with a pattern of greater relative right frontal EEG asymmetry. However, reticent children were rated by their mothers to be more socially fearful and displayed lower cardiac vagal tone than those children who were observed to spend time exploring and constructing on their own while in social company (solitary–passive behavior). In further support of an underlying biological constitution of socially inhibited and reticent behavior, Hastings, Rubin and DeRose (2005) found that observed inhibition, maternal reports of social fearfulness, and cardiac vagal tone loaded on a single factor (with cardiac vagal tone loading negatively) at 2 years of age. Finally, the hypothalamic–pituitary–adrenocortical (HPA) axis is thought be activated during stressful or novel situations. Researchers have demonstrated that elevated cortisol (a stress hormone) is associated with the demonstration of behavioral inhibition (Spangler & Schieche, 1998) and social reticence (Schmidt et al., 1997) in early childhood.

The Contributions of Parents to the Development of Social Withdrawal

Although there is evidence supporting a genetic or biological origin of shy–anxious social withdrawal, there also is evidence implicating distal factors such as parenting style and the quality of the parent–child relationship in the development and maintenance of withdrawn behavioral patterns. Briefly, several researchers have found a contemporaneous and predictive link between insecure attachment status and the display of behaviorally inhibited behavior (e.g., Calkins & Fox, 1992). It bears noting, however, that insecure attachment relationships are also predicted by *maternal* behavior. For example, mothers of insecurely attached "C" babies are overinvolved and overcontrolling compared to mothers of securely attached babies (Erickson, Sroufe, & Egeland, 1985). It is this overcontrolling, intrusive, and overly protective parenting style that is strongly associated, contemporaneously and predictively, with behavioral inhibition (e.g., Rubin et al., 1997; Rubin, Burgess, & Hastings, 2002), and with socially withdrawn and reticent behavior (Coplan et al., 2004; Mills & Rubin, 1998; Rubin, Cheah, & Fox, 2001; Rubin & Mills, 1990, 1991). It has been suggested that such parenting practices not only reinforce anxious–withdrawn behavior but also may negatively impact the child's sense of self-worth and autonomy.

Of course, children's social reticence and anxious–withdrawn behavior may also *cause* parental overprotection and overcontrol (Hastings & Rubin, 1999; Rubin, Nelson, Hastings, & Asendorpf, 1999). Sensing their young child's difficulties in social situations, some parents may try to provide support by manipulating their child's social behaviors in a power assertive, highly directive fashion (telling the child how to act or what to do). Conversely, any expression of social fearfulness in the peer group may evoke parental feelings of concern, sympathy, and perhaps a growing sense of frustration. The parent may begin to believe that their child is vulnerable and must be helped in some way (Rubin & Burgess, 2002). Such a "read" of the child may be guided by a developing belief system that social withdrawal is dispositionally based, that it is accompanied by debilitating child feelings of fear and social anxiety, and that it is accompanied by behaviors that evoke in peers attempts to be socially dominant. The resultant parental behavior, guided by the processing of affect and historically and situationally based information, may be of a "quick fix" variety. To release the child from social discomfort, the parent may simply "take over" by telling the child what to do and how to do it (Rubin et al., 1999). Alternatively, the parent may simply solve the child's social dilemmas by asking other children for information desired by the child, obtaining objects desired by the child, or requesting that peers allow the child to join them in play. These parenting behaviors are likely to reinforce the child's feelings of insecurity, resulting in the maintenance of a cycle of child hopelessness/helplessness and parent overcontrol/overprotection (Mills & Rubin, 1993). Moreover, allowing the child to avoid feared social behaviors may, over time, prevent the child from attaining developmentally appropriate social competencies.

In summary, we have painted a portrait of mothers (and fathers; Rubin et al., 1999) of socially reticent and anxiously withdrawn children as endorsing and practicing intrusive, controlling, and overprotective parenting strategies that are likely detrimental to the child's developing senses of autonomy and social efficacy. Such parenting beliefs and behaviors are not conducive to the development of social competence or positive self-regard. Indeed, research has shown that an overprotective, overly concerned parenting style is associated with submissiveness, dependency, and timidity in early childhood— characteristics that are typical of socially reticent children and that may increase the likelihood of problematic peer relations (Olweus, 1993). We expand on this point in the sections below, wherein we focus on the peer relationships of socially withdrawn children.

Peer Interactions and Relationships

Peer Interactions

Drawing from Hinde's model, the term "interaction" is reserved for dyadic behavior in which participants' actions are interdependent, such that each actor's behavior is both a response to, and stimulus for, the other participant's behavior (Rubin, Bukowski, et al., 2006). At its core, an interaction comprises "such incidents as Individual A shows behavior X to Individual B, or A shows X to B and B responds with Y" (Hinde, 1979, p. 15). Researchers have typically focused on three general forms of interactions: (1) movement toward others, (2) movement against others, and (3) movement away from others (Rubin, Bukowski, et al., 2006). Whereas important individual differences in the extent and nature of social interactions exist at all ages, children who move toward others are considered sociable or outgoing, children who move against others are typically characterized as aggressive (due to the confrontational nature of their behavior), and children who move away from others are considered socially withdrawn (e.g., Caspi, Elder, & Bem, 1988).

By moving away from others, withdrawn children and young adolescents interact less with their peers and spend more time on the periphery of the social scene than do their non-socially-withdrawn counterparts. For example, socially reticent behavior is defined by the frequent display of watching others from afar and aimless wandering when among peers (Coplan, Rubin, Fox, Calkins, & Stewart, 1994). Given that social reticence and withdrawal are often accompanied by felt anxiety in both familiar and unfamiliar social situations (Asendorpf, 1990; Coplan & Rubin, 1998), it should not be surprising that reticent preschoolers and socially withdrawn elementary schoolers direct fewer social overtures to peers than their more sociable counterparts (Chen, DeSouza, Chen, & Wang, 2006; Coplan et al., 1994; Rubin, 1985; Stewart & Rubin, 1995). Also the forms that their overtures take differ from those of nonwithdrawn peers. For instance, it has been shown that withdrawn children are less likely than nonwithdrawn children to make requests of their peers that require them to carry out action requiring both effort and mobility

(Rubin & Borwick, 1984; Rubin & Krasnor, 1986; Stewart & Rubin, 1995). Moreover, withdrawn children are less inclined than children of average sociability to produce socially assertive strategies (e.g., commands) and are more likely to employ subtle, indirect means to attain their social goals (e.g., indirect requests). This pattern of social initiation suggests that children identified as withdrawn are less assertive with, and also less demanding of, their peers than their more sociable counterparts (Rubin, 1985; Rubin & Borwick, 1984; Stewart & Rubin, 1995).

When socially withdrawn children do make requests of their peers, they are more likely than their more sociable agemates to be met by peer refusal and rejection (e.g., Chen et al., 2006; Nelson, Rubin, & Fox, 2005; Rubin & Krasnor, 1986; Stewart & Rubin, 1995). And importantly, as they move from early to middle childhood, withdrawn children become increasingly less assertive, as well as less successful in their attempts to meet their social goals (Stewart & Rubin, 1995). This increasing lack of social assertiveness may be due to repeated peer rejection and/or to a "feedback loop," wherein the initially fearful and withdrawn youngster comes to believe that his or her social failures are internally based, which is strengthened by the increasing failure of his or her social initiatives.

The failure to obtain compliance and collegiality with peers predicts the development of negative *self-perceptions* of social skills and peer relationships (Boivin & Hymel, 1997; Boivin, Hymel, & Bukowski, 1995; Nelson et al., 2005); that is, "real-life" peer rejection (e.g., noncompliance) predicts negative thoughts and feelings about the self. Importantly, socially withdrawn children's self-perceptions are quite accurate; that is, they are well aware of their social difficulties. This is especially true of withdrawn children who are also unpopular (Hymel, Bowker, & Woody, 1993).

The interactional style of anxious–withdrawn children suggests a negative, if not miserable, cycle of anxious attempts to join others, followed by the actual and felt experience of rejection or neglect, followed by reasonable surmising that the self is less than worthy in the company of peers. This cycle suggests also that anxious social withdrawal should be stable over time. It is. Social withdrawal and avoidance has been shown to be reasonably consistent across contexts. Thus, extremely withdrawn children move away from and avoid *both* familiar and unfamiliar peers in settings such as school, home, or community at large (Schneider, Richard, Younger, & Freeman, 2000; Schneider, Younger, Smith, & Freeman, 1998). Furthermore, social withdrawal is stable over time from early to middle childhood and thereafter, into adolescence (e.g., Hymel et al., 1990; Rubin, Chen, et al., 1995; Rubin, Hymel, & Mills, 1989).

Peer Relationships

"Relationships" refer to the meanings, expectations, and emotions that derive from a succession of interactions between two individuals known to each other (Rubin, Bukowski, et al., 2006). Three questions dominate the literature on children's relationships with *friends* (e.g., Hartup, 1996):

1. Does the child have a best friend?
2. Who are the child's friends?
3. What is the quality of the child's friendships?

The extant literature on friendship is reviewed by several authors in this volume. Thus, we focus herein only on the friendships of socially withdrawn children.

Because they remove themselves from the company of peers, socially withdrawn children might be expected to have difficulty making and keeping friends. Indeed, anxious withdrawal has been found to predict negatively the *number* of mutual friendships during middle childhood (Pedersen, Vitaro, Barker, & Borge, 2007). Nevertheless, during middle childhood and early adolescence, socially withdrawn children are as likely as nonwithdrawn children to form and maintain at least *one* close friendship. Rubin, Wojslawowicz, Rose-Krasnor, Booth-LaForce, and Burgess (2006), for instance, reported that approximately 65% of socially withdrawn children age 10–11 years had a mutual best friendship in the fifth grade, a percentage nearly identical to that of their nonwithdrawn counterparts (70%). Furthermore, the majority of these friendships (69%) were stable across the fifth-grade academic year, a finding almost identical to that for nonwithdrawn children (70%). Similar findings have been reported in studies of young withdrawn children (e.g., Ladd & Burgess, 1999).

The friends of socially withdrawn children have been characterized as being similarly withdrawn (e.g., Haselager, Hartup, van Lieshout, & Riksen-Walraven, 1998; Rubin, Wojslawowicz, et al., 2006). Moreover, Rubin and colleagues demonstrated that not only the friends of withdrawn children are similarly withdrawn, but they are also similarly victimized by peers. It also appears to be the case that the quality of withdrawn children's friendships is less than optimal. For example, withdrawn children rate their best friendships as significantly less helpful and intimate, and, in the event of conflict, less likely to result in resolution, than do nonwithdrawn children (Rubin, Wojslawowicz, et al., 2006). Furthermore, the *best friends* of withdrawn children also report their friendships as less fun and helpful than do the friends of nonwithdrawn children. Schneider (1999) found that the friendships of socially withdrawn children were lower in communicative quantity and quality, findings that may begin to explain why the friendships of socially withdrawn children are marked by less intimate disclosure. Given that socially withdrawn children often experience *in vivo* peer rejection, they may engage in self-silencing when in the company of friends. "Self-silencing," a communication style that involves intentional verbal inhibition, is thought to reflect a defensive strategy to protect the self from criticism within the context of close relationships. Importantly, self-silencing has been positively associated with internalizing problems such as depression in samples of adults (e.g., Grant, Beck, Farrow, & Davila, 2007). Although self-silencing has received little attention in studies of children and adolescents (e.g., Harper & Welsh, 2007), a consideration of self-silencing among socially withdrawn children could well enhance our understanding of the ways their inhibitory tendencies and fears of negative evaluation impact qualities and features of their close dyadic relationships.

It is well-known that children's friendships provide important sources of social and emotional support, especially in times of stress or transition (e.g., Berndt, Hawkins, & Jiao, 1999). This protective "power" of friendship has been shown to be particularly helpful for children who have difficulties within the larger peer group (Rubin, Bukowski, et al., 2006). Hodges, Boivin, Vitaro, and Bukowski (1999), for example, demonstrated that simply having a mutual best friendship protected victimized children from increased internalizing and externalizing problems during late childhood. Thus far, there has been limited research on the protective power of friendship for socially anxious and withdrawn children. Oh, Rubin, Burgess, Booth-LaForce, and Rose-Krasnor (2004) employed latent growth curve modeling to investigate the extent to which the perceived supportiveness of friendship served as a protective factor in the maintenance, decrease, or increase of anxious withdrawal over five assessments taken between the fifth and eighth grades (10–13 years of age). The perceived supportiveness of the child's best friendship was a significant predictor for both the initial level of anxious withdrawal and the rate of change in withdrawal over time. Young adolescents who viewed their friendships as highly supportive were less likely to be socially withdrawn in the fifth grade and showed a greater rate of decline in social withdrawal over time.

In a more recent analysis of data from the same sample, Oh and colleagues (2008) used general growth mixture modeling (GGMM) to identify distinct pathways of anxious withdrawal, to differentiate valid subgroup trajectories, and to examine factors that predicted change in trajectories within subgroups. When data were examined across five time points over a period of 4 years, three distinct social withdrawal trajectory classes were discovered: (1) a *low stable* class, in which children were consistently low in social withdrawal; (2) an *increasing* class, comprising children who became increasingly withdrawn over time; and (3) a *decreasing* class, comprising children who initially were highly withdrawn but became less so over time. With regard to friendship factors, children who had a socially withdrawn friend were *more* likely to show an initially high level of social withdrawal at the outset of the study (Fall, fifth grade). In addition, having a socially withdrawn friend after the transition to middle school (Fall, sixth grade) exacerbated children's anxious withdrawal over time, supporting the contention that withdrawn children and their best friends may mutually influence each other's maladaptive behavior, just as is the case for aggressive children and their best friends (e.g., Dishion et al., 1999). Last, for those children who became increasingly more anxiously–withdrawn from fifth to eighth grade, friendlessness and friendship instability, along with peer exclusion and victimization, were significant predictors of *increased* social withdrawal. Taken together, results from these two studies suggest that the benefits of friendship involvement for socially withdrawn children are positive when friendship quality is strong, but are limited or negative when the best friend is likewise withdrawn.

Rejection and Victimization

At the group level of Hinde's social complexity, numerous studies have shown that anxious-solitude and withdrawal are contemporaneously and predictively associated with peer rejection throughout the childhood and early adolescent periods (e.g., Boivin et al., 1995; Hart et al., 2000; Ollendick, Greene, Weist, & Oswald, 1990; Rubin, Chen, & Hymel, 1993). It is argued that the relations between social withdrawal and peer rejection become increasingly strong across the elementary school years, because social solitude becomes increasingly viewed by the peer group as deviant from the norm (e.g., Gavinski-Molina, Coplan, & Younger, 2003; Younger, Gentile, & Burgess, 1993).

Being perceived as anxious and withdrawn while being rejected by the peer group at large may also serve to invite victimization by bullies. At the same time, regular exposure to bullying may lead to increased fear of classmates and further withdrawal from peer interaction and school-related activities. These notions of reciprocal relations between withdrawal and victimization mesh well with suggestions that children characterized by a socially withdrawn demeanor can best be described as "whipping boys" (Olweus, 1993), "easy marks" (Rubin, Wojslawowicz, et al., 2006), physically weak (Hodges et al., 1999; Hodges, Malone, & Perry, 1997), and anxiously vulnerable (Perry, Kusel, & Perry, 1988). Empirical connections between anxious withdrawal and being victimized have been reported by several researchers (e.g., Boivin et al., 1995; Hanish & Guerra, 2004;

Kochenderfer-Ladd, 2003). Importantly, the Oh et al. (2008) study described earlier indicated the significance of peer exclusion and victimization for maintaining, indeed increasing, anxious–withdrawn behavior from childhood through early adolescence.

Social Withdrawal and Intrapersonal Processes

There is considerable evidence that internalizing problems such as loneliness, depression, and social anxiety are both correlates and consequences of social withdrawal throughout childhood and adolescence (e.g., Boivin & Hymel, 1997; Gazelle & Ladd, 2003; Rubin, Chen, et al., 1995). Furthermore, Rubin and colleagues (2003) have argued that as a result of experiences with rejection and victimization, withdrawn children may attribute their social failures to internal causes; that is, over time, they may come to believe that there is something wrong with themselves rather than to attribute their social failures to other people or to situational factors. Supporting these conjectures, Rubin and Krasnor (1986) found that extremely withdrawn children tended to blame social failure on personal, dispositional characteristics rather than on external events or circumstances. These results are in keeping with findings by Wichmann, Coplan, and Daniels (2004), who reported that when 9- to 13-year-old withdrawn children were presented with hypothetical social situations in which ambiguously caused negative events happened to them, they attributed the events to internal and stable "self-defeating" causes. Moreover, withdrawn children suggested that, when faced with such negative situations, they were more familiar with failure experiences and that a preferred strategy was to withdraw and escape. This latter finding with regard to socially withdrawn children's use of avoidant coping in response to negative events was replicated by Burgess, Wojslawowicz, Rubin, Rose-Krasnor, and Booth-LaForce (2006). Given the conceptual associations among social withdrawal, victimization, and peer rejection, these findings by Wichmann et al. (2004) are reminiscent of work by Graham and Juvonen (2001). These latter researchers reported that youngsters who identified themselves as victimized by peers blamed themselves for their peer relationship problems. And Nolen-Hoeksema, Girgus, and Seligman (1992) have argued that self-blame can lead to a variety of negative outcomes of an internalizing nature, such as depression, low self-esteem, and withdrawal, thereby suggesting a self-reinforcing cycle of negative social–emotional functioning.

In recent years, significant *within-group* variation in psychological adjustment has been observed for socially withdrawn children and adolescents; that is, not all withdrawn children report high levels of loneliness, depression, and anxiety (Rubin, Wojslawowicz Bowker, & Oh, 2007). Significantly, heterogeneity in adjustment has been associated with variability in peer exclusion (Boivin et al., 1995; Boivin & Hymel, 1997; Gazelle & Ladd, 2003; Gazelle & Rudolph, 2004). For example, in a longitudinal study, Gazelle and Ladd (2003) reported that shy–anxious kindergartners excluded by peers displayed greater stability in anxious-solitude through the fourth grade and had higher levels of depressive symptoms than shy–anxious peers who did not experience peer exclusion. A diathesis–stress model was suggested, whereby the experience of peer exclusion exacerbates the outcomes associated with anxious-solitude. In a longitudinal study of fifth and sixth graders (10–11 years of age), Gazelle and Rudolph (2004) demonstrated that anxious–withdrawn children who were excluded by their peers maintained or increased the extent of their social avoidance and depression over time. In contrast, increased social approach and decreases in depression among anxious-solitary children resulted from the experience of low exclusion. Taken together, these data strongly suggest that socially withdrawn children's adjustment may be determined in part by the extent to which they experience peer rejection and exclusion.

Other than Gazelle's research noted earlier, there have been few longitudinal investigations of the consequences of social withdrawal vis-à-vis intrapersonal processes. The majority of studies examining the relations between social withdrawal and internalizing problems have been contemporaneous in nature (e.g., Boivin & Hymel, 1997; Rubin et al., 1993). However, in the Waterloo Longitudinal Project, observed and peer-assessed social reticence and passive withdrawal at 7 years of age predicted negative self-regard and loneliness at 9 and 10 years of age (Hymel et al., 1990; Rubin et al., 1989). Moreover, 7-year-olds' social withdrawal predicted self-reported loneliness, depression, and negative self-regard at age 14 years (Rubin, 1993; Rubin, Chen, et al., 1995).

Future Directions of Theory and Research

In the early 1990s, Rubin and colleagues proposed a theoretical model outlining developmental pathways in the etiology of social withdrawal and internalizing problems. This theoretical framework considered the joint influences of child characteristics, parental socialization practices, the quality of relationships outside the family, and macrosystemic forces. Transactional processes were postulated, describing the reciprocal and evolving relations over time between child temperamental predispositions and environmental contexts (see also Rubin et al., 2003; Rubin, Hymel, Mills, & Rose-Krasnor, 1991; Rubin, LeMare, & Lollis, 1990; Rubin & Mills, 1991).

In the past 20 years, researchers have examined the roles of biology and parenting in the etiology of social withdrawal in childhood. We urge researchers not only to continue to explore these areas but also to consider these factors during the middle childhood and adolescent years; there are virtually no such studies of the biological and parent–child concomitants and predictors of social withdrawal during this developmental time frame. Moreover, there is a clear need to consider additional factors that may moderate the relations among biological bases of social withdrawal, the parenting contributions to social withdrawal, and adjustment outcomes over time. Borrowing from Hinde (1987), such additional factors might include social information processing (*individual* factors), social skills (*interactions*), friendships (*relationships*), and peer *group* status (acceptance–rejection; peer perceptions of status—such as an easy mark, a "nerd," an outlier).

As an example of the significance of relationships, during the early adolescent period, children are motivated to become increasingly autonomous, while maintaining suitable and appropriate connections to parents (Collins & Steinberg, 2006). The motivation for increased autonomy, and the demonstration of independent, non-adult-conforming (yet peer-conforming) behavior that reflects such efforts, may play a role in gaining peer acceptance during the early adolescent period. For example, whereas social-conventional reasoning might suggest to adults that bossiness, relational aggression, and risk-taking behavior are less than admirable or acceptable, young adolescents might view such behaviors as within the realm of personal decision-making choices (see Killen, Rutland, & Jampol, Chapter 14, this volume). In turn, such seemingly oppositional behaviors predict perceived popularity in early adolescence (e.g., Rose, Swenson, & Waller, 2004). Put another way, the display of behaviors that suggest a turn toward independence and autonomy are associated with perceived popularity and dominance in the peer group.

But what about socially withdrawn young adolescents? Given the extant literature that such children are overprotected and overdirected, and given that they appear to be adult-dependent during the early years (e.g., Rubin et al., 1997), might it be the case that socially anxious and withdrawn young adolescents do not strive for autonomy to the same extent as their more sociable peers? Relatedly, if overly connected to and reliant on parents, might these relationships provide withdrawn young adolescents with a dysfunctional model for nonfamilial relationships? Might their friendships and romantic relationships be marked by insecurity and overdependence? These are questions that researchers would do well to consider as the literature on social withdrawal moves beyond the years of early and middle childhood.

Recent research has indicated that friendship may serve as protective factors for those young adolescents who have poor parent–child relationships (e.g., Rubin et al., 2004). This being the case, and given what is known about the friendships of socially withdrawn adolescents, might friendship serve as a protective buffer for those whose relationships with parents are less than adequate? Again, this question deserves of some empirical attention.

Another direction to be taken in the future concerns the subtypes of social withdrawal. Since the original contention that not all forms of solitude are "necessarily evil" (Rubin, 1982b), the vast majority of research on the many "faces" or subtypes of social withdrawal has focused on different solitary play behaviors observed in groups of *young* children (for a recent exception, see Coplan, Wilson, Frohlick, & Zelenski, 2006). Although these studies have illustrated the developmental risks associated with certain subtypes of social withdrawal, such as reticence during early childhood, it appears timely to conduct similar studies with older children and young adolescents. To begin with, researchers would do well to inquire about children's motivations for spending time alone rather than in the company of others, or when provided with opportunities to interact with others (e.g., Coplan, Girard, Findlay, & Frohlick, 2007). What are the cognitive or affective underpinnings of various forms of solitary behavior among older children and adolescents (e.g., Bowker, Rubin, Rose-Krasnor, & Booth-LaForce, 2007)?

It is also important that we better understand the ways the concomitants and consequences of social withdrawal in its many forms differ for boys and girls. Although there is some evidence that the negative prognosis for withdrawn boys is greater than that for withdrawn girls, (e.g., Caspi et al., 1988; Coplan, Gavinski-Molina, Lagacé-Séguin, & Wichmann, 2001), additional research is needed that includes a wider range of psychosocial outcomes. For example, withdrawn boys may be at greater risk for *physical* victimization than withdrawn girls; might it be the case that withdrawn girls are at greater risk for *relational* victimization (e.g., Crick & Grotpeter, 1996)? Furthermore, given girls' tendency to co-ruminate in the company of friends (Rose, 2002), perhaps withdrawn girls' friendships represent *risk* contexts as they move into adolescence, at least relative to the friendships of withdrawn boys.

As a final note, it is clear that the etiology of social withdrawal must be considered within cultural contexts. For example, in an extensive series of studies, Chen and colleagues have demonstrated that shy, reticent, reserved behavior in the People's Republic of China is encouraged and accepted by mothers, teachers, and peers, and is positively associated with social competence, peer acceptance, and academic success (e.g., Chen, Hastings, Rubin, Chen, Cen, & Stewart, 1998; Chen, Rubin, & Li, 1995). Chen, Chung, and Hsiao (Chapter 24, this volume) have argued that the collectivistic values found in Chinese culture place a strong emphasis on group cohesion; consequently, shyness and

reservedness are more greatly appreciated than in Western cultures that espouse individualistic beliefs and norms. Although this line of work has consistently found cross-cultural
differences in the prevalence and correlates of socially withdrawn behavior, there is nary
a study of the biological underpinnings of the phenomenon (e.g., EEG, electrocardio-
gram). Importantly for this *Handbook*, there are few, if any, cross-cultural studies of the
prevalence, stability, and quality of socially withdrawn children's *friendships* or *romantic
relationships* during the middle childhood and adolescent years.

Some Final Thoughts

The study of social withdrawal in childhood has garnered an enormous amount of attention in the past two decades. Researchers have examined the developmental origins of
social withdrawal, its contemporaneous and predictive correlates, and its consequences.
It is now known that the social lives of many socially withdrawn children are less than
optimal. Withdrawn children are socially deferential, anxious, lonely, and insecure in the
company of peers, as well as rejected by peers. They recognize their social incapacities,
believing themselves to be deficient in social skills and social relationships. Whether these
factors lead inexorably to the development of psychopathology or clinical disorders is
not yet known. Relatively few longitudinal studies exist; therefore, researchers would do
well to examine the premise that social withdrawal represents a risk factor in childhood
and adolescence. And, certainly, it would behoove researchers to investigate whether the
friendships and group status of socially withdrawn children represent possible protective
and exacerbating factors within and across cultures.

References

Achenbach, T. M., & Edelbrock, C. (1981). Behavioral problems and competencies reported by
     parents of normal and disturbed children aged 4–16. *Monographs of the Society for Research in
     Child Development, 46.*
Asendorpf, J. B. (1990). Development of inhibition during childhood: Evidence for situational
     specificity and two-factor model. *Developmental Psychology, 26,* 721–730.
Asendorpf, J. B. (1993). Beyond temperament: A two-factorial coping model of the development of
     inhibition during childhood. In K. H. Rubin & J. Asendorpf (Eds.), *Social withdrawal, inhibi-
     tion, and shyness in childhood* (pp. 265–289). Hillsdale, NJ: Erlbaum.
Asher, S. R., & Paquette, J. A. (2003). Loneliness and peer relations in childhood. *Current Directions
     in Psychological Science, 12*(3), 75–78.
Berndt, T. J., Hawkins, J. A., & Jiao, Z. (1999). Influences of friends and friendships on adjustment
     to junior high school. *Merrill–Palmer Quarterly, 45,* 13–41.
Boivin, M., & Hymel, S. (1997). Peer experiences and social self-perceptions: A sequential model.
     Developmental Psychology, 33, 135–145.
Boivin, M., Hymel, S., & Bukowski, W. (1995). The roles of social withdrawal, peer rejection, and
     victimization by peers in predicting loneliness and depressed mood in childhood. *Development
     and Psychopathology, 7,* 765–785.
Bowker, J. C., Rubin, K. H., Rose-Krasnor, L., & Booth-LaForce, C. (2007). *Social withdrawal, negative
     emotion, and peer difficulties during late childhood.* Manuscript submitted for publication.
Burgess, K. B., Wojslawowicz, J. C., Rubin, K. H., Rose-Krasnor, L., & Booth-LaForce, C. (2006).
     Social information processing and coping styles of shy/withdrawn and aggressive children:
     Does friendship matter? *Child Development, 77,* 371–383.

Calkins, S. D., & Fox, N. A. (1992). The relations among infant temperament, security of attachment, and behavioral inhibition at twenty-four months. *Child Development, 63,* 1456–1472.

Calkins, S. D., Fox, N. A., & Marshall, T. R. (1996). Behavioral and physiological antecedents of inhibition in infancy. *Child Development, 67,* 523–540.

Caspi, A., Elder, G. H., & Bem, D. J. (1988). Moving away from the world: Life-course patterns of shy children. *Developmental Psychology, 24,* 824–831.

Chen, X., DeSouza, A., Chen, H., & Wang, L. (2006). Reticent behavior and experiences in peer interactions in Canadian and Chinese children. *Developmental Psychology, 42,* 656–665.

Chen, X., Hastings, P. D., Rubin, K. H., Chen, H., Cen, G., & Stewart, S. L. (1998). Child-rearing attitudes and behavioral inhibition in Chinese and Canadian toddlers: A cross-cultural study. *Developmental Psychology, 34,* 677–686.

Chen, X., Rubin, K. H., & Li, Z. (1995). Social functioning and adjustment in Chinese children: A longitudinal study. *Developmental Psychology, 31,* 531–539.

Collins, W. A., & Steinberg, L. (2006). Adolescent development in interpersonal context. In W. Damon, R. M. Lerner, & N. Eisenberg (Eds.), *Handbook of child psychology: Vol. 3. Social, emotional, and personality development* (6th ed., pp. 1003–1067). New York: Wiley.

Coplan, R. J., Gavinski-Molina, M. H., Lagacé-Séguin, D., & Wichmann, C. (2001). When girls versus boys play alone: Gender differences in the associates of nonsocial play in kindergarten. *Developmental Psychology, 37,* 464–474.

Coplan, R. J., Girard, A., Findlay, L. C., & Frohlick, S. L. (2007). Understanding solitude: Young children's attitudes and responses towards hypothetical socially withdrawn peers. *Social Development, 16,* 390–409.

Coplan, R. J., Prakash, K., O'Neil, K., & Armer, M. (2004). Do you "want" to play?: Distinguishing between conflicted shyness and social disinterest in early childhood. *Developmental Psychology, 40*(2), 244–258.

Coplan, R. J., & Rubin, K. H. (1998). Exploring and assessing nonsocial play in the preschool: The development and validation of the preschool play behavior scale. *Social Development, 7*(1), 71–91.

Coplan, R. J., Rubin, K. H., Fox, N. A., Calkins, S. D., & Stewart, S. L. (1994). Being alone, playing alone, and acting alone: Distinguishing among reticence, and passive and active solitude in young children. *Child Development, 65,* 129–138.

Coplan, R. J., Wilson, J., Frohlick, S. L., & Zelenski, J. (2006). A person-oriented analysis of behavioral inhibition and behavioral activation in childhood. *Personality and Individual Differences, 41,* 917–927.

Crick, N. R., & Grotpeter, J. K. (1996). Children's maltreatment by peers: Victims of relational aggression. *Development and Psychopathology, 8,* 367–380.

Damon, W., & Killen, M. (1982). Peer interaction and the process of change in children's moral reasoning. *Merrill–Palmer Quarterly, 28*(3), 347–367.

Dishion, T. J., McCord, J., & Poulin, F. (1999). When interventions harm: Peer groups and problem behavior. *American Psychologist, 54*(9), 755–764.

Dodge, K. A., Coie, J. D., & Lynam, D. (2006). Aggression and antisocial behavior. In N. Eisenberg (Ed.), *Handbook of child psychology: Vol. 3. Social, emotional, and personality development* (pp. 719–788). New York: Wiley.

Erickson, M. F., Sroufe, L. A., & Egeland, B. (1985). The relationship between quality of attachment and behavior problems in preschool in a high-risk sample. *Monographs of the Society for Research in Child Development, 50*(1–2), 147–166.

Fine, G. A. (1987). *With the boys.* Chicago: University of Chicago Press.

Fox, N. A., Henderson, H. A., Rubin, K. H., Calkins, S. D., & Schmidt, L. A. (2001). Continuity and discontinuity of behavioral inhibition and exuberance: Psychophysiological and behavioral influences across the first four years of life. *Child Development, 72,* 1–21.

Fox, N. A., Rubin, K. H., Calkins, S. D., Marshall, T. R., Coplan, R. J., Porges, S. W., et al. (1995). Frontal activation asymmetry and social competence at four years of age. *Child Development, 66,* 1770–1784.

Furman, W., Simon, V. A., Shaffer, L., & Bouchey, H. A. (2002). Adolescents' working models and styles for relationships with parents, friends, and romantic partners. *Child Development, 73*(1), 241–255.

Gavinski-Molina, M. H., Coplan, R. J., & Younger, A. (2003). A closer look at children's knowledge about social isolation. *Journal of Research in Childhood Education, 18*, 93–104.

Gazelle, H., & Ladd, G. W. (2003). Anxious solitude and peer exclusion: A diathesis–stress model of internalizing trajectories in childhood. *Child Development, 74*, 257–278.

Gazelle, H., & Rudolph, K. D. (2004). Moving toward and away from the world: Social approach and avoidance trajectories in anxious solitary youth. *Child Development, 75*, 829–849.

Graham, S., & Juvonen, J. (2001). An attributional approach to peer victimization. In J. Juvonen and S. Graham (Eds.), *Peer harassment in school: The plight of the vulnerable and victimized* (pp. 49–72). New York: Guilford Press.

Grant, D. M., Beck, J. G., Farrow, S. M., & Davila, J. (2007). Do interpersonal features of social anxiety influence the development of depressive symptoms? *Cognition and Emotion, 41*(3), 646–663.

Hanish, L. D., & Guerra, N. G. (2004). Aggressive victims, passive victims, and bullies: Developmental continuity or developmental change. *Merrill–Palmer Quarterly, 50*, 17–38.

Hariri, A. R., Mattay, V., Tessitore, A., Kolachana, B., Fera, F., Goldman, D., et al. (2002). Serotonin transporter genetic variation and the response of the human amygdala. *Science, 297*, 400–403.

Harper, M. S., & Welsh, D. P. (2007). Keeping quiet: Self-silencing and its association with relational and individual functioning among adolescent romantic couples. *Journal of Social and Personal Relationships, 24*, 99–116.

Hart, C. H., Yang, C., Nelson, L. J., Robinson, C. C., Olsen, J. A., Nelson, D. A., et al. (2000). Peer acceptance in early childhood and subtypes of socially withdrawn behaviour in China, Russia and the United States. *International Journal of Behavioral Development, 24*(1), 73–81.

Hartup, W. W. (1996). The company they keep: Friendships and their developmental significance. *Child Development, 67*, 1–13.

Haselager, G. J. T., Hartup, W. W., van Lieshout, C. F. M., & Riksen-Walraven, J. M. A. (1998). Similarities between friends and nonfriends in middle childhood. *Child Development, 69*(4), 1198–1208.

Hastings, P. D., & Rubin, K. H. (1999). Predicting mothers' beliefs about preschool-aged children's social behavior: Evidence for maternal attitudes moderating child effects. *Child Development, 70*(3), 722–741.

Hastings, P. D., Rubin, K. H., & DeRose, L. (2005). Links among gender, inhibition, and parental socialization in the development of prosocial behavior. *Merrill–Palmer Quarterly, 51*(4), 467–493.

Henderson, H. A., Marshall, P. J., Fox, N. A., & Rubin, K. H. (2004). Psychophysiological and behavioral evidence for varying forms and functions of nonsocial behaviors in preschoolers. *Child Development, 75*(1), 251–263.

Hinde, R. A. (1979). *Towards understanding relationships*. London: Academic Press.

Hinde, R. A. (1987). *Individuals, relationships and culture: Links between ethology and the social sciences*. New York: Cambridge University Press.

Hodges, E. V. E., Boivin, M., Vitaro, F., & Bukowski, W. M. (1999). The power of friendship: Protection against an escalating cycle of peer victimization. *Developmental Psychology, 35*, 94–101.

Hodges, E., Malone, M. J., & Perry, D. G. (1997). Individual risk and social risk as interacting determinants of victimization in the peer group. *Developmental Psychology, 33*, 1032–1039.

Hymel, S., Bowker, A., & Woody, E. (1993). Aggressive versus withdrawn unpopular children: Variations in peer and self-perceptions in multiple domains. *Child Development, 64*(3), 879–896.

Hymel, S., Rubin, K., Rowden L., & LeMare, L. (1990). Children's peer relationships: Longitudinal prediction of internalizing and externalizing problems from middle to late childhood. *Child Development, 61*(6), 2004–2021.

Kagan, J., Snidman, N., & Arcus, D. (1993). On the temperamental categories of inhibited and uninhibited children. In K. H. Rubin & J. B. Asendorpf (Eds.), *Social withdrawal, inhibition, and shyness in childhood* (pp. 19–28). Hillsdale, NJ: Erlbaum.

Kochenderfer-Ladd, B. (2003). Identification of aggressive and asocial victims and the stability of their peer victimization. *Merrill–Palmer Quarterly, 49*(4), 401–425.

Ladd, G. W., & Burgess, K. B. (1999). Charting the relationship trajectories of aggressive, withdrawn, and aggressive/withdrawn children during early grade school. *Child Development, 70,* 910–929.

Mead, G. H. (1934). *Mind, self, and society: From the standpoint of a social behaviorist.* Oxford, UK: University of Chicago Press.

Mills, R. S. L., & Rubin, K. H. (1993). Socialization factors in the development of social withdrawal. In K. H. Rubin & J. B. Asendorpf (Eds.), *Social withdrawal, inhibition and shyness in childhood* (pp. 117–148). Hillsdale, NJ: Erlbaum.

Mills, R. S. L., & Rubin, K. H. (1998). Are behavioural and psychological control both differentially associated with childhood aggression and social withdrawal? *Canadian Journal of Behavioural Science, 30*(2), 132–136.

Nelson, L. J., Rubin, K. H., & Fox, N. A. (2005). Social and nonsocial behaviors and peer acceptance: A longitudinal model of the development of self-perceptions in children ages 4 to 7 years. *Early Education and Development, 20,* 185–200.

Nolen-Hoeksema, S., Girgus, J. S., & Seligman, M. E. (1992). Predictors and consequences of childhood depressive symptoms: A 5-year longitudinal study. *Journal of Abnormal Psychology, 101*(3), 405–422.

Oh, W., Rubin, K. H., Bowker, J. C., Booth-LaForce, C. L., Rose-Krasnor, L., & Laursen, B. (2008). Trajectories of social withdrawal middle childhood to early adolescence. *Journal of Abnormal Child Psychology, 36,* 553–556.

Oh, W., Rubin, K. H., Burgess, K., Booth-LaForce, C. L., & Rose-Krasnor, L. (2004, July). *A developmental perspective on social withdrawal across middle childhood and adolescence: Predictions from parental and peer factors.* Poster presented at 18th Biennial Meeting of the International Society for the Study of Behavioral Development, Ghent, Belgium.

Ollendick, T. H., Greene, R. W., Weist, M. D., & Oswald, D. P. (1990). The predictive validity of teacher nominations: A five-year follow up of at-risk youth. *Journal of Abnormal Child Psychology, 18*(6), 699–713.

Olweus, D. (1993). Victimization by peers: Antecedents and long-term outcomes. In K. H. Rubin & J. B. Asendorpf (Eds.), *Social withdrawal, inhibition and shyness in childhood* (pp. 315–341). Hillsdale, NJ: Erlbaum.

Pedersen, S., Vitaro, F., Barker, E., & Borge, A. (2007). The timing of middle-childhood peer rejection and friendship: Linking early behavior to early-adolescent adjustment. *Child Development, 78*(4), 1037–1051.

Perry, D. G., Kusel, S. J., & Perry, L. C. (1988). Victims of peer aggression. *Developmental Psychology, 24*(6), 807–814.

Piaget, J. (1932). *The moral judgment of the child.* Glencoe, IL: Free Press.

Rose, A. (2002). Co-rumination in the friendships of girls and boys. *Child Development, 73,* 1830–1843.

Rose, A. J., Swenson, L. P., & Waller, E. M. (2004). Overt and relational aggression and perceived popularity: Developmental differences in concurrent and prospective relations. *Developmental Psychology, 40,* 378–387.

Rubin, K. H. (1982a). Social and social-cognitive developmental characteristics of young isolate, normal and sociable children. In K. H. Rubin & H. S. Ross (Eds.), *Peer relationships and social skills in childhood* (pp. 353–374). New York: Springer-Verlag.

Rubin, K. H. (1982b). Nonsocial play in preschoolers: Necessarily evil? *Child Development, 53*(3), 651–657.

Rubin, K. H. (1985). Socially withdrawn children: An "at risk" population? In B. Schneider, K. H.

Rubin, & J. Ledingham (Eds.), *Children's peer relations: Issues in assessment and intervention* (pp. 125–139). New York: Springer-Verlag.

Rubin, K. H. (1993). The Waterloo Longitudinal Project: Correlates and consequences of social withdrawal from childhood to adolescence. In K. H. Rubin & J. B. Asendorpf (Eds.), *Social withdrawal, inhibition, and shyness in childhood* (pp. 291–314). Hillsdale, NJ: Erlbaum.

Rubin, K. H., & Asendorpf, J. (1993). *Social withdrawal inhibition, and shyness in childhood.* Hillsdale, NJ: Erlbaum.

Rubin, K. H., & Borwick, D. (1984). The communication skills of children who vary with regard to sociability. In H. Sypher & J. Applegates (Eds.), *Social cognition and communication* (pp. 152–170). Hillsdale, NJ: Erlbaum.

Rubin, K. H., Bukowski, W., & Parker, J. G. (2006). Peer interactions, relationships, and groups. In W. Damon, R. M. Lerner, & N. Eisenberg (Eds.), *Handbook of child psychology: Vol. 3. Social, emotional, and personality development* (6th ed., pp. 571–645). New York: Wiley.

Rubin, K. H., & Burgess, K. (2002). Parents of aggressive and withdrawn children. In M. Bornstein (Ed.), *Handbook of parenting* (2nd ed., Vol. 1, pp. 383–418). Hillsdale, NJ: Erlbaum.

Rubin, K. H., Burgess, K., & Coplan, R. (2002). Social inhibition and withdrawal in childhood. In P. K. Smith & C. Hart (Eds.), *Handbook of childhood social development* (pp. 329–352). London: Blackwell.

Rubin, K. H., Burgess, K. B., & Hastings, P. D. (2002). Stability and social-behavioral consequences of toddlers' inhibited temperament and parenting behaviors. *Child Development, 73,* 483–495.

Rubin, K. H., Burgess, K. B., Kennedy, A. E., & Stewart, S. L. (2003). Social withdrawal in childhood. In E. J. Mash & R. A. Barkley (Eds.), *Child psychopathology* (2nd ed., pp. 372–406). New York: Guilford Press.

Rubin, K. H., Cheah, C. S. L., & Fox, N. A. (2001). Emotion regulation, parenting and display of social reticence in preschoolers. *Early Education and Development, 12*(1), 97–115.

Rubin, K. H., Chen, X., & Hymel, S. (1993). The socio-emotional characteristics of extremely aggressive and extremely withdrawn children. *Merrill–Palmer Quarterly, 39,* 518–534.

Rubin, K. H., Chen, X., McDougall, P., Bowker, A., & McKinnon, J. (1995). The Waterloo Longitudinal Project: Predicting adolescent internalizing and externalizing problems from early and mid-childhood. *Development and Psychopathology, 7,* 751–764.

Rubin, K. H., & Coplan, R. J. (2007). Paying attention to and not neglecting social withdrawal and social isolation. In G. Ladd (Ed.), *Appraising the human developmental sciences: Essays in honor of Merrill–Palmer Quarterly* (pp. 156–185). Detroit: Wayne State University Press.

Rubin, K. H., Coplan, R. J., Fox, N. A., & Calkins, S. D. (1995). Emotionality, emotion regulation, and preschoolers' social adaptation. *Development and Psychopathology, 7*(1), 49–62.

Rubin, K. H., Dwyer, K. M., Booth-LaForce, C. L., Kim, A. H., Burgess, K. B., & Rose-Krasnor, L. (2004). Attachment, friendship, and psychosocial functioning in early adolescence. *Journal of Early Adolescence, 24,* 326–356.

Rubin, K. H., Hastings, P. D., Stewart, S. L., Henderson, H. A., & Chen, X. (1997). The consistency and concomitants of inhibition: Some of the children all of the time. *Child Development, 68*(3), 467–483.

Rubin, K. H., Hymel, S., & Mills, R. S. L. (1989). Sociability and social withdrawal in childhood: Stability and outcomes. *Journal of Personality, 57,* 237–255.

Rubin, K. H., Hymel, S., Mills, R. S. L., & Rose-Krasnor, L. (1991). Conceptualizing different pathways to and from social isolation in childhood. In D. Cicchetti & S. Toth (Eds.), *The Rochester Symposium on Developmental Psychopathology: Vol. 2. Internalizing and externalizing expressions of dysfunction* (pp. 91–122). New York: Cambridge University Press.

Rubin, K. H., & Krasnor, L. R. (1986). Social-cognitive and social behavioral perspectives on problem solving. In M. Perlmutter (Ed.), *Minnesota Symposia on Child Psychology: Vol. 18. Cognitive perspectives on children's social and behavioral development* (pp. 1–68). Hillsdale, NJ: Erlbaum.

Rubin, K. H., LeMare, L. J., & Lollis, S. (1990). Social withdrawal in childhood: Developmental pathways to peer rejection. In S. R. Asher & J. D. Coie (Eds.), *Peer rejection in childhood* (pp. 217–249). New York: Cambridge University Press.

Rubin, K. H., & Mills, R. S. L. (1988). The many faces of social isolation in childhood. *Journal of Consulting and Clinical Psychology, 56*(6), 916–924.

Rubin, K. H., & Mills, R. S. L. (1990). Maternal beliefs about adaptive and maladaptive social behaviors in normal, aggressive, and withdrawn preschoolers. *Journal of Abnormal Child Psychology, 18*, 419–435.

Rubin, K. H., & Mills, R. S. L. (1991). Conceptualizing developmental pathways to internalizing disorders in childhood. *Canadian Journal of Behavioural Science, 19*, 86–100.

Rubin, K. H., Nelson, L. J., Hastings, P. D., & Asendorpf, J. (1999). The transaction between parents' perceptions of their children's shyness and their parenting styles. *International Journal of Behavioral Development, 23*, 937–957.

Rubin, K. H., Wojslawowicz, J. C., Rose-Krasnor, L., Booth-LaForce, C. L., & Burgess, K. B. (2006). The friendships of socially withdrawn and competent young adolescents. *Journal of Abnormal Child Psychology, 34*, 139–153.

Rubin, K. H., Wojslawowicz Bowker, J. C., & Oh, W. (2007). The peer relationships and friendships of socially withdrawn children. In A. S. LoCoco, K. H. Rubin, & C. Zappulla (Eds.), *L'isolamento sociale durante l'infanzia* [Social withdrawal in childhood]. Milan: Unicopli.

Schmidt, L. A., Fox, N. A., Rubin, K. H., Sternberg, E. M., Gold, P. W., Craig, C., et al. (1997). Behavioral and neuroendocrine responses in shy children. *Developmental Psychobiology, 30*, 127–140.

Schmidt, L. A., Fox, N. A., Schulkin, J., & Gold, P. W. (1999). Behavioral and psychophysiological correlates of self-presentation in temperamentally shy children. *Developmental Psychobiology, 35*, 119–135.

Schneider, B. H. (1999). A multi-method exploration of the friendships of children considered socially withdrawn by their peers. *Journal of Abnormal Psychology, 27*, 115–123.

Schneider, B. H., Richard, J. F., Younger, A. J., & Freeman, P. (2000). A longitudinal exploration of the continuity of children's social participation and social withdrawal across socioeconomic status levels and social settings. *European Journal of Social Psychology, 30*, 497–519.

Schneider, B. H., Younger, A. J., Smith, T., & Freeman, P. (1998). A longitudinal exploration of the cross-context stability of social withdrawal in early adolescence. *Journal of Early Adolescence, 18*, 374–396.

Schwartz, C. E., Wright, C. I., Shin, L. M., Kagan, J., & Rauch, S. L. (2003). Inhibited and uninhibited infants "grown up": Adult amygdalar response to novelty. *Science, 300*(5627), 1952–1953.

Selman, R. L., & Schultz, L. H. (1990). *Making a friend in youth: Developmental theory and pair therapy.* Chicago: University of Chicago Press.

Spangler, G., & Schieche, M. (1998). Emotional and adrenocortical responses of infants to the Strange situation: The differential function of emotional expression. *International Journal of Behavioral Development, 22*, 681–706.

Stewart, S. L., & Rubin, K. H. (1995). The social problem solving skills of anxious–withdrawn children. *Development and Psychopathology, 7*, 323–336.

Sullivan, H. S. (1953). *The interpersonal theory of psychiatry.* New York: Norton.

Wichmann, C., Coplan, R. J., & Daniels, T. (2004). The social cognitions of socially withdrawn children. *Social Development, 13*, 377–392.

Younger, A. J., Gentile, C., & Burgess, K. (1993). Children's perceptions of social withdrawal: Changes across age. In K. H. Rubin & J. B. Asendorpf (Eds.), *Social withdrawal, inhibition, and shyness in childhood* (pp. 215–235). Hillsdale, NJ: Erlbaum.

CHAPTER 18

Bullies, Victims, and Bully–Victim Relationships in Middle Childhood and Early Adolescence

CHRISTINA SALMIVALLI
KÄTLIN PEETS

Peer relations can be a source of joy, support, and satisfaction, but they sometimes result in negative experiences and major distress. Being exposed to repeated humiliation and attacks by peers is probably one of the most traumatic experiences a child or adolescent can encounter in the peer context. This phenomenon, "bullying," is the focus of the current chapter. More specifically, we focus on peer-to-peer bullying among children in middle childhood and early adolescence.

The topic of bullying has established its place in the scientific literature during the past decades. Academic attention to the problem started in Scandinavia during the 1970s (Olweus, 1973, 1978) and soon spread to other countries. According to the PsycINFO database, only four studies with "bullying" as a key word ("bully/bullying/bullied") were published during the 1970s. There were 18 such studies during the 1980s and 246 studies in the 1990s. At present, 100–200 new studies on bullying emerge every year.

Not only has the quantity of research increased but so also has the complexity and the depth of questions addressed. As an example of this development, the field is evidencing a shift in focus from study of individual bullies and victims to study of dyadic relationships (i.e., bully–victim dyads; Veenstra et al., 2007). Another line of research is represented by attempts to identify factors at the classroom or school level that might contribute to the problem (Dhami, Hoglund, Leadbeater, & Boone, 2005; Salmivalli & Voeten, 2004). Furthermore, during the past decade, the availability of sophisticated statistical tools (e.g., multilevel modeling) has allowed researchers to understand better the complex interplay between individual, dyadic, and group factors associated with bullying. In terms of research methods and designs, these shifts mean new approaches to collecting data, as well as moving from simple main effect models to the study of interactions and complicated process models at multiple levels of social reality (e.g., individuals, relationships, cliques, classrooms, and schools).

In this chapter, we first take a look at the definitions and operationalizations of bullying and victimization, review different forms of harassment, and review some of the theoretical frameworks used to explain the bullying phenomenon. We then introduce an integrated view of *bullying in context* and review findings concerning the characteristics of individual bullies and victims, as well as the dyadic and group contexts in which bullying occurs. We finish the chapter with some suggestions for future research.

Central Issues

Aggression and Bullying, Victimization and Being Bullied: Is There a Difference?

Being bullied was originally defined by Olweus (1978) as being exposed, repeatedly and over time, to negative actions on the part of one or more other students. Although some researchers have phrased it a bit differently, at least three defining characteristics of bullying seem to be universally accepted: (1) intent to harm, (2) repetition over time,[1] and (3) a power differential (i.e., the victim finds it difficult to defend him- or herself against the perpetrator). Thus, one of the key features of bullying is imbalance of power between the bully and the victim. Power can be defined as "an individual's relative capacity to modify others´ states by providing or withholding resources or administering punishments" (Keltner, Gruenfeld, & Anderson, 2003, p. 265). Therefore, bullying is clearly different from conflicts, quarrels, or fights between two individuals who are equal in terms of psychological or physical strength or social status, regardless of the frequency and severity of such acts.

Although all aggressive encounters taking place at school cannot be regarded as bullying, bullying clearly is a subtype of aggressive behavior. Aggressive behavior is often defined as "any behavior directed toward another individual that is carried out with the proximate (immediate) intent to cause harm. In addition, the perpetrator must believe that the behavior will harm the target and that the target is motivated to avoid the behavior" (see Bushman & Anderson, 2001, p. 274). Although aggression is very often measured only in terms of its behavioral manifestation, without taking into account the intent to harm, there is a widely recognized and used taxonomy based on the underlying goal or motive. "Proactive aggression" is defined as goal-directed, harmful behavior, and it is distinct from "reactive aggression," which is used in response to a perceived threat or social provocation (Dodge, 1991). Because bullying is typically unprovoked and deliberate, it is considered a subtype of proactive aggression.

Another relevant construct used in the peer relations research is "victimization." Because it refers to being a recipient of any kind of aggressive attacks, victimization is usually measured without any reference to the power imbalance between the perpetrator and the victim, or to the repetitive nature of the negative act. Therefore, "victimization" and "being bullied" do not necessarily represent identical constructs. For instance, studies on victimization might ask children to nominate the classmates who are hit, kicked, or called names by others. Such a procedure might generate a number of nominations of children involved in many reciprocated, "symmetrical," aggressive encounters, such as fights between two individuals with equal power. It can also yield high scores for someone who is often the target of reactive aggression. The victimization score derived in this way is not necessarily comparable to the one from another study investigating victimization in the sense of "being bullied." There is also empirical evidence that the overlap between "being bullied" and "victimization" constructs is only moderate (Schäfer, Werner, & Crick, 2002).

Although the distinction between different constructs is acknowledged by scholars, it can be readily forgotten. Controversial findings across studies that might be due to the differences in how bullying/victimization is measured are sometimes mistakenly attributed to differences in cultural context, age, and other sample characteristics. Thus, comparing results across studies that use different operationalizations can create an inaccurate view of the bullying phenomenon.

Forms of Bullying

Similar to aggressive behavior in general, bullying has many faces. Early studies on bullying focused on physical (e.g., hitting, pushing, or kicking) and verbal (verbal ridicule, insulting, threatening) bullying. The early emphasis on direct forms of bullying was associated with a strong research focus on boys. For some time, bullying was considered a "male phenomenon." Olweus (1978, p. 18) wrote: "Aggression variables and the problems to be taken up here can be validly studied for the age groups concerned [sixth to eighth graders] when only the boys of a class take part in the investigation." Today, few investigators would agree with such a view; numerous studies during the past two decades have confirmed that the phenomenon also exists among girls.

Since the late 1980s, research has shifted from examining only physical and verbal aggression (i.e., "direct aggression") to studying more subtle forms of aggression. These involve circuitous, often socially manipulative behaviors, such as spreading nasty rumors or lies about the target ("indirect aggression"; e.g., Björkqvist, Lagerspetz, & Kaukiainen, 1992), harming or threatening to harm the target's relationships ("relational aggression"; Crick & Grotpeter, 1995), or damaging the target's self-esteem or social status by subjecting him or her to social exclusion or insulting facial expressions and gestures ("social aggression"; Underwood, 2003). Although the three forms focus on slightly different aspects, they overlap considerably. In this chapter, we use the term "indirect aggression" to represent all of these subtle forms of bullying.

The original view of indirect aggression as "female aggression" was supported by several studies indicating that it was more common among females than among males (Björkvist et al., 1992; Crick & Grotpeter, 1995). These findings were later challenged by studies that did not find a gender difference (e.g., Galen & Underwood, 1997) or even found that boys used indirect aggression more often than girls (Peets & Kikas, 2006; Salmivalli & Kaukiainen, 2004; Tomada & Schneider, 1997). Although, in an absolute sense, boys often resort to all forms of aggression more frequently than do girls, proportionally, girls seem to use indirect forms more often than direct forms of aggression (i.e., when females do aggress, their preferred mode of aggression is indirect).

Recently, researchers have identified and started to explore several new forms of bullying such as electronic (Raskauskas, 2007) or cyberbullying (Slonje & Smith, 2008). Cyberbullies deliver their harmful acts via electronic communication tools (mobile phones, electronic mail, or Internet Web pages). They may send hurtful text messages and e-mails to their victims, or they may spread insulting material, such as stories, photos, or video clips portraying the victim in embarrassing situations, over the Internet. Although cyberbullying occurs less frequently than traditional forms of bullying, it may be becoming more widespread with the development of new technologies.

It should be noted that although victimization that involves physical violence catches a lot of media attention, and cyberbullying represents a potential new threat to the well-being of children and youth, these are not the most common manifestations of bullying and victimization. Several studies have shown that *the majority of bullying consists of verbal attacks among girls as well as boys* (e.g., Rivers & Smith, 1994). However, whether the harmful acts are in the form of name-calling, hitting, exclusion, or sending nasty e-mails, victimization clearly is a threat to the victim's self-esteem, status, and sense of belongingness within the peer group.

Assessing Bullying and Victimization

Questionnaires are the most prevalent way to gather data about bullying and victimization. Most often, children themselves are utilized as informants. For instance, in self-reports, children are asked how often they bully others/get bullied by others, and in the case of peer-reports, children nominate class- or grademates who bully others/get bullied by others. Questions may be global, such as the previous examples, or they may tap different forms of bullying. Recently, dyadic questions ("Whom do you bully/who bullies you?" or "Who bullies whom in your classroom?") have emerged in studies of bullying.

Utilizing adults, such as parents or teachers, as informants is relatively rare in the age group we discuss in this chapter. Thus, the debate concerning the most reliable and valid method for the assessment of bullying and victimization has concentrated mainly on whether to use self- or peer reports. There are arguments in favor of both methods. From middle childhood onward, peer reports are considered highly reliable, because they can be attained from very many classmates who have observed the behavior of the focal child in a wide range of situations. The composite scores based on reports from several peers include little error variance. A drawback is that peer reports disregard the subjective experience of victimization. However, the child's own perception of being victimized is especially associated with a number of intrapersonal problems that may be considered most detrimental for the individual.

Although numerous studies use only one type of assessment (e.g., peer or self-report), it is suggested that gaining information across different informants is the most comprehensive approach for studying victimization and bullying. The idea is to minimize error variance and possible biases evident in the reports provided by single informants. In a study by Ladd and Kochenderfer-Ladd (2002), a combination of different informants (self-, peer, parent, and teacher reports) for victimization yielded the best prediction of relational adjustment, such as rejection, loneliness, and other social problems, which speaks in favor of utilizing multiple informants.

Another way of thinking is that differences between informants do not represent measurement error but interesting true variance that is worthy of further exploration. Juvonen, Nishina, and Graham (2001, p. 106) have suggested that self- and peer reports of victimization tap different constructs. Whereas self-reports measure the subjective experience of victimization, peer reports assess peer reputation of being victimized. Whereas self-reported victimization is more closely related to intrapersonal problems, such as anxiety, peer-reported victimization is more strongly associated with interpersonal problems, such as peer rejection. Accordingly, the choice of informant should be based on the focus of the study.

Questionnaires are not the only method to gather data on bullying and victimization. Interviews are often necessary with young children (Monks, Smith, & Swettenham,

2005). In addition, direct observations (Schwartz et al., 1998) and daily diaries (Nishina & Juvonen, 2005) have been used. Although many studies still utilize a single method, use of multiple informants and multiple methods has been called for in the bullying literature (e.g., Pellegrini, 2001).

Prevalence of Bullying and Victimization

Solberg and Olweus (2003) have argued that providing a definition of bullying and asking a single question regarding the frequency of being the target of bullying lead to valid prevalence estimates that are comparable across classrooms, schools, or countries. According to them, children who report being bullied at least two to three times or more per month may be categorized as victims. The prevalence of bullied children identified using that method varies considerably across countries (from 5% in Sweden to over 30% in Lithuania), and is on average 11% across the 35 countries involved in the World Health Organization (WHO) *Health Behavior in School-Age Children Survey* (HBSC; Craig & Harel, 2004). Bullies represent another 11% of school-age children. Children who report both bullying others and being bullied by others (i.e., bully-victims) were not identified in the HBSC study, but other studies have shown that by using a similar procedure, approximately 4–6% of children can be classified as bully-victims (Haynie et al., 2001; Nansel et al., 2001). In our recently collected data involving more than 7,000 Finnish students, bully-victims are more frequent among younger children: The frequencies varied from 5.3% (grade 3) to 3.0% (grade 5).

Another way to categorize children into bullies, victims, and bully victims is to use cutoff scores on continuous (often peer-reported) bullying and victimization variables. A standard deviation (*SD*) below or above 1 is often used as a cut point (e.g., Ladd & Kochenderfer-Ladd, 2002). For instance, a child who has a high score on bullying (1 *SD* above the sample mean) and a low score on victimization (1 *SD* below the sample mean) would be classified as a bully. Because cutoff points are more or less arbitrary and are usually based on variables that have already been standardized within the classroom, it is almost impossible to tell the "true" prevalence of bullies and victims based on such a procedure. Categories based on using cutoff scores are beneficial for group comparisons in research settings, but they are not ideal to estimate prevalence rates that would be comparable across studies or across different contexts.

With regard to gender differences, boys are more likely to be bullies and bully-victims than girls (e.g., Pellegrini & Long, 2002; Veenstra et al., 2005). However, gender differences in victimization are less clear. Although boys often score higher on victimization than do girls, some studies indicate no gender differences (for a review, see Rose & Rudolph, 2006) or find that the gender effect is reverse (Veenstra et al., 2005). In addition, the prevalence of victimization is influenced by respondent age. For instance, self-reported victimization tends to decrease as children get older (Smith, Shu, & Madsen, 2001).

Relevant Theory

After decades of research, theoretical explanations of bullying are still scarce. Many early studies on bullying and victimization were descriptive in nature, reporting the prevalence and different forms of bullying, along with the characteristics of children involved. Since then, researchers have tried to understand the mechanisms by which some children become bullies or victims, often turning to the same theories used to explain the development of aggressive behavior more generally, namely, studies on bullying and victimization have relied on biological–genetic explanations, attachment theory, social information processing, social-cognitive learning, and social–ecological theories.

Findings from behavioral genetics indicate that peer difficulties, such as aggression and victimization, are partly heritable (see Brendgen and Boivin, Chapter 25, this volume). Moreover, because genetic effects are influenced by environmental conditions, the heritability estimates change as a function of children's age, as well as characteristics of the social environment. According to attachment theorists, problematic peer relationships, such as bullying and victimization, can be understood as a function of insecure attachment (Troy & Sroufe, 1987).

Furthermore, social information-processing and social-cognitive learning theories have been helpful in understanding different thought processes behind the bullying behavior. Bullying is associated especially with aggression-encouraging social cognitions; that is, children who engage in proactive aggression value instrumental goals (Crick & Dodge, 1996), are more confident in their ability to aggress (Perry, Perry, & Rasmussen, 1986), and evaluate aggression more favorably in terms of its appropriateness (Erdley & Asher, 1998) and expected consequences (Perry et al., 1986).

Most of these theories have been used to explain the behavior of individuals, typically aggressive children or bullies, without considering the social context in which the bullying occurs. However, there have also been attempts to explain the functions of bullying at the peer-group level, without focusing on the individual child. Bukowski and Sippola (2001), for instance, have argued that victimization is "a process by which an individual is forced out of a group because he or she is seen as a threat to the attainment of the group's goals" (p. 363), such as group cohesion, harmony, and movement toward novelty. According to Juvonen and Galván (2008), bullying serves as a means to define and maintain the group's norms. For example, through homophobic bullying, the group members define gay-like behavior as something "*we* do not engage in," and in groups in which less trendy individuals are being harassed, the group creates and enhances the norm of being trendy and good-looking. Garandeau and Cillessen (2006) recently suggested that bullying can provide a common goal and a sense of cohesion for group members, especially in groups with low-quality relationships and a lack of genuine cohesiveness.

More than a decade ago, Pierce and Cohen (1995) called for more contextually oriented research on aggression and victimization. They suggested studying aggressors and victims as *interdependent participants of a relationship* that is *embedded in the larger social context*. They did not talk about bullies exclusively, but because bullies need targets for their coercive behavior, utilizing the dyad as a unit for analysis might be especially relevant. Most definitions of bullying involve a specific target who is attacked "repeatedly and over time," and who has "difficulty in defending him- or herself." The fact that bullying tends to endure makes it especially interesting to study it as a *relationship*, rather than a behavioral tendency or a passing *interaction* between two children.

Bullying Contextualized

Bullying is a form of goal-directed, proactive aggression. In accordance with recent theorizing and empirical findings on bullying, we view "bullying" as an attempt to gain (and maintain) social status within the peer group. According to Keltner et al. (2003), "Status is the outcome of an evaluation of attributes that produces differences in respect and prominence" (p. 266). Thus, status means one's relative visibility, respect, and, indirectly, influence on others. Such goals are by nature *interpersonal*, because they concern what the individual wants to attain, maintain, or avoid not only personally but also *in relation to others* (see Fitzsimons & Bargh, 2003). The view of bullying as a quest for status is not only helpful in understanding the individual child's behavior, but it also serves to explain why some children are targeted by schoolyard bullies, and why and how the larger group gets involved. From the bully's standpoint, the victim can be seen as a means to achieve one's goals, and the group is needed, because status is something that the group assigns to its members, and it exists only in relation to other members in the group.

It is clear that there are individual differences in the likelihood of becoming a bully or a victim. In fact, most children do not ever engage in a bully–victim relationship. We argue that the likelihood for a child to act as a bully, that is, to torment a weaker or a less powerful peer repeatedly is influenced by the individual tendency to value high status. However, other characteristics of an individual may strengthen or weaken the association between status goals and bullying. For instance, whereas aggression-encouraging cognitions, such as efficacy beliefs (i.e., belief in one's capability to engage in bullying behavior) and outcome expectations (e.g., bullying is a way to be admired and respected by others) for bullying, are likely to encourage the bullying behavior, antibullying attitudes and empathy toward the victim are likely to inhibit it. Thus, two children who both value status can actually engage in a very different behavior to achieve their goal.

In addition to individual factors, several contextual factors affect the likelihood of engagement in bullying. These contextual factors may be dyadic, or they may operate at the level of the peer group. Regarding dyadic factors, bullies do not target all their peers with the same probability, but they tend to select victims who serve as "easy" targets; that is, children with personal and interpersonal risk factors, such as physical weakness and lack of (protective) friends, are more likely to become victims of peer abuse. A power differential between two children (e.g., the bully being considerably stronger than the victim) especially increases the likelihood of two children ending up in the bully–victim relationship. In addition, over time, bullies might selectively attend to certain signs, while ignoring others (see also Keltner et al., 2003). For instance, a child's unassertiveness and weakness can automatically trigger social cognitions that promote the bullies' use of aggression to improve their position in the peer group.

Other contextual moderators work at the peer-group level. Bullying is often a classroom phenomenon. Our recently collected data with more than 7,000 children from 400 classrooms indicate that 70–80% of the victims have their tormentors in their own class. Moreover, classmates are often well aware of bullying incidents, and many of them witness the attacks. Research indicates that despite their antibullying attitudes, many peer onlookers give positive feedback to the bully either directly (by assisting) or indirectly (by merely watching). It is understandable that bullies are more likely to use and to continue using coercion as an effective means to achieve status if the social context reinforces their behavior. The characteristics of particular classrooms, such as general attitudes toward bullying (e.g., whether bullying is considered as an accepted way of behaving) and the behavior of onlookers are thus likely to moderate the link between status goals and bullying.

Why would bullying someone lead to high status? Antisocial, tough behavior is often perceived as "cool" even in normative peer cultures (Rodkin, Farmer, Pearl, & Van Acker,

2006), and so is bullying (Juvonen & Galván, 2008). This is especially clear during pre-adolescence and adolescence. It has been suggested that the antisocial and aggressive acts that represent challenges to adult norms and values (Moffit, 1993) become more accepted (or at least less negatively viewed) when children approach adolescence. Furthermore, because bullies do not target all, or even most, of their classmates, but are often selective in their aggression (Card, Isaacs, & Hodges, 2000), many peers never personally experience the most harmful effects of the bullying. Moreover, if other peers actually dislike the victim (which is often the case), bullies might perceive that they are doing a "favor" for others. And even if the majority of classmates disapprove of the bully's behavior, it can still be reinforced by the bully's network of friends, who very often are bullies themselves.

Key Classical and Modern Research Studies

Bullies

In his seminal work, Olweus (1978, p. 136) described the "aggressive personality pattern" of bullies as a driving force behind their behavior. Given the abundance of research on the correlates and predictors of childhood and adolescent aggression long before bullying entered the research agenda, it was quite natural to apply the findings on aggressive behavior to the bullying type of aggression. For a long time, researchers and practitioners regarded bullies as individuals who lack social skills and have low self-esteem, deficiencies in social information processing, low social standing in the peer group, and other adjustment problems. Although many of these factors seem to be associated with aggression in general, or with reactive aggression, there is little empirical support for their being related to bullying specifically.

A glance at some recent titles in the area of bullying, such as "Bullying Is Power" (Vaillancourt, Hymel, & McDougall, 2003), or "It's Easy, It Works, and It Makes Me Feel Good" (Sutton, Smith, & Swettenham, 2001), reveals something about the shift in the way bullying is perceived. In line with the view that bullying is driven by status goals, studies have shown that bullies value dominance (Björkqvist, Ekman, & Lagerspetz, 1982), and that highly agentic goals, such as being respected and admired by peers, are associated with proactive aggression (Salmivalli, Ojanen, Haanpää, & Peets, 2005). Bullying seems to be efficient, at least for some children. Even if bullies are not necessarily personally liked by many classmates, they may be perceived as popular, powerful, and "cool" among their classmates (Juvonen & Galván, 2008; Vaillancourt et al., 2003), especially when they also possess peer-valued characteristics, such as athletic competence, physical attractiveness, or a sense of humor (Vaillancourt & Hymel, 2006). Moreover, bullies are often central members of their peer networks and have friends. They often affiliate with other aggressive peers (Salmivalli, Huttunen, & Lagerspetz, 1997), and thereby derive and provide reinforcement for coercive behavior.

The aggression–low self-esteem hypothesis has received little if any empirical support (Baumeister, Bushman, & Campbell, 2000), and it also is not compatible with the view we present in this chapter. It is unlikely that children and adolescents who are insecure and have low self-esteem would pursue goals of visibility and admiration. To the contrary, research shows that low self-esteem is related to self-protection rather than to self-enhancement goals (Tice, 1993), and children with low self-esteem tend to value goals related to avoiding humiliation, rejection, and other distressing situations (Salmivalli et al., 2005). Although self-esteem per se tends to be unrelated to bullying (Salmivalli, Kaukiainen, Kaistaniemi, & Lagerspetz, 1999), narcissism and high self-esteem combined with a negative view of peers (Salmivalli et al., 2005) are associated with high levels of aggression.

The view of bullies as socially incompetent was challenged by Sutton, Smith, and Swettenham (1999a). They found that 7- to 10-year-old ringleader bullies scored relatively high in tasks designed to assess understanding of others' cognitions and emotions. Accordingly, Kaukiainen et al. (1999) argued that "social intelligence" (e.g., person perception, social flexibility) is a prerequisite for utilizing subtle, indirectly aggressive behaviors, such as manipulating others and turning them against the target. In their study, indirect aggression was positively associated with social intelligence after they controlled for direct aggression. It is not to say that social intelligence is a prerequisite for bullying, but bullies with person perception and social flexibility skills are likely to be more efficient in their bullying behavior. For instance, they might be better at choosing the "right" victims, manipulating other peers to join them, and utilizing other, more prosocial, means to achieve status in the peer group (see also Garandeau & Cillessen, 2006).

Research utilizing social information-processing and social-cognitive learning theories indicates that bullies are guided by distinct thought processes. Studies show that proactively aggressive children hold social cognitions that promote the use of aggression as an effective means to achieve their goals. For instance, bullies feel confident about using aggression, expect positive outcomes for aggression, view aggression as an accepted way of behaving, and have an overall positive view regarding the use of aggression (Tobin, Schwartz, Hopmeyer, & Abou-Ezzeddine, 2005). Whether such tendencies should be regarded as *deficiencies* or merely as *differences* in social-cognitive processing styles has been debated in the literature (Crick & Dodge, 1999; Sutton, Smith, & Swettenham, 1999b). Traditionally, "social competence" has been seen as a socially accepted behavior associated with being liked by others. However, it can be also defined as an ability to be successful at achieving one's goals (LaFontana & Cillessen, 2002; Sutton et al., 1999b). According to the latter view, children who successfully achieve their goals by using either prosocial or coercive strategies may be seen as socially competent. Studies inspired by Hawley's work (e.g., Hawley, Little, & Card, 2007) suggest that many bullies are so-called "bistrategic controllers," who can effectively use both prosocial and coercive strategies to get what they want.

Regarding familial risk factors, there is evidence that bullies (the authors used the label "nonvictimized aggressors") may learn to behave aggressively by observing adult conflict and aggression in preschool years (Schwartz, Dodge, Pettit, & Bates, 1997). Bullies also tend to perceive their parents as authoritarian, punitive, and less supportive (Baldry & Farrington, 2000), and they report less cohesiveness to their parents than do other children (Bowers, Smith, & Binney, 1994). The maladaptive parenting styles can promote the development of proactive type of aggression through social-cognitive processes (e.g., Dodge, 1991). For instance, when children see that their parents get their way by using aggression (or when their parents give in to the child's aggressive control attempts), they may learn that aggression is an effective means to achieve desired outcomes. Moreover, parenting might, at least partly, influence certain goal orientations, such as valuing admiration and dominance, which, in combination with aggression-encouraging cognitions and lack of empathy, can result in proactive type of aggression, such as bullying.

Victims

As we pointed out earlier, bullies do not target all the classmates with the same probability, but tend to select victims who provide them with easy victories. By choosing victims who are submissive (Schwartz et al., 1998), insecure about themselves (Salmivalli & Isaacs, 2005), physically weak (Hodges & Perry, 1999), and rejected by the peer group (Bukowski & Sippola, 2001; Hodges & Perry, 1999; Salmivalli, Lagerspetz, Björkqvist, Österman, & Kaukiainen, 1996), bullies can repeatedly demonstrate their power to the rest of the group, thus renewing their high-status position in the group without having to be afraid of confrontation.

In a meta-analytic review, Hawker and Boulton (2000) showed that victimization is associated with a number of psychosocial problems, such as depression, loneliness, anxiety, and low social and general self-esteem. Personal and interpersonal problems tend to co-occur, and children with internalizing or externalizing problems are more likely to become victimized if they also face interpersonal difficulties (Hodges, Boivin, Vitaro, & Bukowski, 1999; Hodges & Perry, 1999). Thus, a shy and anxious child who is also rejected by classmates, or who has no friends, serves as an ideal target for the bully, because the likelihood of retaliation from the peer group is very low (see Rubin, Bowker, & Kennedy, Chapter 17, this volume). Such a situation creates an even larger power imbalance between the bully and the victim. Many of these risk factors can be understood in the light of bullies' status goals. Children with inter- and intrapersonal difficulties are likely to provide bullies with easy victories, thus increasing the likelihood that bullies receive positive outcomes for their aggressive behavior (e.g., approval by other peers).

Moreover, not only number of friends but also characteristics of friends and friendship quality moderate the association between adjustment and victimization. In other words, behaviorally at-risk children (e.g., children who are shy and anxious) have a higher probability of being victimized, if they have friends who are physically weak and/or disliked by other peers, compared to children who have friends and are strong and/or liked by others (Hodges, Malone, & Perry, 1997).

Examining correlations between victimization and different personal and interpersonal risk variables does not give us the full picture about the heterogeneity of victimized children. Olweus (1978, p. 128) and Perry, Kusel, and Perry (1988) found a zero correlation between victimization and aggression. Moreover, both studies found evidence of the existence of two distinct groups of victims identified as nonaggressive (passive) and aggressive (provocative) victims. This distinction was later acknowledged by many researchers. Whereas passive victims are usually characterized by submissiveness, shyness, and withdrawal, aggressive victims are described as aggressive, hot-tempered, restless, and disruptive (e.g., Schwartz, 2000). Because externalizing behaviors, such as angry outbursts, are often considered non-normative by the peer group, it is understandable why bullies might target peers who demonstrate such behaviors. Moreover, an angry, aggressive outburst on the behalf of the victim is often ineffective and can thereby be rewarding for the bully.

Furthermore, some researchers have identified a group of children who score highly on both bullying and victimization ("bully-victims"; Bowers et al., 1994; Kumpulainen, Räsänen, & Puura, 2001). Whether different types of aggressive victims represent overlapping categories or distinct groups is still unclear. However, there is initial evidence of the existence of three groups: (1) passive victims; (2) reactively aggressive victims; and (3) proactively and, to a lesser extent, reactively aggressive victims (Vermande et al., 2007). It might be that whereas the second group represents the "provocative victims," the third group comprises children who have been labeled bully-victims in the literature.

Differences between aggressive bully-victims and passive victims can be traced back to distinct socialization practices; that is, aggressive victims come from more punitive, hostile, and abusive families than do passive victims (Schwartz et al., 1997). In addition, bully-victims report high levels of parental neglect, overprotection (Bowers et al., 1994), and rejection (Veenstra et al., 2005), as well as low levels of parental monitoring and warmth (Bowers et al., 1994; Veenstra et al., 2005). In contrast, research shows that passive victims tend to enjoy a more positive home environment than do bullies (aggressors) or (aggressive) bully-victims (Bowers et al., 1994; Schwartz et al., 1997; Veenstra et al., 2005).

Research on the Dyadic Context of Bullying

Studies focusing on children's overall levels of bullying and victimization do not provide any insight into who is bullying whom, in other words, into the dynamics of bullying. However, there is growing evidence that aggressive behavior of children and adolescents is not distributed randomly across peers, but is delivered by and toward specific peers. For instance, Dodge, Price, Coie, and Christopoulos (1990), who observed playgroups of boys who were unacquainted with each other, found that 50% of all aggressive acts took place in only 20% of the dyads. They classified the dyads as "mutually aggressive" when aggression was initiated equally by both members of the dyad, and "asymmetric" (i.e., bully-victim) when one of the boys was much more aggressive than the other. Twelve percent of all dyads were asymmetrically aggressive. Whereas these dyads were characterized by high levels of proactive aggression by the bully toward the victim, reactive aggression was more common within symmetrically aggressive dyads (6% of all the dyads).

It is becoming more and more evident that bullies are very selective with regard to their victims. For instance, Card, Isaacs, and Hodges (2000) found that aggressive nonvictims (who could be considered bullies) were selective, delivering their aggression mainly toward children who had a reputation of being victimized. To the contrary, aggressive victims (provocative victims) did not differentiate between their targets, but reported being aggressive toward victims and nonvictims (including aggressive nonvictims). Because bullies can possess protective interpersonal (e.g., friends) and personal characteristics (e.g., physically strong), aggressive victims can put themselves at great risk for a counterattack by an aggressive nonvictim. However, contrary to the perspective of aggressive victims, aggressive nonvictims did not report being victimized by them. This suggests that aggressive victims overestimate their use of aggression or, alternatively, their aggression is viewed as nonharmful by the bullies.

As was already pointed out before, a potential factor influencing involvement and stability of the bully–victim relationship is the power differential between two children. Feeling powerful can increase self-esteem, self-efficacy for aggression, and, as a result, lead to denigration of others. Whereas elevated power increases the probability of having positive affect and representing others as means to one's own ends, reduced power increases the likelihood of negative affect and seeing oneself as a means to others' ends (Keltner et al., 2003). In line with the theory by Keltner and colleagues, a study by Veenstra et al. (2007) demonstrated that the probability of being in a bully–victim relationship was higher if the bully was more dominant than the victim. Similarly, Card and Hodges

(2005) showed that two children who initially differed, for instance, in their physical strength, aggressiveness, and victimization levels, were more apt to become involved in an aggressor–victim relationship than two more similar children. In other words, it is not only submissiveness or low social standing that makes the victim a "good" target. Instead, it is his or her status in relation to the specific bully. This may also explain why some children bully and are bullied by other peers at the same time; that is, they are victimized by their more powerful peers but bully others who have a lower status in relation to them.

Bully–victim relationships characterized by a high degree of power differential are more likely to be stable over time. As might be expected, power differential bears a negative consequence, especially for the victim. For instance, Card and Hodges (2005) found that the larger the difference in physical strength between the bully and the victim, the more likely the victim felt socially less competent over time. Furthermore, because powerful individuals are much more inclined to process information about others in an automatic fashion (Keltner et al., 2003), bullies might act according to the established views of their victims, without paying much attention to immediate cues.

Social-cognitive processes might be one potential mechanism by which the bully–victim relationship is maintained over time. Initially, social information-processing patterns (and consequently, behaviors) were mostly treated as personality-like characteristics (i.e., rather stable over time and over different contexts). However, more resent research shows that social cognitions and behaviors are to a great extent relationship- or target-specific (e.g., Burgess, Wojslawowicz, Rubin, Rose-Krasnor, & Booth-LaForce, 2006; Peets, Hodges, Kikas, & Salmivalli, 2007; Peets, Hodges, & Salmivalli, 2008). For instance, in the study by Hubbard, Dodge, Cillessen, Coie, and Schwartz (2001), relationship-specific reactive aggression was best explained by the attribution of hostility within that relationship (and not by generalized hostile representations of others). However, the results of the same study suggest that dyad-specific proactive aggression is more guided by the characteristics of the aggressor (i.e., aggressiveness of the perpetrator across different dyads) and the victim (i.e., being victimized by peers across different dyads) rather than by the unique relationship between the two.

Moreover, it has been proposed that the emotional valence of the relationship between two individuals affects how the information is processed and, consequently, what behavioral response in enacted (Lemerise & Arsenio, 2000). It is not yet clear whether personal liking or disliking is crucial for the emergence and maintenance of bully–victim dyads. For instance, Dodge et al. (1990) found that whereas the relationship between bullies and victims was not characterized by high levels of dislike, members of mutually aggressive dyads had the highest probability of disliking each other. Thus, bullies might not necessarily have a strong dislike toward the victim. This is concordant with the view that bullying is driven by goals rather than by negative emotions, such as anger. However, Card and Hodges (2007), although not looking at the bullying type of aggression specifically, found that victimization was more likely to come from mutual antipathies than from friends and unilaterally disliked or disliking peers.

The Involvement of the Group

Even when bullying occurs between two children, it is dependent on the larger social context. If the bully is aiming for high status, the group is essential, because status can only be understood within the group, relative to other group members. Furthermore, it is the group that assigns status to its members. Because bullies need witnesses for their power demonstrations, it is understandable that peers are present in most of the bullying incidents (Hawkins, Pepler, & Craig, 2001). Although it is possible that bullying incidents attract spectators, it is highly likely that the attacks are often initiated when a group of peers is already at the spot.

Some studies examining the group aspects of bullying have focused on *how witnessing bullying affects children* who are not directly involved in bullying incidents. Nishina and Juvonen (2005, Study 1) collected 11-year-old children's daily reports of personally experienced and witnessed harassment, and their negative feelings across 4 consecutive days. Just having witnessed bullying was related to increased levels of daily anxiety for children who themselves were not targeted.

However, onlookers are not only influenced by witnessing bullying but can themselves influence the bullying process. Salmivalli et al. (1996) investigated children's different participant roles in bullying situations (victims, bullies, assistants of bullies, reinforcers of bullies, outsiders, and defenders of the victim) and found that rather than supporting the victim, many children acted in ways that encouraged and maintained bullying. For instance, whereas some children reinforced bullies' behavior by laughing or cheering, other children supported the bullying behavior by silently witnessing it.

Although most children have negative attitudes toward bullying, they seldom support the victim or intervene in bullying incidents (O'Connell, Pepler, & Craig, 1999). It is possible that children are afraid that, by siding with the victim, they put themselves at risk for the future attacks from the more powerful bully. In addition, children might not know how to help (Atlas & Pepler, 1998). It has been suggested (Juvonen & Galván, 2008) that at least two motives might prevent children from siding with the victim. First, children want to improve their own social standing by appearing more like the person in power, that is, the bully, and by distancing themselves from the low-status victim. As a consequence, victims tend to become even more rejected as victimization continues (Hodges & Perry, 1999). The second motive is self-protection. By siding with the bully, or at least appearing to accept his or her behavior, the child lowers his or her own risk of becoming the next victim (Juvonen & Galván, 2008). If we think about the typical bullying incident in which there is the powerful (and popular) bully and the weak (socially marginalized) victim, it is understandable that siding with the bully can be adaptive, at least temporarily, for other group members. In the long run, however, such behavior is likely to maintain bullying and harm everyone's well-being.

Because mobilizing bystanders to support victims of bullying might be a promising approach for intervention in bullying (Salmivalli, Kärnä, & Poskiparta, in press), it is important to identify factors associated with assisting and supporting the victim. For instance, "affective empathy" (i.e., the ability to feel vicariously the affective state of another person) and self-efficacy for defending behavior increase the likelihood of defending the victim (Pöyhönen & Salmivalli, 2007). In addition, high-status children are more likely to side with the victim (Salmivalli et al., 1996). Perhaps children who are well-liked by others are more confident about their secure position in the group and are more willing to adopt defending behaviors due to the reduced risk of becoming victims themselves. Furthermore, children who support or defend the victim often believe that their parents and friends expect them to act so (Rigby & Johnson, 2006), and they tend to have friends who also support the victim (Salmivalli et al., 1997).

Whatever role children take in a bullying situation might also depend on their relationship with the bully or the victim (e.g., Ray, Norman, Sadowski, & Cohen, 1999). Children who are friends with, or who like, the bully are probably more likely to assist the bully directly or reinforce his or her behavior. Card and Hodges (2006) found that aggressive adolescents who were friends tended to share their targets for aggression. By aggressing toward the same victim, aggressive friends could model and reinforce each others' bullying behavior. In contrast, children who are friends with the victim might be more prone to support him or her. In addition to individual characteristics of children and their dyadic relationship, how the child acts in bullying situations is also influenced by the norms of the whole classroom. If most of the children in the class think that bullying is a normative behavior, then there is a greater likelihood that children will side with the bully rather than with the victim (Salmivalli & Voeten, 2004).

Furthermore, characteristics of the classroom context might moderate the *consequences of victimization*. For instance, there is evidence that victims are less rejected in classrooms in which victimization is normative, that is, occurring at high levels (Sentse, Scholte, Salmivalli, & Voeten, 2007). In addition, victims have fewer negative feelings in classrooms in which they observe other children also being victimized (Bellmore, Witkow, Graham, & Juvonen, 2004; Nishina & Juvonen, 2005, Study 2). Paradoxically, a "negative" context can serve as a protective factor for the individual victim. Seeing that other children share their plight might make victims feel less bad about their own situation. Furthermore, victims might be less likely to engage in self-blaming attributions in classrooms where many children are victimized.

Future Directions

So far, much of the research on bullying has focused on individual bullies and, to a lesser extent, on victims. The few theories that view bullying as a relationship or group phenomenon are still much "looser" than individual approaches to bullying and victimization. Although studies on dyadic and group aspects of bullying have started to emerge, they are still relatively rare. It is a challenge for future research to incorporate different levels of influence in the same, testable models. For instance, individual risk factors for bullying and victimization are likely to depend on the context. For instance, status goals might lead to bullying behavior only in certain environments, such as classrooms in which bullying is rewarded. By gaining knowledge about how bullying unfolds within different contexts (e.g., dyads, peer groups, classrooms) we will be able to intervene better in bullying and prevent its harmful effects on those who are directly or indirectly involved.

Acknowledgment

We would like to thank Prof. Ernest V. E. Hodges for commenting on a version of the current chapter. The writing of this chapter was supported by the Academy of Finland Grant No. 121091 to Christina Salmivalli.

Note

1. It can be argued that *the threat* of repetition is already sufficient to define an attack as bullying.

References

Atlas, R. S., & Pepler, D. J. (1998). Observations of bullying in the classroom. *Journal of Educational Research, 92*, 86–99.

Baldry, A. C., & Farrington, D. P. (2000). Bullies and delinquents: Personal characteristics and parental styles. *Journal of Community and Applied Social Psychology, 10*, 17–31.

Baumeister, R., Bushman, B., & Campbell, K. (2000). Self-esteem, narcissism, and aggression: Does violence result from low self-esteem or threatened egotism? *Current Directions in Psychological Science, 9*, 26–29.

Bellmore, A., Witkow, M., Graham, S., & Juvonen, J. (2004). Beyond the individual: The impact of ethnic context and classroom behavioral norms on victims' adjustment. *Developmental Psychology, 40*, 1159–1172.

Björkqvist, K., Ekman, K., & Lagerspetz, K. (1982). Bullies and victims: Their ego picture, ideal ego picture and normative ego picture. *Scandinavian Journal of Psychology, 23*, 307–313.

Björkqvist, K., Lagerspetz, K., & Kaukiainen, A. (1992). Do girls manipulate and boys fight?: Developmental trends in regard to direct and indirect aggression. *Aggressive Behavior, 18*, 117–127.

Bowers, L., Smith, P. K., & Binney, V. (1994). Perceived family relationships of bullies, victims and bully/victims in middle childhood. *Journal of Social and Personal Relationships, 11*(2), 215–232.

Bukowski, W., & Sippola, L. (2001). Groups, individuals, and victimization: A view of the peer system. In J. Juvonen & S. Graham (Eds.), *Peer harassment in school: The plight of the vulnerable and victimized* (pp. 355–377). New York: Guilford Press.

Burgess, K. B., Wojslawowicz, J. C., Rubin, K. H., Rose-Krasnor, L., & Booth-LaForce, C. (2006). Social information processing and coping styles of shy/withdrawn and aggressive children: Does friendship matter? *Child Development, 77*, 371–383.

Bushman, B. J., & Anderson, C. A. (2001). Is it time to pull the plug on the hostile versus instrumental aggression dichotomy? *Psychological Review, 108*, 273–279.

Card, N. A., & Hodges, E. V. E. (2005, April). *Power differential in aggressor–victim relationships.* In N. A. Card & E. V. E. Hodges (Chairs), Aggressor–victim relationships: Toward a dyadic perspective. Paper symposium presented at the biennial meeting of the Society for Research in Child Development, Atlanta, GA.

Card, N. A., & Hodges, E. V. E. (2006). Shared targets for aggression by early adolescent friends. *Developmental Psychology, 42*, 1327–1338.

Card, N. A., & Hodges, E. V. E. (2007). Victimization within mutually antipathetic relationships. *Social Development, 3*, 479–496.

Card, N. A., Isaacs, J., & Hodges, E. V. E. (2000, March). *Dynamics of interpersonal aggression in the school context: Who aggresses against whom?* In A. Nishina & J. Juvonen (Chairs), Harassment across diverse contexts. Poster symposium conducted at the 8th biennial meeting of the Society for Research on Adolescence, Chicago, IL.

Craig, W., & Harel, Y. (2004). Bullying, physical fighting, and victimization. In C. Currie, C. Roberts, A. Morgan, R. Smith, W. Settertobulte, O. Samdal, et al. (Eds.), *Young People's Health in Context: International report from the HBSC 2001/02 Survey* (WHO Policy Series: Health Policy for Children and Adolescents, Issue 4). Copenhagen: WHO Regional Office for Europe.

Crick, N., & Dodge, K. (1996). Social information-processing mechanisms on reactive and proactive aggression. *Child Development, 67*, 993–1002.

Crick, N., & Dodge, K. (1999). "Superiority" is in the eye of the beholder: A comment of Sutton, Smith, and Swettenham. *Social Development, 8*, 128–131.

Crick, N., & Grotpeter, J. (1995). Relational aggression, gender, and social-psychological adjustment. Child Development, 66, 710–722.

Dhami, M., Hoglund, W., Leadbeater, B., & Boone, E. (2005). Gender-linked risks for physical and relational victimization in the context of school-level poverty in first grade. *Social Development, 14*, 532–549.

Dodge, K. (1991). The structure and function of reactive and proactive aggression. In D. Pepler & K. Rubin (Eds.), *The development and treatment of childhood aggression* (pp. 201–218). Hillsdale, NJ: Erlbaum.

Dodge, K. A., Price, J. M., Coie, J. D., & Christopoulos, C. (1990). On the development of aggressive dyadic relationships in boys' peer groups. *Human Development, 33,* 260–270.

Erdley, C. A., & Asher, S. R. (1998). Linkages between children's beliefs about the legitimacy of aggression and their behavior. *Social Development, 7,* 321–339.

Fitzsimons, G., & Bargh, J. (2003). Thinking of you: Nonconscious pursuit of interpersonal goals associated with relationship partners. *Journal of Personality and Social Psychology, 84,* 148–163.

Galen, B., & Underwood, M. (1997). A developmental investigation of social aggression among children. *Developmental Psychology, 33,* 589–600.

Garandeau, C., & Cillessen, A. (2006). From indirect aggression to invisible aggression: A conceptual view on bullying and peer group manipulation. *Aggression and Violent Behavior, 11,* 641–654.

Hawker, D., & Boulton, M. (2000). Twenty years' research on peer victimization and psychosocial maladjustment: A meta-analytic review of cross-sectional studies. *Journal of Child Psychology and Psychiatry and Allied Disciplines, 41,* 441–455.

Hawkins, L., Pepler, D., & Craig, W. (2001). Naturalistic observations of peer interventions in bullying. *Social Development, 10,* 512–527.

Hawley, P. H., Little, T. D., & Card, N. A. (2007). The allure of a mean friend: Relationship quality and processes of aggressive adolescents with prosocial skills. *International Journal of Behavioral Development, 31,* 170–180.

Haynie, D., Nansel, T., Eitel, P., Crump, A., Saylor, K., Yu, K., et al. (2001). Bullies, victims, and bully–victims: Distinct groups of at-risk youth. *Journal of Early Adolescence, 21,* 29–49.

Hodges, E. V. E., Boivin, M., Vitaro, F., & Bukowski, W. (1999). The power of friendship: Protection against an escalating cycle of peer victimization. *Developmental Psychology, 35,* 94–101.

Hodges, E. V. E., Malone, M., & Perry, D. (1997). Individual risk and social risk as interacting determinants of victimization in the peer group. *Developmental Psychology, 33,* 1032–1039.

Hodges, E. V. E., & Perry, D. G. (1999). Personal and interpersonal antecedents and consequences of victimization by peers. *Journal of Personality and Social Psychology, 76,* 677–685.

Hubbard, J. A., Dodge, K. A., Cillessen, A. H. N., Coie, J. D., & Schwartz, D. (2001). The dyadic nature of social information processing in boys' reactive and proactive aggression. *Journal of Personality and Social Psychology, 80,* 268–280.

Juvonen, J., & Galván, A. (2008). Peer influence in involuntary social groups: Lessons from research on bullying. In M. J. Prinstein & K. A. Dodge (Eds.), *Understanding peer influence in children and adolescents* (pp. 225–244). New York: Guilford Press.

Juvonen, J., Nishina, A., & Graham, S. (2001). Self-views versus peer perceptions of victim status among early adolescents. In J. Juvonen & S. Graham (Eds.), *Peer harassment in school: The plight of the vulnerable and victimized* (pp. 105–124). New York: Guilford Press.

Kaukiainen, A., Björkqvist, K., Lagerspetz, K., Österman, K., Salmivalli, C., Rothberg, S., et al. (1999). The relationships between social intelligence, empathy, and three types of aggression. *Aggressive Behavior, 25,* 81–89.

Keltner, D., Gruenfeld, D. H., & Anderson, C. (2003). Power, approach, and inhibition. *Psychological Review, 110,* 265–284.

Kumpulainen, K., Räsänen, E., & Puura, K. (2001). Psychiatric disorders and the use of mental health services among children involved in bullying. *Aggressive Behavior, 27,* 102–110.

Ladd, G., & Kochenderfer-Ladd, B. (2002). Identifying victims of aggression from early to middle childhood: Analysis of cross-informant data for concordance, estimation of relational adjustment, prevalence of victimization, and characteristics of identified victims. *Psychological Assessment, 14,* 74–96.

LaFontana, K. M., & Cillessen, A. H. (2002). Children's perceptions of popular and unpopular peers: A multimethod assessment. *Developmental Psychology, 38,* 635–647.

Lemerise, E., & Arsenio, W. (2000). An integrated model of emotion processes and cognition in social information processing. *Child Development, 71*, 107–118.

Moffitt, T. (1993). Adolescence-limited and life-course-persistent antisocial behavior: A developmental taxonomy. *Psychological Review, 100*, 674–701.

Monks, C., Smith, P. K., & Swettenham, J. (2005). Psychological correlates of peer victimization in preschool: Social cognitive skills, executive function and attachment profiles. *Aggressive Behavior, 31*, 571–588.

Nansel, T., Overpeck, M., Pilla, R., Ruan, W., Simon-Morton, B., & Scheidt, P. (2001). Bullying behaviors among U.S. youth: Prevalence and association with psychosocial adjustment. *Journal of the American Medical Association, 285*, 2094–2100.

Nishina, A., & Juvonen, J. (2005). Daily reports of witnessing and experiencing peer harassment in middle school. *Child Development, 76*, 435–450.

O'Connell, P., Pepler, D., & Craig, W. (1999). Peer involvement in bullying: Insights and challenges for intervention. *Journal of Adolescence, 22*, 437–452.

Olweus, D. (1973). *Hackkycklingar och översittare* [Bullies and whipping boys]. Stockholm: Almqvist & Wiksell.

Olweus, D. (1978). *Aggression in schools: Bullies and whipping boys*. Washington, DC: Hemisphere.

Peets, K., Hodges, E., Kikas, E., & Salmivalli, C. (2007). Hostile attributions and behavioral strategies in children: Does relationship type matter? *Developmental Psychology, 43*, 889–900.

Peets, K., Hodges, E., & Salmivalli, C. (2008). Affect-congruent social-cognitive evaluations and behaviors. *Child Development, 79*, 170–185.

Peets, K., & Kikas, E. (2006). Aggressive strategies and victimization during adolescence: Grade and gender differences, and cross-informant agreement. *Aggressive Behavior, 32*, 68–79.

Pellegrini, A. (2001). Sampling instances of victimization in middle school: A methodological comparison. In J. Juvonen & S. Graham (Eds.), *Peer harassment in school: The plight of the vulnerable and the victimized* (pp. 125–144). New York: Guilford Press.

Pellegrini, A. D., & Long, J. D. (2002). A longitudinal study of bullying, dominance, and victimization during the transition from primary school through secondary school. *British Journal of Developmental Psychology, 20*, 259–280.

Perry, D. G., Kusel, S., & Perry, L. (1988). Victims of peer aggression. *Developmental Psychology, 24*, 807–814.

Perry, D. G., Perry, L. C., & Rasmussen, P. (1986). Cognitive social learning mediators of aggression. *Child Development, 57*, 700–711.

Pierce, K., & Cohen, R. (1995). Aggressors and their victims: Toward a contextual framework for understanding children's aggressor–victim relationships. *Developmental Review, 15*, 292–310.

Pöyhönen, V., & Salmivalli, C. (2007, March). *Cognitive and affective factors associated with defending the bullied victims.* Poster presented at the biennial meeting of the Society for Research in Child Development, Boston, MA.

Raskauskas, J. (2007). Involvement in traditional and electronic bullying among adolescents. *Developmental Psychology, 43*, 564–575.

Ray, G. E., Norman, M., Sadowski, C. J., & Cohen, R. (1999). The role of evaluator–victim relationships in children's evaluations of peer provocation. *Social Development, 8*, 380–394.

Rigby, K., & Johnson, B. (2006). Expressed readiness of Australian schoolchildren to act as bystanders in support of children who are being bullied. *Educational Psychology, 26*, 425–440.

Rivers, I., & Smith, P. K. (1994). Types of bullying behaviour and their correlates. *Aggressive Behavior, 20*, 359–368.

Rodkin, P., Farmer, T., Pearl, R., & Van Acker, R. (2006). They're cool: Social status and peer group supports for aggressive boys and girls. *Social Development, 15*, 175–204.

Rose, A., & Rudolph, K. (2006). A review of sex differences in peer relationship processes: Potential trade-offs for the emotional and behavioral development of girls and boys. *Psychological Bulletin, 132*, 98–131.

Salmivalli, C., Huttunen, A., & Lagerspetz, K. (1997). Peer networks and bullying in schools. *Scandinavian Journal of Psychology, 38*, 305–312.

Salmivalli, C., & Isaacs, J. (2005). Prospective relations among victimization, rejection, friendlessness, and children's self- and peer-perceptions. *Child Development, 76*, 1161–1171.

Salmivalli, C., Kärnä, A., & Poskiparta, E. (in press). From peer putdowns to peer support: A theoretical model and how it translated into a national anti-bullying program. In S. Shimerson, S. Swearer, & D. Espelage (Eds.), *The international handbook of school bullying*. Mahwah, NJ: Erlbaum.

Salmivalli, C., & Kaukiainen, A. (2004). "Female aggression" revisited: Variable- and person-centered approaches to studying gender differences in direct and indirect aggression. *Aggressive Behavior, 30*, 158–163.

Salmivalli, C., Kaukiainen, A., Kaistaniemi, L., & Lagerspetz, K. (1999). Self-evaluated self-esteem, peer-evaluated self-esteem, and defensive egotism as predictors of adolescents' participation in bullying situations. *Personality and Social Psychology Bulletin, 25*, 1268–1278.

Salmivalli, C., Lagerspetz, K., Björkqvist, K., Österman, K., & Kaukiainen, A. (1996). Bullying as a group process: Participant roles and their relations to social status within the group. *Aggressive Behavior, 22*, 1–15.

Salmivalli, C., Ojanen, T., Haanpää, J., & Peets, K. (2005). "I'm O.K. but you're not" and other peer-relational schemas: Explaining individual differences in children's social goals. *Developmental Psychology, 41*, 363–375.

Salmivalli, C., & Voeten, M. (2004). Connections between attitudes, group norms, and behaviors associated with bullying in schools. *International Journal of Behavioral Development, 28*, 246–258.

Schäfer, M., Werner, N. E., & Crick, N. R. (2002). A comparison of two approaches to the study of negative peer treatment: General victimization and bully/victim problems among German schoolchildren. *British Journal of Developmental Psychology, 20*, 281–306.

Schwartz, D. (2000). Subtypes of victims and aggressors in children's peer groups. *Journal of Abnormal Child Psychology, 28*, 181–192.

Schwartz, D., Dodge, K., Hubbard, J., Cillessen, A., Lemerise, E., & Bateman, H. (1998). Social-cognitive and behavioral correlates of aggression and victimization in boys' play groups. *Journal of Abnormal Child Psychology, 26*, 431–440.

Schwartz, D., Dodge, K. A., Pettit, G. S., & Bates, J. E. (1997). The early socialization of aggressive victims of bullying. *Child Development, 68*, 665–675.

Sentse, M., Scholte, R., Salmivalli, C., & Voeten, M. (2007). Person–group dissimilarity in involvement in bullying and its relation with social status. *Journal of Abnormal Child Psychology, 35*, 1009–1019.

Slonje, R., & Smith, P. K. (2008). Cyberbullying: Another main type of bullying? *Scandinavian Journal of Psychology, 49*, 147–154.

Smith, P. K., Shu, S., & Madsen, K. (2001). Characteristics of victims of school bullying: Developmental changes in coping strategies and skills. In J. Juvonen & S. Graham (Eds.), *Peer harassment in school: The plight of the vulnerable and the victimized* (pp. 332–351). New York: Guilford Press.

Solberg, M., & Olweus, D. (2003). Prevalence estimation of school bullying with the Olweus Bully/Victim Questionnaire. *Aggressive Behavior, 29*, 239–268.

Sutton, J., Smith, P. K., & Swettenham, J. (1999a). Social cognition and bullying: Social inadequacy or skilled manipulation? *British Journal of Developmental Psychology, 17*, 435–450.

Sutton, J., Smith, P. K., & Swettenham, J. (1999b). Socially undesirable need not be incompetent: A response to Crick and Dodge. *Social Development, 8*, 132–134.

Sutton, J., Smith, P. K., & Swettenham, J. (2001). "It's easy, it works, and it makes me feel good": A response to Arsenio and Lemerise. *Social Development, 10*, 74–78.

Tice, D. (1993). The social motivations of people with low self-esteem. In R. Baumeister (Ed.), *Self-esteem: The puzzle of low self-regard* (pp. 37–53). New York: Plenum Press.

Tobin, R., Schwartz, D., Hopmeyer, A., & Abou-Ezzeddine, T. (2005). Social-cognitive and behavioral attributes of aggressive victims of bullying. *Applied Developmental Psychology, 26*, 329–346.

Tomada, G., & Schneider, B. (1997). Relational aggression, gender, and peer acceptance: Invariance across culture, stability over time, and concordance among informants. *Developmental Psychology, 33*, 601–609.

Troy, M., & Sroufe, L. (1987). Victimization among preschoolers: Role of attachment relationship history. *Journal of Child and Adolescent Psychiatry, 2*, 166–172.

Underwood, M. K. (2003). *Social aggression among girls.* New York: Guilford Press.

Vaillancourt, T., & Hymel, S. (2006). Aggression and social status: The moderating roles of sex and peer-valued characteristics. *Aggressive Behavior, 32*, 396–408.

Vaillancourt, T., Hymel, S., & McDougall, P. (2003). Bullying is power: Implications for school-based intervention strategies. *Journal of Applied School Psychology, 19*, 157–176.

Veenstra, R., Lindenberg, S., Oldehinkel, A. J., De Winter, A. F., Verhulst, F. C., & Ormel, J. (2005). Bullying and victimization in elementary schools: A comparison of bullies, victims, bully/victims, and uninvolved preadolescents. *Developmental Psychology, 41*, 672–682.

Veenstra, R., Lindenberg, S., Zijlstra, B. J. H., De Winter, A. F., Verhulst, F. C., & Ormel, J. (2007). The dyadic nature of bullying and victimization: Testing a dual perspective theory. *Child Development, 78*, 1843–1854.

Vermande, M., Aleva, L., Orobio de Castro, B., Olthof, T., Goossens, F., et al. (2007, June). *Victims of bullying in school: Theoretical and empirical indications for the existence of three categories.* Presentation in Onderwijs Research Dagen, Groningen, the Netherlands.

CHAPTER 19

Adolescent Romantic Relationships and Experiences

WYNDOL FURMAN
W. ANDREW COLLINS

For many years the study of peer relationships focused exclusively on platonic peers. Virtually nothing was known about romantic relationships or romantic experiences prior to age 18 except for a few scattered studies on dating preferences or functions (e.g., Roscoe, Diana, & Brooks, 1987).

That so little was known about these relationships is ironic given the centrality of romantic experiences in adolescents' lives. More than half of adolescents in the United States report having had a special romantic relationship in the past 18 months (Carver, Joyner, & Udry, 2003). High school students typically say that they interact more frequently with their romantic partners than they do with parents, siblings, or friends (Laursen & Williams, 1997). Moreover, even when not interacting with them, adolescents also think about their romantic partners for many hours each week (Richards, Crowe, Larson, & Swarr, 1998). Romantic experiences are believed to play important roles in the development of an identity; the development of close relationships with peers; the transformation of family relationships; sexuality; and scholastic achievement and career planning (Furman & Shaffer, 2003). Mounting evidence indicates that, contrary to widespread skepticism, such experiences are also linked to individual adjustment and may influence the nature of subsequent romantic relationships (Collins, 2003; Furman, 2002; Furman, Ho, & Low, 2007).

We happily report that interest in romantic relationships has blossomed in the last decade. Several edited volumes have been published (Crouter & Booth, 2006; Florsheim, 2003; Furman, Brown, & Feiring, 1999; Shulman & Collins, 1997), and a number of research laboratories are studying the nature of adolescent romantic relationships and experiences. This emerging body of literature on romantic relationships and experiences is the focus of this chapter.

We define "romantic relationships" as mutually acknowledged, ongoing voluntary interactions; in comparison to most other peer relationships, romantic ones typically have a distinctive intensity that is usually marked by expressions of affection and current or anticipated sexual behavior (W. Collins, 2003). Of course, some behaviors are simultaneously affectionate and sexual in nature.

It is important to recognize, however, that the study of adolescent romance entails more than examining the characteristics of specific dyadic relationships. Over time, most people have a number of different romantic relationships. As we discuss subsequently, the number, as well as the characteristics, of romantic relationships has been found to be related to psychosocial development and adjustment. Moreover, romantically relevant experiences occur outside the context of ongoing dyadic relationships. Fantasies and one-sided attractions may occur, as well as interactions with potential romantic partners or brief romantic encounters (e.g., "hooking up" and "dates"; Brown, Feiring, & Furman, 1999). We use the term "romantic experiences" to refer to this broad range of experiences and cognitions, including both those within and outside of particular dyadic relationships. This term incorporates a broad and heterogeneous range of activities and cognitions, but we believe that it has heuristic value by both providing a term for the general domain of romantically relevant experiences and encouraging investigators to examine a wide range of potentially important phenomena.

Our definitions of "romantic relationships" or "romantic experiences" do not refer to the gender of the individuals, because we intend to include both same- and other-gender romantic relationships and experiences. The literature on same-gender romantic experiences is more limited (see Diamond, Savin-Williams, & Dubé, 1999), but we incorporate such literature when available, and note its absence otherwise. The existing literature is also constrained by the fact that almost all of the research has also been conducted in industrialized societies, most typically in North America. Although the experience of love may be universal (Jankowiak & Fischer, 1992), romantic experiences, especially adolescent romantic experiences, are likely to be determined largely by the cultural context in which they occur (see Brown, Larson, & Saraswathi, 2002).

Although we believe that most investigators have similar conceptualizations of romantic relationships, little attention has been given to how romantic relationships should be operationally defined. Typically, investigators have simply asked participants whether they have a romantic relationship, and the participants decide on the basis of their own definition. In some cases, a brief description is provided (e.g., "when you like a guy [girl] and he [she] likes you back"; Giordano, Manning, & Longmore, 2006, p. 131), or a minimal relationship duration is required (e.g., at least a month long). Further attention should be given to the operational definition of romantic relationships, because differences in definition affect estimates of the frequency and duration of romantic relationships, and perhaps even the findings obtained (see Furman & Hand, 2006). For that matter, we know surprisingly little about how adolescents themselves decide whether and when they are in romantic relationships.

In the sections that follow, we discuss key issues in the field, examine relevant theory, and review the empirical literature. Because the topic is still relatively new, we conclude by describing the limitations in our knowledge and identifying important directions for subsequent research and theory.

Central Issues

As noted in the prior section, romantic experiences are believed to influence the course of a number of developmental tasks, such as the development of sexuality, identity development, or the development of close relationships with peers (see Furman & Shaffer,

2003). Adolescents' romantic experiences, however, undoubtedly vary substantially. Whereas some may be extensively involved in romantic relationships, others may have minimal romantic experience. The quality and content of the relationships may vary substantially as well. Consequently, the specific effects of romantic experiences on psychosocial development depend on an adolescent's particular experiences. Thus, a fundamental issue in the field is to identify the dimensions along which romantic experiences can vary. We are guided by a framework that delineates five features of romantic experiences (W. Collins, 2003). The first and most commonly examined feature is romantic involvement or experience, which incorporates elements such as whether a person dates, when he or she began dating, the duration of relationships, and the frequency and consistency of dating and relationships. The second feature is partner selection (i.e., the characteristics of the person the adolescent dates or with whom he or she is having a relationship). The third feature is the content of the relationship—what members of the dyad do (and do not) do together, and how they spend their time. The fourth feature is the quality of the romantic relationship, such as the degree of support or conflict in the relationship. The final features are the cognitive and emotional processes associated with the relationship. The cognitive processes include perceptions; attributions; and representations of oneself, the partner(s), and the relationship(s). Emotional processes include the emotions and moods elicited by and in romantic encounters or relationships, as well as the use of romantic relationships to process (or avoid) emotions elicited by other aspects of one's life. Emotions elicited by the absence or demise of a romantic relationship may also be highly salient. Of course, the cognitive and emotional processes in a relationship are closely related to each other.

Recognition of the variability of romantic experiences leads quite naturally to the three central issues that the theorists and researchers have examined. First, what is the developmental course of romantic experiences? How do the features change or remain the same? Second, what are the causes and consequences of individual differences in romantic experiences? What leads adolescents to have different experiences, and what impact do such differences have on them? Third, how are experiences in other relationships associated with romantic experiences? How do experiences with parents or peers affect romantic experiences? In the sections that follow, we focus on the theory and research relevant to these three central issues.

Relevant Theory

The theoretical formulations that have guided the current flowering of research on adolescent romantic relationships ground romantic relationships in the normative social experiences of adolescence. Three overlapping traditions have been especially important: attachment theory, Sullivanian and behavioral systems approaches, and symbolic interactionism.

Attachment Theory

Attachment formulations emphasize the strong emotional ties between parents and their offspring. The construct of attachment in infant–caregiver relationships refers to a relatively distinct connection that supports infants' efforts to feel safe from threatening conditions and to be regulated emotionally. According to Ainsworth (1989), infant behaviors with attachment partners are prototypes of attachments at every age, including those that occur outside of the biological family. These relationships illustrate four defining criteria for differentiating attachment relationships from other close relationships: proximity seeking; safe-haven behavior (turning first to the other person when facing a perceived threat); secure-base behavior (free exploration in the presence of the other person); and distress over involuntary separations. Attachment theorists propose that committed adult romantic relationships typically meet these criteria (Shaver & Hazan, 1988). In fact, a romantic partner is expected to be the primary attachment figure for most adults. However, adult romantic attachments differ from infant attachments to a caregiver in that the attachments are usually reciprocal, with each person being attached to the other and serving as an attachment figure for the other. Adult romantic attachments also involve sexual behavior. In light of these differences, Shaver and Hazan hypothesized that romantic love involves the integration of the attachment, caregiving, and sexual/reproductive behavioral systems.

Romantic partners are not usually expected to be the primary attachment figure until late adolescence or adulthood, because this shift in attachment objects requires a cognitive and emotional maturity that rarely is achieved before then (Ainsworth, 1989). In fact, most adolescent romantic relationships are unlikely to meet all the criteria of an attachment relationship. At the same time, attachment-related functions begin to be redistributed to close peer relationships, such as friendships or romantic relationships. Hazan and Zeifmann (1994) proposed that attachments are transferred, component by component, from parents to close friends and romantic partners. Specifically, proximity seeking toward close peers first occurs, then safe-haven behavior, and finally separation protest and secure-base behavior.

A key hypothesis of attachment theory is that a history of sensitive, responsive interactions and strong emotional bonds with parents facilitates adaptation during the transitions of adolescence—transitions that simultaneously permit functioning in friendships and romantic relationships, and transform existing bonds with parents into more age-appropriate ones (Allen & Land, 1999). Two largely compatible explanations have been offered for links between attachments with caregivers and those in later extrafamilial relationships. The first is a carry-forward model, in which functions and representations of caregiver–child attachment relationships ("internal working models") organize expectations and behaviors in later relationships (e.g., Waters & Cummings, 2000), including selection of partners congruent with past partners (Sroufe & Fleeson, 1988). The second is the premise that relationships with caregivers prior to adolescence expose individuals to components of effective relating, such as empathy, reciprocity, and self-confidence, that shape interactions in other, later relationships (e.g., W. Collins & Sroufe, 1999; Sroufe & Fleeson, 1988). In turn, childhood and adolescent friendships serve as templates for subsequent close relationships outside of the family (Youniss, 1980). Thus, both processes lead to the expectation that a foundation of emotional and behavioral interdependence in early life is a significant forerunner of one's romantic relationships in adolescence and adulthood. In the subsequent section on key studies, we discuss the research examining continuity across relationships.

Sullivanian and Behavioral Systems Theory

Sullivan (1953) proposed that five basic needs motivate individuals to bring about certain interpersonal situations that promote positive affective states or decrease negative affective states: (1) tenderness, (2) companionship, (3) acceptance, (4) intimacy, and

(5) sexuality. Each need is associated with a key relationship that typically fulfills this need. The need for tenderness emerges in infancy and is met through relationships with parents. In childhood, the need for companionship emerges. Initially, companionship occurs with adults and is subsequently transformed into companionship with peers during the early school years. Additionally, as children become increasingly involved in the peer world, their need for acceptance by peers develops. In preadolescence, the need for intimate exchange emerges and results in the establishment of "chumships," which are typically close, same-gender friendships. Chumships serve as a foundation for later, more sexually charged intimate relationships with romantic partners. According to Sullivan, friendship in preadolescence and adolescence meets a basic psychological need to overcome loneliness—an idea that is similar to the more recent proposal that humans have an evolved need to belong (Baumeister & Leary, 1995). By overcoming loneliness through close friendships with same-gender peers, adolescents develop the psychological capacity to achieve intimacy. With the onset of puberty at adolescence, sexuality, or true genital lust, emerges; moreover, adolescents gradually become interested in achieving intimacy with a romantic partner that is similar to that achieved in chumships. The task of late adolescence is to establish a committed relationship.

Building upon the insights of attachment and Sullivanian theorists, Furman and Wehner's (1994) behavioral systems theory proposes that romantic partners become major figures in the functioning of the attachment, caregiving, affiliative, and sexual/ reproductive behavioral systems. The attachment, caretaking, and sexuality systems have received considerable theoretical attention from attachment theorists, but the affiliative system has not. The "affiliative system" refers to the biological predisposition to interact with known others, and is hypothesized to underlie the capacities to cooperate, collaborate with another, and co-construct a relationship. Initially, affiliation and sexuality are expected to be the central systems in romantic relationships, but eventually the attachment and caregiving system become salient as well.

Behavioral systems theory would expect a moderate degree of consistency between romantic relationships and relationships with peers and parents. When the different behavioral systems are activated, adolescents are likely to be predisposed to respond to romantic partners as they have in other relationships. At the same time, romantic relationships are not expected to be simple replications of other relationships, because the qualitative features of romantic relationships typically differ in some respects from those with friends or parents. Additionally, the adolescent's partner and his or her past and present experiences, as well as those of the adolescent, affect the nature of the relationship (Kelley et al., 1983/2002; Kenny, Kashy, & Cook, 2006; Laursen & Bukowski, 1997; Reis, Collins, & Berscheid, 2000).

Symbolic Interactionism

Symbolic interactionists emphasize that the meanings of romantic experiences emerge from the communication and interactions within romantic relationships (Giordano et al., 2006). These meanings are likely to emerge from the immediate "on site" experiences rather than from prior experiences with peers or parents (Giordano et al., 2006). These distinctive meanings may be quite different from the meanings of prior relationship experiences, because romantic relationship experiences are relatively private and not very scripted. In effect, the adolescent is shaped by these ongoing dynamic processes (Mead, 1934).

In addition to these broad theoretical perspectives, the Furman et al. (1999) edited volume contains a series of conceptual papers focusing on particular facets of romantic experience. Similarly, classic approaches, such as social learning theory or lifespan developmental systems perspectives, have guided some research (e.g., Capaldi, Shortt, & Kim, 2005). At the same time, some theories, such as social exchange theory and evolutionary theory, have been very prominent in research on adult romantic relationships, but as yet have received little attention in research on adolescent relationships (Laursen & Jensen-Campbell, 1999). More generally, it would be fair to say that the development of theories of romantic experiences is still in a rather rudimentary stage. Only a few theories have been proposed, and these have primarily focused on particular issues, such as the links between romantic experiences and other relationship experiences. Further theoretical development is essential to future progress in the area.

Key Studies

The Developmental Course of Romantic Experiences

Romantic experiences and relationships change substantially over the course of development, yet is important to emphasize that there is not a single pattern of romantic development. In most industrialized societies, adolescents vary in terms of when they develop romantic interests, begin to date, or establish a romantic relationship. Not only the timing differs, but also the degree of romantic involvement varies. Some youth may have relatively few or intermittent romantic experiences, whereas others may be seeing someone or having a romantic relationship most all of the time. Even the sequence of romantic experiences varies. Typically, early romantic relationships are relatively short-lived, but some long-term relationships may occur early on. We address the correlates of such variability in romantic involvement in the subsequent section on individual variations.

Romantic Relationship Activity

Variability notwithstanding, adolescent romantic experiences tend to follow a common course. The commonalities were first described in Dunphy's (1963) five-stage model of peer-group development, which invoked the differing types of peer clusters discussed by Brown and Dietz (Chapter 20, this volume). In the first stage, preadolescents and adolescents commonly participate in cliques of four to six same-gender friends. In the second stage, boy and girl cliques begin to interact with each other. In the third stage, a mixed-gender crowd emerges, and the higher status members of the earlier cliques begin to date each other and form mixed-gender cliques. In the fourth stage, the mixed-gender peer crowd is fully developed, and several mixed-gender cliques have emerged as dating becomes more widespread. In the fifth stage, the crowd begins to disintegrate as adolescents pair off and form loosely associated groups of couples. A similar, but less elaborate, three-stage account has been proposed by Connolly, Craig, Goldberg, and Pepler (2004). First, adolescents engage in affiliative activities in a group context (e.g., go to dances and parties). Second, they begin to go out on a "date" with someone as part of a group. Finally, they begin to form dyadic romantic relationships.

Empirical findings on heterosexual adolescents are generally in accord with these models. Prior to adolescence, interactions typically occur with peers of the same gender, and most friendship pairs are of the same gender (Rubin, Bukowski, & Parker, 2006).

Early adolescents think more about members of the other gender, although mixed-gender interactions do not usually occur often until later (Blyth, Hill, & Thiel, 1982; Richards et al., 1998). Consistent with Dunphy's (1963) model, the number of close other-gender friends is predictive of having a larger other-gender network, which is in turn predictive of establishing a romantic relationship (Connolly, Furman, & Konarski, 2000). Although popular adolescents generally date more frequently than other adolescents (Franzoi, Davis, & Vasquez-Suson, 1994), the percentage of adolescents who report having a romantic relationship increases across adolescence (Carver et al., 2003). For example, 36% of 13-year-olds, 53% of 15-year-olds, and 70% of 17-year-olds report having had a "special" romantic relationship in the last 18 months. The proportions are even higher with more inclusive definitions of romantic relationships (e.g., dating, spending time or going out with someone for a month or longer; Furman & Hand, 2006).

Less is known about the developmental course of the romantic experiences of gay, lesbian, and bisexual youth. Approximately 93% of sexual-minority adolescent boys report having had some same-sex activity, and 85% of sexual-minority adolescent girls report having had some same-sex activity (Savin-Williams & Diamond, 2000). Same-gender dating may be uncommon in locations where there are fewer potential partners or fewer who are openly identified as gay, lesbian or bisexual (Diamond et al., 1999), but the number of romantic relationships is comparable to the number for heterosexual youth for those who are involved in organizations for sexual minorities (Diamond & Lucas, 2004). Gender variations are marked. Approximately 42% of girls and 79% of boys report some sexual activity with a member of the other sex (D'Augelli, 1998), and the majority of sexual-minority youth report dating members of the other sex (Savin-Williams, 1996). Such dating can provide either a cover for a minority sexual identity or help to clarify one's identity (Diamond et al., 1999). Finally, the average age of having a "serious" same-gender relationship is 18 years (Floyd & Stein, 2002).

These statistics provide an incomplete picture, however, because substantial variability exists in the timing and sequencing of different experiences. For example, most sexual-minority adolescent males were first sexually rather than emotionally attracted to a male, whereas sexual-minority adolescent females were evenly divided between first having had an emotional or sexual attraction to another female. Boys' same-gender sexual contact was most commonly with a friend, whereas girls' same-gender relationships were with a romantic partner (Savin-Williams & Diamond, 2000). The trajectories and sequencing of experiences also vary substantially within gender (Floyd & Stein, 2002).

A cautionary note is that one's sexual identity and the gender of the person to whom one is attracted can be quite fluid and change over time, especially for women (Diamond, 2000, 2003). In fact, it is important to recognize that same-gender attraction, sexual behavior, and identity do not perfectly correlate with one another (Savin-Williams, 2006). Thus, estimates of the prevalence of homosexuality can range from 1 to 21%, depending upon the definition. Such variability underscores the idea that no simple dichotomy exists between heterosexuality and homosexuality.

Relationship Content, Quality, and Cognitions

In the preceding section, we described common developmental changes in the degree of involvement in romantic experiences and the social context in which such relationships occur (e.g., group dating vs. dyadic dating). Developmental changes also occur in the content and quality of romantic relationships, as do the perceived benefits to the people involved. Consistent with the proposal that relationships are initially affiliation-based (Connolly & Goldberg, 1999; Furman & Wehner, 1994), middle adolescents most commonly report companionship to be the advantage of having a boyfriend or girlfriend (Feiring, 1996), whereas late adolescents and young adults emphasize the possibility of having a special relationship, perhaps one that can become a permanent partnership (Levesque, 1993). Late adolescents also mention companionship and excitement less frequently as advantages (Shulman & Scharf, 2000). On the other hand, attachment, caregiving, and intimacy become more salient in late adolescence or early adulthood. Perceptions of support increase with age (Furman & Buhrmester, 1992), as do interdependence and closeness between romantic partners (Laursen & Williams, 1997; Zimmer-Gembeck, 1999). Adolescents begin to use peers, including romantic partners, as a safe haven, and subsequently as a secure base (Hazan & Zeifman, 1994). Only long-term romantic partners and friends, however, are likely to serve as secure bases (Fraley & Davis, 1997; Hazan & Zeifman, 1994).

Coexisting with these normative transformations within and between relationships are important signs of convergence of cognitions about differing types of relationships. Specifically, representations of parent–adolescent relationships, friendships and romantic relationships are interrelated, and appear to become more interrelated with age (cf. Furman, Simon, Shaffer, & Bouchey, 2002). Perhaps the growing importance of romantic relationships makes the common relationship properties across types of relationships more apparent than before.

With respect to emotions associated with romantic experiences, other-gender peers are the most common source of positive affect for heterosexual youth (Wilson-Shockley, 1985, as cited in Larson, Clore, & Wood, 1999). Such positive emotions are especially likely to occur when socializing on weekend nights with a romantic partner or several other-gender peers (Larson & Richards, 1998). The amount of time spent with other-gender peers and romantic partners in particular increases over the course of adolescence (Laursen & Williams, 1997; Richards et al., 1998).

Emotional feelings of love also seem to change developmentally. In particular, as they get older, adolescents report that they first fell in love at a later age, suggesting that their definition of love has changed (Montgomery & Sorell, 1998; Shulman & Scharf, 2000). Some earlier infatuations or "puppy loves" may no longer be considered true loves, even though they were significant at the time.

As romantic experiences become common, the risks associated with them also increase. Physical and relational aggression by romantic partners increases from early to middle adolescence (Halpern, Oslak, Young, Martin, & Kupper, 2001; Pepler et al., 2006). Similarly, sexual harassment of both same- and other-gender peers increases over early adolescence; these higher levels persist in middle adolescence (McMaster, Connolly, Pepler, & Craig, 2002; Pepler et al., 2006). Finally, sexual victimization is also relatively common throughout much of adolescence, with estimates for girls ranging from 14 to 43% (Hickman, Jaycox, & Aronoff, 2004).

Individual Differences in Romantic Experiences

Individual differences in romantic relationship experiences typically are embedded in experiences in both current close relationships and the history of close relationships that each participant brings to them. The contributions of family and peer relationships to individual differences are especially evident from research on the development of romantic relationship quality, and the cognitive and emotional features of relationships

(Zimmer-Gembeck, Siebenbruner, & Collins, 2001, 2004). For example, the cognitive and behavioral syndrome known as "rejection sensitivity" is believed to arise from experiences of rejection from parents, peers, and, possibly, romantic partners. Rejection sensitivity in turn predicts expectancies of rejection that correlate strongly with both actual rejection and lesser satisfaction in adolescent relationships (Downey, Bonica, & Rincón, 1999). Two strands of literature focus, respectively, on relationships with peers and relationships with parents as significant forerunners of variations in romantic experiences during adolescence.

Relationships with Peers

The potential role of friends in the development of romantic relationships is both fundamental and multifaceted. Friendships and romantic relationships share common ground in that both are voluntary, and relationships with friends function both as prototypes of interactions compatible with romantic relationships and as testing grounds for experiencing and managing emotions in the context of voluntary close relationships (Connolly et al., 2004; Feiring, 1996; Furman, 1999; McNelles & Connolly, 1999; Shulman, Laursen, Kalman, & Karpovsky, 1997; Shulman, Levy-Shiff, Kedem, & Alon, 1997). Friends also serve as models and sources of social support for initiating and pursuing romantic relationships, and for weathering periods of difficulty in them, thus potentially contributing to variations in the qualities of later romantic relationships (Connolly & Goldberg, 1999; Shulman, Levy-Shiff, et al., 1997). The fact that almost half of best friends are romantic partners, from a developmental perspective, is unsurprising (Hendrick & Hendrick, 1993).

Research findings, though not yet extensive, have confirmed the relevance of friendship to individual differences in romantic relationships. Cognitive representations of friendships and the perceived qualities and patterns of interactions in friendships, are associated significantly with corresponding characteristics of romantic relationships (Connolly et al., 2000; Furman & Shomaker, in press; Furman et al., 2002). Hostile talk about women with friends is predictive of later aggression toward female partners (Capaldi, Dishion, Stoolmiller, & Yoerger, 2001).

Less is known about the links between romantic experiences and other aspects of peer relations. Having a larger number of other-sex friends in one's network is linked to dating both currently and in the future (Connolly et al., 2000; Connolly & Johnson, 1996; Kuttler & La Greca, 2004). Those who are liked by many of their peers (i.e., popular and controversial adolescents) date more frequently (Franzoi et al., 1994). Social competence with friends and peers is also a reliable forerunner of romantic relationship involvement in early and middle adolescence, and of romantic relationship quality in early adulthood (Neeman, Hubbard, & Masten, 1985).

Relatively little is known about the links between sexual minorities' peer relationships and romantic relationships. Those who have had more romantic relationships worry more about losing friends, although the size of the network is not predictive of the number of romantic relationships (Diamond & Lucas, 2004).

Relationships with Parents

The unquestionable importance of peers does not preclude other influences on the development of romantic relationships. Parent–adolescent relationships contribute to behavioral, cognitive, and emotional patterns that have been linked to later behavior with romantic partners. Secure working models of parents are linked to early adults' capacity for romantic intimacy (Mayseless & Scharf, 2007), whereas avoidant styles are linked to less positive romantic relationships (N. Collins, Cooper, Albino, & Allard, 2002). Nurturant–involved parenting in adolescence is predictive of warmth, support, and low hostility toward romantic partners in early adulthood (Conger, Cui, Bryant, & Elder, 2000; Donnellan, Larsen-Rife, & Conger, 2005). Similarly, the degree of flexible control, cohesion, and respect for privacy experienced in families is related positively to intimacy in late-adolescent romantic relationships, with especially strong links emerging for women (Feldman, Gowen, & Fisher, 1998). Parent–adolescent conflict resolution is also associated with later conflict resolution with romantic partners (Zimmer-Gembeck et al., 2001).

By contrast, unskilled parenting and aversive family communications are predictive of aggression toward romantic partners in late adolescence (Andrews, Foster, Capaldi, & Hops, 2000; Capaldi & Clark, 1998). Similarly, the degree of negative emotionality in parent–adolescent dyads is predictive of negative emotionality and poor quality interactions with romantic partners in early adulthood (Conger et al., 2000; Kim, Conger, Lorenz, & Elder, 2001; Overbeek, Stattin, Vermulst, Ha, & Engels, 2007). In fact, parenting style in adolescence contributed more substantially to the quality of early adult romantic relationships than did either sibling relationships or the models provided by parents' own relationships (Conger et al., 2000). Family stress and family separation are also risk factors for early romantic involvement (Connolly, Taradash, & Williams, 2001), which is in turn associated with poor adjustment (Aro & Taipale, 1987; Cauffman & Steinberg, 1996; Grinder, 1966; Neeman et al., 1985). The quality of these apparently compensatory early involvements, however, is typically poorer than that of romantic relationships for youth with more beneficent family histories (W. Collins & Van Dulmen, 2006).

A growing number of studies have documented connections between even earlier parent–child relationships and romantic relationships. The history of parent–child relationships in infancy and early childhood significantly predicts the stability and quality of adolescent and young adult romantic relationships (W. Collins & Sroufe, 1999; Simpson, Collins, Tran, & Haydon, 2007). Closeness to parents in childhood is even a forerunner of long-term effects on relationship satisfaction in adulthood and marital stability (e.g., Belt & Abidine, 1996). Thus, a critical mass of findings now implicates familial experiences in childhood and adolescence in the foundations of romantic experiences in the second and third decades of life.

Networks of Relationships

Research that simultaneously examines the contributions of relationships with both parents and peers to adolescent romantic experiences is at a relatively early stage. Similarly, few investigations have examined how all three forms of relationships are linked to development or adjustment, although the number of interesting and potentially important scientific questions that may be addressed by such research attests to the significance of the topic.

The importance of multiple social relationships is apparent in research on social contacts, both human and infrahuman (Reis et al., 2000). Varied relationship partners provide distinctive benefits (Hartup, 1993; Laursen & Bukowski, 1997). Typical exchanges within each of these types of dyads differ accordingly. In comparison to childhood relationships, the diminished distance and greater intimacy in adolescents' peer relationships may both satisfy affiliative needs and contribute to socialization for relations among equals. Intimacy with parents provides nurturance and support but may be less important than friendships for socialization to roles and expectations in late adolescence and early adulthood (W. Collins & Laursen, 2004; Laursen & Bukowski, 1997).

Although each type of relationship is distinct, their features and benefits overlap (Hartup, 1993; Laursen & Bukowski, 1997). Moreover, as the preceding sections illustrate, the links between qualities of friendships and romantic relationships, as well as family and romantic relationships, are equally impressive (W. Collins, Hennighausen, Schmit, & Sroufe, 1997). Because the peer and family domains are linked and often similar in nature, family and peer influences may act in concert with one another (Laursen, Furman, & Mooney, 2006). For example, both a stable family life and a nondeviant peer group reduce the likelihood that a high school youth will have an antisocial partner in early adulthood (Quinton, Pickles, Maughan, & Rutter, 1993). Additionally, family and peer influences may moderate each other; for example, parental support is associated with a reduction in criminality for those without a romantic partner, but the support of a partner is the more important factor for those with a romantic partner (Meeus, Branje, & Overbeek, 2004). Similarly, young adults who make the transition from best friend to romantic partner as the primary intimate relationship show increased and more stable commitment to their partner and display fewer emotional problems (Meeus, Branje, van der Valk, & de Wied, 2007).

The nature and processes of these developmentally significant interrelations of relationships promise to become an increasingly prominent focus of future research. In a recent essay, W. Collins and Laursen (2004, p. 59) proposed that "affiliations with friends, romantic partners, siblings, and parents unfold along varied and somewhat discrete trajectories for most of the second decade of life and then coalesce during the early 20s into integrated interpersonal structures." The initial differentiation process is essential to a range of adolescent developmental achievements—autonomy, individuation, identity, and sexuality—in appropriately distinct settings, whereas the coalescing relationships of the third and fourth decades of life undergird the psychic and social integration that support adult functioning. In this perspective, romantic relationships are not merely reflections of the impact of parent and peer relationships, but are integral to systems in which all three types of relationships mutually influence one another and jointly contribute to developmental outcomes (for a recent example, see Beyers & Seiffge-Krenke, 2007).

Personal Characteristics

Although some researchers have examined the role relationships with peers and parents play in romantic experiences, surprisingly few have looked at how the characteristics of the adolescent are related to romantic experiences. Initial findings imply that adolescent relationships parallel adult relationships in the relevance of individual partners' self-esteem, self-confidence, and physical attractiveness to romantic experiences (e.g., Connolly & Konarski, 1994; Pearce, Boergers, & Prinstein, 2002).

One topic that has received significant attention is the links between psychosocial adjustment and romantic experience. Social competence is related to dating and romantic experience (Furman et al., 2007; Neeman et al., 1985; Davies & Windle, 2000). On the other hand, alcohol and drug use, poor academic performance, externalizing and internalizing symptoms, poor emotional health, and poor job competence are also linked to romantic experience, especially in early adolescence (Aro & Taipale, 1987; Davies &

Windle, 2000; Furman et al., 2007; Thomas & Hsui, 1993). The mixed nature of these correlates may reflect the fact that romantic experiences are embedded in the peer social world, and thus linked to both peer competence and risky behavior. Much of the literature, however, is cross-sectional; thus, it may reflect the effects of romantic experience on adjustment rather than the reverse. In fact, dating or romantic experience in late childhood and early adolescence is predictive of subsequent misconduct and poor academic performance (Neeman et al., 1985); Romantic experience is linked to depression for some youth, such as those with a preoccupied attachment style (Davila, Steinberg, Kachadourian, Cobb, & Fincham, 2004) or those engaging in casual sex (Grello, Welsh, Harper, & Dickson, 2003).

Most of this literature has focused on the amount of romantic experience (or, in some cases, simply whether one has begun dating). Much less is known about the links with other dimensions of romantic experiences. Negative romantic interactions are, however, predictive of depression (La Greca & Harrison, 2005). In fact, a romantic breakup is one of the strongest predictors of depression, suicide attempts, and suicide completions (Brent et al., 1993; Joyner & Udry, 2000; Monroe, Rohde, Seeley, & Lewinsohn, 1999). In one of the few studies to examine multiple dimensions simultaneously, Zimmer-Gembeck et al. (2001) found psychosocial adjustment to be related differently to romantic experience, overinvolvement, and the quality of romantic relationships. Clearly, future studies need to pay greater attention to the different dimensions of romantic relationships and experience.

Future Directions

Research on adolescent romantic relationships and experiences has made great strides in the last decade, yet it is evident that much work remains to be done. Three topics warranting particular attention are partner characteristics, similarities and differences between romantic relationships and other relationships, and the role of context.

Partner Characteristics

Partner characteristics, one of the five features of W. Collins's (2003) framework of romantic experiences, play a still unspecified role in the significance of romantic relationships in adolescent development. Adolescents report that they would like partners who are intelligent, interpersonally skillful, and physically appealing (Regan & Joshi, 2003; Roscoe et al., 1987). Girls tend to have slightly older partners, whereas boys tend to have similar-age partners (Carver et al., 2003); partners are usually similar in race, ethnicity, and other demographic characteristics (Carver et al., 2003; Furman & Simon, 2008). Similarity also exists in attractiveness, adjustment, and peer network characteristics (see Furman & Simon, 2008). Although these studies provide information about what the partner, or desired partner, is like, we know much less about the influence of the partner on the relationship. Only a few studies have examined adolescent couples' interactions, which would provide a means of identifying the potential influence of partner characteristics on romantic relationships (see Furman & Simon, 2006; Galliher, Welsh, Rostosky, & Kawaguchi, 2004; Harper & Welsh, 2007).

In a related vein, a number of studies have examined the links between peer relations or parent–child relationships and romantic experiences, but we know surprisingly little about the influence of romantic relationships on subsequent romantic experiences. Self-reports of the quality of adolescents' relationships with different romantic partners are moderately consistent (Connolly et al., 2000; Seiffge-Krenke, 2003); otherwise, we do not know how much carryover occurs from one adolescent romantic relationship to the next, or how much a new partner may lead to a different experience.

Romantic Relationships and Other Peer Relationships

As described in a prior section, qualities of relationships with peers are predictive of the quality of relationships with romantic partners, but relatively little is known about the similarities and differences in the characteristics of friendships and heterosexual romantic relationships. In early and middle adolescence, same-gender friendships are perceived to be more supportive and intimate than heterosexual romantic partners (Furman & Buhrmester, 1992). Perceptions of the frequency of conflict are similar (Furman & Buhrmester, 1992; Laursen, 1995), although observed rates of conflict in interactions are greater in heterosexual romantic relationships (Furman & Shomaker, in press). Observed affective responsiveness and dyadic positivity are also less in romantic relationships (Furman & Shomaker, in press).

Even less is known about the similarities and differences between other-gender friendships and heterosexual romantic relationships. Early adolescents report that other-gender friendships are primarily characterized by affiliation, whereas romantic relationships are marked by intimacy and passion as well (Connolly, Craig, Goldberg, & Pepler, 1999). Middle adolescents report that companionship, support, and emotional and physical intimacy are more commonly benefits of romantic relationships than of other-gender friendships (Hand & Furman, in press). By contrast, other-gender friendships are more commonly seen as a means of learning about other-gender peers; adolescents may believe that they are expected to know about the other gender when interacting with a romantic partner. With regard to costs, romantic relationships are often seen as limiting autonomy, whereas other-gender friendships can be confusing.

These initial findings are intriguing, but it is important to obtain more information about the similarities and differences in different peer relations as a window into understanding the functions of different relationships in the broad social network. It would be particularly valuable to examine the relationships of sexual-minority youth, both for the sake of inclusiveness and because empirical evidence would help to separate out the influences of relationship type and gender of partner.

Some other forms of seemingly related peer relationships also have been relatively neglected. For instance, passionate friendships have been described as having the emotional intensity of romantic relationships but lacking the sexual activity (Diamond, 1998; Diamond et al., 1999). Such relationships are believed to be particularly significant in the experiences of lesbians and perhaps gay youth (Savin-Williams & Diamond, 2000). Additionally, relatively little is known about "friends with benefits," in which two peers periodically engage in casual sex, without a monogamous relationship or any kind of commitment.

Context

Previously, we noted the absence of research on romantic experiences in different cultures. In fact, relatively little work has examined the role of contextual factors in general. A limited amount of work has examined romantic relationships of African American youth (e.g., Giordano, Manning, & Longmore, 2005); even less is known about other ethnic groups' romantic or interracial relationships (Vaquera & Kao, 2005). Similarly, we know surprisingly little about romantic experiences in rural settings, the role of local neighborhood or community norms, or religious values. The absence of work on contextual factors is particularly ironic, because it is obvious that romantic experiences, especially in adolescence, are strongly influenced by such factors.

A Final Note

As the preceding comments suggest, what we have learned has been based on a relatively select group of adolescents who do not fully represent the range of romantic experiences. Much of the existing work has only examined romantic relationships, and we know less about how these relationships fit into adolescents' social world and overall experiences. Addressing these issues will provide us a more complete picture of adolescent romantic experiences.

Acknowledgments

Preparation of this chapter was supported by Grant No. HD049080 (Wyndol Furman, Principal Investigator) and Grant No. HD 054850 (W. Andrew Collins, Principal Investigator) from the National Institute of Child Health and Human Development.

References

Ainsworth, M. S. (1989). Attachments beyond infancy. *American Psychologist, 44*, 709–716.

Allen, J. P., & Land, D. (1999). Attachment in adolescence. In J. Cassidy & P. R. Shaver (Eds.), *Handbook of attachment: Theory, research, and clinical applications* (pp. 319–335). New York: Guilford Press.

Andrews, J. A., Foster, S. L., Capaldi, D., & Hops, H. (2000). Adolescent and family predictions of physical aggression, communication, and satisfaction in young adult couples: A prospective analysis. *Journal of Consulting and Clinical Psychology, 68*, 195–208.

Aro, H., & Taipale, V. (1987). The impact of timing of puberty on psychosomatic symptoms among fourteen- to sixteen-year-old Finnish girls. *Child Development, 58*, 261–269.

Baumeister, R. F., & Leary, M. R. (1995). The need to belong: Desire for interpersonal attachments as a fundamental human motivation. *Psychological Bulletin, 117*, 497–529.

Belt, W., & Abidine, R. R. (1996). The relation of childhood abuse and early parenting experiences to current marital quality in a non-clinical sample. *Child Abuse and Neglect, 20*, 1019–1030.

Beyers, W., & Seiffge-Krenke, I. (2007). Are friends and romantic partners the "best medicine"?: How the quality of other close relations mediates the impact of changing family relationships on adjustment. *International Journal of Behavioral Development, 31*, 439–448.

Blyth, D. A., Hill, J. P., & Thiel, K. S. (1982). Early adolescents' significant others: Grade and gender differences in perceived relationships with familial and nonfamilial adults and young people. *Journal of Youth and Adolescence, 11*, 425–449.

Brent, D. A., Perper, J. A., Moritz, G., Baugher, M., Roth, C., Balach, L., et al. (1993). Stressful life events, psychopathology, and adolescent suicide: A case–control study. *Suicide and Life-Threatening Behavior, 23*, 179–187.

Brown, B. B., Feiring, C., & Furman, W. (1999). Missing the love boat: Why researchers have shied away from adolescent romance. In W. Furman, B. B. Brown, & C. Feiring (Eds.), *The develop-ment of romantic relationships in adolescence* (pp. 1–16). New York: Cambridge University Press.

Brown, B. B., Larson, R. W., & Saraswathi, T. I. (Eds.). (2002). *The world's youth: Adolescence in eight regions of the globe.* Cambridge, UK: Cambridge University Press.

Capaldi, D. M., & Clark, S. (1998). Prospective family predictors of aggression toward female part-ners for at-risk young men. *Developmental Psychology, 34,* 1175–1188.

Capaldi, D. M., Dishion, T. J., Stoolmiller, M., & Yoerger, K. (2001). Aggression toward female part-ners by at-risk young men. *Developmental Psychology, 37,* 61–73.

Capaldi, D., Shortt, J., & Kim, H. (2005). A life span developmental systems perspective on aggres-sion toward a partner. In W. M. Pinsof & J. L. Lebow (Eds.), *Family psychology: The art of the science* (pp. 141–167). New York: Oxford University Press.

Carver, K., Joyner, K., & Udry, J. R. (2003). National estimates of adolescent romantic relationships. In P. Florsheim (Ed.), *Adolescent romantic relationships and sexual behavior: Theory, research, and practical implications* (pp. 291–329). New York: Cambridge University Press.

Cauffman, E., & Steinberg, L. (1996). Interactive effects of menarcheal status and dating on diet and disordered eating among adolescent girls. *Developmental Psychology, 32,* 631–635.

Collins, N., Cooper, M., Albino, A., & Allard, L. (2002). Psychosocial vulnerability from adolescence to adulthood: A prospective study of attachment style differences in relationship functioning and partner choice. *Journal of Personality, 70,* 965–1008.

Collins, W. A. (2003). More than myth: The developmental significance of romantic relationships during adolescence. *Journal of Research on Adolescence, 13,* 1–25.

Collins, W. A., Hennighausen, K. H., Schmit, D. T., & Sroufe, L. A. (1997). Developmental precur-sors of romantic relationships: A longitudinal analysis. In S. Shulman & W. A. Collins (Eds.), *Romantic relationships in adolescence: Developmental perspectives* (pp. 69–84). San Francisco: Jossey-Bass.

Collins, W. A., & Laursen, B. (2004). Changing relationships, changing youth: Interpersonal con-texts of adolescent development. *Journal of Early Adolescence, 24,* 55–62.

Collins, W. A., & Sroufe, L. A. (1999). Capacity for intimate relationships: A developmental con-struction. In W. Furman, C. Feiring, & B. B. Brown (Eds.), *Contemporary perspectives on adoles-cent romantic relationships* (pp. 123–147). New York: Cambridge University Press.

Collins, W. A., & Van Dulmen, M. (2006). "The course of true love(s) … ": Origins and pathways in the development of romantic relationships. In A. Booth & A. Crouter (Eds.), *Romance and sex in adolescence and emerging adulthood: Risks and opportunities* (pp. 63–86). Mahwah, NJ: Erlbaum.

Conger, R. D., Cui, M., Bryant, C. M., & Elder, G. H., Jr. (2000). Competence in early adult roman-tic relationships: A developmental perspective on family influences. *Journal of Personality and Social Psychology, 79,* 224–237.

Connolly, J., Craig, W., Goldberg, A., & Pepler, D. (1999). Conceptions of cross-sex friendships and romantic relationships in early adolescence. *Journal of Youth and Adolescence, 28,* 481–494.

Connolly, J., Craig, W., Goldberg, A., & Pepler, D. (2004). Mixed-gender groups, dating, and roman-tic relationships in early adolescence. *Journal of Research in Adolescence, 14,* 185–207.

Connolly, J., Furman, W., & Konarski, R. (2000). The role of peers in the emergence of hetero-sexual romantic relationships in adolescence. *Child Development, 71,* 1395–1408.

Connolly, J. A., & Goldberg, A. (1999). Romantic relationships in adolescence: The role of friends and peers in their emergence and development. In W. Furman, B. B. Brown, & C. Feiring (Eds.), *The development of romantic relationships in adolescence* (pp. 266–290). New York: Cam-bridge University Press.

Connolly, J. A., & Johnson, A. M. (1996). Adolescents' romantic relationships and the structure and quality of their close interpersonal ties. *Personal Relationships, 3,* 185–195.

Connolly, J. A., & Konarski, R. (1994). Peer self-concept in adolescence: Analysis of factor structure and of associations with peer experience. *Journal of Research on Adolescence, 4,* 385–403.

Connolly, J. A., Taradash, A., & Williams, T. (2001). *Dating and sexual activities of Canadian boys and girls in early adolescence: Normative patterns and biopsychosocial risks for early onset of heterosexuality* [Working paper series]. Applied Research Branch of Strategic Policy, Human Resources Development Canada, Toronto.

Crouter, A., & Booth, A. (2006). *Romance and sex in adolescence and emerging adulthood: Risks and opportunities.* Mahwah, NJ: Erlbaum.

D'Augelli, A. R. (1998). Lesbian, gay, and bisexual youth and their families: Disclosure of sexual orientation and its consequences. *American Journal of Orthopsychiatry, 68*, 361–371.

Davies, P. T., & Windle, M. (2000). Middle adolescents' dating pathways and psychosocial adjustment. *Merrill–Palmer Quarterly, 46*, 90–118.

Davila, J., Steinberg, S., Kachadourian, L., Cobb, R., & Fincham, F. (2004). Romantic involvement and depressive symptoms in early and late adolescence: The role of a preoccupied relational style. *Personal Relationships, 11*, 161–178.

Diamond, L. M. (1998). Development of sexual orientation among adolescent and adult young women. *Developmental Psychology, 34*, 1085–1095.

Diamond, L. M. (2000). Passionate friendships among adolescent sexual-minority women. *Journal of Research on Adolescence, 10*, 191–209.

Diamond, L. M. (2003). Was it a phase?: Young women's relinquishment of lesbian/bisexual identities over a 5-year period. *Journal of Personality and Social Psychology, 84*, 352–364.

Diamond, L. M., & Lucas, S. (2004). Sexual-minority and heterosexual youths' peer relationships: Experiences, expectations, and implications for well-being. *Journal of Research on Adolescence, 14*, 313–340.

Diamond, L. M., Savin-Williams, R. C., & Dubé, E. M. (1999). Sex, dating, passionate friendships, and romance: Intimate peer relations among lesbian, gay, and bisexual adolescents. In W. Furman, B. B. Brown, & C. Feiring (Eds.), *The development of romantic relationships in adolescence* (pp. 175–210). Cambridge, UK: Cambridge University Press.

Donnellan, M., Larsen-Rife, D., & Conger, R. (2005). Personality, family history, and competence in early adult romantic relationships. *Journal of Personality and Social Psychology, 88*, 562–576.

Downey, G., Bonica, C., & Rincón, C. (1999). Rejection sensitivity and adolescent romantic relationships. In W. Furman, B. B. Brown, & C. Feiring (Eds.), *The development of romantic relationships in adolescence* (pp. 148–174). New York: Cambridge University Press.

Dunphy, D. C. (1963). The social structure of urban adolescent peer groups. *Sociometry, 26*, 230–246.

Feiring, C. (1996). Concepts of romance in 15-year-old adolescents. *Journal of Research on Adolescence, 6*, 181–200.

Feldman, S., Gowen, L. K., & Fisher, L. (1998). Family relationships and gender as predictors of romantic intimacy in young adults: A longitudinal study. *Journal of Research on Adolescence, 8*, 263–286.

Florsheim, P. (2003). *Adolescent romantic relations and sexual behavior: Theory, research, and practical implications.* Mahwah, NJ: Erlbaum.

Floyd, F. J., & Stein, T. S. (2002). Sexual orientation identity formation among gay, lesbian, and bisexual youths: Multiple patterns of milestone. *Journal of Research on Adolescence, 12*, 167–191.

Fraley, R. C., & Davis, K. E. (1997). Attachment formation and transfer in young adolescents' close friendships and romantic relationships. *Personal Relationships, 4*, 131–144.

Franzoi, S. L., Davis, M. H., & Vasquez-Suson, K. A. (1994). Two social worlds: Social correlates and stability of adolescent status groups. *Journal of Personality and Social Psychology, 67*, 462–473.

Furman, W. (1999). Friends and lovers: The role of peer relationships in adolescent romantic relationships. In W. A. Collins & B. Laursen (Eds.), *Relationships as developmental contexts: The 30th Minnesota Symposia on Child Development* (pp. 133–154). Hillsdale, NJ: Erlbaum.

Furman, W. (2002). The emerging field of adolescent romantic relationships. *Current Directions in Psychological Science, 11*(5), 177–180.

Furman, W., Brown, B. B., & Feiring, C. (Eds.). (1999). *The development of romantic relationships in adolescence.* New York: Cambridge University Press.

Furman, W., & Buhrmester, D. (1992). Age and sex differences in perceptions of networks of personal relationships. *Child Development, 63*, 103–115.

Furman, W., & Hand, L. S. (2006). The slippery nature of romantic relationships: Issues in definition and differentiation. In A. Crouter & A. Booth (Eds.) *Romance and sex in adolescence and emerging adulthood: Risks and opportunities* (pp. 171–178). Mahwah, NJ: Erlbaum.

Furman, W., Ho, M. H., & Low, S. M. (2007). The rocky road of adolescent romantic experience: Dating and adjustment. In R. C. M. E. Engels, M. Kerr, & H. Stattin (Eds.), *Friends, lovers, and groups: Key relationships in adolescence* (pp. 61–80). New York: Wiley.

Furman, W., & Shaffer, L. (2003). The role of romantic relationships in adolescent development. In P. Florsheim (Ed.), *Adolescent romantic relations and sexual behavior: Theory, research, and practical implications* (pp. 3–22). Mahwah, NJ: Erlbaum.

Furman, W., & Shomaker, L. (in press). Patterns of interaction in adolescent romantic relationships: Distinct features and associations with other close relationships. *Journal of Adolescence.*

Furman, W., & Simon, V. A. (2006). Actor and partner effects of adolescents' working models and styles on interactions with romantic partners. *Child Development, 77*, 588–604.

Furman, W., & Simon, V. A. (2008). Homophily in adolescent romantic relationships. In M. J. Prinstein & K. A. Dodge (Eds.) *Understanding peer influence in children and adolescents* (pp. 203–224). New York: Guilford Press.

Furman, W., Simon, V. A., Shaffer, L., & Bouchey, H. A. (2002). Adolescents' working models and styles for relationships with parents, friends, and romantic partners. *Child Development, 73*, 241–255.

Furman W., & Wehner, E. A. (1994). Romantic views: Toward a theory of adolescent romantic relationships. In R. Montemayor, G. R. Adams, & G. P. Gullota (Eds.), *Advances in adolescent development: Vol. 6. Relationships during adolescence* (pp. 168–175). Thousand Oaks, CA: Sage.

Galliher, R. V., Welsh, D. P., Rostosky, S. S., & Kawaguchi, M. C. (2004). Interaction and relationship quality in late adolescent romantic couples. *Journal of Social and Personal Relationships, 21*, 203–216.

Giordano, P., Manning, W., & Longmore, M. (2005). The romantic relationships of African-American and white adolescents. *Sociological Quarterly, 46*, 545–568.

Giordano, P., Manning, W., & Longmore, M. (2006). Adolescent romantic relationships: An emerging portrait of their nature and developmental significance. In A. Crouter & A. Booth (Eds.), *Romance and sex in adolescence and emerging adulthood: Risks and opportunities* (pp. 127–150). Mahwah, NJ: Erlbaum.

Grello, C., Welsh, D., Harper, M., & Dickson, J. (2003). Dating and sexual relationship trajectories and adolescent functioning. *Adolescent and Family Health, 3*, 103–112.

Grinder, R. E. (1966). Relations of social dating attractions to academic orientation and peer relations. *Journal of Educational Psychology, 57*, 27–34.

Halpern, C. T., Oslak, S. G., Young, M. L., Martin, S. L., & Kupper, L. L. (2001). Partner violence among adolescents in opposite-sex romantic relationships: Findings from the National Longitudinal Study of Adolescent Health. *American Journal of Public Health, 91*, 1679–1685.

Hand, L. S., & Furman, W. (in press). Other-sex friendships in adolescence: Salient features and comparisons to same-sex friendships and romantic relationships. *Social Development.*

Harper, M., & Welsh, D. (2007). Keeping quiet: Self-silencing and its association with relational and individual functioning among adolescent romantic couples. *Journal of Social and Personal Relationships, 24*, 99–116.

Hartup, W. W. (1993). Adolescents and their friends. In B. Laursen (Ed.), *Close friendships in adolescence* (pp. 3–22). San Francisco: Jossey-Bass.

Hazan, C., & Zeifman, D. (1994). Sex and the psychological tether. In K. Bartholomew & D. Perlman (Eds.), *Advances in personal relationships: Vol. 1. Attachment processes in adulthood* (pp. 151–180). London: Jessica Kingsley.

Hendrick, S. S., & Hendrick, C. (1993). Lovers as friends. *Journal of Social and Personal Relationships, 10*, 459–466.

Hickman, L. J., Jaycox, L. H., & Aronoff, J. (2004). Dating violence among adolescents: Prevalence, gender distribution, and prevention program effectiveness. *Trauma, Violence and Abuse, 5,* 123–142.

Jankowiak, W. R., & Fischer, E. F. (1992). A cross-cultural perspective on romantic love. *Ethos, 31,* 149–156.

Joyner, K., & Udry, J. R. (2000). You don't bring me anything but down: Adolescent romance and depression. *Journal of Health and Social Behavior, 41,* 369–391.

Kelley, H. H., Berscheid, E., Christensen, A., Harvey, J. H., Huston, T. L., Levinger, G., et al. (2002). *Close relationships.* Clinton Corners, NY: Percheron Press. (Original work published 1983)

Kenny, D. A., Kashy, D. A., & Cook, W. L. (2006). *Dyadic data analysis.* New York: Guilford Press.

Kim, K., Conger, R. D., Lorenz, F. O., & Elder, G. H., Jr. (2001). Parent–adolescent reciprocity in negative affect and its relation to early adult social development. *Developmental Psychology, 37,* 775–790.

Kuttler, A., & La Greca, A. (2004). Linkages among adolescent girls' romantic relationships, best friendships, and peer networks. *Journal of Adolescence, 27,* 395–414.

La Greca, A., & Harrison, H. (2005). Adolescent peer relations, friendships, and romantic relationships: Do they predict social anxiety and depression? *Journal of Clinical Child and Adolescent Psychology, 34,* 49–61.

Larson, R. W., Clore, G. L., & Wood, G. A. (1999). The emotions of romantic relationships: Do they wreck havoc on adolescents? In W. Furman, B. B. Brown, & C. Feiring (Eds.), *The development of romantic relationships in adolescence* (pp. 19–49). Cambridge, UK: Cambridge University Press.

Larson, R. W., & Richards, M. (1998). Waiting for the weekend: Friday and Saturday night as the emotional climax of the week. In A. Crouter & R. Larson (Eds.), *Temporal rhythms in adolescence: Clocks, calendars, and the coordination of daily life.* San Francisco: Jossey-Bass.

Laursen, B. (1995). Conflict and social interaction in adolescent relationships. *Journal of Research on Adolescence, 5,* 55–70.

Laursen, B., & Bukowski, W. M. (1997). A developmental guide to the organization of close relationships. *International Journal of Behavioral Development, 21,* 747–770.

Laursen, B., Furman, W., & Mooney, K. S. (2006). Predicting interpersonal competence and self-worth from adolescent relationships and relationship networks: Variable-centered and person-centered perspectives. *Merrill–Palmer Quarterly, 52,* 572–600.

Laursen, B., & Jensen-Campbell, L. A. (1999). The nature and functions of social exchange in adolescent romantic relationships. In W. Furman, B. B. Brown, & C. Feiring (Eds.), *The development of romantic relationships in adolescence* (pp. 50–74). Cambridge, UK: Cambridge University Press.

Laursen, B., & Williams, V. A. (1997). Perceptions of interdependence and closeness in family and peer relationships among adolescents with and without romantic partners. In S. Shulman & W. A. Collins (Eds.), *Romantic relationships in adolescence: Developmental perspectives* (pp. 3–20). San Francisco: Jossey-Bass.

Levesque, R. J. R. (1993). The romantic experience of adolescents in satisfying love relationships. *Journal of Youth and Adolescence, 22,* 219–251.

Mayseless, O., & Scharf, M. (2007). Adolescents' attachment representations and their capacity for intimacy in close relationships. *Journal of Research on Adolescence, 17,* 23–50.

McMaster, L. E., Connolly, J., Pepler, D., & Craig, W. M. (2002). Peer to peer sexual harassment in early adolescence: A developmental perspective. *Development and Psychopathology, 14,* 91–105.

McNelles, L. R., & Connolly, J. A. (1999). Intimacy between adolescent friends: Age and gender differences in intimate affect and intimate behaviors. *Journal of Research on Adolescence, 9,* 143–159.

Mead, G. H. (1934). *Mind, self, and society from the standpoint of a social behaviorist.* Chicago: University of Chicago Press.

Meeus, W., Branje, S., & Overbeek, G. (2004). Parents and partners in crime: A six-year longitudinal study on changes in supportive relationships and delinquency in adolescence and young adulthood. *Journal of Child Psychology and Psychiatry and Allied Disciplines, 45*, 1288–1298.

Meeus, W. Branje, S., van der Valk, I., & de Wied, M. (2007). Relationships with intimate partner, best friends, and parents in adolescence and early adulthood: A study of the saliency of the intimate partnership. *International Journal of Behavioral Development, 31*, 449–460.

Monroe, S. M., Rohde, P., Seeley, J. R., & Lewinsohn, P. M. (1999). Life events and depression in adolescence: Relationship loss as a prospective risk factor for first onset of major depressive disorder. *Journal of Abnormal Psychology, 108*, 606–614.

Montgomery, M. J., & Sorell, G. T. (1998). Love and dating experience in early and middle adolescence: Grade and gender comparisons *Journal of Adolescence, 21*, 677–689.

Neeman, J., Hubbard, J., & Masten, A. S. (1985). The changing importance of romantic relationship involvement to competence from late childhood to adolescence. *Development and Psychopathology, 7*, 727–750.

Overbeek, G., Stattin, H., Vermulst, A., Ha, T., & Engels, R. (2007). Parent–child relationships, partner relationships, and emotional adjustment: A birth-to-maturity prospective study. *Developmental Psychology, 43*, 429–437.

Pearce, M. J., Boergers, J., & Prinstein, M. J. (2002). Adolescent obesity, overt and relational peer victimization, and romantic relationships. *Obesity Research, 10*, 386–393.

Pepler, D. J., Craig, W. M., Connolly, J. A., Yuile, A., McMaster, L., & Jiang, D. (2006). A developmental perspective on bullying. *Aggressive Behavior, 32*, 376–384.

Quinton, D., Pickles, A., Maughan, B., & Rutter, M. (1993). Partners, peers, and pathways: Assortative pairing and continuities in conduct disorder. *Development and Psychopathology, 5*, 763–783.

Regan, P. C., & Joshi, A. (2003). Ideal partner preferences among adolescents. *Social Behavior and Personality, 31*, 13–20.

Reis, H. T., Collins, W. A., & Berscheid, E. (2000). Relationships in human behavior and development. *Psychological Bulletin, 126*, 844–872.

Richards, M. H., Crowe, P. A., Larson, R., & Swarr, A. (1998). Developmental patterns and gender differences in the experience of peer companionship during adolescence. *Child Development, 69*, 154–163.

Roscoe, B., Diana, M. S., & Brooks, R. H. (1987). Early, middle, and late adolescents' views on dating and factors influencing partner selection. *Adolescence, 22*, 59–68.

Rubin, K. H., Bukowski, W. M., & Parker, J. G. (2006). Peer interactions, relationships, and groups. In W. Damon (Series Ed.) & N. Eisenberg (Vol. Ed.), *Handbook of child psychology: Vol. 3. Social, emotional, and personality development* (6th ed., pp. 571–645). New York: Wiley.

Savin-Williams, R. C. (1996). Dating and romantic relationships among gay, lesbian, and bisexual youths. In R. C. Savin-Williams & K. M. Cohen (Eds.), *The lives of lesbians, gays, and bisexuals: Children to adults* (pp. 166–180). Fort Worth, TX: Harcourt Brace.

Savin-Williams, R. C. (2006). Who's gay? Does it matter? *Current Directions in Psychological Science, 15*, 40–44.

Savin-Williams, R. C., & Diamond, L. M. (2000). Sexual identity trajectories among sexual-minority youths: Gender comparisons. *Archives of Sexual Behavior, 29*, 607–627.

Seiffge-Krenke, I. (2003). Testing theories of romantic development from adolescence to young adulthood: Evidence of a developmental sequence. *International Journal of Behavioral Development, 27*, 519–531.

Shaver, P., & Hazan, C. (1988). A biased overview of the study of love. *Journal of Social and Personal Relationships, 5*, 473–501.

Shulman, S., & Collins, W. A. (Eds.). (1997). Romantic relationships in adolescence: Developmental perspectives. *New directions for child development* (pp. 21–36). San Francisco: Jossey-Bass.

Shulman, S., Laursen, B., Kalman, Z., & Karpovsky, S. (1997). Adolescent intimacy revisited. *Journal of Youth and Adolescence, 26*, 597–617.

Shulman, S., Levy-Shiff, R., Kedem, P., & Alon, E. (1997). Intimate relationships among adolescent romantic partners and same-sex friends: Individual and systemic perspectives. In S. Shulman

& W. A. Collins (Eds.), *New directions for child development: Romantic relationships in adolescence: Developmental perspectives* (No. 78, pp. 37–51). San Francisco: Jossey-Bass.

Shulman, S., & Scharf, M. (2000). Adolescent romantic behaviors and perceptions: Age- and gender-related differences, and links with family and peer relationships. *Journal of Research in Adolescence, 10,* 91–118.

Simpson, J. A., Collins, W. A., Tran, S., & Haydon, K. C. (2007). Attachment and the experience and expression of emotions in romantic relationships: A developmental perspective. *Journal of Personality and Social Psychology, 72*(2), 355–367.

Sroufe, L. A., & Fleeson, J. (1988). The coherence of family relationships. In R. A. Hinde & J. Stevenson-Hinde (Eds.), *Relationships within families: Mutual influences* (pp. 27–47). Oxford, UK: Oxford University Press.

Sullivan, H. S. (1953). *The interpersonal theory of psychiatry.* New York: Norton.

Thomas, B. S., & Hsiu, L. T. (1993). The role of selected risk factors in predicting adolescent drug use and its adverse consequences. *International Journal of the Addictions, 28,* 1549.

Vaquera, E., & Kao, G. (2005). Private and public displays of affection among interracial and intraracial adolescent couples. *Social Science Quarterly, 86,* 484–505.

Waters, E., & Cummings, E. M. (2000). A secure base from which to explore close relationships. *Child Development, 71,* 164–172.

Youniss, J. (1980). *Parents and peers in the social environment: A Sullivan–Piaget perspective.* Chicago: University of Chicago Press.

Zimmer-Gembeck, M. J. (1999). Stability, change and individual differences in involvement with friends and romantic partners among adolescent females. *Journal of Youth and Adolescence, 28,* 419–438.

Zimmer-Gembeck, M. J., Siebenbruner, J., & Collins, W. A. (2001). Diverse aspects of dating: Associations with psychosocial functioning from early to middle adolescence. *Journal of Adolescence, 24,* 313–336.

Zimmer-Gembeck, M. J., Siebenbruner, J., & Collins, W. A. (2004). A prospective study of intraindividual and peer influences on adolescents' heterosexual romantic and sexual behavior. *Archives of Sexual Behavior, 33,* 381–394.

CHAPTER 20

Informal Peer Groups in Middle Childhood and Adolescence

B. BRADFORD BROWN
ERIN L. DIETZ

$\mathbf{A}$s they mature, children face an increasingly complex peer social environment. By the time young people reach middle adolescence in most cultures, both the amount of time spent with peers and the types of relationships they must negotiate have expanded dramatically. Aware of this, scholars have devoted considerable attention to studying peer relationships from middle childhood through adolescence. Yet the bulk of this work focuses on dyadic relationships (especially friendship) or individual characteristics salient to peer interaction (Rubin, Bukowski, & Parker, 2006). Remarkably little attention has been paid to *peer-group* relationships (Cairns, Xie, & Leung, 1998), even though they account for a healthy portion of young people's encounters with and concerns about peers (Crockett, Losoff, & Petersen, 1984), and despite evidence that children behave differently in groups than in dyads (Benenson, Nicholson, & Waite, 2001). In this chapter we focus on research devoted to peer-group interactions from middle childhood through adolescence—roughly, ages 6–18. We consider the theoretical and methodological challenges in pursuing this research, the insights that scholarship has yielded to date, and the types of research that ought to be pursued in the future.

We look explicitly at peer *groups*, recognizable subdivisions of a young person's peer context. One can distinguish between "formal" groups, which are organized by adults and occur in adult-supervised settings (school classrooms, afterschool program participants, sports teams, collectives of youth overseen by religious or community organizations, etc.), and "informal" groups, which are initiated and overseen by young people themselves. Informal groups, which are the subject of this chapter, can further be divided into interaction- and reputation-based collectives of young people. Typically, "interaction-based groups" are relatively small (3–10 people) and identify a group of friends or playmates who engage in activities together; they are often labeled "cliques." "Reputation-based groups," most often referred to as "crowds," refer to larger collections of individuals who share the same image or status among peers, even if they fail to spend much time interacting with each other (Brown, Mory, & Kinney, 1994). Typically, these groups are defined by members' abilities (brains), interests and activities (jocks, skaters, druggies), social status (populars, geeks), and ethnic or socioeconomic backgrounds (Asians, farmers). Because they are not based on interaction, they defy a common defining feature of groups, yet we include them because of their obvious significance in the social experiences of many adolescents.

Informal groups are difficult to study in childhood and adolescence because their boundaries are not fixed and their membership is subject to frequent changes, especially in childhood (Kindermann, 2007). Reputation-based groups are especially problematic because there is only moderate consensus about who belongs to each group (Brown, Lamborn, Mounts, & Steinberg, 1993). Yet both types of groups are central to social interaction patterns and the formation of more easily recognized dyadic relationships (friendships and romantic or sexual alliances).

We do not attend to studies that ask respondents to provide global ratings of their friends in general because of evidence that a young person's friendship network can cut across several interaction- or reputation-based groups; in other words, the global ratings do not refer to a functional group (Kiesner, Poulin, & Nicotra, 2003; Urberg, Degirmencioglu, Tolson, & Halliday-Scher, 1995). We also ignore the large corpus of sociometric studies dealing either with standard sociometric categories (popular, neglected, rejected) or peer ratings on specific behaviors or traits (aggression, bullying, etc.). This work addresses important characteristics of young people within a social context, but the unit of analysis in these studies (typically, a school classroom or grade level) is rarely a meaningful group to the young people being examined. In fact, Rodkin, Farmer, Pearl, and Van Acker (2006) presented evidence that the specific peers identified as high in sociometric status (in their study, regarded as "cool") *differed* among members of different peer groups within a classroom.

In this chapter we first identify the central issues that have occupied researchers' interest in young people's informal peer groups over the past 15 years, then review major theoretical or conceptual frameworks that underlie this corpus of research. Next, we discuss classic studies, as well as more exemplary recent studies of informal peer groups, before turning our attention to key directions for future research.

Central Issues

Much of the research about child and adolescent peer groups can be placed in one of four major domains: issues of definition and measurement, group structure, group functioning, and the impact of membership on individual outcomes. We overview issues in each domain.

Definitions and Measurement

Compared to other aspects of young people's peer relationships, research on peer groups is limited. One reason for this is the lack of consensus among scholars on how to define or measure peer groups. Different definitions or understandings of interaction-based groups are apparent in the four major methods that have been used to identify these collectives. One method is to ask respondents to list all of their closest peer associates within a circumscribed network (most often, a school classroom or grade level), then use various statistical procedures arising from social network analysis (e.g., factor analysis or the Negative Entropy program [NEGOPY]) to identify the most common linkages among network members (e.g., Bagwell, Coie, Terry, & Lochman, 2000). This approach creates cliques that comprise interconnected dyadic friendships. A second method, social-cognitive mapping (SCM; Cairns, Perrin, & Cairns, 1985), involves asking a subset of individuals within a social network to name all the groupings of three or more person who "hang out" together, then generating a co-occurrence matrix to determine which sets of individuals are consistently described by raters. This approach treats peer groups as collectives that routinely interact, regardless of their affective ties (e.g., strength of friendship) with one another.

Studies indicate that the cliques young people identify through SCM correspond substantially with observer ratings of groupings within classrooms (Gest, Farmer, Cairns, & Xie, 2003). Nevertheless, fearing that young people's ratings will be skewed by their biases about certain peers or their inclination to overstate their own status or connections, some investigators prefer to rely on their own observations of peer interactions to identify cliques within the social network (e.g., Eder, 1985). This, too, assumes that peer groups encompass common coparticipants in social interactions but further constrains interactions to what adult observers can see. A final alternative is simply to ask respondents to think about peers who are part of their group and to answer questions on a self-report survey in terms of that group (e.g., Kiesner, Cadinu, Poulin, & Bucci, 2002). The basis of the peer group in these studies is subjective and certainly meaningful to the respondent but unknown to the investigator and probably variable among respondents.

Among studies of larger, reputation-based peer groups ("crowds"), many investigators employ a common definition of the groups, namely, clusters of individuals who display similar behaviors, or who share a common image or reputation among peers, whether or not they commonly interact with each other. In some cases, however, respondents report their crowd affiliation themselves, whereas in other studies, investigators rely upon peer ratings (see Sussman, Pokhrel, Ashmore, & Brown, 2007), and there is evidence that the two methods do not correlate very strongly (Brown, Von Bank, & Steinberg, in press; Urberg, Degirmencioglu, Tolson, & Halliday-Scher, 2000). Moreover, self-ratings sometimes direct respondents to select the group with which they identify the most, and other times, the group with which they would be most closely associated by peers. In some cases, raters or respondents can select just one crowd; in other cases, they can indicate membership in multiple groups.

From a theoretical perspective, it may be reasonable for investigators to maintain these separate methods of identifying peer groups, but they make it difficult to compare findings across studies and to draw meaningful conclusions about the nature of young people's peer-group affiliations and interactions. Even in their recent review of research on young people's peer relations, Rubin et al. (2006) offer two distinct definitions of peer groups, one focusing on the nature of relationships and interactions among group members, and the other emphasizing the capacity of group members to influence each other.

If investigators can reach agreement on the way to define and operationalize peer groups, they can proceed to a more daunting challenge: deriving methods to map peer groups and observe group interaction that can adjust to the changing social context that many young people encounter as they move from middle childhood through adolescence. In many nations, young people move from neighborhood elementary schools, featuring self-contained classrooms, to communitywide secondary schools, requiring hourly shifts to new classrooms and new sets of peers. Entry into community-based activities (e.g., European sports clubs) can also broaden the base for peer-group formation. The emergence of mixed-gender groups and romantic relationships at some point in adolescence further complicates the social network. Classroom based procedures for defining peer groups, especially those that are gender-specific, lose their value and meaning in the face of such transitions, which is certainly one reason for the paucity of studies of clique patterns among middle adolescents. Another is that as the social context from which peer groups are formed expands in size (from the classroom to grade level or school, or from the neighborhood to the community), it strains the capabilities of statistical programs used to identify groups.

Peer-Group Structure

Beyond efforts to define peer groups and to delineate a strategy for measuring them, researchers have endeavored to identify their structure or organization, focusing on issues such as group size and stability, homogeneity, and rates of participation. Of course, these features vary according to how groups are defined.

Participation

With regard to participation rates, for example, when asked whether they belonged to a clique, virtually all of the Italian sixth and seventh graders in Kiesner et al.'s (2002) study claimed membership in such a group at school, and 85% belonged to an out-of-school clique. Similarly, Bagwell et al. (2000) located nearly all of their fourth-grade American respondents in cliques, using an admittedly liberal set of statistical criteria for identifying groups based on student lists of close friends. Using an SCM procedure, Kindermann (1993) placed 85% of his fourth-grade sample into a clique. On the other hand, Espelage, Holt, and Henkel (2003) classified less than 70% of their eighth-grade sample as clique members, and with more stringent requirements for peer groups, Henrich, Kuperminc, Sack, Blatt, and Leadbeater (2000) found that less than 20% of the middle school youth in their sample were part of a clique. Membership in peer crowds is similarly variable among studies (Sussman et al., 2007), although it tends to be higher when based on peer ratings rather than self-report.

Group Size

In contrast to incidence rates, there is substantial agreement about the average size of interaction-based groups. Most investigators report a median group size of between five and eight members for cliques, roughly the same as Dunphy (1963) noted in his classic observational study of Australian youth half a century ago. Again, however, there are methodological challenges. SCM requires raters to recall freely all members of each clique they name, possibly leading to an underspecification of members, and some of the statistical routines used to derive clique structures from lists of friendship nominations are inclined to limit the size of groups, or are prevented from fully articulating clique membership because of missing data from some network members. Based on observations of children's play groups, Ladd (1983) found that boys tended to have larger cliques than girls, and sociometrically popular youth had larger groups than average or, especially, rejected children. Others have also observed that boys are drawn to larger playgroups than are girls in the early portion of middle childhood (Benenson, Apostoleris, & Parnass, 1998). Whether this persists across adolescence is difficult to determine because the playground no longer serves as a viable observation context for older youth.

Reputation-based groups are much more variable in size, not only across different crowd types but also within type across schools or communities (Garner, Bootcheck, Lorr, & Rauch, 2006; Thurlow, 2001). Crowd size is also very sensitive to research method. Among U.S. teenagers, the "normal" crowd is much larger, and the "loner" or "outcast" group is much smaller, when information is gathered via self-report rather than peer ratings (Brown et al., in press). Group size increases if individuals are allowed to claim membership in more than one crowd.

Stability

One reason for the difficulty in specifying group size is that membership is in a relatively constant state of flux. The consensus seems to be that clique membership is reasonably stable over the short term (less than a month) but quite unstable over longer time periods (3 or more months) (Kindermann, 1993, 2007). However, although young people may shift from one clique to another or witness frequent changes in the membership of their clique across childhood, they will likely continue to associate with the same types of peers in terms of traits such as aggressiveness or academic engagement (Cairns & Cairns, 1994) and retain similar status positions (as central or peripheral members of groups) across their peer-group transitions. The stability of crowd affiliations in adolescence is unclear because these affiliations have rarely been measured at more than one time point. In one U.S. sample (Kinney, 1993), crowds became much more clearly delineated with the transition from middle school to high school, but the boundaries between crowds blurred in the final year or two of high school. This suggests the possibility of multiple or partial group memberships among young people.

Exclusivity

In Verkooijen, deVries, and Nielson's (2007) sample of Dutch adolescents, nearly half of those who acknowledged belonging to any crowd claimed membership in two or more groups. Peer ratings of crowd affiliation based on social-type rating (STR) procedures (Brown et al., 1993; Schwendinger & Schwendinger, 1985) are rarely unanimous and often are divided between two or three groups. One solution is to give an individual continuous scores on all crowds, representing the proportion of raters assigning the person to each group (e.g., Brown et al., 1993). The notion that individuals can be partial members of multiple crowds may undermine many people's notion of a peer group, but it seems to be a more accurate depiction of adolescents' experiences with peers.

The possibility of multiple group memberships is acknowledged more directly in studies of interaction based groups that differentiate group members from "liaisons" (those whose friendships seem to connect them to two or more groups) and "isolates" (those with no reciprocated friendships with members of discernible cliques). Liaisons constituted over a third of Henrich et al.'s (2000) ethnically and socioeconomically diverse sample of U.S. middle school students. Shrum and Cheek's (1987) classic study of clique positions indicated that the percentage of liaisons swelled from less than 10% of third graders to 40% of high school students. Although it is sensible that clique (and crowd) members vary in their centrality and that groups vary in how tightly knit or exclusive they are (Eder, 1985), it is not clear that statistically identified liaisons actually connect members of two peer groups in any meaningful way. Likewise, isolates are often not truly isolated; an isolate may have a strong friendship bond with one member of the peer social system or extensive bonds with peers outside the social system being evaluated. When evaluation of clique positions is confined to an arbitrarily defined social system (e.g., a school classroom), the group structure that investigators identify may not adequately capture the peer experiences of young people, whose peer relationships often extend beyond this social system.

Homogeneity

The final structural issue concerns the degree of similarity among group members. Consistent with the notion that "birds of a feather flock together," throughout middle childhood and into adolescence, most cliques comprise youth of the same gender and school grade level, although this homogeneity diminishes in middle adolescence. Reports about clique homogeneity in ethnicity (in multiethnic social contexts), socioeconomic status (SES), or other demographic characteristics are less consistent. One might expect that most cliques are homogeneous in behavioral characteristics or sociometric status. Farmer et al. (2002), however, found that aggressive, sociometrically rejected, and deviant youth all were distributed broadly among cliques in a social network, although the relative concentration of these youth in a given clique did affect the clique's influence on its members. Clique homogeneity may also be contingent on its demographic composition. Henrich et al. (2000) found less variability among members of middle school girls' than among boys' cliques on measures of academic performance, internalizing, and friendship quality.

Studies suggest that member similarity is an important predictor of the initiation and maintenance of dyadic relationships (friends or romantic partners). To date, researchers have not examined this issue in the context of peer groups, nor have they considered whether member homogeneity on specific characteristics is especially predictive of group stability.

Generally, then, although scholars have explored numerous aspects of peer-group structure, several issues remain uncertain. Some of these are contingent on clarifying the definition of "cliques" or "crowds," or the ways that group membership is measured. Others require researchers to be more attentive to developmental issues—to the fact that group structure may change over the course of the group's existence and/or differ as a function of members' ages.

Peer-Group Functioning

The ultimate concern of parents, educators, and policymakers may be how peer groups affect members' attitudes and behaviors, but to understand these effects, one must first examine how these groups operate. Some investigators have concentrated on intragroup dynamics, whereas others have been concerned with intergroup dynamics. We briefly summarize issues in both areas.

Intragroup Dynamics

There is an extensive literature, much of it laboratory based, examining the dynamics of dyadic relationships in childhood and adolescence. A similar literature on peer groups has yet to emerge, especially if one focuses on naturally occurring groups rather than groups arbitrarily conceived by researchers (e.g., a collection of peers brought together for an experimental session in a research laboratory). The logistics of identifying interaction-based groups, then coordinating schedules to bring the group together for study are admittedly daunting, especially in middle childhood when group composition frequently changes. Intragroup processes within reputation-based groups are even more challenging, because they do not necessarily center on observable interactions among group members. Many of the most insightful studies of group processes involve intensive ethnographic analyses; some of these are highlighted in a later section of this chapter. The key issues for investigators to address are (1) the major emergent roles within a group that are vital to group functioning, (2) how specific members come to occupy these roles, and (3) how group activities serve to maintain (or, in some cases, undermine) the integrity of the group and the attitudes or behavior of group members. These are standard issues in small-group research, but they are complicated by developmental issues within the target population. By late childhood, clique dynamics seem to be influenced by the emerging crowd structure, in that young people may interpret the behavior of groupmates in terms of the larger social system in which the clique is located.

Intergroup Dynamics

One danger of concentrating too closely on processes within a clique of young people is that its activities may be heavily influenced by its relationships with other cliques. Much of the research on intergroup dynamics has applied principles of social identity theory (Tajfel & Turner, 1979) to assess the extent to which children or adolescents favor their own group over other groups of peers. In many cases they employ experimental or survey methods to study "minimal groups," clusters of youth that essentially are created for the study and have little meaning beyond it. This focus on the dynamics of ingroup favoritism and outgroup derogation is important, if one believes that peer influence emanates primarily from fellow group members rather than from the larger collective of agemates.

With the emergence of a peer crowd system in early adolescence, however, young people seem to become more preoccupied with peer status. According to ethnographic studies of American youth, ingroup favoritism can easily give way to desires to be part of cliques from higher status crowds (Eder, 1985; Merten, 1996). By middle adolescence, the sharp status distinctions between crowds can galvanize cliques into bitter rivalries (Eckert, 1989; Willis, 1977), in which ingroup favoritism is still visible but defensive in tone. However, Kinney (1993) offered evidence that status distinctions among crowds are actually tempered with the proliferation of peer groups that can occur as children transition to public high schools, and Larkin (1979) observed a dissipation of crowd boundaries toward the end of high school that allowed for broader mixing of cliques.

The consequences of these transformations for the sort of intergroup dynamics predicted by social identity theory need to be examined more closely. Moreover, one must be cautious about generalizing ethnographic findings because they are often based on observations of highly visible and cohesive cliques, whose members seem to be more highly identified with their group than is typical of most peer groups in a social system. Tarrant (2002) reported that ingroup favoritism and outgroup derogation among British teenagers, especially males, was enhanced by strong identification with one's clique. Thus, ethnographies may be prone to present extreme cases of intergroup dynamics.

Group Influences on Individuals' Behavior

Whereas social psychologists may be drawn to the study of peer groups because of the intriguing interpersonal processes that occur between and within groups, developmental psychologists are more likely to be interested in the potential of groups to influence young people's behavior and psychological adjustment. Documenting peer group influence is obfuscated by the opportunity of young people to choose freely most of their peer groups. This allows them to seek out or form groups with like-minded or "like-behaviored" associates, so that similarities between self and group norms, or group members' characteristics, are a function of "selection" rather than "socialization." Carefully designed longitudinal studies can control for selection effects to derive a more accurate estimate of peer-group influence. The most reliable evidence of influence processes comes from experimental designs, but it may be difficult for such a methodology to address the full range of influence mechanisms that occur within peer groups (Brown, Bakken, Ameringer, & Mahon, 2008). They must be complemented by longitudinal, ethnographic observations of peer-group interactions in natural contexts (e.g., Adler & Adler, 1995; Eder, 1985).

At this point, scholars still do not have a clear idea about which personal characteristics are most amenable to peer-group influence, or what factors moderate the type or level of influence that peer groups can exert on children and adolescents. For example, Ellis and Zarbatany (2007) found that short-term (3-month) effects of group membership on behaviors of Canadian early adolescents depended upon the group's position within the peer social system. Using a modified SCM method to identify cliques, the investigators found that group level of deviance predicted individual change in deviance, but only for those who belonged to groups that were low in social preference (e.g., whose members were generally disliked by peers). Prosocial behaviors increased for respondents belonging to groups high in centrality (i.e., forming the core of the peer social system) but decreased for those in groups low in centrality. Adolescents' commitment to the peer group also seems to be an important factor. In a sample of British ninth graders, Tarrant, MacKenzie, and Hewitt (2006) found that the more strongly youth identified with their friendship group, the stronger was their self-esteem in several domains. Verkooijen et al. (2007) reported that strong identification with one of the risk-prone crowds in a sample of Danish 16- to 20-year-olds was associated with higher rates of substance use.

Thus, group status, group characteristics, and member commitment are all factors to be considered in assessing peer-group effects on member behavior. One might also question whether an individual's status within the group affects the group's ability to influence behavior. Are peripheral members more susceptible to influence, because they strive to conform to group norms to prove their loyalty and improve their position in the group, or are central members (group leaders) most susceptible because their leadership depends upon their being strong models of group norms (see Pearson & Michell, 2000; Wiseman, 2002)?

In addition to exploring factors that might moderate peer-group influences on young people, some investigators have considered how peer-group affiliation itself may modify influences *outside* of the group on members' behavior. For example, Lansford, Criss, Pettit, Dodge, and Bates (2003) collected data at several time points over a 2-year period with a sample of American middle school youth. They found that strong identification with a peer clique was able to temper the ill effects of negative parenting on early adolescents' behavioral adjustment. Such research serves as an important reminder that peer groups do not operate independently of other social contexts that young people must negotiate, and peer-group interactions may moderate or be moderated by features of these other contexts.

An additional challenge for those studying peer-group influence is to create models and methods that account for the "interactive" nature of influence—the fact that group members influence the group and are at the same time influenced by it. Kindermann (1993) examined changes in achievement motivation from fall to spring in a sample of U.S. fourth and fifth graders. Using SCM to identify cliques in participating classrooms, he found that average levels of achievement motivation in the group predicted individuals' changes in motivation, but the opposite was true as well.

Theoretical Considerations

The study of child and adolescent peer groups operates at the intersection of two distinct disciplines: developmental psychology and social psychology or sociology. Each has different theoretical traditions that serve as a foundation for research. Theories of small-group behavior are especially pertinent for studies of intragroup dynamics (e.g., Festinger, Schachter, & Back, 1950). These theories focus on the influence structures that exist within groups and the ways in which group members' actions enhance or undermine group cohesion.

Much of the work on intergroup dynamics stems from social identity theory (Tajfel & Turner, 1979) or one of its derivatives. A product of symbolic interactionist perspectives on social relationships, this theory posits that individuals are motivated to favor their own group and to denigrate other groups as a means of self-image enhancement; they also tend to perceive outgroup members in more generic terms (Brewer, 1993). This process may be the basis for prejudice and discrimination directed at outgroup members (Aboud, 2003), which encourages investigators to regard intergroup relations in adversarial terms.

Studies of adolescent crowds also draw from symbolic interactionist theories, especially fundamental notions such as the impact of reflected appraisals on self-understanding (Cooley, 1902). Additionally, these studies consider more developmental conceptualizations of identity (Erikson, 1968), as well as the extensions of symbolic interactionist theories that address issues of status and intergroup competition (Tajfel & Turner, 1979).

The challenge for researchers from more sociological or social-psychological traditions is to come to grips with the developmental features of peer groups. This includes the evanescent and constantly evolving nature of clique structures in middle childhood, and the emergence of more heterosocial peer structures with the transition to adolescence. The appearance of peer crowds in many societies, usually in early adolescence, further complicates the study of clique dynamics. Although it does not appear that all cliques are squarely situated within specific crowds, as Dunphy (1963) claimed (Urberg et al., 1995), crowd structures do alter individuals' access to peers who might become part of a friendship clique (Brown et al., 1994; Kinney, 1993). They also affect individuals' inclinations to associate with cliques whose members are linked with more or less desirable crowds within the peer system (Eder, 1985). The connection between cliques and crowds may itself be a developmental phenomenon, growing stronger between middle childhood and early adolescence, only to fade as adolescence progresses (Kinney, 1993; Larkin, 1979).

To date, however, there is little theory to guide the integration of developmental and sociological or social-psychological perspectives on peer groups across middle childhood and adolescence. The challenge is to consider how group dynamics that are well articulated in sociological or social-psychological models are modulated by aspects of individual development of group members. In the next section we highlight a few studies that are moving the field in this direction.

Exemplary Studies

The most common theme in research on interaction-based groups during childhood and adolescence concerns ingroup favoritism in intergroup relations, perhaps because this theme is easily adapted from studies of older populations. Many investigators employ experimental or survey methods to study "minimal groups," clusters of youth that are essentially created for the study and have little meaning beyond it. For example, Abrams, Rutland, and Cameron (2003) presented a sample of British youth, ages 5–11, with profiles of hypothetical peers who either were fans of England's or Germany's national soccer team and made statements that seemed either to bolster or to undermine the team that they favored. After establishing that respondents all favored the English team, the investigators asked how acceptable respondents thought the hypothetical peers would be to other English or German team fans (the "ingroup" and "outgroup," respectively, from the respondents' point of view). Children viewed a hypothetical peer who supported his or her own team (normative peer-group member) as more acceptable to the group than one who seemed to support the other team (deviant group member). They also judged normative ingroup and deviant outgroup members as more likable and more easily accepted by the "English" peer group than other hypothetical peers. These inclinations increased across age, presumably because of older respondents' more sophisticated social-cognitive skills.

Nesdale and Flesser (2001) entered status into the equation by leading a sample of 5- or 8-year-old Australian children to believe they were part of a group judged by experts to have either high or low ability at drawing pictures. When asked to compare their group to an outgroup (judged to have a level of drawing ability opposite that of their group), children claimed to like their ingroup members more than outgroup peers, but especially if they were in the high-status group. However, when children in a low-status group were told that they might be able to change to the other (high-status) group, respondents said they had less in common with ingroup members and more desire to switch groups than when they were led to believe that their ingroup was high in status or the outgroup was unreceptive to new members. This suggests that even young children appreciate status differences among groups.

To examine status effects in a more concrete setting, Bigler, Brown, and Markell (2001) distributed blue and yellow T-shirts randomly to children (ages 7–11) in a summer learning program. They created conditions in which attention was or was not drawn to the T-shirts (teachers did or did not use T-shirt color as a basis for classroom activities, such as lining up for recess), and status was or was not accorded to one T-shirt color (via the presence or absence of posters in the classroom depicting students with yellow T-shirts as frequent winners of classroom competitions the previous year). The investigators found that in classrooms lacking status markers but featuring group activities organized by T-shirt color, students expressed more favorable attitudes about their ingroup than about the outgroup, reflecting similar dynamics to Sherif, Harvey, White, Hood, and Sherif's (1961) classic observations of children's intergroup dynamics in a summer camp.

In classrooms that also featured status differentials between groups, high-status group members still displayed ingroup favoritism, but the low-status group rated ingroup and outgroup members more equally.

These studies illustrate a progression in research design toward examining intergroup dynamics in more realistic ways. Yet ecological validity remains doubtful, because investigators have not yet found a way to assess the dynamics in observations of *actual* cliques in school classrooms or other contexts of children's social interactions. Researchers studying intragroup dynamics have been more successful in this regard, using either experimental or ethnographic methods. For example, in an effort to determine how adolescents are influenced by peers during an effort to "break in" to an interaction-based group, Cohen and Prinstein (2006) involved a sample of U.S. high school males of average social status in what subjects were led to believe was a chat room encounter with e-confederates who appeared to be either high or low in social status. The researchers used previous information collected on students in the school to construct groups of e-confederates whose identity (though not revealed) the subjects could infer. The e-confederates displayed aggressive and health-risk behaviors, and the experimenters tracked the degree to which subjects conformed to e-confederates' behavior. Subjects modeled this behavior when it emanated from ostensibly high-status peers but actually rejected the same behavior when it came from what appeared to be low-status peers.

In an ethnographic study, Adler and Adler (1995) used their role as parents to observe pre-adolescent groups closely over a period of several years. They discovered that the multiple roles occupied by group members were organized into a hierarchy of authority among these roles, reminiscent of the dominance structure that Savin-Williams (1979) found in groups of boys of comparable ages in a summer camp environment. Interactions were careful and stress-laden, relationships were cautious, and violations of group norms were quickly addressed by individuals of higher status than the offender in the group hierarchy. Other investigators offer similar portraits of high-status cliques among early adolescent girls (Eder, 1985; Wiseman, 2002). The study suggests that cliques may be highly differentiated and carefully regulated environments.

Results from another ethnographic study, however, caution against overgeneralizing findings from assessments of youth in only one portion of the peer-group system. Finders (1997) followed two female cliques, one high and the other low in social status. Although the high-status group conformed to interaction patterns observed in previous studies, the low-status group came from more economically disadvantaged backgrounds and focused on school achievement rather than peer popularity and influence. The low-status group members concentrated their social interactions on family and kin rather than peers, and approached peer interactions in a calmer, more supportive manner. The interaction style among this group's members resembled Eckert's (1989) depiction of older, mixed-sex groups in the "burnout" crowd, also hailing from less economically advantaged circumstances. Although interactions among groups lower in social and/or SES may be less emotionally charged, they still serve the central mission of establishing and enforcing group norms. Eder (1993) described how extensive group conversation, derogation of outgroup members, and occasional teasing of group members serve to affirm and maintain group expectations about relationships with the other sex in a clique of middle school girls.

Exemplary studies of adolescent crowds are more challenging to identify, partly because they are as much a cognitive as a concrete phenomenon. Ethnographers tend to focus on a single, central clique within a crowd, whose dynamics may not be typical of crowd membership as a whole. It seems prudent to regard crowds as playing a moderating role on the dynamics observed in interaction-based groups, as is suggested by Finders's (1997) and Eckert's (1989) results. Moreover, because crowd affiliations do not necessarily involve persistent and exclusive daily interaction with crowd members, young people can more easily sidestep their influence. Brown et al. (in press) charted changes in self-esteem and social self-concept over a 1-year period among members of different peer crowds in a large sample of U.S. adolescents. Drawing from symbolic interaction theory principles of reflected appraisals, the authors reasoned that members of low-status crowds (established through peer ratings) might escape the blow to their self-concept stemming from such a reflected appraisal by claiming membership in a higher status group or in no crowd at all. Conversely, youth perceived by peers to be in high-status crowds might not advance in self-esteem if they did not acknowledge their association with a highly esteemed crowd. Analyses provided modest support for these hypotheses, suggesting that crowd influences can be moderated by members' cognitions or level of group identification.

Virtually all of the studies of child and adolescent peer groups, even the exemplary cases that we have cited, follow groups and their members over short periods of time—no more than a year. This is simply not sufficient time to understand either the normative effects of groups on members or the range of individual (member) differences in such effects. Although investigators are improving in their ability to interpret study results within the context of the developmental period from which their respondents are sampled, there still is little effort to replicate studies across age groups to examine developmental trajectories in peer-group structures, functions, or influence processes.

Future Research Directions

Our understanding of peer-group processes has increased dramatically over the past 15 years, but there is still much to be learned. We have already urged investigators to develop and to apply more comprehensive, interdisciplinary conceptual models, and to seek new methods that can adjust to developmental changes in the organization of peer groups. Researchers should address five additional objectives.

1. *Consider cultural issues more carefully.* Studies of peer-group dynamics are derived from fairly diverse populations in several nations on two continents, but European or European American youth still dominate samples. Cultures that deemphasize peer interactions in childhood and adolescence deserve closer attention, and more attention should be paid to the dynamics of peer-group formation and interaction in multicultural settings. This will help investigators identify ways in which cultural forces shape the nature of peer-group relations, as well as how peer-group norms may precipitate changes in young people's other social relationships in contexts outside of middle-class European or European American youth.

2. *Extend the time frame of longitudinal studies.* Few studies examine the organization and operation of peer groups at more than two time points, and very few consider peer-group dynamics in middle adolescence (ages 15–18). Longer term studies with more frequent data collection points post daunting logistical and methodological challenges, but they are sorely needed to address several important questions: Is there a curvilinear trajectory in the stability of clique and crowd affiliations (reaching an apex at the begin-

ning of middle adolescence)? What makes some cliques or crowds more stable than others, and how does this stability affect the peer group's capacity to exert influence over individuals? How do peer groups adapt to oscillating memberships as individuals move in and out of romantic relationships?

3. *Develop more coordinated assessments of the two levels of peer-group interaction.* Rather than considering the study of interaction- and reputation-based groups as independent lines of investigation, researchers should attempt to bridge these two topics with more coordinated studies. Are cliques nested within crowds or wholly independent of them, or does this vary among crowds or across different social contexts? Is the organization or operation of cliques markedly different when dominated by members of one crowd versus another, or when members are drawn from several crowds instead of just one? Is clique membership more constrained when crowds are organized by ascribed rather than achieved characteristics?

4. *Pay more attention to individuals' positions within a clique.* Ethnographic studies suggest that central and peripheral group members, leaders, and followers have different experiences within cliques (Adler & Adler, 1995; Wiseman, 2002), but beyond the differentiation of clique members, liaisons, and isolates, other investigators have paid little attention to within-group position in their studies of peer-group dynamics. Young people's drive to be fully integrated into cliques or to be engaged only modestly in peer groups should be considered more carefully in attempts to chart peer-group effects on members.

5. *Consider peer-group aspirations, as well as group memberships.* Kiesner et al. (2002) cautioned that isolates who view themselves as part of a clique may still be affected by the group's norms. Likewise, we suspect that young people who are members of one peer group but aspire to membership in another may be influenced more strongly by their "reference group" than by their "membership group" and, as a consequence, may be disruptive to the smooth operation of their clique or crowd. Peer-group aspirations may account for the constant state of flux that seems to characterize childhood peer groups, and it may be a critical missing variable in our understanding of peer influence processes.

Researchers are just beginning to capture the complex dynamics of child and adolescent peer-group relations. As more sophisticated conceptual models and measurement strategies are developed, they are likely to unveil the critical role that cliques and crowds play in the social lives of this age group.

References

Aboud, F. E. (2003). The formation of in-group favoritism and out-group prejudice in children: Are they distinct attitudes? *Developmental Psychology, 39,* 48–60.

Abrams, D., Rutland, A., & Cameron, L. (2003). The development of subjective group dynamics: Children's judgments of normative and deviant in-group and out-group individuals. *Child Development, 74,* 1840–1856.

Adler, P. A., & Adler, P. (1995). Dynamics of inclusion and exclusion in preadolescent cliques. *Social Psychology Quarterly, 58,* 145–162.

Bagwell, C. L., Coie, J. D., Terry, R. A., & Lochman, J. E. (2000). Peer clique participation and social status in preadolescence. *Merrill–Palmer Quarterly, 46,* 280–305.

Benenson, J. F., Apostoleris, N., & Parnass, J. (1998). The organization of children's same-sex peer relationships. In W. M. Bukowski & A. H. Cillessen (Eds.), *Sociometry then and now* (pp. 5–23). San Francisco: Jossey-Bass.

Benenson, J. F., Nicholson, C., & Waite, A. (2001). The influence of group size on children's competitive behavior. *Child Development, 72*, 921–928.

Bigler, R. S., Brown, C. S., & Markell, M. (2001). When groups are not created equal: Effects of group status on the formation of intergroup attitudes in children. *Child Development, 72*, 1151–1162.

Brewer, M. B. (1993). Social identity, distinctiveness, and in-group homogeneity. *Social Cognition, 11*, 150–164.

Brown, B. B., Bakken, J. P., Ameringer, S. W., & Mahon, S. D. (2008). A comprehensive conceptualization of the peer influence process in adolescence. In M. J. Prinstein & K. A. Dodge (Eds.), *Understanding peer influence in children and adolescents* (pp. 17–44). New York: Guilford Press.

Brown, B. B., Lamborn, S. L., Mounts, N. S., & Steinberg, L. (1993). Parenting practices and peer group affiliation in adolescence. *Child Development, 64*, 467–482.

Brown, B. B., Mory, M., & Kinney, D. A. (1994). Casting adolescent crowds in relational perspective: Caricature, channel, and context. In R. Montemayor, G. R. Adams, & T. P. Gullotta (Eds.), *Advances in adolescent development: Vol. 6. Personal relationships during adolescence* (pp. 123–167). Newbury Park, CA: Sage.

Brown, B. B., Von Bank, H. G., & Steinberg, L. (in press). Smoke in the looking glass. Effects of discordance between self- and peer rated crowd affiliation on adolescent anxiety, depression, and self-esteem. *Journal of Youth and Adolescence.*

Cairns, R. B., & Cairns, B. D. (1994). *Lifelines and risks: Pathways of youth in our time.* New York: Cambridge University Press.

Cairns, R. B., Perrin, J. E., & Cairns, B. D. (1985). Social structure and social cognition in early adolescence: Affiliative patterns. *Journal of Early Adolescence, 5*, 339–355.

Cairns, R. B., Xie, H., & Leung, M.-C. (1998). The popularity of friendship and the neglect of social networks: Toward a new balance. In W. M. Bukowski & A. H. Cillessen (Eds.), *Sociometry then and now* (pp. 25–53). San Francisco: Jossey-Bass.

Cohen, G. L., & Prinstein, M. J. (2006). Peer contagion of aggression and health risk behavior among adolescent males: An experimental investigation of effects on public conduct and private attitudes. *Child Development, 77*, 967–983.

Cooley, C. H. (1902). *Human nature and social order.* New York: Scribners.

Crockett, L., Losoff, M., & Petersen, A. C. (1984). Perceptions of the peer group and friendship in early adolescence. *Journal of Early Adolescence, 4*, 155–181.

Dunphy, D. C. (1963). The social structure of urban adolescent peer groups. *Sociometry, 26*, 230–246.

Eckert, P. (1989). *Jocks and burnouts: Social categories and identity in the high school.* New York: Teachers College Press.

Eder, D. (1985). The cycle of popularity: Interpersonal relations among female adolescents. *Sociology of Education, 58*, 154–165.

Eder, D. (1993). "Go get ya a French!": Romantic and sexual teasing among adolescent girls. In Tannen, D. (Ed.), *Gender and conversational interaction* (pp. 17–31). New York: Oxford University Press.

Ellis, W. E., & Zarbatany, L. (2007). Peer group status as a moderator of group influence on children's deviant, aggressive, and prosocial behavior. *Child Development, 78*, 1240–1254.

Erikson, E. H. (1968). *Identity, youth, and crisis.* New York: Norton.

Espelage, D. L., Holt, M. K., & Henkel, R. R. (2003). Examination of peer-group contextual effects on aggression during early adolescence. *Child Development, 74*, 205–220.

Farmer, T. W., Leung, M., Rodkin, P. C., Cadwallader, T. W., Pearl, R., & Van Acker, R. (2002). Deviant or diverse peer groups?: The peer affiliations of aggressive elementary students. *Journal of Educational Psychology, 94*, 611–620.

Festinger, L., Schachter, S., & Back, K. (1950). *Social pressures in informal group*. Stanford, CA: Stanford University Press.

Finders, M. J. (1997). *Just girls: Hidden literacies and life in junior high*. New York: Teachers College Press.

Garner, R., Bootcheck, J., Lorr, M., & Rauch, K. (2006). The adolescent society revisited: Cultures, crowds, climates, and status structures in seven secondary schools. *Journal of Youth and Adolescence, 35*, 1023–1035.

Gest, S. D., Farmer, T. W., Cairns, B. D., & Xie, H. (2003). Identifying children's peer social networks in school classrooms: Links between peer reports and observed interactions. *Social Development, 12*, 513–529.

Henrich, C. C., Kuperminc, G. P., Sack, A., Blatt, S. J., & Leadbeater, B. J. (2000). Characteristics and homogeneity of early adolescent friendship groups: A comparison of male and female clique and nonclique members. *Applied Developmental Science, 4*, 15–26.

Kiesner, J., Cadinu, M., Poulin, F., & Bucci, M. (2002). Group identification in early adolescence: Its relation with peer adjustment and its moderator effect on peer influence. *Child Development, 73*, 196–208.

Kiesner, J., Poulin, F., & Nicotra, E. (2003). Peer relations across contexts: Individual–network homophily and network inclusion in and after school. *Child Development, 74*, 1328–1343.

Kindermann, T. A. (1993). Natural peer groups as contexts for individual development: The case of children's motivation in school. *Developmental Psychology, 29*, 970–977.

Kindermann, T. A. (2007). Effects of naturally existing peer groups on changes in academic engagement in a cohort of sixth graders. *Child Development, 78*, 1186–1203.

Kinney, D. (1993). From "nerds" to "normals": Adolescent identity recovery within a changing social system. *Sociology of Education, 66*, 21–40.

Ladd, G. W. (1983). Social networks of popular, average, and rejected children in school settings. *Merrill–Palmer Quarterly, 29*, 283–307.

Lansford, J. E., Criss, M. M., Pettit, G. S., Dodge, K. A., & Bates, J. E. (2003). Friendship quality, peer group affiliation, and peer antisocial behavior as moderators of the link between negative parenting and adolescent externalizing behavior. *Journal of Research on Adolescence, 13*, 161–184.

Larkin, R. W. (1979). *Suburban youth in cultural crisis*. New York: Oxford University Press.

Merten, D. E. (1996). Visibility and vulnerability: Responses to rejection by nonaggressive junior high school boys. *Journal of Early Adolescence, 16*, 5–26.

Nesdale, D., & Flesser, D. (2001). Social identity and the development of children's group attitudes. *Child Development, 72*, 506–517.

Pearson, M., & Michell, L. (2000). Smoke rings: Social network analysis of friendship groups, smoking, and drug-taking. *Drug Addictions, Prevention, and Policy, 7*, 21–37.

Rodkin, P. C., Farmer, T. W., Pearl, R., & Van Acker, R. (2006). They're cool: Social status and peer group supports for aggressive boys and girls. *Social Development, 15*, 175–204.

Rubin, K. H., Bukowski, W. M., & Parker, J. G. (2006). Peer interactions, relationships, and groups. In W. Damon & R. M. Lerner (Series Eds.) & N. Eisenberg (Vol. Ed.), *Handbook of child psychology: Social, emotional, and personality development* (6th ed., Vol. 3, pp. 571–645). New York: Wiley.

Savin-Williams, R. C. (1979). Dominance hierarchies in groups of early adolescents. *Child Development, 50*, 923–935.

Schwendinger, H., & Schwendinger, J. S. (1985). *Adolescent subcultures and delinquency*. New York: Praeger.

Sherif, M., Harvey, O. J., White, B. J., Hood, W. R., & Sherif, C. W. (1961). *Intergroup conflict and cooperation: The Robbers Cave experiment*. Norman, OK: University Book Exchange.

Shrum, W., & Cheek, N. H. (1987). Social structure during the school years: Onset of the degrouping process. *American Sociological Review, 52*, 218–223.

Sussman, S., Pokhrel, P., Ashmore, R. D., & Brown, B. B. (2007). Adolescent peer group identification and characteristics: A review of the literature. *Addictive Behaviors, 32*, 1602–1627.

Tajfel, H., & Turner, J. C. (1979). An integrative theory of intergroup conflict. In W. G. Austin & S. Worschel (Eds.), *The social psychology of intergroup relations* (pp. 178–234). New York: Brooks/Cole.

Tarrant, M. (2002). Adolescent peer groups and social identity. *Social Development, 11*, 110–123.

Tarrant, M., MacKenzie, L., & Hewitt, L. A. (2006). Friendship group identification, multidimensional self-concept, and experience of developmental tasks in adolescence. *Journal of Adolescence, 29*, 627–640.

Thurlow, C. (2001). The usual suspects?: A comparative investigation of crowds and social-type labelling among young British teenagers. *Journal of Youth Studies, 4*, 319–334.

Urberg, K. A., Degirmencioglu, S. M., Tolson, J. M., & Halliday-Scher, K. (1995). The structure of adolescent peer networks. *Developmental Psychology, 31*, 540–547.

Urberg, K. A., Degirmencioglu, S. M., Tolson, J. M., & Halliday-Scher, K. (2000). Adolescent social crowds: Measurement and relationship to friendships. *Journal of Adolescent Research, 15*, 427–445.

Verkooijen, K. T., deVries, N. K., & Nielson, G. A. (2007). Youth crowds and substance use: The impact of perceived group norm and multiple group identification. *Psychology of Addictive Behaviors, 21*, 55–61.

Willis, P. E. (1977). *Learning to labour*. Farnborough, UK: Saxon House.

Wiseman, R. (2002). *Queen bees and wannabes*. New York: Three Rivers Press.

CHAPTER 21

Sex Differences in Peer Relationships

AMANDA J. ROSE
RHIANNON L. SMITH

In recent years, many parents, teachers, and other caregivers have worked to socialize children in a non-sex-typed manner, which includes promoting a wide variety of skills and competencies. Nevertheless, sex remains a powerful factor in organizing and shaping the behaviors of children, including those that occur within the peer context. Our aims in this chapter are to review theories regarding the development of sex differences that are relevant to the peer context and empirical evidence regarding sex differences in peer relationships. Finally, we propose future directions for advancing our understanding of the role of sex in children's peer relationships.

Relevant Theory

There is much theoretical work related to the development of sex differences. Less theoretical work focuses on sex differences in the peer domain in particular; however, the more general theories can be applied to the understanding of peer relationships. In this section, we review theoretical work regarding sex differences, with a focus on applications to peer relationships. Theories regarding how children develop sex-typed behavior have been summarized in several excellent reviews (Golombok & Hines, 2002; Leaper & Friedman, 2007; Ruble, Martin, & Berenbaum, 2006). The following discussion draws heavily on these.

Biological theories emphasize the role of hormones in the development of sex-typed behavior, including behavior in the peer context. Support for these theories comes from animal and human research. For example, studies with rats link testosterone to male-typed behavior such as rough-and-tumble play and high activity levels (see Golombok & Hines, 2002). Although hormone levels are not experimentally manipulated in humans, a natural experiment is provided by girls with congenital adrenal hyperplasia (CAH), who were exposed prenatally to high levels of androgens. Although findings are not completely consistent across studies, research suggests that girls with CAH may exhibit greater male-typed behavior in peer contexts than do typically developing girls, including an increased preference for toys typically preferred by boys (e.g., Berenbaum & Hines, 1992) and for male playmates (e.g., Hines & Kaufman, 1994; for reviews, see Golombok & Hines, 2002; Ruble et al., 2006).

A primary cognitive theory of the development of sex differences is gender schema theory. Different theorists have had different emphases, but all highlight the active role of the child in sex role development (see Martin, Ruble, & Szkrybalo, 2002; Ruble et al., 2006). Children are thought to actively form schemas or mental representations about gender, including the behaviors typical of each sex. Thereafter, they are motivated to match their own behavior to their gender-related schemas. In support of this theory, researchers have demonstrated that when toys are labeled as being for girls or for boys, or are labeled as liked by girls or boys, children actively use that information to guide their behavior toward sex-typed activities (see Martin et al., 2002).

Socialization theories also address how children acquire sex-typed behaviors. Social learning theory and social-cognitive theories (e.g., Bussey & Bandura, 1999) suggest that children develop sex-typed behavior by modeling same-sex others and through differential reinforcement that works to increase sex-typed and to decrease cross-sex behaviors. Moreover, children are most likely to model behaviors that are especially valued and judged to be rewarded when others do them. Adults, including parents and teachers, are thought to be of particular importance in shaping the development of sex-typed behavior (see Ruble et al., 2006). However, peers also serve as important models (see Leaper & Friedman, 2007) and agents of reinforcement (see Ruble et al., 2006). Compared to the role of adults, the role of peers in the development of sex-typed behavior is understudied. However, in a later section of this chapter, we describe existing work indicating that, in social contexts, children do shape the sex-typed behavior of peers.

Also, whereas many theories focus on individual-difference factors that contribute to sex-typed behavior, others focus on the role of context in eliciting sex differences. Deaux and Major (1987) integrated the role of individual differences and context effects by suggesting that whether people engage in sex-typed behavior depends on the interplay of their gender self-systems and the characteristics of the context (e.g., whether the situation activates gender schemas; the gender beliefs of others in the interaction). In the peer domain, it has been suggested that differences in the contexts in which girls versus boys spend the most time (e.g., dyadic vs. group contexts) may help to account for sex differences in particular behaviors, including self-disclosure (which may emerge most naturally in dyadic interactions; Leaper, 1994; Underwood, 2004) and competition (which may emerge most naturally in group interactions; Benenson, Gordon, & Roy, 2000; Benenson, Maiese, et al., 2002). The role of context is considered further in the later section on future research directions.

Last, other theoretical perspectives focus on the role of the same-sex peer group. Group-related processes, such as attraction to other ingroup members and devaluing of outgroup members (Tajfel, 1982), likely apply to children's identification with the same-sex peer group (Maccoby, 1988; Ruble et al., 2006). Maccoby (1988, 1998) has argued that these processes contribute to children's tendency to segregate by sex. Moreover, these group processes may strengthen children's individual identification with their female or male identities, which may further strengthen the self-socialization processes described in regard to gender schema theory.

Notably, there is considerably more theoretical work regarding how children come to behave in sex-typed ways than theoretical work that attempts to predict or explain the content of these differences. One relevant theory in this latter regard is evolutionary theory. For instance, Geary, Byrd-Craven, Hoard, Vigil, and Numtee (2003) proposed that because males in our evolutionary history formed coalitions that competed with one another for resources and status, boys should be more likely than girls to play in groups that compete with one another to develop these skills. Wood and Eagly (2002) modify these ideas with their biosocial model. They proposed that certain psychological/behavioral traits, such as competitiveness, are not evolved. Instead, they propose that sex differences in the likelihood of fulfilling certain roles (e.g., warrior, infant caregiver) emerged due to sex differences in size/strength and the biological necessity that women be close to home for birthing and nursing. Biosocial theory suggests that these roles are then socially constructed as male or female roles, and boys and girls are socialized to acquire skills for these roles (e.g., competitiveness for boys, nurturance for girls) regardless of whether the role is a good fit for a particular individual (e.g., in the case of weak males or childless females). Although it is not possible to obtain unequivocal evidence to confirm or refute these theories, both theories provide useful frameworks for thinking about the consistent patterns of sex differences in peer relationships that we describe below.

Key Studies of Sex Differences in Peer Relationships

Although the theoretical work regarding sex differences in peer relationships has focused largely on the development of sex differences, the bulk of empirical studies has documented sex differences in the content of peer relationships. In fact, the pattern of sex differences in peer relationships is strong and consistent enough that some have referred to girls' and boys' peer groups as separate worlds or cultures (Maccoby, 1990; Maltz & Borker, 1982; Tannen, 1990; Thorne, 1986). However, others have argued that this view is too extreme (Thorne, 1993; Underwood, 2003; Zarbatany, McDougall, & Hymel, 2000). In the following subsection, a review of differences in girls' and boys' peer relationships is provided. In the next subsection, the question of whether girls and boys exist in separate peer worlds or cultures is addressed.

Review of Sex Differences in Peer Relationships

The review of sex differences in girls' and boys' peer relationships draws on the writings of Rose and Rudolph (2006). Consistent with distinctions made by them and by Rose (2007), the first subsection of the review focuses on the *structure* of peer relationships (e.g., number of friends, peer group size), and the second focuses on the *content* of peer relationships (e.g., rough-and-tumble play, competitive games, self-disclosure). This review also builds on Rose and Rudolph's (2006) review by including constructs that were not considered therein (e.g., number of friends, peer competition, physical and indirect–relational–social aggression). This review also gives more detail about individual studies, highlighting particular investigations that have made especially significant contributions.

Structure

One of the most robust findings involves the tendency of children to segregate by sex in their peer groups. Children tend to interact primarily with same-sex peers (e.g., Fabes, Martin, & Hanish, 2003; Maccoby & Jacklin, 1987; Martin & Fabes, 2001; Sroufe, Bennett, Englund, Urban, & Shulman, 1993) and they tend to form dyadic friendships with same-sex peers (e.g., Kovacs, Parker, & Hoffman, 1996; Rose, Swenson, & Carlson, 2004). For example, in terms of interactions, in a classic study, Maccoby and Jacklin (1987) found that preschool children played with same-sex peers about three times more often than they played with other-sex peers, and by first grade, the ratio of same-sex to other-sex interaction was about 11:1. To illustrate this point in terms of friendships, Kovacs et al. (1996) found that only about 15% of children in a sample of third and fourth graders had a cross-sex reciprocal friend.

In terms of these same-sex groups, there is a widespread belief that boys' groups are larger than girls' groups. There is some support for this idea, but results vary based on whether general peer interactions or dyadic friendships are considered. In terms of interactions, although observational studies of preschool children are mixed regarding whether there is a sex difference in children's frequency of playing in groups (Benenson, 1993; Fabes et al., 2003; Martin & Fabes, 2001), the tendency of boys to play in groups more than girls increases from ages 4–6 (Benenson, Apostoleris, & Parnass, 1997). By middle childhood, boys' playgroups tend to be larger than girls' groups (Ladd, 1983; Lever, 1976, 1978). Insofar as friendships in middle childhood are concerned, researchers generally do not find a sex difference in the number of reciprocal friends that children have (Kovacs et al., 1996; Rose & Asher, 1999, 2004; Zarbatany et al., 2000); some recent studies have even reported that girls have more reciprocal friends than do boys (Lee, Howe, & Chamberlain, 2007; Rudolph, Ladd, & Dinella, 2007).

One possibility is that girls have as many friends as boys but tend to interact with them sequentially, whereas boys tend to interact with their friends simultaneously in larger groups. If this is the case, boys' friendship networks should be more interconnected than girls' networks, which means that boys' friends would be more likely than girls' friends to be friends with one another. In fact, studies do generally indicate that boys' networks are denser or more interconnected than girls' networks (Benenson, 1990, 1993; Parker & Seal, 1996).

In this light, it is somewhat surprising that boys generally are not found to have larger networks when network size is based on peer nominations of who hangs around together with whom (Bagwell, Coie, Terry, & Lochman, 2000; Cairns, Leung, Buchanan, & Cairns, 1995). It may be that there is some methodological ambiguity regarding the threshold required for nominating classmates as "hanging around" together. For example, a group of four boys who are nominated by classmates as hanging around together may, in fact, be friends with one another and spend most of their time together as a unified group. Classmates also may report that four girls hang around together, even if the girls split their time between being together as a quartet and in two separate dyads.

Content

Sex differences also emerge in how children spend their time with peers. One strong and consistent finding is that boys engage in more rough-and-tumble play than do girls in early and middle childhood (e.g., Fabes et al., 2003; Martin & Fabes, 2001; Blatchford, Baines, & Pellegrini, 2003). For example, in a classic study of preschoolers, DiPietro (1981) found that boys were observed to engage in more wrestling and playful physical assaults (e.g., playful hitting, grabbing, or pushing enacted without intent to harm) than were girls.

Boys also are more likely than girls to engage in competitive activities, such as sports, with peers (e.g., Mathur & Berndt, 2006; Zarbatany et al., 2000). Recent research with children in kindergarten and in fourth grade regarding feelings of discomfort during competition (Benenson, Roy, et al., 2002) may help to explain this sex difference. In a first experiment in which children were placed in groups of four, girls exhibited more discomfort than did boys during the process of choosing a group leader. In a second experiment, children played a game in which they competed with a same-sex peer. Girls exhibited more discomfort while waiting for the winner to be announced and just after the winner was announced. Interestingly, girls did not express more discomfort playing the game when separated from one another by a barrier. Benenson and colleagues suggested that girls' greater discomfort with face-to-face competition might be one reason they are less likely than boys to engage in competitive sports and games.

Other activities are more common among girls. In particular, conversation and disclosure are more common in girls' than in boys' peer interactions. In observational studies of middle childhood youth, girls have been found to spend more time than boys talking with peers (Ladd, 1983; Moller, Hymel, & Rubin, 1992; Blatchford et al., 2003). Girls in middle childhood and adolescence also reported spending more time talking to friends in person and on the telephone (Raffaelli & Duckett, 1989). Self-report studies of personal disclosure have produced mixed results in early to middle childhood (e.g., Buhrmester & Furman, 1987; Parker & Asher, 1993; Patterson, Kupersmidt, & Griesler, 1990), but findings more consistently favor girls among youth in the sixth grade and older (e.g., Buhrmester & Furman, 1987; Camarena, Sarigiani, & Petersen, 1990; Lempers & Clark-Lempers, 1993; for a more thorough review in support of this conclusion, see Rose & Rudolph, 2006). In fact, within single studies, sex differences in self-disclosure have been found to strengthen with age around the transition to adolescence (e.g., Rose, 2002; Zarbatany et al., 2000).

Moreover, some of the most interesting studies of sex differences in peer talk have involved detailed analyses of peer conversations. Whereas some of these studies have been ethnographic (e.g., Tannen, 1990; Sheldon, 1990), others have been quantitative (e.g., Leaper, 1991; Leaper, Tenenbaum, & Shaffer, 1999; Strough & Berg, 2000). For example, in a study of 5- and 7-year-olds, Leaper (1991) compared the conversations of male–male, female–female, and cross-sex dyads. Sex differences were most pronounced among the 7-year-old same-sex dyads, with 7-year-old girl dyads using more collaborative speech and less controlling speech compared to boys. Such findings are consistent with a recent meta-analysis of children's talk with peers (Leaper & Smith, 2004), which found that girls use more affiliative speech than boys, and boys use more assertive speech than girls. Notably, the sex difference for affiliative speech was greater for preadolescents and adolescents than for younger children.

These findings regarding sex differences in language use with peers suggest that girls may be more prosocial with peers than are boys. This question has been addressed in the context of dyadic friendships with studies that examine children's reports of helping in their friendships. The findings are not completely consistent across studies; however, studies with relatively large samples do tend to find a sex difference favoring girls (e.g., Bukowski, Hoza, & Boivin, 1994; Parker & Asher, 1993).

Finally, in terms of content, consider the ways in which children aggress. Sex differences are well documented in terms of physical aggression, with boys consistently found to physically aggress more than do girls (see Archer, 2004; Coie & Dodge, 1998). These findings emerge across methodological approaches, including observation (e.g., Ostrov & Keating, 2004), peer report (e.g., Coie, Dodge, & Copottelli, 1982), and self-report (e.g., Delveaux & Daniels, 2000).

Research is more mixed regarding whether there are sex differences in more subtle forms of aggression. Early studies focused on indirect (Lagerspetz, Bjorkqvist, & Peltonen, 1988) and social (Cairns, Cairns, Neckerman, Ferguson, & Gariépy, 1989) aggression. "Indirect aggression" involves covert aggressive behaviors that are not easily attributed to the perpetrator, because they inflict harm through other peers (e.g., convincing others not to like a peer; Lagerspetz et al., 1988). "Social aggression" refers to exclusion and other behaviors that purposefully damage a peer's reputation (Cairns et al., 1989). This definition was later expanded to include explicitly negative nonverbal behaviors (Galen & Underwood, 1997).

In addition, much of the recent research on more subtle aggression forms focuses on the related construct of "relational aggression" (Crick et al., 1999), which involves aggressive behaviors aimed at harming others' social relationships, such as excluding and threatening to withdraw friendship (Crick & Grotpeter, 1995). In the first study of relational aggression, third- through sixth-grade children nominated peers who displayed relationally aggressive behavior, and results indicated that girls were more relationally aggressive than boys (Crick & Grotpeter, 1995). Since that first study of relational aggression, many additional studies have been conducted.

Despite the increased interest, results are mixed regarding whether there are sex differences in indirect, relational, or social aggression, and different conclusions have been drawn (Crick et al., 1999; Underwood, 2003). A complicating factor is that these studies have differed in terms of the constructs assessed (indirect, relational, or social aggression), the assessment approach used (peer report, self-report, or observation), the age of the participants, and the analytic approach (controlling or not controlling for overt/physical aggression when examining sex differences). Findings may be inconsistent across studies in part because of the different approaches used (Archer, 2004; Underwood, 2003). For example, a recent review of studies examining peer reports of indirect, relational, and social aggression revealed that sex differences are more likely to emerge for adolescents than for children and when overt aggression is controlled in analyses (Smith, Rose, & Schwartz-Mette, 2008). New empirical evidence from a single sample presented in the Smith et al. (2008) paper also indicated that sex differences in relational aggression were stronger for adolescents than for children and when overt aggression was controlled. These findings suggest that one should take into account the different methods used when attempting to draw conclusions about sex differences in nuanced forms of aggression (see also Archer, 2004; Underwood, 2003).

There is more agreement regarding sex differences in terms of the hurtfulness of these more subtle forms of aggression. Studies indicate that girls perceive indirect, relational, and social aggression as more hurtful than do boys (Coyne, Archer, & Eslea, 2006; Crick, 1995; Galen & Underwood, 1997; Paquette & Underwood, 1999). For example, in the study by Paquette and Underwood, young adolescents described recent incidents in which they had been the victim of social aggression, such as a time when they were the target of gossip. Girls reported more negative affect in response to social aggression than did boys and reported thinking about the incidents more than did boys. These find-

ings highlight the importance of examining sex differences in the correlates and consequences of these more subtle aggression forms, in addition to mean-level sex differences
in the aggressive acts per se.

Two Worlds/Cultures Revisited

As noted, the pattern of sex differences in peer relationships is strong and consistent
enough that some have referred to girls and boys as occupying separate worlds (Thorne,
1986) or cultures (Maccoby, 1990; Maltz & Borker, 1982; Tannen, 1990). More recently,
though, criticisms of the two worlds/cultures framework have been raised (Thorne, 1993;
Underwood, 2003, 2004; Zarbatany et al., 2000). Even when significant sex differences for
social behaviors in the peer context emerge, the distributions of girls' and boys' scores
overlap. It has been argued that the two worlds/cultures framework leads to an exaggerated view of sex differences by implying that all girls share a single, homogeneous interaction style, as do boys, and that these styles clearly distinguish girls from boys (Thorne,
1993; Zarbatany et al., 2000; for a similar argument regarding sex difference research in
general, see Hyde, 2005). It has been argued that the framework contributes to thinking about girls and boys in stereotypical ways (e.g., all girls are nice, and all boys are
rough; Underwood, 2004), and that it ignores important within-sex variation in behavior
(Thorne, 1993; Zarbatany et al., 2000). Additionally, critics suggest that the two worlds/
cultures framework ignores the important influence of context on girls' and boys' behavior (Thorne, 1993; Zarbatany et al., 2000), including the existence of contexts in which
girls and boys interact together comfortably (but for an early discussion of the effects of
context on cross-sex interaction, see Thorne, 1986).

Is it reasonable, then, to think of girls and boys as belonging to separate worlds or
cultures? First, if these analogies are considered in a literal sense, then girls and boys do
not occupy separate worlds (e.g., such as Venus and Mars, as has been suggested in the
popular literature; Gray, 1992). However, the two cultures analogy may be reasonable.
Triandis (1994) explains that there may be notable variation among members of a single
culture, and that individuals from different cultures tend to be more similar than different given the many universal human behaviors and perceptions. Although culture has
been defined in a variety of ways, many definitions focus on shared behaviors, norms, and
values (see Matsumoto, 1997; Triandis, 1994). As reviewed, children within a single sex
have behavioral styles that are similar enough to one another and different enough from
children of the other sex to result in conceptually meaningful patterns of sex differences.
In regard to norms and values, other reviews highlight consistent mean-level sex differences in social cognitions related to interpersonal behavior (see Rose & Rudolph, 2006;
Cross & Madson, 1997). As such, despite considerable within-sex variation and overlap in
the behaviors and values of girls and boys, the analogy of girls and boys as representing
different cultures may be reasonable.

Perhaps a more important question, however, is how the framework and recent
criticisms can guide future research (see Underwood, 2004). Work guided by the two
worlds/cultures framework has largely been aimed at identifying mean-level sex differences in peer relationships. Although continuing to document mean-level sex differences
is important, the field also needs to move toward more complex ways of thinking about
the role of sex in peer relationships (see also Underwood, 2003, 2004). Accordingly, the
recent criticisms are useful for guiding future work. In particular, future studies considering within-sex variation would be especially useful, including studies that examine the

correlates and socioemotional outcomes for youth who engage in behavior that is more typical of the other sex (for examples of this type of work, see Crick, 1997; Moller et al., 1992). Also, as we consider in detail in the next section, the role of context is especially useful for providing a more detailed and nuanced understanding of girls' and boys' peer interactions.

Future Directions

There are many possible future directions in regard to understanding better the role of sex in children's peer relationships. We discuss three of them in this section. The first two involve theories of the development of sex differences that we discussed briefly in the first section. In particular, the role of context in eliciting sex differences is considered, then the role of peers as socialization agents. The third direction involves understanding better the psychological and relationship outcomes of sex-typed peer relationship styles.

Context

Although social psychologists often have focused on the role of context in understanding sex differences (Deaux & Major, 1987; Eagly, 1995), developmental scientists have tended to focus on individual-difference factors that contribute to the development of sex differences. Nevertheless, ideas related to context have increasingly been incorporated in peer relations research. Intimate disclosure and competition are two peer behaviors for which sex differences may be better understood by considering context. In terms of disclosure, girls' tendency to interact in smaller dyadic contexts may help to account for girls' greater self-disclosure, in that dyadic contexts may lend themselves more naturally to intimate disclosure (Lansford & Parker, 1999; Leaper, 1994; Underwood, 2004). In contrast, larger group contexts, which are more common among boys, may lend themselves to competition. Consider, for example, a recent study (Benenson, Maiese, et al., 2002) in which third- and fourth-grade children played a competitive game either in groups or in dyads. In this game, children could acquire beads they needed to win the game by either taking beads from a box (a noncompetitive strategy) or taking beads from another child (a competitive strategy). Children were more competitive (i.e., took more beads from other children) in the group context than in the dyadic context. Extrapolating from these results, it seems possible that the greater time they spend in larger peer groups may help to account for boys' greater involvement in activities such as competitive games and sports (Benenson et al., 2000; Benenson, Maiese, et al., 2002). Future studies should examine further how characteristics of contexts that are more typical of girls or boys (e.g., playing close to the teacher) may contribute to sex differences in behaviors in the peer domain.

Also, although it is certainly plausible that girls and boys participating in different social contexts contribute to differences in social behavior, the other direction of effect should be considered as well; that is, it also is possible that preferences for particular behaviors drive children's tendency to participate in certain contexts (Benenson & Heath, 2006; Underwood, 2004). For example, it may be that girls' enjoyment of self-disclosure leads them to seek out dyadic contexts that fit well with this behavior. Likewise, boys' enjoyment of competitive games and sports may lead them to seek out groups, which are necessary for these activities.

Zakriski, Wright, and Underwood (2005) argued that it is useful not only to consider sex differences in the frequency with which children encounter different social contexts, but it is also important to examine whether girls and boys respond differently to the same social contexts. For instance, sex differences in a behavior could occur because one sex encounters a particular context that elicits the behavior more frequently and/or because one sex responds more strongly to the context with that behavior. For instance, Zakriski and colleagues found that the older boys in their sample (mean age of 13 years) encountered peer provocation situations more frequently than did girls and were more likely than girls to respond with physical aggression in this context. The result was an overall sex difference in physical aggression favoring boys. Interestingly, even when girls and boys engage in behaviors at the same frequency, taking the social contexts into account can reveal important sex differences. As an example, in the Zakriski et al. study, there was no overall sex difference in withdrawn behavior for the older children in the sample. However, girls were more likely than boys to withdraw in peer provocation contexts. Girls' greater tendency to withdraw in this context did not result in their exhibiting greater withdrawn behavior overall, because boys were more likely than girls to encounter peer provocation. Accordingly, the finding of no overall sex difference in withdrawn behavior masked interesting differences between girls and boys. In future research, it would be beneficial for researchers to adopt the method used by Zakriski and colleagues, which provides an especially nuanced view of the role of sex in peer relationships.

Peer Socialization

As noted earlier, parents and other adults have been studied as socialization agents to a greater degree than have peers. Nevertheless, some theorists have highlighted the role of peers in socialization (e.g., Harris, 1995). In fact, although the two worlds/cultures framework is not always discussed in this way, the framework can be seen as a peer socialization model, suggesting that girls and boys selectively learn sex-typed interpersonal behaviors in the same-sex groups in which they are immersed (Ruble et al., 2006).

Recent research supports the idea that sex segregation contributes to the development of sex-typed peer interaction styles. Early research suggested that there were not stable individual differences in children's tendencies to interact with same-sex peers (Maccoby & Jacklin, 1987), which meant that children's tendency to segregate by sex was an unlikely candidate for explaining individual differences in sex-typed peer behavior. However, more recent work (Martin & Fabes, 2001) has indicated that there are stable individual differences in preschoolers' tendency to segregate by sex. Most importantly, Martin and Fabes found that a tendency to associate with same-sex peers predicted increases in sex-typed peer behavior over time. For example, greater same-sex exposure predicted increasing rough-and-tumble play, active play, and aggression over time for boys, and more time spent playing close to the teacher for girls.

Demonstrating that same-sex peer exposure contributed to increased sex-typed peer behavior was very important in regard to working toward a better understanding peer socialization of sex-typed behavior. Future research must now address the processes through which same-sex peer exposure leads to sex-typed peer relationship styles (Zarbatany et al., 2000). Early observational studies of preschoolers conducted primarily by Fagot (1977, 1985) suggest that differential reinforcement by peers of sex-typed and cross-sex-typed behavior may be of significance. However, future studies must demonstrate that such processes mediate the link between same-sex peer exposure and increasing sex-typed behavior over time. The lack of such research is an important gap in the literature. Moreover, very little is known about peer socialization of sex-typed behavior after the period of early childhood. Given the intensification of sex-typed behavior that is seen at the transition to adolescence (Hill & Lynch, 1983), the effects of same-sex peer exposure and the processes that help to explain such effects among older children and adolescents require examination.

Trade-Offs

As a final future direction, it will be important to learn more about the outcomes for children who have sex-typed peer relationships styles. Theorists have proposed that the interpersonal styles of girls in general (Keenan & Shaw, 1997), and in peer contexts in particular (Crick & Zahn-Waxler, 2003; Rose & Rudolph, 2006), have trade-offs in that they serve as protective factors for some problems but risk factors for others. For example, Rose and Rudolph (2006) proposed that girls' interpersonal styles with peers benefit their peer relationships in some ways and protect them from the development of externalizing problems but put them at risk for the development of internalizing problems. Rose and Rudolph argued that an important direction for future research is to use longitudinal mediational designs to test directly the idea that sex-typed peer processes contribute to adjustment trade-offs for girls and boys.

Moreover, it was proposed that identifying single relationship processes that have adjustment trade-offs will be especially useful. One such process is "co-rumination," which refers to discussing problems excessively with a relationship partner (Rose, 2002). Co-rumination in friendship, which is more common among girls than boys, is related both to positive friendship quality and to internalizing symptoms concurrently and over time (Rose, 2002; Rose, Carlson, & Waller, 2007). Identifying other, single sex-typed relationship processes related to both positive and negative adjustment outcomes may be useful for informing intervention efforts; that is, it may be difficult to move youth away from peer relationship styles that predict negative adjustment outcomes if these same styles also predict positive outcomes that youth find reinforcing.

Finally, consider the idea that sex-typed relationship styles may lead to a trade-off in terms of communication with same- versus other-sex relationship partners. Specifically, individuals with sex-typed relationship styles may communicate well with same-sex relationship partners but have trouble communicating with people of the other sex. In fact, it has been argued that developing a sex-typed communication style with peers in childhood may lead to difficulties in communication with other-sex relationship partners later in life, in both personal and professional contexts (Leaper, 1994; Maccoby, 1990, 1998, Maltz & Borker, 1982).

However, an alternative hypothesis is that individuals who are especially successful at interacting with same-sex peers in childhood will be successful in their adolescent and adulthood cross-sex relationships. It may be that children with successful same-sex relationships develop these relationships because they are especially socially competent. For example, they may have particularly good social perspective-taking skills and the flexibility to alter their interpersonal styles as needed to facilitate smooth interaction. If this is the case, they may be able to alter their interpersonal styles as needed when they are older to form successful cross-sex relationships. Consistent with this hypothesis, the quality of adolescents' same-sex friendships is predictive of the quality of their romantic relationships prospectively over 1 year (Connolly, Furman, & Konarski, 2000). Future research with longer prospective designs is needed that systematically tracks individuals' communication styles with same- and other-sex relationship partners from childhood through adulthood.

Conclusions

Peer relations researchers have effectively documented mean-level sex differences in peer relationships. Regardless of whether these differences are sufficiently large to justify thinking of girls and boys as inhabiting different peer cultures, the consistent patterns of sex differences in peer relationships are at least as large as those found in many other areas of developmental and social psychology. Researchers also have begun more consistently to move beyond examining mean-level sex differences, and this is an important trend for future research. Future research should further examine the role of context, which includes examining girls' and boys' responses to the same social context. Further consideration of peers as socialization agents and of the outcomes of sex-typed peer styles also will move the field further. Through these and other lines of inquiry, we will learn much more regarding the powerful role of peers in the development of sex-typed relationship styles, as well as regarding the important psychological and relationship outcomes of these styles.

Acknowledgments

During the preparation of this chapter, Amanda J. Rose was partially supported by National Institute of Mental Health Grant No. R01 MH 073590 and Rhiannon L. Smith was supported by a Ridgel Fellowship from the University of Missouri–Columbia.

References

Archer, J. (2004). Sex differences in aggression in real-world settings: A meta-analytic review. *Review of General Psychology, 8*, 291–322.

Bagwell, C. L., Coie, J. D., Terry, R. A., & Lochman, J. E. (2000). Peer clique participation and social status in preadolescence. *Merrill–Palmer Quarterly, 46*, 280–305.

Benenson, J. F. (1990). Gender differences in social networks. *Journal of Early Adolescence, 10*, 472–495.

Benenson, J. F. (1993). Greater preference among females than males for dyadic interaction in early childhood. *Child Development, 64*, 544–555.

Benenson, J. F., Apostoleris, N. H., & Parnass, J. (1997). Age and sex differences in dyadic and group interaction. *Developmental Psychology, 33*, 538–543.

Benenson, J. F., Gordon, A. J., & Roy, R. (2000). Children's evaluative appraisals of competition in tetrads versus dyads. *Small Group Research, 31*, 635–652.

Benenson, J. F., & Heath, A. (2006). Boys withdraw more in one-on-one interactions, whereas girls withdraw more in groups. *Developmental Psychology, 42*, 272–282.

Benenson, J. F., Maiese, R., Dolenszky, E., Dolenszky, N., Sinclair, N., & Simpson, A. (2002). Groups size regulates self-assertive versus self-deprecating responses to interpersonal competition. *Child Development, 73*, 1818–1829.

Benenson, J. F., Roy, R., Waite, A., Goldbaum, S., Linders, L., & Simpson, A. (2002). Greater discomfort as a proximate cause of sex differences in competition. *Merrill–Palmer Quarterly, 48,* 225–247.

Berenbaum, S. A., & Hines, M. (1992). Early androgens are related to childhood sex-typed toy preferences. *Psychological Sciences, 3,* 203–206.

Blatchford, P., Baines, E., & Pellegrini, A. (2003). The social context of school playground games: Sex and ethnic differences, and changes over time after entry to junior school. *British Journal of Developmental Psychology, 21,* 481–505.

Buhrmester, D., & Furman, W. (1987). The development of companionship and intimacy. *Child Development, 58,* 1101–1113.

Bukowski, W. M., Hoza, B., & Boivin, M. (1994). Measuring friendship quality during pre- and early adolescence: The development and psychometric properties of the friendship qualities scale. *Journal of Social and Personal Relationships, 11,* 471–484.

Bussey, K., & Bandura, A. (1999). Social cognitive theory of gender development and differentiation. *Psychological Review, 106,* 676–713.

Cairns, R. B., Cairns, B. D., Neckerman, H. J., Ferguson, L. L., & Gariépy, J. (1989). Growth and aggression: I. Childhood to early adolescence. *Developmental Psychology, 25,* 320–330.

Cairns, R. B., Leung, M., Buchanan, L., & Cairns, B. D. (1995). Friendships and social networks in childhood and adolescence: Fluidity, reliability, and interrelations. *Child Development, 66,* 1330–1345.

Camarena, P. M., Sarigiani, P. A., & Petersen, A. C. (1990). Gender specific pathways to intimacy in early adolescence. *Journal of Youth and Adolescence, 19,* 19–32.

Coie, J. D., & Dodge, K. A. (1998). Aggression and antisocial behavior. In W. Damon (Series Ed.) & N. Eisenberg (Vol. Ed.), *Handbook of child psychology: Vol. 3. Social, emotional, and personality development* (5th ed., pp. 779–862). New York: Wiley.

Coie, J. D., Dodge, K. A., & Copottelli, H. (1982). Dimensions and types of social status: A cross-age perspective. *Developmental Psychology, 18,* 557–570.

Connolly, J., Furman, W., & Konarski, R. (2000). The role of peers in the emergence of heterosexual romantic relationships in adolescence. *Child Development, 71,* 1395–1408.

Coyne, S. M., Archer, J., & Eslea, M. (2006). "We're not friends anymore! Unless … ": The frequency and harmfulness of indirect, relational, and social aggression. *Aggressive Behavior, 32,* 294–307.

Crick, N. R. (1995). Relational aggression: The role of intent attributions, feelings of distress, and provocation type. *Development and Psychopathology, 7,* 313–322.

Crick, N. R. (1997). Engagement in gender normative versus nonnormative forms of aggression: Links to social-psychological adjustment. *Developmental Psychology, 33,* 610–617.

Crick, N. R., & Grotpeter, J. K. (1995). Relational aggression, gender, and social-psychological adjustment. *Child Development, 66,* 710–722.

Crick, N. R., Werner, N. E., Casas, J. F., O'Brien, K. M., Nelson, D. A., Grotpeter, J. K., et al. (1999). Childhood aggression and gender: A new look at an old problem. In D. Bernstein (Ed.), *Nebraska Symposium on Motivation: Vol. 45. Gender and motivation* (pp. 75–141). Lincoln: University of Nebraska Press.

Crick, N. R., & Zahn-Waxler, C. (2003). The development of psychopathology in females and males: Current progress and future challenges. *Development and Psychopathology, 15,* 719–742.

Cross, S. E., & Madson, L. (1997). Models of the self: Self-construals and gender. *Psychological Bulletin, 122,* 5–37.

Deaux, K., & Major, B. (1987). Putting gender into context: An interactive model of gender related behaviors. *Psychological Review, 94,* 369–389.

Delveaux, K. D., & Daniels, T. (2000). Children's social cognitions: Physically and relationally aggressive strategies and children's goals in peer conflict situations. *Merrill–Palmer Quarterly, 46,* 672–692.

DiPietro, J. A. (1981). Rough and tumble play: A function of gender. *Developmental Psychology, 17,* 50–58.

Eagly, A. H. (1995). The science and politics of comparing women and men. *American Psychologist, 50*, 145–158.

Fabes, R. A., Martin, C. L., & Hanish, L. D. (2003). Young children's play qualities in same-, other-, and mixed-sex peer groups. *Child Development, 74*, 921–932.

Fagot, B. (1977). Consequences of moderate cross-gender behavior in preschool children. *Child Development, 48*, 902–907.

Fagot, B. (1985). Beyond the reinforcement principle: Another step toward understanding sex role development. *Developmental Psychology, 21*, 1097–1104.

Galen, B. R., & Underwood, M. K. (1997). A developmental investigation of social aggression among children. *Developmental Psychology, 33*, 589–600.

Geary, D. C., Byrd-Craven, J., Hoard, M. K., Vigil, J., & Numtee, C. (2003). Evolution and development of boys' social behavior. *Developmental Review, 23*, 444–470.

Golombok, S., & Hines, M. (2002). Sex differences in social behavior. In P. K. Smith & C. H. Hart (Eds.), *Blackwell handbook of childhood social development* (pp. 117–136). Malden, MA: Blackwell.

Gray, J. (1992). *Men are from Mars, women are from Venus: The classic guide to understanding the opposite sex*. New York: HarperCollins.

Harris, J. R. (1995). Where is the child's environment?: A group socialization theory of development. *Psychological Review, 102*, 458–489.

Hill, J. P., & Lynch, M. E. (1983). The intensification of gender-related role expectations during early adolescence. In J. Brooks-Gunn & A. C. Petersen (Eds.), *Girls at puberty: Biological and psychosocial perspectives* (pp. 201–228). New York: Plenum Press.

Hines, M., & Kaufman, F. (1994). Androgen and the development of human sex-typed behavior: Rough-and-tumble play and sex of preferred playmates in children with congenital adrenal hyperplasia (CAH). *Child Development, 65*, 1042–1053.

Hyde, J. S. (2005). The gender similarities hypothesis. *American Psychologist, 60*, 581–592.

Keenan, K., & Shaw, D. (1997). Developmental and social influences on young girls' early problem behavior. *Psychological Bulletin, 121*, 95–113.

Kovacs, D. M., Parker, J. G., & Hoffman, L. W. (1996). Behavioral, affective, and social correlates of involvement in cross-sex friendship in elementary school. *Child Development, 67*, 2269–2286.

Ladd, G. W. (1983). Social networks of popular, average, and rejected children in school settings. *Merrill–Palmer Quarterly, 29*, 283–307.

Lagerspetz, K. M. J., Bjorkqvist, K., & Peltonen, T. (1988). Is indirect aggression typical of females?: Gender differences in aggressiveness in 11- to 12-year old children. *Aggressive Behavior, 14*, 403–414.

Lansford, J. E., & Parker, J. G. (1999). Children's interactions in triads: Behavioral profiles and effects of gender and patterns of friendships among members. *Developmental Psychology, 35*, 80–93.

Leaper, C. (1991). Influence and involvement in children's discourse: Age, gender, and partner effects. *Child Development, 62*, 797–811.

Leaper, C. (1994). Exploring the consequences of gender segregation on social relationships. In *Childhood gender segregation: Causes and consequences* (New Directions for Child Development, No. 65, pp. 67–86). San Francisco: Jossey-Bass.

Leaper, C., & Friedman, C. K. (2007). The socialization of gender. In J. E. Grusec & P. D. Hastings (Eds.), *Handbook of socialization: Theory and research* (pp. 561–587). New York: Guilford Press.

Leaper, C., & Smith, T. E. (2004). A meta-analytic review of gender variations in children's language use: Talkativeness, affiliative speech, and assertive speech. *Developmental Psychology, 40*, 993–1027.

Leaper, C., Tenenbaum, H. R., & Shaffer, T. G. (1999). Communication patterns of African American girls and boys from low-income, urban backgrounds. *Child Development, 70*, 1489–1503.

Lee, L., Howe, C., & Chamberlain, B. (2007). Ethnic heterogeneity of social networks and cross-ethnic friendships of elementary school boys and girls. *Merrill–Palmer Quarterly, 53*, 325–346.

Lempers, J. D., & Clark-Lempers, D. S. (1993). A functional comparison of same-sex and opposite-sex friendships during adolescence. *Journal of Adolescent Research, 8*, 89–108.

Lever, J. (1976). Sex differences in the games children play. *Social Problems, 23*, 478–487.

Lever, J. (1978). Sex differences in the complexity of children's play and games. *American Sociological Review, 43*, 471–483.

Maccoby, E. E. (1988). Gender as a social category. *Developmental Psychology, 24*, 755–765.

Maccoby, E. E. (1990). Gender and relationships: A developmental account. *American Psychologist, 45*, 513–520.

Maccoby, E. E. (1998). *The two sexes: Growing up apart, coming together.* Cambridge, MA: Harvard University Press.

Maccoby, E. E., & Jacklin, C. N. (1987). Gender segregation in childhood. In H. W. Reese (Ed.), *Advances in child development and behavior* (Vol. 20, pp. 239–287). New York: Academic Press.

Maltz, D. N., & Borker, R. A. (1982). A cultural approach to male–female miscommunication. In J. A. Gumperz (Ed.), *Language and social identity* (pp. 195–216). New York: Cambridge University Press.

Martin, C. L., & Fabes, R. A. (2001). The stability and consequences of young children's same-sex peer interactions. *Developmental Psychology, 37*, 431–446.

Martin, C. L., Ruble, D. N., & Szkrybalo, J. (2002). Cognitive theories of early gender development. *Psychological Bulletin, 128*, 903–933.

Mathur, R., & Berndt, T. J. (2006). Relations of friends' activities to friendship quality. *Journal of Early Adolescence, 26*, 365–388.

Matsumoto, D. (1997). *Culture and modern life.* Pacific Grove, CA: Brooks/Cole.

Moller, L. C., Hymel, S., & Rubin, K. H. (1992). Sex typing in play and popularity in middle childhood. *Sex Roles, 26*, 331–353.

Ostrov, J. M., & Keating, C. F. (2004). Gender differences in preschool aggression during free play and structured interactions: An observational study. *Social Development, 13*, 255–277.

Paquette, J. A., & Underwood, M. K. (1999). Gender differences in young adolescents' experiences of peer victimization: Social and physical aggression. *Merrill–Palmer Quarterly, 45*, 242–266.

Parker, J. G., & Asher, S. R. (1993). Friendship and friendship quality in middle childhood: Links with peer group acceptance and feelings of loneliness and social dissatisfaction. *Developmental Psychology, 29*, 611–621.

Parker, J. G., & Seal, J. (1996). Forming, losing, renewing, and replacing friendships: Applying temporal parameters to the assessment of children's friendship experiences. *Child Development, 67*, 2248–2268.

Patterson, C. J., Kupersmidt, J. B., & Griesler, P. C. (1990). Children's perception of self and of relationships with others as a function of sociometric status. *Child Development, 61*, 1335–1349.

Raffaelli, M., & Duckett, E. (1989). "We were just talking … ": Conversations in early adolescence. *Journal of Youth and Adolescence, 18*, 567–582.

Rose, A. J. (2002). Co-rumination in the friendships of girls and boys. *Child Development, 73*, 1830–1843.

Rose, A. J. (2007). Structure, content, and socioemotional correlates of girls' and boys' friendships: Recent advances and future directions. *Merrill–Palmer Quarterly, 53*, 489–506.

Rose, A. J., & Asher, S. R. (1999). Children's goals and strategies in response to conflicts within a friendship. *Developmental Psychology, 35*, 69–79.

Rose, A. J., & Asher, S. R. (2004). Children's strategies and goals in response to help-giving and help-seeking tasks within a friendship. *Child Development, 75*, 749–763.

Rose, A. J., Carlson, W., & Waller, E. M. (2007). Prospective associations of co-rumination with friendship and emotional adjustment: Considering the socioemotional trade-offs of co-rumination. *Developmental Psychology, 43*, 1019–1031.

Rose, A. J., & Rudolph, K. D. (2006). A review of sex differences in peer relationship processes: Potential trade-offs for the emotional and behavioral development of girls and boys. *Psychological Bulletin, 132*, 98–131.

Rose, A. J., Swenson, L. P., & Carlson, W. (2004). Friendships of aggressive youth: Considering the influences of being disliked and of being perceived as popular. *Journal of Experimental Child Psychology, 88*, 25–45.

Ruble, D. N., Martin, C. L., & Berenbaum, S. A. (2006). Gender development. In W. Damon & R. M. Lerner (Series Eds.) & N. Eisenberg (Vol. Ed.), *Handbook of child psychology: Vol. 3. Social, emotional, and personality development* (6th ed., pp. 858–932). Hoboken, NJ: Wiley.

Rudolph, K. D., Ladd, G., & Dinella, L. (2007). Gender differences in the interpersonal consequences of early-onset depressive symptoms. *Merrill–Palmer Quarterly, 53*, 461–488.

Sheldon, D. (1990). Pickle fights: Gendered talk in preschool disputes. *Discourse Processes, 13*, 5–31.

Smith, R. L., Rose, A. J., & Schwartz-Mette, R. A. (2008). *Relational and overt aggression in childhood and adolescence: Clarifying mean-level gender differences and associations with peer acceptance.* Manuscript submitted for publication.

Sroufe, L. A., Bennett, C., Englund, M., Urban, J., & Shulman, S. (1993). The significance of gender boundaries in preadolescence: Contemporary correlates and antecedents of boundary violation and maintenance. *Child Development, 64*, 455–466.

Strough, J., & Berg, C. A. (2000). Goals as a mediator of gender differences in high-affiliation dyadic conversations. *Developmental Psychology, 36*, 117–125.

Tajfel, H. (1982). Social psychology of intergroup relations. *Annual Review of Psychology, 33*, 1–39.

Tannen, D. (1990). Gender differences in topical coherence: Creating involvement in best friends' talk. *Discourse Processes, 13*, 73–90.

Thorne, B. (1986). Girls and boys together … but mostly apart: Gender arrangements in elementary schools. In W. W. Hartup & Z. Rubin (Eds.), *Relationships and development* (pp. 167–184). Hillsdale, NJ: Erlbaum.

Thorne, B. (1993). *Gender play: Girls and boys in school.* New Brunswick: Rutgers University Press.

Triandis, H. C. (1994). *Culture and social behavior.* New York: McGraw-Hill.

Underwood, M. K. (2003). *Social aggression among girls.* New York: Guilford Press.

Underwood, M. K. (2004). Gender and peer relations: Are the two gender cultures really all that different? In J. B. Kupersmidt & K. A. Dodge (Eds.), *Children's peer relations: From development to intervention* (pp. 21–36). Washington, DC: American Psychological Association.

Wood, W., & Eagly, A. H. (2002). A cross-cultural analysis of the behavior of women and men: Implications for the origins of sex differences. *Psychological Bulletin, 128*, 699–727.

Zakriski, A. L., Wright, J. C., & Underwood, M. K. (2005). Gender similarities and differences in children's social behavior: Finding personality in contextualized patterns of adaptation. *Journal of Personality and Social Psychology, 88*, 844–855.

Zarbatany, L., McDougall, P., & Hymel, S. (2000). Gender-differentiated experience in the peer culture: Links to intimacy in preadolescence. *Social Development, 9*, 62–79.

CHAPTER 22

Race and Ethnicity
in Peer Relations Research

SANDRA GRAHAM
APRIL Z. TAYLOR
ALICE Y. HO

As we began to gather the relevant empirical literatures for this *Handbook* chapter, we were reminded of an article that S. Graham (1992) published, with the title, "Most of the Subjects Were White and Middle Class." That article reported a 20-year (1970–1989) content analysis of empirical studies in six journals of the American Psychological Association in which African Americans were represented as participants. The representation was small, hovering around 4%, which led to the conclusion that psychology had not established an adequate empirical base to understand the psychological functioning of African American children and adults.

When it comes to the peer relations literature, the situation is not much better today. To illustrate, we conducted a literature search on PsycINFO, with the key words "peer relations," "peer networks," "friendships," "peer nominations," or "sociometrics" in age groups that spanned childhood and adolescence. We specified 20 years (1986–2006) and journal articles only, to exclude dissertations or other unpublished works. The search yielded 1,495 articles that met the selection criteria. We then did an additional search of these articles, selecting PsycINFO key words that included "race," "ethnicity," the specific racial/ethnic groups (i.e., "African American/black," "Latino/Hispanic," "Asian American," "American Indian") or related terms such as "racial and ethnic attitudes" and "racial relations." Of the 1,495 citations. only 111, or 7%, addressed race and ethnicity as indicated by mention of any of these key words.

This brief content analysis tells us something important. Much of the extant peer relations research has been conducted in urban school contexts that represent multiple ethnic groups, but little of that research has systematically examined ethnicity-related variables. This is disappointing, because the formation and maintenance of friendships, the dynamics of peer acceptance and rejection, and the factors that exacerbate aggression and victimization are likely to be influenced by contextual factors, such as the ethnic composition of schools and neighborhoods, as well as the social and ethnic identities that are most significant to youth.

The absence of a strong empirical base made organizing this chapter a challenge—how to select topics that had been adequately studied, and that fit within the disciplinary boundaries of peer relations research. Following the lead of other reviews that focused on peer interactions at increasing levels of complexity (e.g., Rubin, Bukowski, & Parker, 2006), we divided this chapter into three main sections. We begin at the dyadic level with the literature on cross-racial friendships. Next, we focus on peer processes to consider how race and ethnicity inform research on the characteristics of students who enjoy positive status in the peer group and those who endure disdain (e.g., victimization) or fall under the influence of deviant peers. In the third section we turn to group-level analyses in which membership is defined by race or ethnicity. Here we focus on challenges that youth of color may confront from outgroup members in the form of prejudice and discrimination, and from ingroup members who may question their allegiance to the presumed norms of their particular racial/ethnic group. Although selective in our topics, we needed to cast a broad conceptual net that recognizes the historical and cultural forces that continue to shape the experiences of ethnic minority youth in the United States. Those forces often result in social and economic marginality that positions some minority groups at the bottom of a status hierarchy. We acknowledge the structural inequality that affects the peer experiences of youth of color, although we realize that we cannot do justice to it in this chapter. Rather, our goal is to discuss the unique challenges of children from different racial and ethnic groups as they forge social bonds with peers.

We use the terms "race" and "ethnicity" throughout the chapter. In theory, race is an ascribed category, with a "race" being a group of persons with shared genetic, biological, and physical features. Using that definition and the U.S. census designations, black/African Americans, whites, and Asians represent different races, and we refer to them as such in this chapter. "Ethnicity," on the other hand, is a category, either ascribed or voluntary, that reflects a group's common history, nationality, geography, language, and culture. With common origins in Mexico, Latin America, or the Caribbean, Latinos/Hispanics can be of any racial group, and the construct of ethnicity allows us to define their shared identity. We prefer the term "Latino" to "Hispanic," because it better captures that group's non-Western European ancestry. We acknowledge that race is more socially constructed than biologically determined, in that the meaning of racial group membership changes across time and context. For that reason some scholars prefer to only use the label "ethnicity," because it is less reductionist (Blaine, 2007), whereas others advocate consolidating "race" and "ethnicity" into a single identifier for the sake of clarity (Phinney, 1996). We maintain the distinction but use the terms in tandem in this chapter, except when referring to distinct research literatures (e.g., cross-racial friendships between whites and blacks vs. cross-ethnic friendships between whites and Latinos).

Friendships across Different Racial and Ethnic Groups

There is a robust empirical literature on the role of race and ethnicity in children's friendships, although that research has been carried out more by sociologists of education than by developmental psychologists with expertise on peer relations. Beginning with the school desegregation literature of the 1970s, researchers have been asking to what extent children prefer friends from their same racial or ethnic group, the conditions under which they become receptive to interracial friendships, whether same-race and cross-race friendships are similar or different in quality, and whether there are psychological benefits to crossing racial and ethnic boundaries in friendship choices.

Interracial friendships in school have been studied at virtually all developmental periods, including preschool (e.g., Lederberg, Chapin, Rosenblatt, & Vandell, 1986), early elementary school (e.g., Finkelstein & Haskins, 1983; Singleton & Asher, 1979), middle and late elementary grades (e.g., Aboud, Mendelson, & Purdy, 2003; Graham & Cohen, 1997), middle school (e.g., Damico & Sparks, 1986; DuBois & Hirsch, 1990), and high school (e.g., Hamm, Brown, & Heck, 2005). In most of these studies, respondents either selected their close friends from a class or school roster or rated all of the rostered schoolmates on friendship closeness. Observational studies that track close interactions between students of different ethnic groups have also been carried out during nonacademic time in classrooms (Schofield & Francis, 1982), on playgrounds (Finkelstein & Haskins, 1983), and in cafeterias during lunch (Schofield & Sagar, 1977; Zisman & Wilson, 1992).

In choosing friends, do students show a preference for same-race/ethnicity peers over different race/ethnicity peers? The answer to this question is a resounding "yes" for all racial/ethnic groups and developmental periods studied. A strong ingroup preference has been documented regardless of whether friendship choices are derived from sociometric nominations, ratings of classmates, or observational techniques, and whether the studies sample only a few classrooms in a single school (e.g., Sagar, Schofield, & Snyder, 1983) or several thousand students across multiple schools, as in nationally representative samples such as the National Longitudinal Study of Adolescent Health (Add Health; e.g., Mouw & Entwisle, 2006). In studies that calculate frequencies or odds ratios of same-race to cross-race choices, same-race close friendships are at least twice as likely as cross-race friendships to be endorsed (Moody, 2001). Moreover, strong within racial/ethnic group preference appears to increase as children get older (Singleton & Asher, 1979; Shrum, Cheek, & Hunter, 1988). Most of the interracial friendship research has been restricted to African American and white respondents, but studies that do include multiple ethnic groups report that Latino and Asian youth also prefer ingroup peers as friends (e.g., Hamm et al., 2005). It should be expected that students prefer same-ethnicity peers as friends, because one of the major determinants of friendship selection is "homophily," or the degree of similarity between potential friends (see Rubin et al., 2006). However, the robustness of the ingroup preference was somewhat surprising.

Quality of Interracial Friendships

Studies that directly tap quality indicators such as closeness and support report some differences in favor of same ethnicity dyads, but the differences tend to be small (Aboud et al., 2003; Schneider, Dixon, & Udvari, 2007). This makes sense, in that cross-ethnic friendships are harder to come by and can therefore be expected to be of relatively high quality. In one study reporting indirect evidence of quality, Lease and Blake (2005) found that elementary school-age children with a mutual interracial friendship who were also members of the majority racial group in their classroom (black or white) were reported to be more popular, more self-confident, and better leaders than their majority group peers without an interracial friend, suggesting that the friendship promoted the development of positive qualities. On the other hand, a recent Add Health study (Kao & Joyner, 2004) that used reported activities in the last week (e.g., getting together after school, talking on the phone) as a measure of quality found that cross-racial and ethnic best friendships were lower in quality (involved fewer activities) than within-group friendships.

Another index of friendship quality is stability; a small longitudinal literature has examined the endurance of interracial compared to intraracial friendship dyads. The findings are fairly consistent in documenting less stability when children befriend a peer of a different race (Aboud et al., 2003; Hallinan & Williams, 1987; Schneider et al., 2007). For example, Hallinan and Williams (1987) reported that cross-race friendships were less likely to endure for more than 6 weeks in their fourth- to seventh-grade sample, but that contextual factors moderated the stability findings. Black students' choices of a white friend were less stable in classrooms where teachers emphasized academic performance, suggesting that academic status differences between blacks and whites can be a deterrent to friendship maintenance.

Friendships and the Ethnic Composition of Schools

The public discourse in support of *Brown v. Board of Education* always maintained that racially integrated schools increase the opportunity for cross-race friendships. Probably the most cited research on racial composition and interracial friendships in integrated schools is the series of studies conducted by Hallinan and colleagues during the 1980s (e.g., Hallinan & Smith, 1985; Hallinan & Teixeira, 1987). Hallinan et al. examined same- and cross-race friendships of black and white fourth- to seventh-grade students selected from 20–40 classrooms that varied in racial composition (i.e., majority white, balanced, majority black). Findings supported the "opportunity hypothesis": As the proportion of minority group (white or black) students increased in a classroom, majority group students were more likely to befriend them.

More recent studies of cross-ethnic friendships focusing on racial/ethnic composition have benefited from the much larger and ethnically diverse samples available in the national panel studies such as Add Health. With about 100,000 seventh to twelfth graders from multiple ethnic groups, the Add Health sample was drawn from more than 100 U. S. middle schools and high schools that represent a full range of ethnic diversity (from ethnically homogeneous to heterogeneous). Add Health is also amenable to more sophisticated multilevel modeling techniques that allow researchers to assess whether the probability of endorsing cross-ethnic friendships is equal to the opportunity for such relationships based on ethnic composition of the school. Like the earlier and smaller scale research with younger children, studies using Add Health data report that increasing racial/ethnic homogeneity at the school level does lead to more cross-ethnic friendships (e.g., Kao & Joyner, 2004; Moody, 2001; Mouw & Entwisle, 2006). However, the rate of increase does not keep pace with the opportunity for such friendships based on the ethnic composition of schools. Ironically, the likelihood of befriending a peer from another ethnicity actually *decreases* at moderate levels of ethnic diversity, with only two groups that are about equally represented at 50% each (Moody, 2001). It has been suggested that two groups of equal size exacerbate perceptions of "us" versus "them," which can then lead to greater ingroup favoritism and outgroup derogation.

Friendships and the Organization of Schools

Imagine a multiethnic school with African American, white, Asian, and Latino students all fairly well represented. This level of racial/ethnic diversity theoretically should maximize the opportunity for students to form friendships outside of their own group. However, if schools adopt organizational practices, such as academic tracking, that limit the mixing opportunities of students, then the possible benefits of exposure to multiple ethnic groups will be compromised. Because African American and Latino students are more likely to be placed in lower ability tracks, whereas white and Asian students are more likely to be placed in higher ability tracks (e.g., Oakes, 1995), tracking can resegregate students by limiting cross-ethnic exposure even in ethnically diverse schools. Many studies, both older and more recent, have documented the negative effects of academic tracking on cross-ethnic friendships (e.g., Damico & Sparks, 1986; Kubitschek & Hallinan, 1998; Moody, 2001; Schofield & Sagar, 1977). Furthermore, academic tracking appears to particularly inhibit the willingness of white students to form friendships with African American students (Damico, Bell-Nathaniel, & Green, 1981; Hallinan & Teixeira, 1987) and for Asian students to befriend anyone else but whites (Hamm et al., 2005). Clearly, the opportunities for cross-ethnic interaction that are facilitated by numerical balance among racial/ethnic groups in diverse schools are superseded by the numerical imbalance among racial/ethnic groups that academic tracking brings.

Friendships and Intergroup Attitudes

One reason for the interest in cross-race friendships is the role that friendships are presumed to play in the improvement of intergroup relations in schools. A core feature of the social scientist's argument in support of *Brown v. Board of Education* was that closer contact between members of different races (i.e., through school desegregation) promotes positive racial attitudes. The development of friendships was presumed to be one mechanism for the maintenance of sustained contact (see Pettigrew, 1998).

Hundreds of studies with child and adult populations have examined whether interracial contact improves intergroup attitudes. In a recent meta-analysis of this vast literature, Pettigrew and Tropp (2006) concluded that contact does indeed reduce prejudice. However, only a few of those contact studies actually measured interracial friendships, and even fewer were carried out with children and adolescents (e.g., Damico et al., 1981). Moreover, because cross-race friendship studies are mainly correlational, it is not possible to determine whether, indeed, cross-race friendships lead to improved intergroup attitudes, in support of the contact hypothesis, or whether more positive attitudes increase one's receptivity to crossing racial boundaries in friend selection. Only two studies—one with college students (Levin, van Laar, & Sidanius, 2003), the other with a sample of adolescents and adults (Eller & Abrams, 2003)—examined changes in friendship and intergroup attitudes longitudinally. For example, Levin et al. (2003) documented that cross-ethnic friendships in the second and third year of college predict better racial attitudes during the fourth year of college, even when controlling for precollegiate and freshman-year attitudes and cross-ethnic friendships.

Summary

A very robust finding in the interracial friendship literature is that children and adolescents show a preference for same-race/ethnicity friendships. Within-group friendships also appear to be of higher quality, although only a few studies have examined differences between same-race and cross-race friendships on this dimension. More ethnic diversity in schools increases the opportunity for cross-ethnic friendships; however, instructional practices, such as academic tracking, limit the mixing opportunities of students of different ethnic groups even in diverse schools. Cross-ethnic friendships are related to improved intergroup attitudes, but the needed longitudinal studies to establish causal relationships have not been conducted.

Peer Processes

Social Acceptance and Popularity

Concurrent with the study of cross-ethnic friendships in the 1970s and the increasing use of peer nomination techniques to identify friends, researchers also became interested in the behavioral profiles of socially accepted or popular ethnic minority (primarily African American) youth. In one of the first studies to examine multiple social status types based on peer nominations (Coie, Dodge, & Coppotelli, 1982), third- to eighth-grade children who had reputations as well liked were also perceived to be leaders, although this relation was stronger for white than African American children. For African American youth, perceived leadership was more strongly associated with having a reputation as controversial (i.e., many *liked most* and *liked least* nominations). In a similar study with third to fifth graders (Kistner, Metzler, Gatlin, & Risi, 1993), sociometric popularity among white youth was correlated with a high prosocial and low aggressive reputation whereas among black youth, low aggression did not predict popularity. Such findings intimated that the social consensus about what it means to be popular might be different for African American youth.

The most consistent evidence for racial differences in the meaning of popularity has focused on the relationship between social acceptance and having a reputation as aggressive. Beginning in the 1990s, a number of studies using variants of peer nomination procedures have documented a positive relationship between popularity and aggressive status among African American youth (Luthar & McMahon, 1996; Meisinger, Blake, Lease, Palaedy, & Olejnik, 2007; Rodkin, Farmer, Pearl, & Van Acker, 2000) For example, applying cluster analysis to peer nominations and teacher reports of the behavioral characteristics of fourth- to sixth-grade African American and white boys, Rodkin et al. (2000) identified an aggressive and popular subgroup that they labeled as "tough" boys, in contrast to a popular and prosocial group, classified as "model" boys. These authors reported that African American boys were more likely than their white peers to be in the tough cluster, especially when they were a numerical minority in their classroom, a context in which their antisocial behavior might have been more prominent. Based on peer nominations in fourth- to sixth-grade classrooms that were majority white or majority African American, Meisinger et al. (2007) reported that aggression predicted popularity only in majority African American classrooms, suggesting that the peer norms supporting aggression were higher when there were more African American students in a classroom. These latter studies are among the very few in the peer relations literature documenting that the racial composition of classrooms might be an important contextual factor shaping social reputations.

Based on comparative racial analyses, such as those cited earlier, it has been suggested that aggression may be more accepted, tolerated, or even admired among urban African American youth, particularly males, many of whom must cope with the challenges of growing up in economically disadvantaged communities (e.g., Luthar & McMahon, 1996). Other evidence, however, calls into question whether a popular–aggressive reputation relationship is unique, or even stronger, in youth of color. First, studies that examine within–racial group peer preferences document much heterogeneity among African American respondents in the degree to which antisocial youth enjoy positive regard (e.g., Farmer, Estell, Bishop, O'Neal, & Cairns, 2003; Xie, Li, Boucher, Hutchins, & Cairns, 2006). In the eyes of black youth, there are both popular and unpopular antisocial peers and popularity is just as likely to be associated with prosocial as with antisocial characteristics. Second, studies that have attempted to track the developmental course of popularity–aggression linkages have documented that it is quite normative for all children in late childhood and early adolescence to associate popularity with both prosocial and antisocial tendencies (see Asher & McDonald, Chapter 13, this volume). In many studies with white, as well as with ethnic minority youth, peers who are rated highly on popularity are not only athletic and smart but also physically and relationally aggressive. As researchers have attempted to distinguish between sociometric popularity (nominations for *like* vs. *dislike*) and perceived popularity, we know that popularity is more closely associated with visibility (notoriety?) and dominance than with being liked or disliked, and it is quite consistent with developmental analyses to document that antisocial youth in general enjoy short-term popularity (e.g., Moffitt, 1993).

Negative Peer Regard: Victimization

"Peer victimization," also labeled as peer "harassment" or "bullying," has been defined as physical, verbal, or psychological abuse of a victim by one or more perpetrators who intend to cause the victim harm (Olweus, 1994). The critical features that distinguish victimization from simple conflict between peers are the intention to cause harm and an imbalance of power between perpetrator and victim. Hitting, name-calling, intimidating gestures, racial slurs, spreading of rumors, and social exclusion by powerful others are all examples of behaviors that constitute peer victimization. These kinds of behaviors at school are widespread and have detrimental effects on the lives of many youth (see S. Graham, 2006).

North American research on peer victimization that has addressed race or ethnicity is predictably sparse. Of the extant empirical literature, generally two types of studies have been conducted. One group of studies, largely descriptive and guided by a public health model, has examined the prevalence of victimization in particular racial/ethnic groups during adolescence (Juvonen, Graham, & Schuster, 2003; Nansel et al., 2001; Peskin, Tortolero, & Markham, 2006; Storch, Nock, Masia-Warner, & Barlas, 2003). Findings from these studies are inconsistent. For example, Juvonen et al. (2003) reported that Latinos were the least victimized among the four major racial/ethnic groups of sixth graders; Nansel et al. (2001) documented that Latinos were the most victimized in their sample of sixth to tenth graders from the same ethnic groups; Peskin et al. (2006) documented that Africans Americans were more victimized than Latinos in sixth to twelfth grade; and Storch et al. (2003) found no differences in victim status between African American and Latino fifth and sixth graders. Based on these comparative analyses, there is no generalizable support for the notion that ethnicity, in and of itself, is a risk factor for peer victimization.

A second type of peer victimization research that includes multiethnic samples has focused on the ethnic composition of classrooms and schools. Rather than restricting analyses to comparisons between different racial/ethnic groups, these studies have examined whether students are in the numerical majority or minority in their school context, and have documented that victimized students are more likely to be members of ethnic minority groups (S. Graham & Juvonen, 2002; Hanish & Guerra, 2000). Such findings are consistent with theoretical analyses of victimization as involving an imbalance of power between perpetrator and victim (Olweus, 1994). Numerical majority versus minority status is one form of asymmetrical power relations. Elaborating the study of ethnic context, S. Graham and colleagues have documented that members of the ethnic majority group face their own unique challenges (see S. Graham, 2006). For example, students with reputations as victims who are also members of the ethnic majority group feel especially anxious and lonely, in part because they deviate from what is perceived as normative for their numerically more powerful group (i.e., to be aggressive and dominant). Deviation from the norm can then result in more self-blame for being a victim ("It must be *me*").

If there are risks associated with being a member of the minority or majority ethnic group, then this has implications for the kinds of ethnic configurations that limit both the amount and impact of victimization. It could be, for example, that the best configuration is an ethnically diverse context in which no one group holds the numerical balance of power. Consistent with this hypothesis, Juvonen, Nishina, and Graham (2006) documented that greater ethnic diversity at both the classroom and school level was related to less perceived vulnerability among sixth-grade students, including less self-reported victimization. The authors proposed that power relations are more balanced in ethnically diverse schools with multiple ethnic groups, and that shared power, in turn, reduces incidents of harassment. Thus, it is not so much ethnicity per se as it is the ethnic composition of classroom and schools that shapes the experience of victimization.

Deviant Peer Influences

We would be remiss if we did not consider at least briefly the influence of deviant peers (see Dishion & Piehler, Chapter 32, this volume). For example, do aggressive youth tend to affiliate with antisocial peers? Are youth at increased risk for delinquency if their peer group comprises primarily antisocial members? Such questions are particularly relevant to understanding peer relations of youth of color, particularly African American children and adolescents, in part because of the known correlations between gender, race, and antisocial behavior in the United States. African American boys are more likely than any other racial/ethnic group to be labeled as aggressive by teachers and peers, to be suspended or expelled from school for antisocial behavior, and to penetrate the deepest levels of the juvenile justice system (see Noguera, 2003). This is not the place for us to take up the issue of why such racial disproportionality surrounding antisocial behavior exists; rather, we note it as an empirical reality that shapes peer relations researchers' thinking about the impact of deviant peers on African American youth.

One well-documented finding in the deviant peer literature is that affiliating with antisocial or aggressive peers is associated with increased antisocial behavior (Dodge, Coie, & Lynam, 2006). The public discourse accompanying this robust finding presumes that because African American youth engage in more documented antisocial behavior, they must be more vulnerable to negative peer influences. We could not uncover any substantive literature documenting that African American delinquent or nondelinquent youth were more susceptible to pressure from their peers to behave in particular ways. To the contrary, we identified two comparative racial/ethnic studies—one involving interviews (Giordano, Cernkovich, & Pugh, 1986), the other using a self-report measure (Steinberg & Monahan, 2007)—documenting *greater* resistance to peer pressure among African American youth compared to other racial/ethnic groups. The Steinberg and Monahan study is noteworthy, because the large multiethnic sample was drawn from four distinct studies that included both delinquent and nondelinquent respondents ranging in age from early adolescence to young adulthood.

A promising approach to understanding the processes underlying deviant peer influences that may be particularly relevant to ethnic minority youth is the work by Dishion,

Dodge, and colleagues on "deviancy training" (Dishion, McCord, & Poulin, 1999; Dodge, Dishion, & Lansford, 2006), which refers to increases in endorsement of rule-breaking and other antisocial behavior that can occur when aggression-prone youth are grouped together. As youth reinforce and promote one another's antisocial postures and endorsement of rule breaking ("talking trash"), antisocial group norms can quickly materialize. It has been suggested that deviancy training occurs widely, not only in informal and unsupervised peer networks but also in highly structured, adult-directed therapeutic or intervention settings that aggregate antisocial youth, or where the ratio of deviant to nondeviant youth is high (Dodge, Dishion, et al., 2006). Examples of such settings are group homes, alternative schools for suspended or expelled students, wilderness camps, long-term incarceration in juvenile detention facilities, and academic tracking that isolates behavior-problem youth in low-ability tracks. Meta-analyses of a large number of mental health education and juvenile justice interventions have documented that aggregating high-risk youth together often produces iatrogenic treatment effects (Dodge, Dishion, et al., 2006). These findings are particularly relevant for the focus of this chapter, inasmuch as youth of color, African American youth in particular, are overrepresented in virtually all of the intervention settings in which deviant peer contagion has been documented. Thus, for researchers interested in how the processes of deviant peer influences unfold in ethnic minority youth at greatest risk for delinquency, these interventions settings are a good place to begin.

Summary

Social reputation and peer norms are important components of peer processes, and there may be some misconceptions about the nature of these processes in ethnic minority youth. There is no strong evidence that popularity is more associated with aggression in children of color, that some ethnic groups are more vulnerable to peer victimization than others, or that African American youth are especially prone to deviant peer influences. Comparative racial research involving aggression has focused more on *rates* of antisocial behavior in different racial/ethnic groups rather than on processes leading to these outcomes. Research on deviancy training provides a good context for studying these processes.

Ethnic Identity and Peer Relations at the Group Level

People construct individual identities ("Who am *I*?"), as well as social identities ("Who are *we*?"). For youth of color, one of the most important social identities is that related to race or ethnicity. Ethnic identity is a person's sense of belonging to his or her ethnic group and the meaning attached to that group membership (e.g., Phinney, 1990). The meaning dimension is particularly important, and it distinguishes between personal feelings about group membership (e.g., the extent to which one feels pride vs. shame or psychological closeness to vs. distance from other members of one's ethnic group) and beliefs about how others judge one's ethnic group (e.g., with respect vs. disdain). Defining the meaning dimension of one's ethnic identity and balancing it with other emergent social identities can be challenging, especially during adolescence, and may affect peer relations in significant ways. In this section, we focus on challenges from outgroup members in the form of stereotypes and perceived discrimination, as well as challenges from the ingroup, as individuals attempt to negotiate their identities as both good students and members of their racial/ethnic group.

Challenges from the Outgroup: Stereotypes and Discrimination

"Stereotypes" are culturally shared beliefs, both positive and negative, about the characteristics and behaviors of particular groups. The study of stereotypes is important in a chapter of race and ethnicity in peer relations, because racial stereotypes are pervasive; are endorsed by both youth and adults, including youth of color (e.g., Hudley & Graham, 2001); and influence how both perceivers and the targets of stereotypes interact with one another.

Most of the racial stereotype literature in the United States has focused on African Americans, and there is much evidence that the cultural stereotypes of that group remain largely negative. Numerous studies employing a variety of methods document that respondents associate being black (and male) with low intelligence, hostility, aggressiveness, and violence (see Blaine, 2007). Similarly negative, the much smaller stereotype literature on Latinos often portrays them as illegal immigrants who prefer menial jobs and have little personal ambition (e.g., Kao, 2000). Unlike African Americans and Latinos, the cultural stereotype about Asians is that they are a "model minority"—hardworking and intellectually gifted high achievers who are especially competent in math and science (e.g., Kao, 2000). Coping with such stereotypes can put strains on mental health. For example, the stereotype threat literature (Aronson & Steele, 2005) documents how awareness of the cultural consensus associating blackness with intellectual inferiority can be particularly debilitating for African American students in highly evaluative contexts if they worry about confirming those stereotypes (e.g., "What does my performance say about *me* or about members of my racial group?"). Similarly, for Asian American students, there are well-documented psychological and emotional costs associated with trying to live up to the perception of their group as academic superstars (Lee, 1994).

Stereotypes often lead to experiences of "discrimination," or perceived unfair treatment based on race or ethnicity. Many studies document that such perceptions are quite common among youth of color, particularly in school settings and from both peers and authority figures (Rosenbloom & Way, 2004; Greene, Way, & Pahl, 2006; Fisher, Wallace, & Fenton, 2000). The most prevalent kinds of unfair treatment reported by ethnic minority youth include receiving a lower grade than deserved from teachers; being the recipient of unusually harsh discipline from authority figures; and being the target of verbal, psychological, or physical abuse from peers. Some data indicate that African American and Latino youth are especially likely to report discrimination from adults in the school, whereas Asian students feel more harshly treated by peers, especially peers of color (Rosenbloom & Way, 2004; Fisher et al., 2000). It has been suggested that the privileged position among teachers that Asian students enjoy (as "model" minorities) can elicit anger from Black and Latino students who perceive their preferential treatment as unfair (Conchas & Noguera, 2004). The fact that schools often limit the mixing opportunities of Asian students with other students of color through academic tracking practices that derive from racial stereotypes about ability can contribute to ethnic tensions between groups.

Research on the consequences of perceived race-based discrimination among adolescents has focused almost exclusively on mental health, including depression, anxiety, and perceived self-worth. For example, we know that discrimination is predictive of depression and low self-esteem, but that a strong racial identity can buffer those negative consequences (Greene et al., 2006; Sellers, Copeland-Linder, Martin, & Lewis, 2006). However, much less is known about how prevalent experiences with discrimination affect peer relations and social adjustment. The cross-ethnic friendship literature revealed that friendships become more segregated along racial/ethnic lines as youth approach adolescence, which is also the developmental period when racial stereotypes about intelligence and antisocial behavior become widely known. Some adolescents of color may respond to stereotypes and discrimination by turning toward same-race peers for social support, particularly if they are numerical minorities in their school context (e.g., Tatum, 1997). Other youth may react by cultivating relationships with other-ethnicity peers as a way to disconfirm anticipated discrimination or to align themselves with a more powerful group (e.g., Mendoza-Denton, Page-Gould, & Pietrzak, 2006). There are trade-offs to each of these strategies. We believe that the effects of perceived discrimination on peer relations are greatly understudied and are likely to have stronger effects on long-term adjustment than the short-term mental health outcomes that typically are studied.

Challenges from the Ingroup: Oppositional Identity

"Oppositional identity" is a construct that emerged from anthropological analyses that take into account the historical circumstances that have shaped the experiences of ethnic minorities in this country. African Americans are what anthropologist John Ogbu calls an "involuntary minority," that is, a group that has become part of the American fabric not by choice, but as a result of slavery, conquest, or colonization (Fordham & Ogbu, 1986). For involuntary minorities, a legacy of slavery and resultant perceived barriers to opportunity may communicate to group members that certain behaviors and symbols associated with the dominant group are threatening to their social identity ("us" vs. "them"). Particularly during adolescence, African American youngsters may adopt oppositional identities whereby they show relative indifference, or even disdain, toward achievement behaviors that are valued by the larger society. Included in those behaviors are being on time for school, bringing books to class, participating in class discussions, completing assignments, and getting good grades. Based on their interviews with gifted high school students, Fordham and Ogbu coined the term "acting white" to describe African American high school students' perceptions of their same-race peers who work hard to do well in school. Antiachievement peer group pressure from involuntary minorities can take many forms, including being labeled an "Oreo" or "sellout," social ostracism, and even physical assault (Kao, 2000).

The discourse surrounding oppositional identity during adolescence has become very lively among researchers, in part because it provides a motivational explanation for the achievement gap between black and white students. One would be hard-pressed to find an article in the last decade on the relations between peer groups and achievement strivings in African American adolescents that does not explicitly or implicitly make reference to oppositional identity. Most of the research in support of the phenomenon has been based on ethnographic studies that describe in vivid detail how high achieving black youth sometimes conceal their accomplishments or adopt a "raceless" identity to avoid rejection and outright ridicule from same-race peers (Fordham, 1996). Case studies of youth of Mexican descent (Matute-Bianchi, 1991) and even of Asian American youth document similar findings. For example, Lee (1994) reported that some Asian-identified students, labeled as "New Wavers," showed disdain for academic achievement, in part as a reaction to the model minority stereotype, and in part because they associated being popular with academic disengagement.

Aside from the ethnographic studies, however, there is less empirical support for widespread oppositional identity among ethnic minority youth. For example, two studies (Ainsworth-Darnell & Downey, 1998; Cook & Ludwig, 1997) tested hypotheses about oppositional identity using data from the National Education Longitudinal Study (NELS), a nationally representative panel study of 25,000 ethnically diverse students assessed in the 8th, 10th, and 12th grades. Neither study found clear evidence for attitudes resembling oppositional identity in African American high school students. In these studies, black students were *more* likely than white students to endorse positive school attitudes and just as likely to hold high educational aspirations and to be among the most popular students in their school.

More recent qualitative studies do not find that high-achieving African American and Latino adolescents are rejected by the peer group (Bergin & Cooks, 2002; Datnow & Cooper, 1997; Flores-Gonzalez, 2005; Horvat & Lewis, 2003). For example, the high-achieving African American high school students in the ethnography conducted by Horvat and Lewis learned to manage their academic and social lives by affiliating with multiple peers groups and acknowledging or camouflaging their academic achievements selectively depending on norms of the peer group. When these students downplayed their academic achievements, it was not so much to avoid ostracism as to protect their less successful peers from having their feelings hurt.

Sense of Belonging

Sense of belonging at school may be an antidote to the challenges from outgroups and ingroups discussed earlier. By "belonging," we mean feelings of being included, accepted, supported, and respected by teachers and peers (Juvonen, 2006). A large body of empirical research has documented that students have more positive attitudes about school, are more motivated, and achieve better outcomes as feelings of belonging increase (Österman, 2000). In comparative studies, ethnic minority youth have lower sense of belonging than do white youth, with the greatest differences involving African American youth (e.g., Faircloth & Hamm, 2005). Underscoring this racial asymmetry, Benner and Graham (2007) reported that black students, more so than other ethnic groups, experienced a greater decline in feelings of belonging across the transition to high school when the numerical representation of their racial group dropped from middle school to high school. Thus, moving to a school context in which there are significantly fewer same-race schoolmates may heighten African American students' concerns about being a numerical ethnic minority and the target of others' prejudice.

Even a relatively simple experimental manipulation can have significant impact on African American students' perceived social fit. Walton and Cohen (2007) had black and white undergraduates generate a list of either eight friends or two friends in the computer science department at their university. Generating eight friends was especially difficult and led black students to question their social connectedness to the computer science field (e.g., "People like me do not belong here"). In a second study, Walton and Cohen created an attributional intervention designed to deracialize doubts about social belonging. Black and white first-year college students were randomly assigned to a condition that portrayed worry about school belonging as a temporary phenomenon, common among many racial/ethnic groups, or to a no-attribution control condition.

African American students in the intervention reported less stress and showed more improvement in sophomore year grade point average (GPA) compared to controls. Although a few interventions have been designed to increase school belongingness among school-age children and adolescents (e.g., Battistich, Schaps, & Wilson, 2004), none has focused on the particular challenges of youth of color that can be traced to their racial/ethnic group membership. We view such interventions as a useful direction for future research.

Summary

Membership in a particular racial or ethnic group affects the ways in which peers relate to one another. Outgroup members are likely to endorse stereotypes about intellectual ability and antisocial behavior, which then influences their willingness to interact with the targets of those stereotypes. Ingroup peers may be rejecting if they perceive that individuals deviate from the peer norms for that group. Although empirical support for the construct of oppositional identity is limited, there is general agreement that many ethnic minority adolescents experience conflict between achievement strivings and being accepted by same-ethnicity peers. Enhanced feelings of belonging may mitigate the identity challenges from both outgroup and ingroup members.

Future Directions for Research

Ways to Study Race and Ethnicity

There are many approaches to incorporating race and ethnicity in developmental research (see Steinberg & Fletcher, 1998). Peer relations researchers interested in race and ethnicity have primarily taken a comparative approach in which ethnicity is treated as an independent variable, and different groups are then contrasted on the peer variable of interest. Many scholars have written about the shortcomings of this approach in developmental psychology research (e.g., Garcia-Coll et al., 1996). All too often, social class is not accounted for, and the emphasis is on deficits or deviance when the behavior of the majority (white) group is considered normative and important within-group variability is ignored.

We believe that there is a role for comparative racial/ethnic analyses in peer relations research, if they are carried out with methodological rigor and can shed light on developmental process. For example, in the popularity and aggression literature, what began as a set of empirical findings that suggested aggressive youth may enjoy more social status among African American peers (e.g., Luthar & McMahon, 1996) in part stimulated peer relations researchers to articulate conceptual and empirical distinctions between sociometric acceptance and perceived popularity, and to document as a general developmental process that, by adolescence, popular youth have both prosocial and antisocial characteristics (Asher & McDonald, Chapter 13, this volume). Similarly, the oppositional identity literature associated with involuntary minorities has encouraged a more thoughtful analysis of adolescents' endorsement of antiachievement attitudes to gain peer approval as a robust developmental phenomenon (e.g., Ainsworth-Darnell & Downey, 1998). Peer relations researchers should be alerted to other systematic patterns of differences between ethnic groups in peer processes that might also have broad generalizability.

With the emergence of more sophisticated strategies to test mediation and moderation, the time also seems ripe for studies of how peer processes might account for well-documented racial/ethnic differences on important outcomes (mediation), or how basic peer processes might be different in one racial/ethnic group compared to others (moderation). Regarding mediation, for example, based on studies of feelings of belonging at school (e.g., Walton & Cohen, 2007), a testable hypothesis is that ethnic differences in academic engagement are in part explained by differences in the degree to which members of different racial/ethnic groups feel accepted, respected, and supported by peers and teachers at school. In studies of moderation, one could hypothesize that the effect of peer victimization on maladjustment would be weaker in ethnically diverse classrooms and in schools where there is a shared numerical balance of power (S. Graham, 2006), or that cross-race friendships are less predictive of improved intergroup relations in contexts of academic tracking that limit the mixing opportunities of students from different ethnic groups (Moody, 2001). Moderation analyses are especially promising, in that the presence of differences can lead to theory refinement, whereas the absences of differences can contribute to theory generality.

The Need for a Multidisciplinary Perspective

As race and ethnicity assume a more important role in peer relations research, there will be a need to draw on the contributions of other disciplines. The theoretical underpinnings of many of the topics examined in this chapter are just as much the intellectual terrain of sociologists and anthropologists as they are of developmental social psychologists. Because race and ethnicity are integrally linked to social status, we need the perspective of sociologists to help us understand how social inequality shapes peer experiences, such as the opportunity for cross-racial experiences, exposure to deviant peers, or vulnerability to stereotypes and discrimination. Most peer relations research takes place in schools, yet sociologists seem to be much more sophisticated than developmental psychologists in thinking about schools as social structures that promote or impede the development of children. Anthropological approaches inform peer relations researchers about the historical and cultural forces that impact the peer ecology of youth of color. The qualitative methods of anthropology also allow for a rich and nuanced description of the everyday lives of ethnic minority youth. The type of conflict that some ethnic minority adolescents experience between achievement strivings and the desire to be accepted by same-ethnicity peers is probably best captured by the ethnographic studies that followed the research of Fordham and Ogbu (1986).

Beyond Black and White

Like psychology in general, most of the subjects in peer relations research are still white and middle class (cf. S. Graham, 1992). When research has crossed racial boundaries, the focal group has been African Americans. Historically, this is understandable. Until recently, African Americans were the largest racial/minority group in the United States, and most social-psychological research on children of color emerged from school desegregation literature that was almost exclusively concerned with the school experiences of black and white children.

The changing demography of the last generation, driven largely by immigration and revealed by Census 2000, has redefined the racial and ethnic landscape in the United

States. Although whites are still the majority group, African Americans have been surpassed by Latinos as the largest ethnic minority group, and Latinos and Asians are now the fastest growing ethnic groups in the United States. A K–12 population that was 80% white a generation ago has dropped to 57% white, and public schools will soon be the first social institution without a clear racial/ethnic majority group (Orfield & Lee, 2007).

Peer relations research will need to cast a broader methodological net to encompass more ethnically diverse samples. These efforts will require addressing complex issues related to language, culture, and generational status that were not an issue when African Americans were the predominant racial/minority sample. For example, a growing literature on the psychosocial adjustment of Latino and Asian youth as a function of immigrant history documents poorer adjustment across successive generations of residence in the United States (e.g., Suarez-Orozco & Suarez-Orozco, 2001). This research on "new immigration" has primarily focused on school achievement, physical health, and psychological well-being as outcomes. Complementing that work with studies of how peer relations are shaped by generational status will be an important next step. For example, it is known that first- and second-generation immigrant youth have a strong sense of family obligation that entails a sense of duty to help one another and to take into account family needs when making personal decisions (Fuligni, Tseng, & Lam, 1999). Even during adolescence, loyalties to parents may override those to peers, such that it is more important to be a dutiful son or daughter than to be popular at school.

In this chapter, we have discussed research on Asian and Latino youth as if those racial/ethnic groups were homogeneous. As with the study of African Americans, it will be important for researchers to be sensitive to within-ethnic-group variation, especially that related to country of origin. In addition, with growing housing segregation and decreasing presence of white students in urban schools, peer relations researchers will have opportunities to test novel hypotheses in studies with multiethnic samples that do not include white youth and are therefore less vulnerable to criticisms about the presumed normative comparison group.

Peer Relations and the Psychosocial Benefits and Challenges of Ethnic Diversity in Schools

As we stated earlier, most peer relations research is conducted in school settings, even though many researchers do not have an interest in schooling issues per se. We encourage more integration of the study of basic peer processes, with schools as contexts that vary in racial/ethnic composition. Virtually all of the peer processes discussed in this chapter—friendships, social reputations, experiences with victimization and discrimination, and social belonging—vary as a function of whether an individual is a member of a majority or minority ethnic group in nondiverse contexts, in comparison to relatively more diverse settings without clear numerical majorities and minorities. We need a systematic mapping of particular types of ethnic diversity onto different peer outcomes. For example, we cited evidence that African American students experience decreases in feelings of belonging when they transition from middle schools to high schools, where there are fewer members of their racial group (Benner & Graham, 2007). This suggests that there must be a critical mass of same-ethnicity peers in any school context to ease the challenges of finding one's niche and fitting in. What that critical mass might be is of interest to researchers, as well as to policymakers, who must judge the legitimacy of both affirmative action in higher education and race-conscious policies in the assignment of K–12 students to school (National Research Council, 2007). Greater diversity, as measured by the presence of multiple ethnic groups with relatively equal representation, has been related to positive outcomes such as more cross-ethnic friendships (Moody, 2001) and less perceived victimization (Juvonen et al., 2006). These studies represent a starting point for a fuller exploration of the psychosocial benefits of greater diversity in American schools.

This is a critical period in the history of American public schools, which are more racially and ethnically segregated now than they have been in the last 30 years (Orfield & Lee, 2007). Researchers in our field are well-positioned to explore how peer relations are shaped by the school ethnic contexts in which they unfold, and to use that knowledge to aid our understanding of a complex social problem of great significance.

References

Aboud, F., Mendelson, M., & Purdy, K. (2003). Cross-race peer relations and friendship quality. *International Journal of Behavioral Development, 27*, 165–173.

Ainsworth-Darnell, J., & Downey, D. (1998). Assessing the oppositional culture explanation for racial/ethnic differences in school performance. *American Sociological Review, 63*, 536–553.

Aronson, J., & Steele, C. (2005). Stereotypes and the fragility of academic competence, motivation, and self-concept. In A. Elliot & C. Dweck (Eds.), *Handbook of competence and motivation* (pp. 436–456). New York: Guilford Press.

Battistich, V., Schaps, E., & Wilson, N. (2004). Effects of an elementary school intervention on students' "connectedness" to school and social adjustment during middle school. *Journal of Primary Prevention, 24*, 243–262.

Benner, A., & Graham, S. (2007). Navigating the transition to multi-ethnic urban high schools: Changing racial/ethnic congruence and adolescents' school-related affect. *Journal of Research on Adolescence, 17*, 207–220.

Bergin, D., & Cooks, H. (2002). High school students of color talk about accusations of "acting white." *Urban Review, 34*, 113–134.

Blaine, B. (2007). *Understanding the psychology of diversity*. Los Angeles: Sage.

Coie, J., Dodge, K., & Coppotelli, H. (1982). Dimensions and types of social status: A cross age perspective. *Developmental Psychology, 18*, 557–570.

Conchas, G., & Noguera, P. (2004). Understanding the exceptions: How small schools support the achievement of academically successful black boys. In N. Way & J. Chu (Eds.), *Adolescent boys: Exploring diverse cultures of boyhood* (pp. 317–337). New York: New York University Press.

Cook, P., & Ludwig, J. (1997). Weighing the "burden of 'acting white'": Are there race differences in attitudes toward education? *Journal of Policy Analysis and Management, 16*, 256–278.

Damico, S., Bell-Nathaniel, A., & Green, C. (1981). Effects of school organizational structure on interracial friendships in middle school. *Journal of Educational Research, 74*, 388–393.

Damico, S., & Sparks, C. (1986). Cross-group contact opportunities: Impact on interpersonal relationships in desegregated middle schools. *Sociology of Education, 59*, 113–123.

Datnow, A., & Cooper, R. (1996). Peer networks of African American students in independent schools: Affirming academic success and racial identity. *Journal of Negro Education, 66*, 56–72.

Dishion, T., McCord, J., & Poulin, F. (1999). When interventions harm: Peer groups and problem behavior. *American Psychologist, 54*, 755–764.

Dodge, K., Coie, J., & Lynam, D. (2006). Aggression and antisocial behavior in youth. In N. Eisenberg (Ed.), *Handbook of child psychology: Vol. 3. Social emotional, and personality development* (6th ed., pp. 719–788). Hoboken, NJ: Wiley.

Dodge, K., Dishion, T., & Lansford, J. (Eds.). (2006). *Deviant peer influences in programs for youth.* New York: Guilford Press.

DuBois, D., & Hirsch, B. (1990). School and neighborhood friendship patterns of blacks and whites in early adolescence. *Child Development, 62,* 524–536.

Eller, A., & Abrams, D. (2003). "Gringos" in Mexico: Cross-sectional and longitudinal effects of language school-promoted contact on intergroup bias. *Group Processes and Intergroup Relations, 6,* 55–75.

Faircloth, B., & Hamm, J. (2005). Sense of belonging among high school students representing four ethnic groups. *Journal of Youth and Adolescence, 34,* 293–309.

Farmer, T., Estell, D., Bishop, J., O'Neal, K., & Cairns, B. (2003). Rejected bullies or popular leaders?: The social relations of aggressive subtypes of rural African American early adolescents. *Developmental Psychology, 39,* 992–1004.

Finkelstein, N., & Haskins, R. (1983). Kindergarten children prefer same-color peers. *Child Development, 54,* 502–508.

Fisher, C., Wallace, S., & Fenton, R. (2000). Discrimination distress during adolescence. *Journal of Youth and Adolescence, 29,* 679–694.

Flores-Gonzalez, N. (2005). Popularity versus respect: School structure, peer groups, and Latino academic achievement. *International Journal of Qualitative Studies in Education, 18,* 625–642.

Fordham, S. (1996). *Blacked out.* Chicago: University of Chicago Press.

Fordham, S., & Ogbu, J. (1986). Black students' school success: Coping with the "burden of 'acting White.'" *Urban Review, 18,* 176–206.

Fuligni, A., Tseng, V., & Lam, M. (1999). Attitudes toward family obligation among American adolescents with Asian, Latin American, and European backgrounds. *Child Development, 70,* 1030–1044.

Garcia-Coll, C., Lamberty, G., Jenkins, R., McAdoo, H., Crnic, K., Wasik, B., et al. (1996). An integrative model of developmental competencies in minority children. *Child Development, 67,* 1891–1914.

Giordano, P., Cernkovich, S., & Pugh, M. (1986). Friendship and delinquency. *American Journal of Sociology, 91,* 1170–1202.

Graham, J., & Cohen, R. (1997). Race and sex as factors in children's sociometric ratings and friendship choices. *Social Development, 6,* 353–370.

Graham, S. (1992). "Most of the subjects were white and middle class": Trends in published research on African Americans in selected APA journals, 1970–1989. *American Psychologist, 47,* 629–639.

Graham, S. (2006). Peer victimization in school: Exploring the ethnic context. *Current Directions in Psychological Science, 15,* 317–320.

Graham, S., & Juvonen, J. (2002). Ethnicity, peer harassment and adjustment in middle school: An exploratory study. *Journal of Early Adolescence, 22,* 173–199.

Greene, M., Way, N., & Pahl, N. (2006). Trajectories of perceived adult and peer discrimination among Black, Latino, and Asian American adolescents: Patterns and psychological correlates. *Developmental Psychology, 42,* 218–238.

Hallinan, M., & Smith, S. (1985). The effects of classroom racial composition on students' interracial friendliness. *Social Psychology Quarterly, 48,* 3–16.

Hallinan, M., & Teixeira, R. (1987). Opportunities and constraints: Black–white differences in the formation of interracial friendships. *Child Development, 58,* 1358–1372.

Hallinan, M., & Williams, R. (1987). The stability of students' interracial friendships. *American Sociological Review, 52,* 653–664.

Hamm, J., Brown, B., & Heck, D. (2005). Bridging the ethnic divide: Student and school characteristics in African American, Asian-descent, Latino, and white adolescents' cross-ethnic friend nominations. *Journal of Research on Adolescence, 15,* 21–46.

Hanish, L., & Guerra, N. (2000). The roles of ethnicity and school context in predicting children's victimization by peers. *American Journal of Community Psychology, 28*, 201–223.

Horvat, E., & Lewis, K. (2003). Reassessing the "burden of acting white": The importance of peer groups in managing academic success. *Sociology of Education, 76*, 265–280.

Hudley, C., & Graham, S. (2001). Stereotypes of achievement strivings among early adolescents. *Social Psychology of Education, 5*, 201–224.

Juvonen, J. (2006). Sense of belonging, social bonds, and school functioning. In P. Alexander & P. Winne (Eds.), *Handbook of educational psychology* (pp. 655–674). Mahwah, NJ: Erlbaum.

Juvonen, J., Graham, S., & Schuster, M. (2003). Bullying among young adolescents: The strong, the weak, and the troubled. *Pediatrics, 112*, 1231–1237.

Juvonen, J., Nishina, A., & Graham, S. (2006). Ethnic diversity and perceptions of safety in urban middle schools. *Psychological Science, 17*, 393–400.

Kao, G. (2000). Group images and possible selves among adolescents: Linking stereotypes to expectations by race and ethnicity. *Sociological Forum, 15*, 407–430.

Kao, G., & Joyner, K. (2004). Do race and ethnicity mater among friends?: Activities among interracial, interethnic, and intraethnic adolescent friends. *Sociological Quarterly, 45*, 557–573.

Kistner, J., Metzler, A., Gatlin, D., & Risi, S. (1993). Classroom racial proportions and children's peer relations: Race and gender effects. *Journal of Educational Psychology, 85*, 446–452.

Kubitschek, W., & Hallinan, M. (1998). Tracking and students' friendships. *Social Psychology Quarterly, 62*, 1–15.

Lease, A. M., & Blake, J. (2005). A comparison of majority-race children with and without a minority-race friend. *Social Development, 14*, 20–41.

Lederberg, A., Chapin, S., Rosenblatt, V., & Vandell, D. (1986). Ethnic, gender, and age preferences among deaf and hearing preschool peers. *Child Development, 57*, 375–386.

Lee, S. (1994). Behind the model-minority stereotype: Voices of high- and low-achieving Asian American students. *Anthropology and Education Quarterly, 25*, 413–429.

Levin, S., van Laar, C., & Sidanius, J. (2003). The effects of ingroup and outgroup friendships on ethnic attitudes in college: A longitudinal study. *Group Processes and Intergroup Relations, 6*, 76–92.

Luthar, S., & McMahon, T. (1996). Peer reputation among inner-city adolescents: Structure and correlates. *Journal of Research on Adolescence, 6*, 581–603.

Matute-Bianchi, M. (1991). Situational ethnicity and patterns of school performance among immigrant and nonimmigrant Mexican-descent students. In M. Gibson & J. Ogbu (Eds.), *Minority status and schooling: A comparative study of immigrant and involuntary minorities* (pp. 205–247). New York: Garland Press.

Meisinger, E., Blake, J., Lease, A., Palaedy, G., & Olejnik, S. (2007). Variant and invariant predictors of perceived popularity across majority-black and majority-white classrooms. *Journal of School Psychology, 45*, 21–44.

Mendoza-Denton, R., Page-Gould, E., & Pietrzak, J. (2006). Mechanisms of coping with status-based rejection expectations. In S. Levin & C. van Laar (Eds.), *Stigma and group inequality* (pp. 151–170). Mahwah, NJ: Erlbaum.

Moffitt, T. (1993). Adolescence-limited and life-course persistent antisocial behavior: A developmental taxonomy. *Psychological Review, 100*, 674–701.

Moody, J. (2001). Race, school integration, and friendship segregation in America. *American Journal of Sociology, 107*, 679–716.

Mouw, T., & Entwisle, B. (2006). Residential segregation and interracial friendship in schools. *American Journal of Sociology, 112*, 394–441.

Nansel, T. R., Overpeck, M., Pilla, R. S., Ruan, W. J., Simons-Morton, B., & Scheidt, P. (2001). Bullying behaviors among U.S. youth: Prevalence and association with psychosocial adjustment. *Journal of the American Medical Association, 285*, 2094–2100.

National Research Council. (2007). *Race conscious policies for assigning students to schools: Social science research and the Supreme Court cases.* Washington, DC: National Academy Press.

Noguera, P. (2003). The trouble with black boys: The role and influence of environmental and cultural factors on the academic performance of African American males. *Urban Education, 38,* 431–459.

Oakes, J. (1995). Two cities' tracking and within-school segregation. *Teachers College Record, 96,* 681–690.

Olweus, D. (1994). Bullying at school: Basic facts and effects of a school-based intervention program. *Journal of Child Psychology and Psychiatry and Allied Disciplines, 35,* 1171–1190.

Orfield, G., & Lee, C. (2007). *Historic reversals, accelerating resegregation, and the need for new integration strategies.* Los Angeles: Civil Rights Project.

Österman, K. (2000). Students' need for belonging in the school community. *Review of Educational Research, 70,* 323–367.

Peskin, M., Tortolero, S., & Markham, C. (2006). Bullying and victimization among black and Hispanic adolescents. *Adolescence, 41,* 467–484.

Pettigrew, T. (1998). Intergroup contact theory. *Annual Review of Psychology, 49,* 65–85.

Pettigrew, T., & Tropp, L. (2006). A meta-analytic test of intergroup contact theory. *Journal of Personality and Social Psychology, 90,* 751–783.

Phinney, J. (1990). Ethnic identity in adolescents and adults: Review of research. *Psychological Bulletin, 108,* 499–514.

Phinney, J. (1996). When we talk about American ethnic groups, what do we mean? *American Psychologist, 51,* 918–927.

Rodkin, P., Farmer, T., Pearl, R., & Van Acker, R. (2000). Heterogeneity of popular boys: Antisocial and prosocial configurations. *Developmental Psychology, 36,* 14–24.

Rosenbloom, S., & Way, N. (2004). Experiences of discrimination among African American, Asian American, and Latino adolescents in an urban high school. *Youth and Society, 35,* 420–451.

Rubin, K., Bukowski, W., & Parker, J. (2006). Peer interactions, relationships, and groups. In N. Eisenberg (Ed.), *Handbook of child psychology: Vol. 3. Social emotional, and personality development* (6th ed., pp. 571–645). Hoboken, NJ: Wiley.

Sagar, H., Schofield, J., & Snyder, H. (1983). Race and gender barriers: Preadolescent peer behavior in academic classrooms. *Child Development, 54,* 1032–1040.

Schneider, B., Dixon, K., & Udvari, S. (2007). Closeness and competition in the inter-ethnic and co-ethnic friendships of early adolescents in Toronto and Montreal. *Journal of Early Adolescence, 27,* 115–138.

Schofield, J., & Francis, W. (1982). An observational study of peer interaction in racially mixed "accelerated" classrooms. *Journal of Educational Psychology, 74,* 722–732.

Schofield, J., & Sagar, A. (1977). Peer interaction patterns in an integrated middle school. *Sociometry, 40,* 130–138.

Sellers, R., Copeland-Linder, N., Martin, P., & Lewis, R. (2006). Racial identity matters: The relationship between racial discrimination and psychological functioning in African American adolescents. *Journal of Research on Adolescence, 16,* 187–216.

Shrum, W., Cheek, N., & Hunter, S. (1988). Friendship in school: Gender and racial homophily. *Sociology of Education, 61,* 227–239.

Singleton, L., & Asher, S. (1979). Racial integration and children's peer references: An investigation of developmental and cohort differences. *Child Development, 50,* 936–941.

Steinberg, L., & Fletcher, A. (1998). Data analytic strategies in research on ethnic minority youth. In V. McLoyd & L. Steinberg (Eds.), *Studying minority adolescents* (pp. 279–294). Mahwah, NJ: Erlbaum.

Steinberg, L., & Monahan, K. (2007). Age differences in resistance to peer influence. *Developmental Psychology, 43,* 1531–1543.

Storch, E., Nock, M., Masia-Warner, C., & Barlas, M. (2003). Peer victimization and social-psychological adjustment in Hispanic and African American children. *Journal of Child and Family Studies, 12*, 439–452.

Suarez-Orozco, C., & Suarez-Orozco, M. (2001). *Children of immigration*. Cambridge, MA: Harvard University Press.

Tatum, B. (1997). *Why are all the black kids sitting together in the cafeteria?: And other conversations about race*. New York: Basic Books.

Walton, G., & Cohen, G. (2007). A question of belonging: Race, social fit, and achievement. *Journal of Personality and Social Psychology, 92*, 82–96.

Xie, H., Li, Y., Boucher, S., Hutchins, B., & Cairns, B. (2006). What makes a girl (or a boy) popular (or unpopular)?: African American children's perceptions and developmental differences. *Developmental Psychology, 42*, 599–612.

Zisman, P., & Wilson, P. (1992). Table hopping in a cafeteria: An exploration of "racial" integration in early adolescent social groups. *Anthropology and Education Quarterly, 23*, 199–220.

CHAPTER 23

Neighborhood Contexts of Peer Relationships and Groups

HÅKAN STATTIN
MARGARET KERR

Adolescent behavior is embedded in a social context. When parents move to a particular neighborhood, all family members are in some way affected. The community and neighborhood provide the good and bad settings that adolescents encounter in everyday life. Neighborhood effects on social adjustment have been the focus of a fair amount of research in criminology aimed at understanding delinquency development (e.g., Beyers, Loeber, Wikström, & Stouthamer-Loeber, 2001; Brody et al., 2001; Leventhal & Brooks-Gunn, 2000), and the effects can be considered direct and indirect. The direct effects involve exposure to deviant peers and problem behaviors. In economically impoverished neighborhoods, the pool of peers involved in delinquency, substance abuse, and violence is higher than that in more affluent neighborhoods; consequently, exposure to these problems is more likely in poor than in affluent neighborhoods (Brody et al., 2001; Roosa et al., 2005). Influences on attitudes and norms are also direct effects (e.g., Sampson & Groves, 1989; Sampson, Raudenbush, & Earls, 1997). The indirect effects include undermining of parenting, educational aspirations, and school connectedness (Chung & Steinberg, 2006; Sameroff, Peck, & Eccles, 2004). Thus, neighborhoods influence adolescents' development directly and indirectly in many different ways.

In this chapter, however, we look at contexts *within* communities and neighborhoods where youths come into contact with their peers. This domain has not received much attention in developmental studies. Neighborhood contexts in this chapter refer to the physical settings in neighborhoods or communities in which youths spend time, perform various activities, and interact with their peers. These physical contexts might be youth clubs, sports places, and localities where youths are involved in hobbies, religious activities, music, theater, art, and politics, or they can be shopping malls, street corners, arcades, and public drinking places. We deal with the peer processes that take place within those settings.

Central Issues

Perhaps the most central issue in this area of research is selection and socialization, broadly conceptualized. One conceptualization of selection and socialization involves explaining behavioral similarities between youths and their friends. Similarity might appear because youths choose friends who are already similar to them (selection), or because youths become similar to their friends through social influence processes (socialization). Ideally, research designs should try to tease apart these explanations. Another conception of selection and socialization concerns explaining why youths who spend time in some kinds of activities are better adjusted than those who spend time in other activities. Here, again, well-adjusted adolescents might choose certain types of activities, whereas poorly adjusted youths choose others, but youths might also be influenced by others in the activities, once chosen. In this chapter, we rely on both these conceptualizations of selection and socialization. Our main arguments rest on ideas about why youths choose certain types of settings, the implications of those reasons relative to socialization into problematic behavior in certain types of settings, and individual characteristics that put some youths more at risk than others for negative socialization by peers. These issues arise because adolescents in Western societies have much more freedom than younger children to select their leisure-time settings.

Adolescents spend a substantial part of their waking time in different leisure activities, and they have much leeway to choose their own settings for activities. Another central issue involves the important characteristics of different settings, and whether and how youths are affected by the settings they choose. Two main types of contexts that adolescents frequent during their leisure time have been considered in the literature: structured, adult-controlled contexts and unstructured, peer-controlled contexts.

Structured contexts are commonly viewed as settings in which adults are present as leaders, mentors or facilitators, in which there are scheduled meeting times, goal-directed activities, and an emphasis on skills building (Eccles & Gootman, 2002; Mahoney & Stattin, 2000). Conversely, unstructured contexts are settings in which adults typically are not present or do not have a leadership role. Participation in these contexts typically occurs more spontaneously, and activities are not primarily associated with skills building. Participation in structured and unstructured activities varies with age. The majority, perhaps as many as 60–80% of early adolescents, are part of one or several structured activities, and the proportion gradually decreases over adolescence. In part, this probably reflects normative developmental changes (e.g., Hendry, Glendinning, & Schucksmith, 1996), but dropping out of structured activities is also linked to changes in social adjustment (Persson, Kerr, & Stattin, 2007). Hence, more attention should be paid to staying in versus quitting structured activities.

Studies show that well-adjusted adolescents are more actively involved in structured leisure-time activities and settings, such as organized sports, hobbies, religious activities, music, theater, art, and politics, whereas less well-adjusted adolescents are more likely to hang out on the streets or in shopping malls, arcades, and public drinking places. These activities may facilitate adjustment problems and antisocial behavior (e.g., Hirschi, 1969; McCord, 1978; Shannahan & Flaherty, 2001). Thus, understanding adolescents' choices of activities, and how activities and association with peers in these settings relate to adolescent adjustment is critical.

Relevant Theories

The theoretical bases for research on structured activities largely differ from those found in research on unstructured activities, but there is some overlap. Much of the thinking in research on structured activities is based on the notion of intrinsic motivation. The idea is that, with increasing autonomy, adolescents can choose to spend time on things that genuinely interested them—music or sports, for instance. According to Deci and Ryan's (1985) self-determination theory, adolescents engage in these activities because they satisfy their needs for autonomy, competence, and relatedness. Autonomy concerns doing activities that express the adolescent's interests rather than what others say is interesting. Competence concerns the need to feel capable and good at something, and relatedness is the need to be with others and to feel connected. When their activities satisfy these needs, adolescents feel good about themselves and others.

Studies on structured activities also rely, implicitly or explicitly, on classical social learning theory, which is where we see the overlap with work on unstructured activities. In structured activities, adolescents learn through observation and practice how to give and take praise and criticism, regulate their behaviors, communicate skillfully, and work as a group (Dworkin, Larson, & Hansen, 2003). Research on unstructured activities is also based on the classical principles of social learning theory. But the main arguments in this research about context come from social control theory (Sampson & Laub, 1993; Thornberry, 1987). According to this theory, people are inclined to behave antisocially unless they are stopped from doing so; therefore, the likelihood is high that adolescents will engage in problem behaviors if they spend time in social settings away from adults' social control. School and family are the main sources of social control in adolescence, and parents' supervision protects youths from engaging with deviant peers, but friends and adults in the neighborhood might also function as informal social controls. In short, theories of intrinsic motivation have been used in research on structured activities, whereas social control theory has been used in research on unstructured activities. Social learning theory has been used in both.

Key Classical and Modern Research Studies

This is a relatively new area of research. Virtually all of the relevant studies have been published during the last 10–15 years. Therefore, none of these studies is classical in the normal sense of the word, and most of this literature would be considered modern. Many of these studies, however, have contributed important, basic knowledge in the area. We begin with an overview of the literature on community contexts and adjustment, and how scholars have thought about the mechanisms linking the two. Then, we consider how peer relationships fit into this picture.

Structured Activities and Good Adjustment

A growing body of empirical studies suggests that participation in structured activities, such as sports, music, arts, and school activities, is beneficial for positive development. Participation in these kinds of activities is linked to better academic achievement (Cooper, Valentine, Nye, & Lindsay, 1999; Eccles & Barber, 1999; Fredricks & Eccles, 2006; Jordan & Nettles, 1999; Marsh, 1992), lower rates of school dropout (Mahoney, 2000;

Mahoney & Cairns, 1997), lower delinquency and externalizing problems (Landers & Landers, 1978; Mahoney, 2000), less alcohol and drug use (Darling, 2005; Fredricks & Eccles, 2006), and less depression (Barber, Eccles, & Stone, 2001; Fredricks & Eccles, 2004; Mahoney, Schweder, & Stattin, 2002). Whereas extracurricular activities have been found to be valuable for adolescents generally, participation seems to be especially beneficial for multiproblem (Mahoney & Cairns, 1997) and low socioeconomic status (SES) youths (Fredricks & Eccles, 2006). Thus, a sizable literature with robust findings shows that youths who participate in structured activities are better adjusted than those who do not.

Participation in structured activities is largely voluntary. Hence, self-selection and preexisting differences can explain behavioral differences between the adolescents who decide to spend time in these activities and those who do not. Studies show that well-adjusted adolescents tend to choose structured activities, such as organized sports, hobbies, religious activities, music, theater, art, and politics, whereas less well-adjusted adolescents tend to choose unstructured activities, such as hanging out on the streets or in shopping malls, arcades, and public drinking places (Feinstein, Bynner, & Duckworth, 2006). But even when controlling for relevant confounding factors, participation in structured activities is associated with good adjustment (Darling, Caldwell, & Smith, 2005; Fredricks & Eccles, 2004, 2006). Perhaps the most convincing evidence comes from longitudinal studies in which self-selection can be controlled by associating activity participation with changes in the outcome variable (Fredricks & Eccles, 2006), and it is also possible to examine variability in participation in structured activities over ages (Darling, 2005). These studies clearly show increases in positive outcomes and decreases in negative outcomes as consequences of participation. Participation in structured activities can have long-term effects. Greater civic engagement in young adulthood was found for adolescents who had participated in school clubs or prosocial extracurricular activities in 11th grade (Fredricks & Eccles, 2004), and better age-30 outcomes, in terms of health, economy, and civic engagement, were reported by Feinstein et al. (2006) for adolescents who took part in sports, uniformed youth associations, and church clubs. Thus, although the effect sizes are modest, experiences in structured activities seem to change adolescents for the better.

There is one exception to this general picture of beneficial consequences of structured activities. Participants in team sports often report drinking alcohol more frequently than do other youths (Eccles & Barber, 1999; Fredricks & Eccles, 2004). In some cases, though, they report lower use of alcohol (Fredricks & Eccles, 2006). All in all, however, higher drinking levels seem to be the more robust finding, and this raises the possibility that all structured activities should not necessarily be thought of as equal. Also, there are indications that higher levels of alcohol drinking might precede sports involvement (Feinstein et al., 2006), which suggests that there might be essential differences between team sports and other activities in the experiences they offer *or* the people who choose them.

There are many reasons to believe that structured activities might produce good adjustment. One is that being in an adult-controlled setting reduces the time spent in peer-oriented settings and strengthens the ties with school (McNeal, 1995). Researchers from different perspectives have also argued that to be involved in organized leisure-time activities can reduce adjustment problems among adolescents by imposing structure on their daily lives, linking them to competent adults and peers, building their skills and interests, and creating opportunities for them to feel competent and accepted within a social system (Mahoney & Stattin, 2000). The work by Larson and colleagues on what adolescents experience and learn when they attend structured activities is particularly informative. Using experience sampling (Csikszentmihalyi & Larson, 1984), focus groups (Dworkin et al., 2003), and qualitative interviews (Larson, Walker, & Pearce, 2005), their findings suggest that participation has benefits in the personal, emotional, cognitive, and social domains. Taking part in structured activities may help youths develop initiative, defined as an intrinsic motivation to plan, carry through, and achieve a valued goal. In the words of Larson (2000):

> The capacity for initiative is essential for adults in our society and will become more important in the 21st century. The context best suited to the development of initiative appears to be that of structured voluntary activities, such as sports, arts, and participation in organizations, in which youths experience the rare combination of intrinsic motivation in combination with deep attention. (p. 170)

Thus, the findings on the benefits of structured activities are both robust and intuitively appealing.

Despite these insights, we should mention that ideas about what adolescents get out of structured activities have not been subjected to empirical testing. Despite clear theoretical ideas, the empirical evidence is weak concerning which features of structured activities contribute to positive development (Larson, 2000; Eccles, Barber, Stone, & Hunt, 2003). With few exceptions, empirical studies have used simple designs comparing adjustment of adolescents who participate in various afterschool activities with those who do not participate. What is going on in these activities is largely unknown. It is possible that once proposed mechanisms are included in evaluation designs, better prediction of the effects of participation and higher effect sizes might be found.

All in all, what we can say is that there is growing evidence that youths involved in structured, adult-led activities are better adjusted in a number of respects than those who are not involved (see Mahoney, Larson, & Eccles, 2005). In part, this is because better adjusted youths choose these activities, but the activities also seem to contribute to good adjustment.

Unstructured Activities and Poor Adjustment

Traditionally, peer associations in certain kinds of neighborhood contexts have been viewed as posing a risk for the development of problem behaviors. Specifically, the argument is that when peer groups gather in unstructured settings without adult leadership, the lack of control allows deviant behaviors to emerge in the group. Empirical studies attest to these conclusions. Participation in unstructured, unsupervised activities has been associated with antisocial behavior and substance use (Mahoney, Stattin, & Lord, 2004; Osgood, Wilson, O'Malley, Bachman, & Johnston, 1996; Persson, Kerr, & Stattin, 2004; Stattin, Kerr, Mahoney, Persson, & Magnusson, 2005).

Apart from the general notion that "idle hands" are problematic, there have been few attempts to develop a theoretical model linking participation in unstructured settings to social adjustment. There is one exception. The routine activity perspective (Osgood et al., 1996) is a theoretical model developed in criminology to explain how adolescents' experiences in certain leisure settings are associated with the development of deviant behavior. According to the routine activity idea, when adolescents are in unstructured leisure settings, away from adult supervision and interacting with peers, deviant activities are more likely than in other types of settings. The lack of social control and structure increases the *opportunities* for deviance. The more adolescents spend their time in such settings, the higher the risk for deviant behavior. In a 2005 study, Haynie and Osgood argued even more strongly that spending time in unstructured leisure settings with peers, rather than associating with deviant peers per se, should be linked to delinquency.

Routine activity theory seeks to explain deviant behavior in situational terms. A problem is that the theory does not explain why some adolescents choose to spend time in these settings in the first place and others do not. Is it something about the adolescents who spend most of their time in these settings rather than being part of structured leisure activities? Another problem is that the perspective does not account for individual differences. According to the theory, much unsupervised time spent socializing in unstructured settings with peers should increase the likelihood for deviance uniformly. The theory does not explain why increased deviance is true for some but not other adolescents who spend time in unstructured settings. In their empirical study, Osgood and coworkers (1996) found that unsupervised activities, such as riding in a car for fun, going to parties, and spending most evenings out, predicted changes in criminal behavior and heavy use of alcohol, marijuana, and other illicit drugs, which they interpreted as supportive of the situational explanation. We should mention, however, that although the links to problem behavior were statistically significant, they did not explain much variance in deviant behavior. So it seems that more than routine exposure to unstructured, unsupervised settings with peers—is needed to explain deviant behavior.

Conclusions about Structured–Unstructured Contexts and Adjustment

Two conclusions can be drawn about research on unstructured and structured activities. First, unstructured and structured activities are often framed as polar opposites. Unstructured, unsupervised time spent with peers is often referred to as *risky*, whereas time spent in structured activities and with the family is considered *protective* (e.g., Richards et al., 2004). In unstructured settings, adolescents are not supervised by their parents and are at risk of being exposed to bad peers and drawn into deviant activities. In structured setting, they are directly supervised by adults or by the parents themselves, and these adults can steer adolescents away from bad influences and provide a setting for personal growth and positive social experiences.

In reality, this dichotomy is less clear. On one hand, it is true that antisocial adolescents meet their friends at the friends' homes, at cafés, parties, discotheques, street corners, sport places, playgrounds, neighborhood parks, community gardens, pool halls, shopping malls, arcades, and other places. Dishion, McCord, and Poulin (1999) have argued that association with deviant peers in these normal, everyday settings is perhaps the major reason for escalation in deviant behavior in early adolescence. On the other hand, nondelinquent adolescents also interact with their peers in many of these same settings. In fact, one of the most salient features of normative adolescent social development is the increase in time spent away from home and in the company of peers. Interacting informally with peers—talking and doing things together—is fun and enjoyable. In unstructured settings adolescents make new friends, learn what is going on in the neighborhood, gossip and share information, and develop social skills. These settings provide contexts for identity exploration. What would a normal adolescent's life be like without any of this kind of "down time"—with every moment structured? Thus, because virtually all adolescents spend some part of their free time in unstructured settings, conceptualizing structured versus unstructured activities as polar opposites limits understanding of peer relationships in everyday contexts.

A second conclusion that may be drawn about research on unstructured and structured activities is that research has focused primarily on relating participation or nonparticipation to behavioral outcomes, but experiences in those activities and their effects on the outcomes have seldom been investigated. What happens in structured and unstructured settings is often brought up theoretically but seldom is transformed into empirical research. Most studies focus only on participation effects. In Bronfenbrenner's (1986) terminology, this is research on "social addresses," where the activity is the object of study, but what happens in the activity is largely unknown. For this reason, we should not be surprised to find that participating in a particular type of setting, whether unstructured or structured, yields low predictions of specific behavior (e.g., Goldstein, Davis-Kean, & Eccles, 2005). Youths who spend time in certain settings have different personalities, different prior experiences, and react to the experiences of the settings in their own ways. For example, in sports, some will be "stars" and others will be "bench warmers." Surely these two groups of youths will have different experiences and outcomes. In most research, however, people with different characteristics, motivations, and reasons for participating are merged together under the label of participant. This limits prediction of specific outcomes in terms of social adjustment. In short, what is largely missing is an understanding of the processes that operate in structured and unstructured settings.

How Peer Relationships Fit In

In the literatures linking unstructured contexts with poor adjustment and structured contexts with good adjustment, explanatory mechanisms, including the role of peer relationships, have not yet been thoroughly investigated. The causal explanations focus very much on adult control, or the lack thereof, and keeping youths busy versus allowing them idle time in which to get into trouble. We advance an argument that peer relationships are important parts of the explanation for the links between structured or unstructured contexts and adjustment. We build our argument in two steps. First, we argue that youths choose their contexts. Structured contexts attract mainly well-adjusted youths, whereas unstructured contexts attract both well-adjusted and deviant youths, albeit for different reasons. In the second step, we argue that not all youths who spend time in unstructured contexts are negatively affected, but for those who are, the explanation likely involves the influence of deviant peers.

Youths Choose Contexts

In the literature that exists, little attention has been paid to youth's choices of activities. Selection effects are confounds in studies of the effects of structured and unstructured contexts. In our view, these effects should be seen as part of the explanation rather than simply as a problem.

Research in North America and Sweden suggests that the vast majority of youths are involved in some organized activity when they enter adolescence (Eccles & Barber, 1999; Persson et al., 2007; U.S. Department of Education, 1995), so the question is why some stay involved while others drop out and enter into unstructured activities. These choices are unlikely to be random, but they are also unlikely to be singly determined. There might be many different reasons within and across adolescents.

Concerning adult-led, structured activities such as organized sports, talents and abilities are likely to play an important role in youths' choices. Those who have athletic talent are likely to enter sports and stay involved because of intrinsic and extrinsic rewards. For instance, developing a skill might bring intrinsic rewards, and the recognition from parents, coaches, and peers that results from excellent athletic performance might provide extrinsic rewards. Research also suggests that parents' encouragement of activity participation plays a role in youths' choices of structured activities (Anderson, Funk, Elliot, & Hull Smith, 2003). These are explanations for choices of the activity, but youths might choose the *context* as much as the activity.

There are at least three logical explanations for youths' choices between adult-controlled, structured contexts and peer-controlled, unstructured contexts. One is that youths want to do what their friends are doing, and they stay in structured activities or drop out depending on their friends' choices (Persson et al., 2007). Thus, the activity itself might be less important to adolescents than being in the same context as their friends.

A second explanation of why adolescents would choose an unstructured, peer-controlled context over a structured, adult-controlled context involves their basic temperamental qualities. Oppositional, anger-prone temperament is identifiable very early in life, and it is also linked in longitudinal studies to later conduct problems and criminal behavior (Caspi, Henry, McGee, Moffitt, & Silva, 1995; Stoolmiller, 2001). We know of no empirical test of this, but it is reasonable to expect that youths who oppose adult restrictions would steer away from contexts in which adults are setting the rules and requiring compliance. This explanation also suggests that poorly adjusted youths, or those who are oppositional and have developed, or will develop, conduct problems, including criminality, should be overrepresented in peer contexts in which adults are not in control. This is only suggestive evidence, but in one longitudinal study, 10th graders reported which character they were most like in the popular film *The Breakfast Club* (Eccles et al., 2003). About half of all youths who said they were most like the *criminal* were in team sports in 10th grade, but 70% dropped out before 12th grade. This represented the highest drop-out rate of all groups in the study. To the extent that oppositional temperament played a role in self-identifying with the *criminal*, this supports our hypothesis that youths with oppositional temperament should be underrepresented in structured, adult-led activities and overrepresented in unstructured, peer-controlled activities.

A third explanation for youths' choices of structured or unstructured contexts rests on the emotions they have connected to other adult-controlled settings. This "context-choice" model says that if youths have negative experiences in one adult-controlled setting (e.g., the home), then their negative emotions might generalize to other adult-controlled settings (for a detailed account of proposed mechanisms, see Kerr, Stattin, Biesecker, & Ferrer-Wreder, 2003). Specifically, parental behaviors such as angry outbursts, derisive comments, or inconsistent discipline, might make children feel unvalued, disrespected, and not in control of their circumstances, and the negative emotions connected with these kinds of experiences could become conditioned to fundamental aspects of the home context, such as having adults present and more or less in control. If so, then, when youths are old enough to choose their leisure contexts, they steer away from adult-led, structured contexts and toward unstructured, peer-defined contexts. Two studies have shown support for this idea. In one, girls who often engaged in unstructured leisure activities had poorer relationships with their parents and more negative emotions connected with the home setting than those who were not involved in unstructured activities (Persson et al., 2004). In the other study, which was a direct test of the context choice idea, youths' self-reported negative feelings in the family context and negative interactions with parents predicted switching from structured activities to loitering on the streets—an unstructured activity in which youths are not supervised by adults—controlling for age, delinquency, gender, and family structure (Persson et al., 2007). Thus, there is mounting evidence that youths who have negative experiences at home avoid adult-controlled, structured leisure contexts and opt for unstructured contexts.

A final explanation for youths' choices of unstructured leisure contexts is that these contexts allow them to socialize on their own terms, free from adult interference. Most youths spend a certain amount of time hanging out in cafés, public parks, downtown streets, or malls, just because it is fun to socialize with other adolescents and make new contacts—often romantic contacts (Silbereisen, Noack, & von Eye, 1992). A few studies have shown that going to discos and pubs in later adolescence can also be instrumental in developing close friendships and romantic relationships (Engels & Knibbe, 2000; Silbereisen et al., 1992). Thus, although not all adolescents spend time in structured, adult-controlled contexts, most spend at least some time in unstructured, unsupervised contexts.

What this line of reasoning suggests is that, unstructured contexts have more diverse populations than structured, adult-controlled contexts. Youths who have bad home experiences and those who are temperamentally oppositional and prone to anger probably spend much time in unstructured contexts, but most other adolescents spend at least some time in them as well. This heterogeneity in unstructured contexts allows for a wide variety of peer relationships to form, and we argue that it underlies the link between unstructured contexts and poor adjustment.

Peers Help Explain Why Contexts Are Linked to Adjustment

Concerning structured activities and good adjustment, many researchers have suggested that the positive effects are partly due to social network composition—making friends with well-adjusted peers (e.g., see Eccles et al., 2003). To our knowledge, this has not yet been tested in longitudinal studies of changes in peer network composition following entry into extracurricular activities. Studies in this area tend to rely on youths' reports of their friends' behavior and characteristics, which have been shown to reflect the false belief that people are more alike than they are (Ross, Greene, & House, 1977), thus inflating similarity to peers (Iannotti, Bush, & Weinfurt, 1996). In a study using peers' own reports, however, youths who participated in extracurricular activities experienced less negative outcomes only if members of their social networks were also engaged in school activities (Mahoney, 2000). Overall, however, there is a lack of direct empirical study of the role peer relationships play in youths' structured activity experiences.

Concerning the link between unstructured contexts and poor adjustment, few studies have tried to investigate the mechanisms. An exception is a series of studies examining the development of deviance in a particular unstructured context: neighborhood youth recreation centers. These centers exist all over Sweden and are ideal for studying peer socialization in unstructured contexts, because they are low in structure and they gather adolescents with problematic adjustment and well-adjusted adolescents.

Youth Recreation Centers: An Unstructured Context

The Swedish youth centers were designed to give adolescents not interested in organized sports or other activities a place to go, where they would be off the streets and in the presence of adults. These government-supported centers open around dinnertime and close around 11:30 P.M. Adolescents can go there to socialize with their friends in an unstructured setting. There are adults present at the centers, but they do not direct the youths' activities or place any demands on them. The adolescents decide what they want to do among the available options. Typically, they can play pool, video games, ping-pong, or darts, watch TV, listen to music, or drink coffee. Because the ratio of adults to adolescents is extremely low and the philosophy is nondirective, it is likely that much goes on outside of the awareness of the youth center leaders.

Youth centers exist in some form in many European countries and in the United States. The European Confederation Youth Clubs comprise approximately 18,000 centers serving 3.5 million youths throughout Europe. Boys' and Girls' Clubs of America are different, in that they offer structured programs, but similar in that youths do not have to enroll in the programs. If they do not, they can go to the Clubs and have essentially the same experience as youths at the Swedish centers—the experience of a context in which adults are present but do not structure the activities. Mahoney, Stattin, and colleagues designed a series of studies to test theoretical ideas about when unstructured settings do and do not influence problematic adjustment of youths.

An Initial, Cross-Sectional Test

In the first study, Mahoney and Stattin (2000) simply looked at whether the youth recreation centers tended to have visitors with higher than average levels of adjustment problems. They compared four groups of 15-year-olds: (1) youths who often visited the centers and were not members of any club or organization; (2) youths who often visited the centers but were at the same time members of one or more clubs or organizations; (3) youths who seldom or never visited the centers, and did not belong to any clubs or organizations; and (4) youths who seldom or never visited the centers but were members of one or more clubs or organizations. Youths who often visited the centers and were not members of clubs or organizations had higher incidences of: drinking alcohol, delinquency, smoking, violence, depression, psychosomatic problems; having friends who often stayed out late at night and had been caught by the police; poor school adjustment and teacher relationships; and failure expectations and poor self-esteem than other groups. According to their parents' reports, these youths withdrew more than the other groups from demands and disclosed little about their leisure-time activities. As a consequence, parents had little knowledge about these youths' activities away from home, they had little trust in these youths, they seldom engaged in the youths' leisure activities, and they reported more delinquency in the youths. Overall, the findings showed conclusively that adolescents who visited the youth recreation centers and were not members of clubs or associations had more problems than other adolescents. The question, however, was whether problematic youths gravitated to these centers, as suggested above, or whether their problem behaviors emerged as a result of their experiences in the unstructured setting. To answer this, longitudinal data were required.

A Longitudinal Perspective

In a second study, an all-boy, longitudinal sample was used to determine whether problem behaviors developed before or after boys started attending the youth recreation centers (Mahoney, Stattin, & Magnusson, 2001). Adolescents younger than age 13 were not allowed to attend the youth centers, so teacher ratings of children's aggressiveness, hyperactivity, peer preference, and school achievement at age 10 were used as measures of pre-existing behavior problems. These measures had been linked to adult delinquency in an earlier study (Bergman & Magnusson, 1994), so boys who scored high on these measures could be considered at risk. At age 13, boys reported how often they attended the centers. The outcome measure was registered criminal offenses from ages 13–30. The results revealed that the higher the boys' preexisting problems, the greater the likelihood of attending the centers. All of the teacher-rated problems correlated significantly with frequency of center attendance, and person-centered analyses showed that 30% of boys with very low levels of all the preexisting problem measures attended the centers, whereas 60% of those with high levels of all the problem measures attended. So problematic boys did seem to gravitate to the centers, even though the heterogeneity of the center population also came through in the results. It was clear, however, that additional problems emerged for those who attended the centers, regardless of their levels of earlier problems. Controlling for parents' reports of concerns, marital status, and SES, and teachers' ratings of aggressiveness, hyperactivity, peer preference, and school achievement, youth center participation predicted future registered criminal activity and was a stronger predictor than any of the other measures. In addition, person-centered analyses revealed that the effects associated with center attendance were equally strong for those who had very high and very low levels of all the problem behavior measures at age 10. Additional analyses showed that the differences in registered criminality were not limited to adolescence, but continued from ages 18–30, and that the same pattern of results appeared for 13 of the 14 individual youth centers in the sample. Overall, the results showed that whether boys scored high or low on preexisting behavior problems, the risk for future delinquency was almost doubled if they often attended the youth recreation centers in early adolescence. In short, then, problematic youths tended to gravitated to this unstructured context, but problem behaviors tended to emerge for both problematic and nonproblematic youths who spent time in this unstructured setting.

These results do not apply only to Swedish conditions. A study that followed more than 11,000 participants in the 1970 British Birth Cohort from ages 16–30 (Feinstein et al., 2006) showed similar results for British youths who spent time in youth clubs. These authors examined the relation between taking part in various leisure activities in mid-adolescence (sports and community centers, youth clubs, uniformed youth associations, church clubs) and social adjustment problems (poor economy, criminality, health, family situation) at age 30. They controlled for a wide spectrum of potentially confounding family, SES, and individual factors. Attending youth clubs was associated with being an offender, a serious offender, or a victim of crime at the age of 30; not voting; being a single parent; and having a low income. As extra controls, Feinstein and colleagues in a next step included drinking alcohol and delinquency at the time when the youths were attending the different activities. Even then, attending youth clubs was associated with being an offender or a serious offender, not voting, and having a low income. Thus, the British findings are consistent with the findings reviewed above. Even with strict controls, spending time in these settings implies higher risk for future social problems.

Perhaps the most pressing question that these studies left unanswered was whether the development of criminal activity actually occurred at the youth centers. From the results of these studies, one knows only that youths who attended the centers at one point in time developed more problems than they had had earlier—problems that those who did not attend were less likely to develop. To begin, one would like to see whether the increase in problem behaviors could be linked temporally to youth center attendance.

Short-Term Changes

These studies were followed up with a short-term longitudinal study over 18 months to determine whether problems start when youths begin attending the youth centers and end when they stop (Mahoney et al., 2004). All 15-year-olds in one community who were in the eighth grade were selected and followed up after 18 months, when they finished the ninth grade. The sample was divided into four groups: (1) *nonattenders*: those who seldom or never went to the youth centers in grades 8 and 9; (2) *joiners*: those who did not go regularly in grade 8 but did so in grade 9; (3) *dropouts*: those who visited the centers regularly in grade 8 but not in grade 9; and (4) *stable attenders*: those who visited the centers in both grade 8 and grade 9. The dropouts did not change in problem behavior, but the joiners showed a marked increase in violence, delinquency, drinking, and use of marijuana from grade 8 to grade 9. In follow-up analyses, the 13 centers that youths in the sample attended were categorized according to the numbers of delinquent youths who reported attending regularly (few, some, or many). Results revealed that the increase in problem behaviors among the joiners was concentrated entirely in the youth centers categorized as having many delinquent participants. Thus, problems in various domains seemed to be linked in time with starting to visit youth centers, specifically, youth centers with many delinquent peers in attendance.

Again, because the study was designed to examine the changes that occurred over time for a normal sample of midadolescents, causal interpretations cannot be made, and like much of the literature, these studies do not reveal the mechanisms linking youth centers and behavioral problems. This series of studies involved boys and girls, youth centers in countryside and city neighborhoods, and cohorts as far apart as 20 years. The results are consistent; where youth recreation centers create an impact, it is negative. Nonetheless, this study was limited in that it did not show negative peer socialization in the unstructured, youth-center setting. Like much of the literature, this study did not include measures that would allow an investigation of actual peer processes.

Explaining the Mechanisms

What are the mechanisms through which deviance develops in unstructured leisure contexts? To date, there is little research that provides insights into this. An exception is the groundbreaking work of Dishion and colleagues. In a series of studies, these scholars convincingly argued for a "deviancy training" mechanism, in which deviant youths reinforce each other's comments about deviant behaviors by chuckling, laughing, or otherwise showing approval. These exchanges, taken from taped dyadic interactions between youths and friends they brought to the lab, have been linked longitudinally to increased probability of the initiation of substance use (Dishion, Capaldi, Spracklen, & Li, 1995), increased delinquency (Dishion, Spracklen, Andrews, & Patterson, 1996), and increased violent behavior (Dishion, Eddy, Haas, Li, & Spracklen, 1997). As Dodge, Dishion, and Lansford (2006) pointed out, many programs for treating high-risk or already delinquent youths involve bringing them together in one way or another, and this is likely to result in iatrogenic effects through the reinforcement of deviant talk and other possible mechanisms (see also Dishion, McCord, & Poulin, 1999). To date, only the deviant talk mechanism has been tested empirically. These demonstrations have been critically important, however, for understanding the role of unstructured contexts and their links to the development of problem behaviors. An important finding was that nondeviant youths did not reinforce deviant talk; the reinforcement occurred among deviant youths. This suggests that unstructured contexts alone will not produce problem behavior without the aggregation of problematic youths. In other words, it argues against a situational interpretation of the link between unstructured contexts and problem behavior.

The question is whether these negative effects of youth center attendance can be attributed to peer socialization, as the work of Dishion and colleagues would suggest, rather than to the situation, as Osgood's (see Osgood et al., 1996) theory suggests. Furthermore, why would a certain proportion of youths with no risk factors end up developing criminal records after attending youth centers, as seen in the long-term longitudinal study described above (Mahoney et al., 2001). We argue that to understand this phenomenon, one must take into account individual differences that might predispose nonproblematic youths to become involved with the problematic youths at the centers. In other words, one must consider the person, as well as the context and the process.

The Context, the Process, and the Person

The youth center studies described above considered the context and the process, but specifically ignored the person by controlling for characteristics associated with delinquency. However, in two studies of youth center attendance and problem behavior in girls, we examined a peer socialization explanation for the effect of youth center attendance and then tried to explain why some girls and not others attend the youth centers and are influenced by deviant peers (Persson et al., 2004; Stattin et al., 2005).

The Context

As a starting point, we examined whether the same effects of youth center attendance found earlier for boys would apply to girls. In analyses similar to those described above for boys, but using adolescent norm-breaking behaviors as the outcome instead of registered criminality, girls who attended youth recreation centers at age 13 were more likely to engage in norm-breaking activities such as getting drunk, shoplifting, and vandalizing property (Stattin et al., 2005). This link was found at both age 13 and age 15, and it could not be explained by age-10 behavior, such as aggression and hyperactivity, or by age-10 family factors, such as parent concern and SES. Thus, for girls, the link between youth center attendance and problem behavior was similar to that for boys. Girls who spent time in the context developed problem behaviors that could not be explained by their earlier problems.

The Process

We tested a peer socialization explanation for this increase. We reasoned that only under conditions that increase the likelihood of involvement with deviant peers should we find increases in girls' norm-breaking behavior. In general, boys engage in more norm breaking than do girls, and both boys and girls who attend the centers engage in more norm breaking than those who do not. Thus, we reasoned that heavy involvement with friends at the centers and involvement in heterosexual relationships would mean involvement with peers who, on average, engaged in more norm breaking that the ordinary 13-year-old girl. We examined peer involvement with a scale that assessed girls' numbers of friends outside of school and the amount of free time girls spent away from home and with friends.

We found an interaction between center attendance and peer involvement in predicting norm breaking. Essentially, only when girls were heavily involved with peers *and* attended the youth centers was norm breaking high. Heavy peer involvement outside of the centers was not linked to norm breaking, nor was center attendance without heavy peer involvement. This is consistent with the explanation that the friends the girls made at the youth centers were engaged in more norm breaking and drew them into those behaviors. The weak link in the logic, however, was we could not be certain that heavy peer involvement meant involvement with peers who attended the centers. Using data from another sample, however, we were able to show that girls more often shoplifted, got drunk, and talked about illegal things with best friends who, by their own accounts, often visited the youth centers than with best friends who did not, which strengthens the argument for a peer socialization explanation of the higher norm breaking among center attenders.

The results for heterosexual relationships were similar. A significant interaction between heterosexual involvement and center attendance showed that heterosexual involvement was linked to somewhat higher norm breaking overall, but to much higher levels for girls who went often to the youth centers than for those who did not. The same was true for registered delinquency up to age 35. Again, with data from another sample, we tested the assumption that associations with boys involve more norm breaking than do associations with girls. Girls who named a boy rather than a girl as their most important peer relationship reported doing more of a number of norm-breaking activities with that peer: playing hooky, getting drunk, keeping secrets from parents, talking about illegal things, and doing things other than shoplifting for which one could be arrested. Taken together, these findings showed that center attendance per se did not usher in problem behavior. It was only linked to higher levels of problems for girls who were the most involved with peers and boys—presumably at the centers where deviant youth tend to congregate. This supports the peer socialization explanation of the process through which youths who attend the centers increase in problem behavior.

The Person

But why would some girls more than others become involved with peers and boys at the youth centers and get drawn into delinquent behavior? We tested explanations involving family relationships and the girls' characteristics. In the context choice theory described above, bad experiences at home spur youths to choose unstructured contexts with little adult control, and exposure to deviant peers happens as a consequence, because oppositional youths have also chosen unstructured contexts with little adult control. In this explanation, girls with poor family relationships should choose to go to the youth centers. Consistent with this idea, those who went to the youth centers had more negative experiences at home than those who did not, and center attendance was a substantial predictor of peer and heterosexual involvement. Negative experiences at home did not predict peer and heterosexual involvement directly, though. So it seems that girls with bad home experiences chose the unstructured context, then the peers with whom they came into contact had a negative socializing effect.

We also considered that girls' adventurous personalities might play one of several roles. Adventurousness (defined as thrill-seeking and impulsivity) could be a reason for choosing the unstructured context, because girls with these characteristics might want to be free of adult control. These same characteristics might underlie the pursuit of peer and heterosexual relationships, and might explain norm breaking, apart from any peer socialization effect. Thus, what appears to be a peer socialization effect might be a spurious effect produced by adventurousness. Adventurousness did seem to be involved in girls choosing to spend their free time in the youth center context and forming associations with problematic peers and boys, but even though it also partly explained norm breaking, it did not explain why girls who chose the youth centers and became involved with peers and boys engaged in more norm breaking. Thus, adventurousness explains why girls go to the centers and why they get involved there with peers (both boys and girls), but it does not explain the links between these peer associations and norm breaking. It seems that in the unstructured youth centers (the context), negative socialization takes place though involvement with deviant peers (the process), but adventurousness (the person) determines which girls choose the unstructured context and seek out peer associations. The context, the process, and the person are all necessary parts of the explanation.

Future Directions

To understand peer relationships in neighborhood contexts presents several interrelated challenges for future research. First, peers' behaviors and youths' joint activities and interactions with their peers must be captured better than they are with the typical measures presently used in research, and these activities and interactions must be contextualized. Studies on deviant and prosocial peer association have typically used global measures of adolescents' perceptions of how many of their friends are involved in delinquent activities or engage in prosocial activities, ranging from none to all of their friends. In fact, based largely on findings from this type of perception measure, delinquent peers have been referred to as the best predictor of delinquency. As discussed earlier in this chapter, these measures have been shown to overestimate similarity to a youth's own behavior; therefore, whether they validly capture peers' behaviors may be questionable. In addition, these measures do not capture the contextual conditions under which youths affiliate with these peers or how their interactions play out. In short, global characterizations of peers are of questionable validity and say little about the contexts or specifics of peer interactions. In future research, better ways will have to be developed to capture these phenomena.

Another challenge for future research will be to specify and test the processes through which youths are influenced, for better or worse, when they take part in structured or unstructured activities, and particularly what role peer interactions play in those effects. In the current literature, effects of participation have been reported and speculations have been made about the processes that explain those effects, but this is largely a black box. With a few exceptions, which we described earlier in the chapter, little has been done to hypothesize about and directly test the processes, including the peer processes involved. Thus, a challenge for future research will be to open the black box.

Yet another challenge will be to understand the role of choices of activities relative to the youth as a person. Much of the research has been designed to covary out individual characteristics to detect other influences on behavior, but a more nuanced understanding of the effects of leisure contexts will include individual characteristics—their role in youths' choices of contexts and in the processes that play out in the context. In short, if the context, the process, and the person are all necessary to explain the roles neighborhood contexts of peer relationships play in development, then future research must move in the direction of better capturing their joint contributions.

References

Anderson, J. C., Funk, J. B., Elliot, R., & Hull Smith, P. (2003). Parental support and pressure and children's extracurricular activities: Relationships with amount of involvement and affective experience of participation. *Applied Developmental Psychology, 24*, 241–257.

Barber, B. L., Eccles, J. S., & Stone, M. R. (2001). Whatever happened to the jock, the brain, and the princess? Young adult pathways linked to adolescent activity involvement and social identity. *Journal of Adolescent Research, 16*, 429–455.

Bergman, L. R., & Magnusson, D. (1994). Stability and change in patterns of extrinsic adjustment problems. In D. Magnusson, L. R. Bergman, G. Rudinger, & B. Törestad (Eds.), *Problems and methods in longitudinal research: Stability and change* (pp. 323–346). New York: Cambridge University Press.

Beyers, J. M., Loeber, R., Wikström, P.-O. H., & Stouthamer-Loeber, M. (2001). What predicts adolescent violence in better-off neighborhoods? *Journal of Abnormal Child Psychology, 29*, 369–381.

Brody, G. H., Ge, X., Conger, R., Gibbons, F. X., McBride, M. V., Gerrard, M., et al. (2001). The influence of neighbourhood disadvantage, collective socialization, and parenting on African American children's affiliation with deviant peers. *Child Development, 72*, 1231–1246.

Bronfenbrenner, U. (1986). Ecology of the family as a context for human development: Research perspectives. *Developmental Psychology, 22*, 723–742.

Caspi, A., Henry, B., McGee, R., Moffitt, T., & Silva, P. (1995). Temperamental origins of child and adolescent behavior problems: From age 3 to age 15. *Child Development, 66*, 55–68.

Chung, H. L., & Steinberg, L. (2006). Relations between neighborhood factors, parenting behaviors, peer deviance, and delinquency among serious juvenile offenders. *Developmental Psychology, 42*, 319–331.

Cooper, H., Valentine, J. C., Nye, B., & Lindsay, J. J. (1999). Relationships between five after-school activities and academic achievement. *Journal of Educational Psychology, 91*, 369–378.

Csikszentmihalyi, M., & Larson, R. (1984). *Being adolescent.* New York: Basic Books.

Darling, N. (2005). Participation in extracurricular activities and adolescent adjustment: Cross-sectional and longitudinal findings. *Journal of Youth and Adolescence, 34*, 493–505.

Darling, N., Caldwell, L. I., & Smith, R. (2005). Participation in school-based extracurricular activities and adolescent adjustment. *Journal of Leisure Research, 37*, 51–76.

Deci, E. L., & Ryan, R. M. (1985). *Intrinsic motivation and self-determination in human behavior.* New York: Plenum Press.

Dishion, T. J., Capaldi, D. M., Spracklen, K. M., & Li, F. (1995). Peer ecology of male adolescent drug use. *Development and Psychopathology, 7*, 803–824.

Dishion, T. J., Eddy, J. M., Haas, E., Li, F., & Spracklen, K. (1997). Friendships and violent behavior during adolescence. *Social Development, 6*, 207–223.

Dishion, T. J., McCord, J., & Poulin, F. (1999). When interventions harm: Peer groups and problem behavior. *American Psychologist, 9*, 755–764.

Dishion, T. J., Spracklen, K. M., Andrews, D. W., & Patterson, G. R. (1996). Deviancy training in male adolescent friendships. *Behavior Therapy, 27*, 373–390.

Dodge, K. A., Dishion, T. J., & Lansford, J. E. (2006). Deviant peer influences in intervention and public policy for youth. *Social Policy Report: Giving Child and Youth Development Knowledge Away, 20*, 3–19.

Dworkin, J. B., Larson, R., & Hansen, D. (2003). Adolescents' accounts of growth experiences in youth activities. *Journal of Youth and Adolescence, 32*, 17–26.

Eccles, J. S., & Barber, B. L. (1999). Student council, volunteering, basketball, or marching band: What kind of extracurricular involvement matters? *Journal of Adolescent Research, 14*, 10–43.

Eccles, J. S., Barber, B. L., Stone, M., & Hunt, J. (2003). Extracurricular activities and adolescent development. *Journal of Social Issues, 59*, 865–889.

Eccles, J. S., & Gootman, J. A. (Eds.). (2002). *Community programs to promote youth development.* Washington, DC: National Academy Press.

Engels, C. M. E., & Knibbe, R. A. (2000). Alcohol use and intimate relationships in adolescence: When love comes to town. *Addictive Behaviors, 25,* 435–439.

Feinstein, L., Bynner, J., & Duckworth, K. (2006). Young people's leisure contexts and their relation to adult outcomes. *Journal of Youth Studies, 9,* 305–327.

Fredricks, J. A., & Eccles, J. S. (2004). Developmental benefits of extracurricular involvement: Do peer characteristics mediate the link between activities and youth outcomes? *Journal of Youth and Adolescence, 34,* 507–520.

Fredricks, J. A., & Eccles, J. S. (2006). Is extracurricular participation associated with beneficial outcomes?: Concurrent and longitudinal relations. *Developmental Psychology, 42,* 698–713.

Goldstein, S. E., Davis-Kean, P. E., & Eccles, J. S. (2005). Parents, peers, and problem behavior: A longitudinal investigation of the impact of relationship perceptions and characteristics on the development of adolescent problem behavior. *Developmental Psychology, 41,* 401–413.

Haynie, D. L., & Osgood, D. W. (2005). Reconsidering peers and delinquency: How do peers matter? *Social Forces, 84,* 1109–1130.

Hendry, L. B., Glendinning, A., & Shucksmith, J. (1996). Adolescent focal theories: Age-trends in developmental transitions. *Journal of Adolescence, 19,* 307–320.

Hirschi, T. (1969). *Causes of delinquency.* Berkeley: University of California Press.

Iannotti, R. J., Bush, P. J., & Weinfurt, K. P. (1996). Perceptions of friends' use of alcohol, cigarettes, and marijuana among urban schoolchildren: A longitudinal analysis. *Addictive Behaviors, 21,* 615–632.

Jordan, W. J., & Nettles, S. M. (1999). How students invest their time outside of school: Effects on school-related outcomes. *Social Psychology of Education, 3,* 217–243.

Kerr, M., Stattin, H., Biesecker, G., & Ferrer-Wreder, L. (2003). Relationships with parents and peers in adolescence. In R. M. Lerner, M. A. Easterbrooks, & J. Mistry (Eds.), *Handbook of psychology: Vol. 6. Developmental psychology* (pp. 395–422). Hoboken, NJ: Wiley.

Landers, D. M., & Landers, D. M. (1978). Socialization via interscholastic athletics: Its effects on delinquency. *Sociology of Education, 51,* 299–303.

Larson, R. W. (2000). Toward a psychology of positive youth development. *American Psychologist, 55,* 170–183.

Larson, R. W., Walker, K., & Pearce, N. (2005). A comparison of youth-driven and adult-driven youth programs: Balancing inputs from youth and adults. *Journal of Community Psychology, 33,* 57–74.

Leventhal, T., & Brooks-Gunn, J. (2000). The neighborhoods they live in: The effects of neighborhood residence on child and adolescent outcomes. *Psychological Bulletin, 126,* 309–337.

Mahoney, J. L. (2000). School extracurricular activity participation as a moderator in the development of antisocial patterns. *Child Development, 71,* 502–516.

Mahoney, J. L., & Cairns, R. B. (1997). Do extracurricular activities protect against early school dropout? *Developmental Psychology, 33,* 241–253.

Mahoney, J. L., Larson, R., & Eccles, J. S. (2005). *Organized activities as contexts of development: Extracurricular activities, after-school and community programs.* Mahwah, NJ: Erlbaum.

Mahoney, J. L., Schweder, A. E., & Stattin, H. (2002). Structured after-school activities as a moderator of depressed mood for adolescents with detached relations to their parents. *Journal of Community Psychology, 30,* 69–86.

Mahoney, J. L., & Stattin, H. (2000). Leisure time activities and adolescent antisocial behavior: The role of structure and social context. *Journal of Adolescence, 23,* 113–127.

Mahoney, J. L., Stattin, H., & Lord, H. (2004). Unstructured youth recreation centre participation and antisocial behaviour development: Selection influences and the moderating role of antisocial peers. *International Journal of Behavioral Development, 28,* 553–560.

Mahoney, J. L., Stattin, H., & Magnusson, D. (2001). Youth recreation centre participation and criminal offending: A 20-year longitudinal study of Swedish boys. *International Journal of Behavioral Development, 25*, 509–520.

Marsh, H. W. (1992). Extracurricular activities: Beneficial extension of the traditional curriculum or subversion of academic goals? *Journal of Educational Psychology, 84*, 553–562.

McCord, J. (1978). A 30-year follow-up of treatment effects. *American Psychologist, 33*, 284–289.

McNeal, R. B. (1995). Extracurricular activities and high school dropouts. *Sociology of Education, 68*, 62–81.

Osgood, D. W., Wilson, J. K., O'Malley, P. M., Bachman, J. G., & Johnston, L. D. (1996). Routine activities and individual deviant behavior. *American Sociological Review, 61*, 635–655.

Persson, A., Kerr, M., & Stattin, H. (2004). Why a leisure context is linked to normbreaking for some girls and not others: Personality characteristics and parent–child relations as explanations. *Journal of Adolescence, 27*, 583–598.

Persson, A., Kerr, M., & Stattin, H. (2007). Staying in or moving away from structured activities: Explanations involving parents and peers. *Developmental Psychology, 43*, 197–207.

Richards, M. H., Larson, R., Miller, B. V., Luo, Z., Sims, B., Parrella, D. P., et al. (2004). Risky and protective contexts and exposure to violence in urban African American young adolescents. *Journal of Clinical Child and Adolescent Psychology, 33*, 138–148.

Roosa, M. W., Deng, S., Ryu, E., Burrell, G. L., Tein, J.-Y., Jones, S., et al. (2005). Family and child characteristics linking neighborhood context and child externalizing behavior. *Journal of Marriage and the Family, 67*, 515–529.

Ross, L., Greene, D., & House, P. (1977). The false consensus effect: An egocentric bias in social perception and attribution processes. *Journal of Experimental Social Psychology, 13*, 279–301.

Sameroff, A. J., Peck, S. C., & Eccles, J. S. (2004). Changing ecological determinants of conduct problems from early adolescence to early adulthood. *Development and Psychopathology, 16*, 873–896.

Sampson, R. J., & Groves, W. B. (1989). Community structure and crime: Testing social disorganization theory. *American Journal of Sociology, 94*, 774–802.

Sampson, R. J., & Laub, J. H. (1993). *Crime in the making: Pathways and turning points through life.* Cambridge, MA: Harvard University Press.

Sampson, R. J., Raudenbush, S. W., & Earls, F. (1997). Neighborhoods and violent crime: A multilevel study of collective efficacy. *Science, 277*, 918–924.

Shannahan, M. J., & Flaherty, B. P. (2001). Dynamic patterns of time use in adolescence. *Child Development, 72*, 385–401.

Silbereisen, R. K., Noack, P., & von Eye, A. (1992). Adolescents' development of romantic friendship and change in favorite leisure contexts. *Journal of Adolescent Research, 7*, 80–93.

Stattin, H., Kerr, M., Mahoney, J., Persson, A., & Magnusson, D. (2005). Explaining why a leisure context is bad for some girls and not for others. In J. L. Mahoney, R. W. Larson, & J. S. Eccles (Eds.), *Organized activities as contexts of development: Extracurricular activities, after-school and community programs* (pp. 211–244). Mahwah, NJ: Erlbaum.

Stoolmiller, M. (2001). Synergistic interaction of child manageability problems and parent-discipline tactics in predicting future growth in externalizing behavior for boys. *Developmental Psychology, 37*, 814–823.

Thornberry, T. P. (1987). Toward and interactional theory of delinquency. *Criminology, 25*, 863–892.

U.S. Department of Education. (1995). *The condition of education.* Washington, DC: U.S. Government Printing Office.

CHAPTER 24

Peer Interactions and Relationships from a Cross-Cultural Perspective

XINYIN CHEN
JANET CHUNG
CELIA HSIAO

Research on children's peer interactions and peer relationships has traditionally been conducted in Western, particularly North American, cultures (e.g., Asher & Coie, 1990). In the past two decades, however, there has been increased interest in peer relationships in different cultures. The findings of various studies have consistently supported the view that children's peer experiences are likely to be affected by cultural norms and values. For example, children's interactions with peers may vary in quality across cultures. Moreover, cultural values may provide guidance for social judgments and interpretations with regard to specific social behaviors, thus imparting "meanings" to the behaviors. Children in different cultures may also develop different types of dyadic and group relationships, and hold different beliefs about the functions and organization of peer relationships. In this chapter, we review and discuss the literature on the role of culture in children's social functioning in peer interactions, relationships, and groups.

The main theme of the chapter is the understanding of peer experiences in cultural context. We first discuss theoretical issues concerning cultural values, children's social functioning, and peer relationships. Then, we review the literature on children's social behaviors in peer interactions in different societies. In the following sections, we review and discuss how cultural factors may be involved in determining the structural features and functional roles of friendships and peer groups. Researchers have recently been interested in the impact of macro-level social, economic, and cultural changes on children's social functioning and relationships. We review the findings in this area in the next section. Our chapter concludes with a discussion of future directions in the study of culture and peer relationships.

Central Issues and Theory

According to Hinde (1987), children's social and psychological functioning may be analyzed at the intrapersonal, interactional, relationship, and group network levels. The different levels of individual and social experiences are embedded within an all-reaching cultural system. Harris (1995) argues that cultural norms, either adopted from existing cultural systems or created by children themselves, serve as a basis for children's peer interactions and mutual socialization. Similarly, sociocultural theory (Cole, 1996; Vygotsky, 1978) emphasizes cultural influence on human activities. According to this theory, children internalize external signs, along with their cultural meanings, during collaborative or guided learning, in which more experienced peers or adults act as both skilled tutors or representatives of the culture and co-constructivists (e.g., Rogoff, 2003) in assisting the child to understand and perform tasks. Participation in cultural practices (e.g., schooling) and interpersonal cooperation play a particularly important role in the development of competence.

Based on these arguments, Chen and his colleagues (e.g., Chen & French, 2008) have recently proposed a contextual–developmental perspective, which is reflected by a conceptual framework concerning cultural context and socioemotional functioning, and a process model focusing on how social evaluations and responses in interactions are guided by cultural beliefs and values and, at the same time, regulate individual behavior and development. According to Chen, Wang, and DeSouza (2006), social initiative and self-control, as manifestations of the fundamental temperamental dimensions of reactivity and regulation (Rothbart & Bates, 2006), are two distinct systems that may account for individual and group differences in social interactional styles. "Social initiative" refers to the tendency to initiate and maintain social interactions. High social initiative is driven by the child's approach motive and is reflected by high interest in social activities. In contrast, internal anxiety, or feelings of insecurity, may impede spontaneous engagement in social participation, leading to a low level of social initiative (Asendorpf, 1990). "Self-control" represents the regulatory ability to modulate behavioral and emotional reactivity, which is closely related to the maintenance of the socially appropriate behaviors during social interactions and is particularly concerned with children's "fitting in with others."

Different societies may place different values on social initiative and norm-based behavioral control in children and adolescents (Chen, Wang, et al., 2006). In Western, self-oriented or individualistic cultures, where acquiring autonomy and assertive skills is an important socialization goal, social initiative is viewed as a major index of social maturity. Although self-regulation and control are encouraged, the cultural emphasis on individual decision making allows individuals to maintain a balance between the needs of the self and those of others. Consequently, behavioral control is often regarded as less important, especially when it is in conflict with the attainment of individual goals (Triandis, 1995). In group-oriented societies, such as many East Asian and Latin American societies, social initiative may not be highly appreciated or valued, because it may not facilitate harmony and cohesiveness in the group. To maintain interpersonal and group harmony, individuals need to restrain personal desires in an effort to address the needs and interests of others. Thus, self-control may be emphasized in a more consistent and absolute manner; the lack of control is often regarded as a serious problem during childhood and adolescence (Triandis, 1995).

Different cultural values pertaining to social initiative and self-control may have a direct impact on the social interpretations and evaluations of specific socioemotional characteristics including aggression–disruption (based on high social initiative and low control), shyness–inhibition (based on low social initiative and adequate control to constrain behavioral and emotional reactivity toward self rather than others), and different aspects of adaptive social functioning, such as sociability and prosocial–cooperative behavior (Chen & French, 2008). The social and developmental processes involving culturally directed social evaluations and responses and the active participation of the child in interactions are illustrated in a model presented in Figure 24.1.

According to the process model, there may exist individual and group biases in early disposition that constitute a major developmental origin of socioemotional functioning. Peers and adults may evaluate socioemotional characteristics in manners that are consistent with cultural belief systems in the society. Moreover, peers and adults in different cultures may respond differently to these socioemotional characteristics and express different attitudes (e.g., acceptance, rejection) toward children who display the characteristics in social interactions. Social evaluations and responses may in turn regulate children's behaviors and, ultimately, the developmental patterns of social functioning. Cultural norms and values, which are changing themselves, provide a basis for the social processes. At the same time, children actively engage in interactions by displaying their reactions to social influence and participating in construction of cultural norms for social

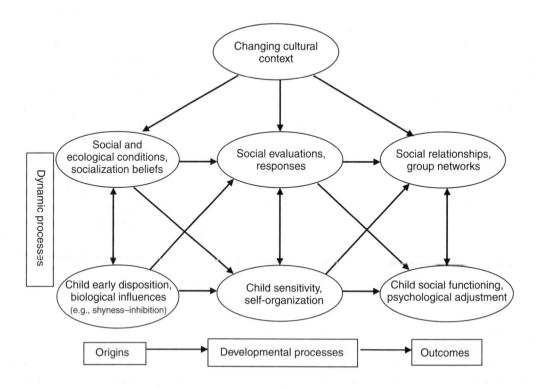

FIGURE 24.1. A process model concerning the mediating role of social interaction in cultural influence on socioemotional development.

evaluations and other peer-group activities. Thus, the social processes are bidirectional and transactional in nature.

In the following sections, we discuss children's social functioning in peer interactions representing social initiative (sociability and shyness–social inhibition) and behavioral control (cooperation and aggression–defiance) in cultural context. We also discuss how cultural values of initiative and control affect the quality and function of peer relationships, such as friendships. Our discussion is guided by the contextual–developmental perspective focusing on cultural context for peer interactions and the role of the social interaction processes in the development of peer relationships, and social and psychological adjustment.

Relevant Research

Social Functioning and Peer Interaction in Cultural Context

Cultural values may affect the exhibition and the meaning of social functioning and peer interaction styles. Social interpretations and evaluations in interactions, which are guided by cultural values, play an important role in shaping the social experiences of children with particular characteristics.

Sociability and Peer Interaction

Peer interaction may be a fundamental part of human development in most societies. Even in cultures where children are required to spend much of their time helping with family duties, such as caring for their younger siblings, children often do this in the company of peers (Tietjen, 2006). However, levels of social participation or sociability seem to be related to cultural and social conditions; cultures that value social initiative tend to facilitate children's social interactions (Parmar, Harkness, & Super, 2004). Edwards (2000), for example, found that children in relatively open communities (e.g., Taira in Okinawa and Orchard Town in the United States), in which peer interactions were encouraged, had significantly higher scores than children in more "close" and agricultural communities (e.g., Nyansongo in Kenya and Khalapur in India) on overall social engagement. Relatively low social interaction has also been found among Chinese and Indonesian children compared with their North American counterparts (Chen, DeSouza, Chen, & Wang, 2006; Farver & Howes, 1988).

Self-Expression in Peer Interaction

Culture may affect not only overall social engagement but also the nature or characteristics of peer interaction. A particular form of peer interaction that varies across cultures is socio-dramatic play. The ability to engage in socio-dramatic behavior and pretense is considered to represent the mastery of skills that promote the coordination of decontextualized and substitutive activities (Rubin, Fein, & Vandenberg, 1983). As indicated by Farver, Kim, and Lee (1995) and Edwards (2000), however, this type of social behavior requires children to control their social-evaluative anxiety, to express their inner interests and personal styles, and to engage in self-explanation and negotiation. Cultural values of assertiveness and self-expression may be related to the display of socio-dramatic behavior in children's social interactions.

In North American societies, children are socialized to behave in a self-directive and assertive manner, and are encouraged to exhibit personal styles (e.g., Triandis, 1995). As a result, North American children tend to engage in more socio-dramatic play behaviors than children in many other, particularly group-oriented cultures. It has been found that children in Maya (Gaskins, 2000), Bedouin Arabia (Ariel & Sever, 1980), Kenya, Mexico, and India (Edwards, 2000) engage in little socio-dramatic activity. Farver et al. (1995) also found that Korean American preschool children display less social and pretend play than Anglo-American children. Moreover, Korean children's pretend play contained more everyday and family role activities and less fantastic themes (i.e., actions performed by fantasy characters; Farver & Shin, 1997). Farver et al. (1995) argued that the cross-cultural differences might be related to the cultural beliefs about social competence that guided the structuring of the environment for children's social interactions.

Sociability and Social and Psychological Adjustment

Children who are active and assertive in their peer interactions are regarded as socially competent by peers and adults in North America (e.g., Rubin, Burgess, & Coplan, 2002). Due to the cultural endorsement, North American sociable children are likely to be accepted by peers and to achieve success in social and emotional areas (Rubin, Bukowski, & Parker, 2006). Sociability appears to be less valued and associated with less positive outcomes in group-oriented cultures. In a longitudinal study, Chen, Li, Li, Li, and Liu (2000) found that sociability in Chinese children positively predicted social impact or salience in the peer group, but not social acceptance or preference. Moreover, after its overlap with prosocial behavior was controlled, sociability did not predict social or academic outcomes, and it *positively* predicted later externalizing problems. Nevertheless, sociability was found to be associated positively with self-regard and negatively with internalizing symptoms, such as loneliness. Active social participation of sociable children may facilitate the formation of interpersonal support systems that help these children cope with psychological difficulties under adverse circumstances.

Shyness–Inhibition

Shyness–inhibition, derived from internal anxiety and lack of self-confidence, is manifested in wary, vigilant, and sensitive behavior in challenging social situations. Children who display shy and wary behaviors are often viewed as socially incompetent and immature in Western cultures (e.g., Rubin et al., 2002). Empirical findings indicate that shy–inhibited children, especially during the school years, are likely to experience low peer acceptance and poor social adjustment in the West (e.g., Coplan, Prakash, O'Neil, & Armer, 2004). When they become aware of their social difficulties through negative social feedback, shy–inhibited children tend to develop negative self-perceptions and emotions, such as depression (e.g., Rubin et al., 2002).

Shyness–inhibition is not necessarily perceived as incompetent or associated with adjustment problems in societies where social initiative and assertiveness are not valued. Cultural values may influence the prevalence and functional significance of shy–inhibited behavior. Indeed, cross-cultural differences in the display of shyness–inhibition have been reported in childhood and adolescence (e.g., Farver & Howes, 1988; Kagan, Kearsley, & Zelazo, 1978; Lee, Okazaki, & Yoo, 2006). Farver et al. (1995), for example, found that Korean American children displayed more shy and reticent behaviors than European American children in a naturalistic peer interaction setting. Rubin, Hemphill, et al. (2006) also reported that Korean and Chinese toddlers exhibited higher inhibition than Italian and Australian toddlers in laboratory free-play sessions. Chen et al. (1998) found that, relative to Canadian toddlers, Chinese toddlers stayed closer to their mothers and were less likely to explore in free-play sessions. Moreover, Chinese toddlers displayed more anxious and vigilant behaviors when interacting with a stranger, as indicated by their higher scores on the latency to approach the stranger and to touch the toys when they were invited to do so.

Peer Attitudes and Responses toward Shyness–Inhibition

Shy–inhibited behavior may be evaluated and responded to differently by peers in different cultures. Chen, DeSouza, et al. (2006) found that when shy–inhibited Canadian children made passive and low-power social initiations, they were more likely than others to receive fewer positive responses and more rejection from peers. However, shy–inhibited Chinese children who displayed the same behavior were more likely than others to receive positive responses. These peer responses to shy–inhibited children's social bids may reflect varying cultural values and socialization goals. In traditional Chinese culture, shy and wary behavior is thought to be associated with virtuous qualities, such as modesty, cautiousness, and self-control. Socially sensitive and restrained behavior is often regarded as indicating accomplishment, and shy–sensitive children are perceived to be well-behaved and understanding.

Shyness, Peer Relationships, and Adjustment

In North America, shy children, particularly boys, are likely to experience difficulties in peer relationships and life adjustment (e.g., Caspi, Elder, & Bem, 1988). Shy children in China, however, are accepted by peers and perform well socially and academically in childhood and adolescence (e.g., Chen, Rubin, & Li, 1995). Moreover, shy Chinese children perceive themselves positively and do not feel lonely or depressed (e.g., Chen, He, et al., 2004).

It should be noted that the construct of shyness–inhibition is different from those representing various types of social withdrawal, such as social solitude, social disinterest, and unsociability (e.g., kids who are often alone or who would rather be alone). Social disinterest and preference for solitude or aloneness are inconsistent with the collectivistic orientation. Children who prefer solitude and intentionally stay away from the group may be regarded as anticollective and selfish, which likely leads to negative reactions from others in group-oriented cultures. Thus, whereas shy, sensitive, and inhibited children may adjust well, socially solitary or withdrawn children are clearly rejected by peers and experience extensive socioemotional problems in China (Chang et al., 2005; Chen, 2008). It should also be noted that as China is undergoing dramatic reforms toward a market economy, the adaptive value of shyness–inhibition has been declining in urban children (Chen, Cen, Li, & He, 2005). Recent findings indicate that shyness is still associated with social and psychological adjustment among children in rural areas of China (Chen & Wang, 2006), but the association will likely change rapidly as the massive transformation expands to these areas.

There is evidence that shyness is viewed as less deviant and problematic in some other Asian cultures as well (e.g., Indonesia: Eisenberg, Pidada, & Liew, 2001; Korea: Farver et al., 1995). Shyness has also been linked with fewer negative outcomes in Swedish than in American youth. In a study of children born in Sweden in the mid-1950s, Kerr, Lambert, and Bem (1996) found that although shyness predicted later marriage and parenthood, it did not affect adulthood education and careers, which differed from Caspi et al.'s findings (1988) for U.S. youth. According to Kerr et al. (1996), the social welfare and support systems that evolved from the egalitarian values in Sweden ensured that people did not need to be assertive or competitive to achieve career success. Interestingly, because similar social support systems were not available for girls during the period in which the study was conducted, shy Swedish girls appeared to attain lower levels of education than nonshy girls. Kerr et al. expected that shy and nonshy girls would not differ in Sweden today.

Cooperation–Compliance

The cross-cultural differences in children's cooperative–compliant behavior have been observed in many studies (e.g., Whiting & Edwards, 1988). The differences are believed to be associated with the extent to which the culture emphasizes social obligation, group harmony, and family interdependence. Children in societies where extended families live together in traditional styles, and where children are required to assume family responsibilities, tend to display more prosocial–cooperative and compliant behaviors than children in economically complex societies with class structures and occupational division of labor (Edwards, 2000). Graves and Graves (1983), for example, found that Aituaki (Cook Islands) children from rural and extended families displayed more cooperative and compliant behavior than their urban counterparts in both family and peer interactions. Kagan and Knight (1981) found that Mexican American children were more cooperative than children from urban and Westernized cultures. Finally, children in China, India, and Korea tend to display more cooperative and compliant behaviors than children in the West (e.g., Farver et al., 1995; Orlick, Zhou, & Partington, 1990). Orlick et al., for example, found remarkable differences in cooperation between Chinese and Canadian children; 85 and 22% of the social behaviors displayed by kindergarten children were cooperative in China and Canada, respectively.

Cultural Values of Responsibility, Socialization, and Prosocial-Cooperative Behavior

The cooperative tendency of children toward others in some Asian countries may be due to the great emphasis that the society puts on socializing children to strive for group, rather than individual, accomplishment. Miller (1994) argues that individuals in sociocentric societies view responsiveness to the needs of others to be a fundamental commitment, whereas individuals in Western societies attempt to maintain a balance between prosocial concerns and individual freedom of choice. Thus, interpersonal cooperation and prosocial behavior are seen in Western cultures as a personal decision based on factors such as how much one likes the target person (s) (Greenfield, Suzuki, & Rothstein-Fisch, 2006). In societies that value group harmony, however, there is considerable pressure on children to view prosocial–cooperative behavior as obligatory (e.g., Miller, 1994). In these societies, socialization of responsibility and cooperation often emerges in the early years, with an emphasis on children's self-control and regulation.

Cross-cultural differences in the socialization of regulation and responsibility have been found in early childhood. Keller et al. (2004), for example, found that rural Cameroonian Nso mothers were higher than Costa Rican mothers, who in turn were higher than middle-class Greek mothers, on a proximal parenting style (body contact, body stimulation), which was believed to facilitate child obedience and regulation. Accordingly, Cameroonian Nso toddlers displayed more regulated behaviors, as indicated by their compliance with maternal requests and prohibitions, than their counterparts in the other two groups. Costa Rican toddlers also had higher regulation scores than Greek toddlers. Chen, Rubin, et al. (2003) found that Chinese mothers attempted to help their toddlers to exert a higher level of behavioral regulation than did Canadian mothers. Moreover, children in China displayed more mature forms of self-control than did children in Canada in the early years. It has been argued that early self-regulatory ability may be a basis for the internalization of social norms and rules (Eisenberg, Zhou, Liew, Champion, & Pidada, 2006). Indeed, researchers have found that children's self-regulation in many cultures, such as China, Indonesia, and France, is predictive of adaptive social functioning, particularly prosocial–cooperative behavior in peer interactions (Eisenberg et al., 2006).

Prosocial–Cooperative Behavior, Peer Relationships, and Adjustment

Prosocial–cooperative behavior is associated robustly with peer acceptance in a variety of cultures (e.g., Casiglia, Lo Coco, & Zappulla, 1998; Chen et al., 2000; Eisenberg et al., 2001). Children who display prosocial–cooperative behaviors are generally liked by peers and obtain a high status in the peer group. Researchers have found little cultural variation in the linkage between prosocial–cooperative behavior and the quality of peer relationships, suggesting that social behavior based on the consideration of the interests of others or the group may be a universal antecedent of peer acceptance.

Nevertheless, prosocial–cooperative behavior may have a more extensive impact on children's adjustment, including psychological well-being, in group- than in self-oriented cultures. It was found, for example, that prosocial behavior served as a protective factor for children who experienced difficulties in emotional adjustment in China (Chen et al., 2000). Prosocial behavior was positively associated with later perceived self-worth and negatively associated with later loneliness and depression, particularly for children who experienced heightened psychological and emotional distress. It is possible that given its particular importance for group functioning, prosocial–cooperative behavior helps children improve their overall social conditions, which, in turn, changes their negative attitudes and feelings about self and the world.

Aggression and Defiance

Cultural context may facilitate or inhibit the expression of aggressive and defiant behaviors (Whiting & Edwards, 1988). In general, cultures that value competitiveness and the pursuit of personal goals seem to allow for more coercive and aggressive behavior, whereas cultures that emphasize group harmony and personal control tend to inhibit aggressive behavior (Bergeron & Schneider, 2005; Weisz et al., 1988). Consistent with this argument, it has been found that children in Asian countries, such as China, Korea, Thailand, in Australia, and in some European nations, such as Sweden and the Netherlands, tend to display relatively fewer aggressive and externalizing behaviors compared with their North American counterparts (e.g., Bergeron & Schneider, 2005; Farver et al., 1995; Russell, Hart, Robinson, & Olsen, 2003; Weisz et al., 1988).

Cultural Norms, Individual Attitudes, and Aggressive Behaviors

Cultural influences may occur during the socialization process through the shaping of individual beliefs and attitudes about aggressive behaviors, because these beliefs and attitudes constitute a basis for attributions and the activation of scripts about aggressive acts. This is illustrated by Cole and associates' studies on anger and aggression of Brahman and Tamang children in rural Nepal (Cole, Bruschi, & Tamang, 2002; Cole, Tamang, & Shrestha, 2006). Brahmans are high-caste Hindus who value hierarchy and dominance in the caste. In contrast, Tamangs, with a background of Tibetan Buddhism, value social equality, compassion, modesty, and nonviolence. Accordingly, Brahman children are more likely than Tamang children to endorse anger and aggressive behaviors. Moreover, Brahman children react to difficult social situations, such as peer conflict, with anger and other negative emotions more often than do Tamang children (Cole et al., 2002). In addition, Zahn-Waxler, Friedman, Cole, Mizuta, and Hiruma (1996) found that Japanese children showed less anger and less aggressive behavior than U.S. children in their responses to conflict and distress in hypothetical situations.

Aggressive Behavior, Peer Status, and Psychological Adjustment

In Western individualistic cultures, despite the general discouragement of aggression, aggressive children and adolescents may receive social support from peers and are sometimes even perceived as "stars" in their groups (e.g., Cairns & Cairns, 1994). As a result, aggressive children often have biased self-perceptions, overestimate their social competence, and do not report internalizing psychological problems (e.g., Hoza, Molina, Bukowski, & Sippola, 1995). Unlike their Western counterparts, aggressive children in China experience pervasive social and psychological difficulties, including low social status, poor quality of peer relationships, negative self-perceptions, and feelings of loneliness and depression (e.g., Chen, He, et al., 2004). The psychological problems of aggressive children in China may be related to the regular collective and public evaluations in schools. During these activities, children are required to evaluate themselves in the group in terms of whether their behaviors reach the school standards, and whether they have made improvement over time. Peers and teachers provide feedback on the child's self-evaluations. This social-interactive process makes it difficult for aggressive children to develop inflated or "biased" self-perceptions of their competence and social status. Therefore, culturally directed peer-group attitudes and social-evaluative processes may to a large extent determine the developmental patterns of aggressive behavior.

Friendship and the Peer Group in Cultural Context

A major developmental outcome of social behaviors in peer interactions is children's success in developing and maintaining relationships with peers (Rubin, Bukowski, et al., 2006). The indices of success with peer relationships include becoming integrated into social networks and establishing friendships with others. There appear to be cultural differences in the extent to which group integration or development of friendships is encouraged (e.g., Sharabany & Wiseman, 1993). Moreover, cultural beliefs and expectations about socialization may affect the structural and organizational aspects of peer relationships.

Involvement in peer relationships increases in North American children from childhood to early adolescence, which may derive from the desire of youth to become autonomous from the family (Rothbaum, Pott, Azuma, Miyake, & Weisz, 2000). Once they enter the peer world, children are encouraged to learn to be independent and self-directed, while maintaining positive relationships with others, and are expected eventually to acquire a sense of self-identity (Brown, 1990). Thus, peer relationships provide a social context for children to understand themselves in relation to others and to experience self-validation (Sullivan, 1953). Group-oriented cultures emphasize conformity to others and commitment to social relationships. In these cultures, children are expected and encouraged to maintain strong social affiliations and to identify with the group (Sharabany, 2006). Different cultural expectations regarding individual independence and group commitment may exert a significant impact on children's and adolescents' peer experiences, which may be reflected in the qualities of peer relationships and the functions that they serve in daily activities (Chen & French, 2008; Tietjen, 1989).

Friendship in Cultural Context

In some societies, involvement with agemates typically occurs within extended family networks of siblings and cousins, leaving little opportunity for relationships with nonkin (e.g., the Yucatan Mayan; Gaskins, 2006). Sharabany and Wiseman (1993) also reported that children in Israeli kibbutz communities focus on group involvement and have few dyadic friendships. In many contemporary societies, however, schools bring together large numbers of nonkin, same-age children, thus providing opportunities to form close friendships.

In general, most children and adolescents in most societies have reciprocal friends (e.g., French, Jansen, Riansari, & Setiono, 2003; Schneider, Fonzi, & Tani, 1997). Across cultures, more girls than boys form mutual friendships, and girls' friendships tend to be more stable over time (e.g., Benenson, Apostoleris, & Parnass, 1997; Schneider et al., 1997). Children who have mutual friendships are more competent in social, school, and emotional areas than are children without mutual friendships (see Berndt & McCandless, Chapter 4, this volume).

Functions of Friendship: Enhancement of Self-Worth and Instrumental Assistance

The support of friends may be an important mechanism for children in Western cultures to accomplish the socialization goal of developing confidence and positive views about the self (Sullivan, 1953). Chen and French (2008) argue, however, that the role of friendship in promoting self-worth may be less salient in many non-Western cultures, where the development of the self is not considered a major developmental task. For example, Chinese (e.g., Chen, Kaspar, Zhang, Wang, & Zheng, 2004; Cho, Sandel, Miller, & Wang, 2005) and Indonesian (French, Pidada, & Victor, 2005) children, and children with Arab and Caribbean background (Dayan, Doyle, & Markiewicz, 2001), often do not report the enhancement of self-worth as an important function of friendship.

In contrast to self-validation, instrumental aid appears to be particularly important for friendships of children in many group-oriented cultures (Tietjen, 1989). Way (2006) found that sharing money and protecting friends from harm were salient aspects of the friendships of low-income black and Hispanic adolescents in the United States. Instrumental assistance has also been documented to be a highly salient feature of friendships in Asian nations, such as China (Chen, Kaspar, et al., 2004), Indonesia (French et al., 2005), South Korea (French, Lee, & Pidada, 2006), the Philippines (Hollnsteiner, 1979), and in Latino societies, such as Cuba (Gonzalez, Moreno, & Schneider, 2004) and Costa Rica (DeRosier & Kupersmidt, 1991). In these societies, instrumental assistance may be reflected in broad areas, such as helping others solve problems and learn social skills. For example, a theme that has emerged from interviews with Chinese adolescents in China, Taiwan, and the United States is the high appreciation of mutual assistance of friends in learning and school achievement (Chen, Kaspar, et al., 2004; Way, 2006).

Intimacy in Friendship

Understanding friendship intimacy across cultures is a challenging task, because intimacy is closely associated with constructs such as sensitivity, mutual understanding, exclusivity, attachment, emotional closeness, and trust. Moreover, the extent to which these different aspects of intimacy are emphasized may differ across cultures (Chen & French, 2008). Triandis, Bontempo, Villareal, Asai, and Lucca (1988) have argued that friendships in collectivistic cultures tend to be more intimate than those in individualistic cultures. Sharabany (2006), however, has suggested that in some collectivistic societies, friendships are characterized as low in intimacy because of the availability of other sources of emotional support, reduced privacy inherent in collectivistic lifestyles, and the potential threat of exclusive dyadic friendships to the cohesiveness of the larger group.

Empirically, researchers have found that friendships of South Korean children and adolescents are highly intimate (French, Lee, et al., 2006; French, Bae, Pidada, & Lee, 2006). Intimate friendships in Korean children and adolescents are often represented by high exclusivity and strong boundaries between close friends and nonfriends. In addition, children in Central and Southern Italy report more close and harmonious friendships than do Canadian children (Schneider et al., 1997; Schneider, Fonzi, Tomada, & Tani, 2000). Within the United States, it has been found that Latino and black adolescents perceive their friendships as more intimate and closer than do adolescents in European American and other cultural groups (Gonzalez et al., 2004; Way, 2006). These results appear to be consistent with the Triandis et al. (1988) argument.

Relatively low intimacy has been found in children's friendships in some other group-oriented societies, which is consistent with the Sharabany (2006) argument. For example, youth in Indonesian, rural Arab, and Israeli kibbutz cultures report lower intimacy than their North American counterparts (e.g., French et al., 2005; French, Lee, et al., 2006; Sharabany, 2006). Anthropological findings suggest that compared with U.S. students, Indonesian students are less likely to develop close friendships, because they are encouraged to focus on integration into general peer networks and the larger community (Jay, 1969). Similarly, in a study concerning parental values of friendship, Beit-Hallahmi, Sharabany, Dana-Engelstein, Rabin, and Regev (1982) found that kibbutz adults preferred a large number of superficial or "shallow" friends to a few close, in-depth friends.

The nature and quality of children's friendships may depend on complex social, historical, and ecological factors. For example, emotional expressivity, especially in conveying warmth and affection in social interactions, is typically encouraged in Latino cultures. It is possible that relatively intimate social relationships in Latino youth are related to the cultural values of emotional expressivity. In addition, French and his colleagues (2005) argue that the salience of loyalty and exclusivity in friendships in Korea and other Asian countries may largely be due to the Confucian values of trust and obligation between friends. Thus, future research on friendship should take into account specific social circumstances, and broad cultural and historical factors.

The Peer Group across Cultures

Like North American children (e.g., Cairns & Cairns, 1994; Kindermann, 1993), most school-age children in non-Western societies are affiliated with a peer group (e.g., D'Hondt & Vandewiele, 1980; Kiesner, Poulin, & Nicotra, 2003; Leung, 1996; Salmivalli, Huttunen, & Lagerspetz, 1997). Peer groups often comprise same-sex members, with more mixed-sex groups appearing in late adolescence. The size of groups tends to increase with age. Studies of youth in many countries, including China, Japan, Singapore, Senegal, and the United States, indicate that boys are more likely to belong to groups and are more susceptible to peer pressure than girls and that boys' groups tend to be larger than girls' groups (e.g., Benenson et al., 1997; Dekovic, Engels, Shirai, De Kort, & Anker, 2002; D'Hondt & Vandewiele, 1980; Salmivalli et al., 1997; Sim & Koh, 2003). Gender differences have not been reported in several studies in China and the United States (e.g., Cairns, Leung, Buchanan, & Cairns, 1995; Chen, Chang, & He, 2003).

Specific social–ecological circumstances may be related to the formation and maintenance of peer groups. Corsaro and Molinari (2005), for example, have noticed that Italian elementary schools are structured to allow children to stay together with the same teachers for multiple years, and to encourage extensive peer discussion and interaction in the classroom. The educational policy and school settings may lead to relatively weak differentiations and boundaries among peer groups in Italian schools.

Group Homogeneity

Peer groups are likely to be homogenous on social and behavioral attributes. In North America, groups are homogeneous on such deviant behaviors as aggression, smoking, drinking, and drug use (e.g., Cairns & Cairns, 1994). Group members are also similar in joining clubs, dating frequency, academic motivation, and self-perceptions (e.g., Kindermann, 1993). In a study of peer networks in Finland, Salmivalli et al. (1997) found that children who behaved in similar or complementary roles in bullying situations (bullies, assistants/reinforcers, victims, defenders, and outsiders) formed networks with each other. Chen, Chang, et al. (2003) found that peer groups among Chinese children were most homogeneous on leadership status, aggression, and learning problems. In Chinese schools, leadership status represents an important aspect of social competence, whereas aggression and learning problems are major indices of maladaptation. Taken together, it appears that children form groups on the basis of similar social and behavioral attributes that are significant in the culture.

Culture and Peer-Group Functioning

In North American youth, intensive interaction within the small clique appears to be the major form of peer activity in childhood; this tends to decline from middle childhood to adolescence, when affiliation with multiple groups and larger crowds becomes more salient (e.g., Brown, 1990). During adolescence, a variety of peer groups can be identified, including those labeled as "jocks," "brains," "populars," "greasers," "partyers," "druggies," "nerds," "loners," and "burnouts" (Brown, 1990). The diversity of peer groups is interesting and reflects the individualistic values in American societies: Children and adolescents form groups based mainly on their particular individual interests. As adolescents increasingly seek independence and attempt to avoid group restrictions, there is a general loosening of group ties, and children's sense of belongingness declines steadily with age (see Rubin, Bukowski, et al., 2006). Researchers have found that peer groups, particularly deviant groups, may contribute to individual social and psychological adjustment, such as school dropout, academic motivation, early pregnancy, substance use, and antisocial behavior, in Western cultures (e.g., Espelage, Holt, & Henkel, 2003; Kiesner et al., 2003; Kindermann, 2007). In general, however, the role of peer groups is often highlighted as a major social resource for fulfilling individual psychological needs, such as the formation of self-identity and the development of positive self-perceptions and self-feelings.

In collectivistic societies, the tension between the pursuit of independence and personal identity, and the commitment to group undertaking may be less evident than in Western cultures. Thus, children may maintain strong group affiliations across different developmental periods in collectivistic cultures. In these cultures, there is often great pressure on group members to conform to group norms (Sharabany, 2006). Moreover, peer groups may be valued mainly according to their socialization functions in helping children learn social standards and develop socially acceptable behaviors. Children and adolescents in China, for example, tend to describe group activities in terms of how they are in accord with adults' social requirements and standards, such as maintaining interpersonal cooperation and collective well-being (Chen, Kaspar, et al., 2004). The culture pays particular attention to the *nature* of peer groups, in terms of whether group activities are guided by the "right" social goals, and whether these activities are beneficial to children's social and school achievement.

The Contextual Effects of the Peer Group

Developmental theorists have long been interested in the peer group as a social context for children's social and cognitive functioning. The contextual nature of the group has not been adequately examined, largely due to methodological difficulties in assessing the different levels of social complexity (group vs. individual levels). In several recent studies with North American children using statistical analyses such as hierarchical linear modeling (HLM); researchers found significant group main effects on individual social behaviors such as aggression, but failed to find moderating effects of group context on developmental patterns (e.g., Espelage et al., 2003).

Chen, Chang, et al. (2003) found that group academic context in Chinese children not only made direct contributions to individual social functioning but also affected the significance of individual academic achievement for social development. In groups that function on the basis of academic achievement as a major standard, children evaluate each other according to their attitudes and achievement in academic areas. At the same time, group members are sensitive to the feedback from group peers on their academic performance. Within the group, children who perform better on academic subjects are more likely to receive social and emotional support from others and to have more opportunities to learn from others. In low-achieving groups, however, the common negative attitudes toward academic achievement lead to group approval and support for deviant behaviors, such as violation of school rules. This group context exacerbates the social and behavioral problems of academically poor children, thus placing them at particular risk for maladaptive social development. It has also been found that the social norms of the peer group may moderate the effects of parental socialization efforts; whereas prosocial–cooperative groups serve to facilitate parental socialization efforts to help children develop social and school competencies, antisocial–destructive groups tend to undermine the contributions of supportive parenting to child development (Chen, Chang, He, & Liu, 2005).

The comprehensive effects of the peer group on social and academic development in Chinese children may be related to the cultural values in the society. Collectivistic values of individual conformity and commitment to the group may reinforce the regulatory effect of group norms on children's behaviors. In a study with Senegalese youth, D'Hondt and Vandewiele (1980) noticed that peer groups were organized on social and moral principles, such as solidarity, unity, and struggle against social injustices. It will be interesting to investigate how these group values affect individual attitudes and behaviors. It will also be interesting to examine the significance of peer groups in other cultures that may highly endorse peer-group affiliation (Azmitia & Cooper, 2004).

The Impact of Social and Cultural Changes on Peer Interactions and Relationships

Major changes in political and economic conditions and cultural values may affect the development of various aspects of social functioning, including self-control and social initiative. The urbanization of traditional rural societies (Graves & Graves, 1983), for example, has resulted in children having fewer interactions with their extended kin group and a decrease in cooperative and obedient behaviors. Reduced opportunities to learn and practice nurturance and responsibility by performing family labor and household work, such as caring for younger siblings, may be a main contributing factor to children's behavioral changes (e.g., Graves & Graves, 1983).

Modernization may not necessarily weaken interpersonal support and interdependence in group-oriented societies (Kagitcibasi, 2005). Due to the enduring influence of the culture of relatedness, social relationships may continue to play a significant role in social and psychological adjustment. Nevertheless, urban lifestyles, increased affluence, and new cultural values, such as individual autonomy, that are promoted by modernization may affect social relationships. Social relationships seem to serve a more utilitarian function in societies where relying on others for basic needs is essential (Guthrie, 2006). Increased value of personal independence and social initiative during modernization may undermine the utilitarian function of relationships and enhance their role in providing emotional support. Consistently, Tamis-LeMonda et al. (2008) have noticed that the traditional utilitarian and instrumental type of relationship, *Guan Xi*, is losing significance in China as the society moves toward a market economy and stronger legal infrastructure. Adults and children increasingly appreciate the function of peer relationships in fulfilling individual psychological needs.

Little, Brendgen, Wanner, and Krappmann (1999) found that, compared to children in West Berlin, children in the former East Berlin reported less fun and enjoyment within their friendships, largely due to the adult control of children's interactions with friends. With the changes in the education system after German unification, peer interactions and group activities among children in East Berlin are based more on personal choices and are less controlled by adults. As a result, children may be more likely to engage in playful and intimate interactions with friends, and to experience greater enjoyment in their friendships.

Since the 1980s, there has been a dramatic change from a command economy to a market economy in China. This has had a considerable impact on children's peer relationships and social behaviors, particularly those (e.g., shyness–inhibition) that are incompatible with the requirement of assertiveness in the challenging market-oriented society. The transformations in social structure and organization, and the introduction of individualistic values such as liberty and individual freedom may have led to the decline in the adaptive value of shy–inhibited behavior. In the new competitive environment, shy–inhibited behavior that may impede self-expression and active exploration is no longer regarded as adaptive and competent (Chang et al., 2005; Hart et al., 2000).

Chen, Cen, et al. (2005) examined relations between shyness–inhibition and adjustment in Chinese children in three urban cohorts (1990, 1998, and 2002), which represented different phases of the social and economic reform in China. Shyness was perceived positively by peers and adults and was associated with peer acceptance, leadership, and school adjustment in the 1990 cohort. In contrast, shyness was associated with peer rejection, school problems, and depression in the 2002 cohort. The relations between shyness, and peer relationships and adjustment variables were either nonsignificant or mixed in the 1998 cohort. Interestingly, Chen, Cen, et al. found that shyness was positively associated with both peer acceptance and peer rejection in the 1998 cohort, indicating mixed attitudes of peers toward shy–inhibited children, which may reflect the cultural conflict between imported Western values of social initiative and autonomy and traditional Chinese values on self-control.

Conclusions and Future Directions

Cross-cultural research has indicated the involvement of cultural factors in virtually all aspects of children's peer interactions and relationships. Cultural norms and values may affect the display and significance of children's social behaviors in peer interactions, the structural and functional features of friendships, and the organization of peer groups. In addition, macro-level social, economic, and cultural changes may have pervasive implications for children's social behaviors and relationships.

In this chapter, we focused on different values that self- and group-oriented cultures place on two main dimensions of social functioning in peer relationships—social initiative and behavioral control. It is important to note that cultural exchanges and interactions may lead to the merging and coexistence of diverse value systems (Kagitcibasi, 2005). Moreover, within-culture variability is likely to be increased during this process. There is substantial evidence that subcultures related to social class, religion, and ethnicity within a society may influence peer relationships (e.g., Graves & Graves, 1983). These within-culture factors should receive greater attention in the future.

According to the contextual–developmental perspective (Chen & French, 2008), cultural influence on individual functioning is a dynamic social process. From middle childhood, peer relationships provide a milieu in which children negotiate with each other to adopt existing cultural standards and values, and to create their own peer cultures. How peer interaction processes, particularly mutual evaluations and responses in group activities, serve to transmit and construct cultures and to regulate children's social behaviors needs to be examined thoroughly in the future.

Finally, cross-cultural issues in peer relationships need to be examined from a developmental perspective. A comprehensive and in-depth understanding of the cultural meanings of individual behaviors and social relationships requires systematic investigations of developmental antecedents, concomitants, and outcomes, as well as developmental patterns. Developmental research can also offer important information about the transactional processes between culture and development, and the active role of the child in the processes.

Acknowledgment

During the preparation of this chapter, Xinyin Chen was partially supported by grants from the Social Sciences and Humanities Research Council of Canada.

References

Ariel, S., & Sever, I. (1980). Play in the desert and play in the town: On play activities of Bedouin Arab children. In H. B. Schwartzman (Ed.), *Play and culture* (pp. 164–175). West Point, NY: Leisure Press.

Asendorpf, J. (1990). Beyond social withdrawal: Shyness, unsociability, and peer avoidance. *Human Development, 33,* 250–259.

Asher, S. R., & Coie, J. D. (1990). *Peer rejection in childhood.* New York: Cambridge University Press.

Azmitia, M., & Cooper, C. R. (2004). Good or bad?: Peer influences on Latino and European American adolescents' pathways through school. *Journal of Education for Students Placed at Risk, 6,* 45–71.

Beit-Hallahmi, B., Sharabany, R., Dana-Engelstein, H., Rabin, A. I., & Regev, E. (1982). Patterns of interpersonal attachment: Sociability, friendship and marriage. In A. I. Rabin & B. Beit-Hallahmi (Eds.), *Twenty years later: Kibbutz children grow up* (pp. 119–144). New York: Springer.

Benenson, J. F., Apostoleris, N. H., & Parnass, J. (1997). Age and sex differences in dyadic and group interaction. *Developmental Psychology, 33,* 538–543.

Bergeron, N., & Schneider, B. H. (2005). Explaining cross-national differences in peer-directed aggression: A quantitative synthesis. *Aggressive Behavior, 31,* 116–137.

Brown, B. B. (1990). Peer groups and peer cultures. In S. S. Feldman & G. R. Elliott (Eds.), *At the threshold: The developing adolescent* (pp. 171–196). Cambridge, MA: Harvard University Press.

Cairns, R. B., & Cairns, B. D. (1994). *Lifelines and risks: Pathways of youth in our time.* New York: Cambridge University Press.

Cairns, R. B., Leung, M. C., Buchanan, L., & Cairns, B. D. (1995). Friendships and social networks in childhood and adolescence: Fluidity, reliability, and interrelations. *Child Development, 66,* 1330–1345.

Casiglia, A. C., Lo Coco, A., & Zappulla, C. (1998). Aspects of social reputation and peer relationships in Italian children: A cross-cultural perspective. *Developmental Psychology, 34,* 723–730.

Caspi, A., Elder, G. H., Jr., & Bem, D. J. (1988). Moving away from the world: Life-course patterns of shy children. *Developmental Psychology, 24,* 824–831.

Chang, L., Lei, L., Li, K. K., Liu, H., Guo, B., Wang, Y., et al. (2005). Peer acceptance and self-perceptions of verbal and behavioural aggression and withdrawal. *International Journal of Behavioral Development, 29,* 49–57.

Chen, X. (2008). Shyness and unsociability in cultural context. In A. S. LoCoco, K. H. Rubin, & C. Zappulla (Eds.), *L'isolamento sociale durante l'infanzia* [Social withdrawal in childhood] (pp. 143–160). Milan, Italy: Unicopli.

Chen, X., Cen, G., Li, D., & He, Y. (2005). Social functioning and adjustment in Chinese children: The imprint of historical time. *Child Development, 76,* 182–195.

Chen, X., Chang, L., & He, Y. (2003). The peer group as a context: Mediating and moderating effects on the relations between academic achievement and social functioning in Chinese children. *Child Development, 74,* 710–727.

Chen, X., Chang, L., He, Y., & Liu, H. (2005). The peer group as a context: Moderating effects on relations between maternal parenting and social and school adjustment in Chinese children. *Child Development, 76*, 417–434.

Chen, X., DeSouza, A., Chen, H., & Wang, L. (2006). Reticent behavior and experiences in peer interactions in Canadian and Chinese children. *Developmental Psychology, 42*, 656–665.

Chen, X., & French, D. (2008). Children's social competence in cultural context. *Annual Review of Psychology, 59*, 591–616.

Chen, X., Hastings, P., Rubin, K. H., Chen, H., Cen, G., & Stewart, S. L. (1998). Childrearing attitudes and behavioral inhibition in Chinese and Canadian toddlers: A cross-cultural study. *Developmental Psychology, 34*, 677–686.

Chen, X., He, Y., De Oliveira, A. M., Lo Coco, A., Zappulla, C., Kaspar, V., et al. (2004). Loneliness and social adaptation in Brazilian, Canadian, Chinese and Italian children. *Journal of Child Psychology and Psychiatry, 45*, 1373–1384.

Chen, X., Kaspar, V., Zhang, Y., Wang, L., & Zheng, S. (2004). Peer relationships among Chinese and North American boys: A cross-cultural perspective. In N. Way & J. Chu (Eds.), *Adolescent boys in context* (pp. 197–218). New York: New York University Press.

Chen, X., Li, D., Li, Z., Li, B., & Liu, M. (2000). Sociable and prosocial dimensions of social competence in Chinese children: Common and unique contributions to social, academic and psychological adjustment. *Developmental Psychology, 36*, 302–314.

Chen, X., Rubin, K. H., & Li, Z. (1995). Social functioning and adjustment in Chinese children: A longitudinal study. *Developmental Psychology, 31*, 531–539.

Chen, X., Rubin, K. H., Liu, M., Chen, H., Wang, L., Li, D., et al. (2003). Compliance in Chinese and Canadian toddlers. *International Journal of Behavioral Development, 27*, 428–436.

Chen, X., & Wang, Z. (2006, July). *Social and cultural changes and the development of social functioning.* Presented at the 19th Biennial Meeting of the International Society for the Study of Behavioral Development, Melbourne, Australia.

Chen, X., Wang, L., & DeSouza, A. (2006). Temperament and socio-emotional functioning in Chinese and North American children. In X. Chen, D. French, & B. Schneider (Eds.), *Peer relationships in cultural context* (pp. 123–147). New York: Cambridge University Press.

Cho, G. E., Sandel, T. L., Miller, P. J., & Wang, S. (2005). What do grandmothers think about self-esteem? American and Taiwanese folk theories revisited. *Social Development, 14*, 701–721.

Cole, M. (1996). *Cultural psychology.* Cambridge, MA: Harvard University Press.

Cole, P. M., Bruschi, C., & Tamang, B. L. (2002). Cultural differences in children's emotional reactions to difficult situations. *Child Development, 73*, 983–996.

Cole, P. M., Tamang, B. L., & Shrestha, S. (2006). Cultural variations in the socialization of young children's anger and shame. *Child Development, 77*, 1237–1251.

Coplan, R. J., Prakash, K., O'Neil, K., & Armer, M. (2004). Do you "want" to play? Distinguishing between conflicted-shyness and social disinterest in early childhood. *Developmental Psychology, 40*, 244–258.

Corsaro, W. A., & Molinari, L. (2005). *I compagni: Understanding children's transition from preschool to elementary school.* New York: Teachers College Press.

Dayan, J., Doyle, A. B., & Markiewicz, D. (2001). Social support networks and self-esteem of idiocentric and allocentric children and adolescents. *Journal of Social and Personal Relations, 18*, 767–784.

Dekovic, M., Engels, R. C. M. E., Shirai, T., De Kort, G., & Anker, A. L. (2002). The role of peer relations in adolescent development in two cultures: The Netherlands and Japan. *Journal of Cross-Cultural Psychology, 33*, 577–595.

DeRosier, M. E., & Kupersmidt, J. B. (1991). Costa Rican children's perceptions of their social networks. *Developmental Psychology, 27*, 656–662.

D'Hondt, W., & Vandewiele, M. (1980). Adolescents' groups in Senegal. *Psychological Reports, 47*, 795–802.

Edwards, C. P. (2000). Children's play in cross-cultural perspective: A new look at the Six Culture Study. *Cross-Cultural Research, 34*, 318–338.

Eisenberg, N., Pidada, S., & Liew, J. (2001). The relations of regulation and negative emotionality to Indonesian children's social functioning. *Child Development, 72*, 1747–1763.

Eisenberg, N., Zhou, Q., Liew, J., Champion, C., & Pidada, S. (2006). Emotion, emotion-related regulation, and social functioning. In X. Chen, D. French, & B. Schneider (Eds.), *Peer relationships in cultural context* (pp. 170–197). New York: Cambridge University Press.

Espelage, D. L., Holt, M. K., & Henkel, R. R. (2003). Examination of peer-group contextual effects on aggression during early adolescence. *Child Development, 74*, 205–220.

Farver, J. M., & Howes, C. (1988). Cultural differences in social interaction: A comparison of American and Indonesian children. *Journal of Cross-Cultural Psychology, 19*, 203–315.

Farver, J. M., Kim, Y. K., & Lee, Y. (1995). Cultural differences in Korean- and Anglo-American preschoolers' social interaction and play behaviors. *Child Development, 66*, 1088–1099.

Farver, J. M., & Shin, Y. L. (1997). Social pretend play in Korea- and Anglo-American preschoolers. *Child Development, 68*, 544–556.

French, D. C., Bae, A., Pidada, S., & Lee, O. (2006). Friendships of Indonesian, S. Korean and U.S. college students. *Personal Relationships, 13*, 69–81.

French, D. C., Jansen, E. A., Riansari, M., & Setiono, K. (2003). Friendships of Indonesian children: Adjustment of children who differ in friendship presence and similarity between mutual friends. *Social Development, 12*, 605–621.

French, D. C., Lee, O., & Pidada, S. (2006). Friendships of Indonesian, South Korean and United States youth: Exclusivity, intimacy, enhancement of worth, and conflict. In X. Chen, D. French, & B. Schneider (Eds.), *Peer relationships in cultural context* (pp. 379–402). New York: Cambridge University Press.

French, D. C., Pidada, S., & Victor, A. (2005). Friendships of Indonesian and United States youth. *International Journal of Behavioral Development, 29*, 304–313.

Gaskins, S. (2000). Children's daily activities in a Mayan village: A culturally grounded description. *Cross-Cultural Research, 34*, 375–389.

Gaskins, S. (2006). The cultural organization of Yucatec Mayan children's social interactions. In X. Chen, D. French, & B. Schneider (Eds.), *Peer relationships in cultural context* (pp. 283–309). New York: Cambridge University Press.

Gonzalez, Y., Moreno, D. S., & Schneider, B. H. (2004). Friendship expectations of early adolescents in Cuba and Canada. *Journal of Cross-Cultural Psychology, 35*, 436–445.

Graves, N. B., & Graves, T. D. (1983). The cultural context of prosocial development: An ecological model. In D. L. Bridgeman (Ed.), *The nature of prosocial development* (pp. 795–824). San Diego: Academic Press.

Greenfield, P. M., Suzuki, L. K., & Rothstein-Fisch, C. (2006). Cultural pathways through human development. In K. A. Renninger & I. E. Sigel (Eds.), *Handbook of child psychology: Vol. 4. Child psychology in practice* (pp. 655–699). New York: Wiley.

Guthrie, D. (2006). *China and globalization: The social, economic, and political transformation of Chinese society.* New York: Routledge.

Harris, J. R. (1995). Where is the child's environment?: A group socialization theory of development. *Psychological Review, 102*, 458–489.

Hart, C. H., Yang, C., Nelson, L. J., Robinson, C. C., Olson, J. A., Nelson, D. A., et al. (2000). Peer acceptance in early childhood and subtypes of socially withdrawn behaviour in China, Russia and the United States. *International Journal of Behavioral Development, 24*, 73–81.

Hinde, R. A. (1987). *Individuals, relationships and culture.* Cambridge, UK: Cambridge University Press.

Hollnsteiner, M. R. (1979). Reciprocity as a Filipino in value. In M. R. Hollnsteiner (Ed.), *Culture and the Filipino* (pp. 38–43). Quezon City, Phillippines: Atteneo de Manila University.

Hoza, B., Molina, B. G., Bukowski, W. M., & Sippola, L. K. (1995). Peer variables as predictors of later childhood adjustment. *Development and Psychopathology, 7*, 787–802.

Jay, R. R. (1969). *Javanese villagers: Social relations in rural Modjokuto.* Cambridge, MA: MIT Press.

Kagan, J., Kearsley, R. B., & Zelazo, P. R. (1978). *Infancy: Its place in human development.* Cambridge, MA: Harvard University Press.

Kagan, S., & Knight, G. P. (1981). Social motives among Anglo-American and Mexican-American children: Experimental and projective measures. *Journal of Research in Personality, 15,* 93–106.

Kagitcibasi, C. (2005). Autonomy and relatedness in cultural context: Implications for self and family. *Journal of Cross-Cultural Psychology, 36,* 403–422.

Keller, H., Yovsi, R., Borke, J., Kartner, J., Jensen, H., & Papaligoura, Z. (2004). Developmental consequences of early parenting experiences: Self-recognition and self-regulation in three cultural communities. *Child Development, 75,* 1745–1760.

Kerr, M., Lambert, W. W., & Bem, D. J. (1996). Life course sequelae of childhood shyness in Sweden: Comparison with the United States. *Developmental Psychology, 32,* 1100–1105.

Kiesner, J., Poulin, F., & Nicotra, E. (2003). Peer relations across contexts: Individual–network homophily and network inclusion in and after school. *Child Development, 74,* 1328–1343.

Kindermann, T. A. (1993). Natural peer groups as contexts for individual development: The case of children's motivation in school. *Developmental Psychology, 29,* 970–977.

Kindermann, T. A. (2007). Effects of naturally existing peer groups on changes in academic engagement in a cohort of sixth graders. *Child Development, 78,* 1186–1203.

Lee, M. R., Okazaki, S., & Yoo, H. C. (2006). Frequency and intensity of social anxiety in Asian Americans and European Americans. *Cultural Diversity and Ethnic Minority Psychology, 12,* 291–305.

Leung, M. C. (1996). Social networks and self enhancement in Chinese children: A comparison of self reports and peer reports of group membership. *Social Development, 5,* 147–157.

Little, T. D., Brendgen, M., Wanner, B., & Krappmann, L. (1999). Children's reciprocal perceptions of friendship quality in the sociocultural contexts of East and West Berlin. *International Journal of Behavioral Development, 23,* 63–89.

Miller, J. G. (1994). Cultural diversity in the morality of caring: Individually oriented versus duty-based interpersonal moral codes. *Cross-Cultural Research, 28,* 3–39.

Orlick, T., Zhou, Q. Y., & Partington, J. (1990). Co-operation and conflict within Chinese and Canadian kindergarten settings. *Canadian Journal of Behavioral Science, 22,* 20–25.

Parmar, P., Harkness, S., & Super, C. M. (2004). Asian and Euro-American parents' ethnotheories of play and learning: Effects on preschool children's home routine and school behaviour. *International Journal of Behavioral Development, 28,* 97–104.

Rogoff, B. (2003). *The cultural nature of human development.* New York: Oxford University Press.

Rothbart, M. K., & Bates, J. E. (2006). Temperament. In N. Eisenberg (Ed.), *Handbook of child psychology: Vol. 3. Social, emotional, and personality development* (pp. 99–166). New York: Wiley.

Rothbaum, F., Pott, M., Azuma, H., Miyake, K., & Weisz, J. (2000). The development of close relationships in Japan and the United States: Paths of symbiotic harmony and generative tension. *Child Development, 71,* 1121–1142.

Rubin, K. H., Bukowski, W., & Parker, J. G. (2006). Peer interactions, relationships, and groups. In N. Eisenberg (Ed.), *Handbook of child psychology: Vol. 3. Social, emotional, and personality development* (pp. 571–645). New York: Wiley.

Rubin, K. H., Burgess, K. B., & Coplan, R. J. (2002). Social withdrawal and shyness. In P. K. Smith & C.H. Hart (Eds.), *Blackwell handbook of childhood social development* (pp. 330–352), Malden, MA: Blackwell.

Rubin, K. H., Fein, G. G., & Vandenberg, B. (1983). Play. In E. M. Hetherington (Ed.), *Handbook of child psychology* (Vol. 4, 4th ed., pp. 693–774). New York: Wiley.

Rubin, K. H., Hemphill, S. A., Chen, X., Hastings, P., Sanson, A., LoCoco, A., et al. (2006). A cross-cultural study of behavioral inhibition in toddlers: East–west–north–south. *International Journal of Behavioral Development, 30,* 219–226.

Russell, A., Hart, C. H., Robinson, C. C., & Olsen, S. F. (2003). Children's sociable and aggressive behavior with peers: A comparison of the US and Australia, and contributions of temperament and parenting styles. *International Journal of Behavioral Development, 27*, 74–86.

Salmivalli, C., Huttunen, A., & Lagerspetz, K. (1997). Peer networks and bullying in schools. *Scandinavian Journal of Psychology, 38*, 305–312.

Schneider, B. H., Fonzi, A., & Tani, F. (1997). A cross-cultural exploration of the stability of children's friendships and the predictors of their continuation. *Social Development, 6*, 322–333.

Schneider, B. H., Fonzi, A., Tomada, G., & Tani, F. (2000). A cross-national comparison of children's behavior with their friends in situations of potential conflict. *Journal of Cross-Cultural Psychology, 31*, 259–266.

Sharabany, R. (2006). The cultural context of children and adolescents: Peer relationships and intimate friendships among Arab and Jewish children in Israel. In X. Chen, D. French, & B. Schneider (Eds.), *Peer relationships in cultural context* (pp. 452–478). New York: Cambridge University Press.

Sharabany, R., & Wiseman, H. (1993). Close relationships in adolescence: The case of the kibbutz. *Journal of Youth and Adolescence, 22*, 671–695.

Sim, T. N., & Koh, S. F. (2003). Domain conceptualization of adolescent susceptibility to peer pressure. *Journal of Research on Adolescence, 13*, 58–80.

Sullivan, H. S. (1953). *The interpersonal theory of psychiatry*. New York: Norton.

Tamis-LeMonda, C. S., Way, N., Hughes, D., Yoshikawa, H., Kalman, R. K., & Niwa, E. (2008). Parents' goals for children: The dynamic co-existence of collectivism and individualism in cultures and individuals. *Social Development, 17*, 183–209.

Tietjen, A. (1989). The ecology of children's social support networks. In D. Belle (Ed.), *Children's social networks and social support* (pp. 37–69). New York: Wiley.

Tietjen, A. (2006). Cultural influences on peer relations: An ecological perspective. In X. Chen, D. French, & B. Schneider (Eds.), *Peer relationships in cultural context* (pp. 52–74). New York: Cambridge University Press.

Triandis, H. C. (1995). *Individualism and collectivism*. Boulder, CO: Westview Press.

Triandis, H. C., Bontempo, R., Villareal, M. J., Asai, M., & Lucca, N. (1988). Individualism and collectivism: Cross-cultural perspectives on self-ingroup relationships. *Journal of Personality and Social Psychology, 54*, 323–333.

Vygotsky, L. S. (1978). *Mind in society: The development of higher psychological processes* (M. Cole, V. John-Steiner, S. Scribner, & E. Souberman, Eds.). Cambridge, MA: Harvard University Press.

Way, N. (2006). The cultural practice of close friendships among urban adolescents in the United States. In X. Chen, D. French, & B. Schneider (Eds.), *Peer relationships in cultural context* (pp. 403–425). New York: Cambridge University Press.

Weisz, J. R., Suwanlert, S., Chaiyasit, W., Weiss, B., Walter, B. R., & Anderson, W. W. (1988). Thai and American perspectives on over-and undercontrolled child behavior problems: Exploring the threshold model among parents, teachers, and psychologists. *Journal of Consulting and Clinical Psychology, 56*, 601–609.

Whiting, B. B., & Edwards, C. P. (1988). *Children of different worlds*. Cambridge: Harvard University Press.

Zahn-Waxler, C., Friedman, R. J., Cole, P. M., Mizuta, I., & Hiruma, N. (1996). Japanese and United States preschool children's responses to conflict and distress. *Child Development, 67*, 2462–2477.

PART VI

Proximal Correlates of Children's Social Skills and Peer Relationships

CHAPTER 25

Genetic Factors
in Children's Peer Relations

MARA BRENDGEN
MICHEL BOIVIN

Peers are believed to play a central role in child development (Bukowski, Brendgen, & Vitaro, 2007). They provide contexts for the acquisition of new social skills, the validation of the self-concept, and the learning of social roles, norms, and processes involved in interpersonal relationships (Boivin, Vitaro, & Poulin, 2005). Peer relations can also have negative effects. They may impede healthy development by reinforcing inappropriate behaviors and lead to undesirable outcomes, such as delinquency and substance abuse (Boivin et al., 2005; Bukowski et al., 2007). Accordingly, numerous studies have documented significant associations between children's peer relations and diverse aspects of child adjustment (Bukowski et al., 2007).

A major challenge for peer relations research lies in the difficulty of testing specific hypotheses about the developmental processes underlying the association between peer relations and child adjustment. For example, studies based on simple correlations cannot indicate whether affiliation with deviant peers causes a child's antisocial behavior. Experimental manipulations could be used to test causal hypotheses but are precluded by ethical concerns. As an alternative, researchers can take advantage of (1) randomized intervention studies to test causal links, and the mediating mechanisms underlying these links (Vitaro, Brendgen, & Tremblay, 2001), or (2) behavioral-genetics designs. Although behavioral-genetics designs cannot provide direct and conclusive proof of causation, "they are a useful addition to the toolkit for testing environmental causation" (Moffitt, 2005, p. 534). For example, by disentangling genetic from nongenetic sources of interindividual variation, behavioral genetics can evaluate to what extent the child's inherent genetic factors account for the involvement in deviant peer affiliation. Such a finding might indicate that an active selection process based on heritable personal characteristics is involved. In other words, behavioral-genetics studies may test for possible "child effects" on specific (i.e., measured) features of peer relations. Behavioral-genetics designs also permit the assessment of other theoretical models of the association between peer experiences and child behavior. For example, in line with the diathesis–stress model of psychopathology, behavioral-genetics analyses may test for a possible gene–environment interaction linking peer victimization and emotional adjustment. A gene–environment interaction would be indicated if the effect of peer victimization on child emotional adjustment were conditioned by the level of genetic risk for such problems.

Compared with behavioral-genetics studies on children's behavioral or cognitive characteristics, genetically informed research on children's peer relations is still in its infancy. Nevertheless, the findings so far offer important insights into the development of children's peer experiences and the processes linking these experiences with behavior, development, and adjustment. In this chapter, we first provide an overview of the basic logic underlying behavioral-genetics methods. We then review extant empirical evidence from behavioral-genetics studies on peer relations and discuss their significance for our understanding of the developmental role of peer relations. We conclude with a discussion of future directions.

Theoretical Overview
of the Behavioral–Genetics Method

Behavioral-genetics methods are typically based on the assumption that interindividual differences in a measured behavior (i.e., a phenotype) can be decomposed into three different sources of variance: "genetic" (or heritable) factors, "shared" (or common) environmental factors, and "nonshared" (or unique) environmental factors (Petrill, 2002). In most behavioral-genetics studies these three variance components are generally conceived as latent (i.e., unmeasured) variables. Phenotypic variance is decomposed into genetic and environmental sources of influence by examining the degree of phenotypic similarity among family members according to their level of genetic relatedness. For example, genetic factors are thought to be at play if children are "phenotypically" more similar to their biological siblings, with whom they share 50% of genetic relatedness (on average), than to their adopted or stepsiblings, with whom they are not genetically related in principle. Similarly, genetic factors are implicated if identical or monozygotic (MZ) twins, who share 100% of their genetic makeup, are more similar to each other than are same-sex fraternal or dizygotic (DZ) twins, who share on average only 50% of their genes. In a mixed twin and nontwin sibling design, genetic effects are indicated by the following pattern of similarity: MZ twins > DZ twins = full siblings > half-siblings > unrelated (e.g., adopted or step-) siblings.

"Shared" environment refers to environmental factors, both inside and outside of the family, that make members of the same family unit (i.e., living together) similar to each other. Shared environment encompasses geographical or social neighborhood characteristics (e.g., crime level), family characteristics (e.g., socioeconomic scale [SES], parental mental health), school-related characteristics (e.g., academic track), and other features of the physical and social environment to which members of the family are jointly exposed. Shared environment is implicitly involved when children are similar to their adopted or stepsiblings, although they are genetically unrelated. In twin designs, shared environment is indicated when (1) MZ, as well as DZ, twin pairs are similar to each other, *and* (2) the degree of similarity among DZ twins is comparable to that of MZ twins. In a mixed twin and nontwin sibling design, shared environmental effects are suggested when twin and nontwin sibling pairs are similar to each other regardless of their degree of genetic relatedness.

In contrast with shared environment, "nonshared" environment refers to environmental factors that account for differences among members of the same family. Thus, because MZ twins "share" the same home and 100% of their genes, any within-pair differences among MZ twins can only be accounted for by nonshared environmental factors (and measurement error). More generally, nonshared environmental factors implicitly refer to experiences within or outside the family that make children of the same family grow apart. For example, although siblings may be raised together in the same family, parents may treat them differently (Dunn, Stocker, & Plomin, 1990). Siblings' differential treatment by parents has been related to differences in siblings' behavior (Conger & Conger, 1994; Dunn et al., 1990; McHale, Crouter, McGuire, & Updegraff, 1995).

The most important nonshared environmental influences, however, are likely those experienced outside the family (Dunn & Plomin, 1990). A particularly relevant source of nonshared environmental influence in this context may be children's experiences with peers (Harris, 1998), because many children do not affiliate with the same friends as their cosiblings (Pike & Atzaba-Poria, 2003; Rose, 2002; Thorpe & Gardner, 2006). Nevertheless, even extrafamilial experiences, such as those with peers, may not necessarily be purely environmental features that are completely independent of a child's genetic disposition.

Central Issue:
Do Peers Constitute a "Pure" Environmental Factor?

Features that are "environmental," in the sense that they are external to the individual, are not necessarily independent of genetic factors. Indeed, it is possible that individuals evoke their environment as a function of heritable traits (Scarr & McCartney, 1983). For example, aggressive behavior in children is to a significant extent explained by genetic factors (DiLalla, 2002), and aggressive behaviors are a proximal determinant of peer relations difficulties (Boivin et al., 2005). Thus, it is possible that children with a genetic disposition toward aggressive behavior may elicit rejection or victimization from the peer group as a function of their genetic disposition. Similarly, children may actively seek out friends with similar behavioral characteristics based on their own genetic disposition toward aggressive behavior. Genetically informative designs typically estimate the proportions of genetic and environmental sources of variance on a measured behavioral characteristic (e.g., aggression). This type of analysis can also be extended to measured "environmental" aspects, such as peer relations, to evaluate the extent to which these peer relations are shared or uniquely experienced by siblings, and whether they may have been induced by genetically influenced child characteristics. Most genetically sensitive studies on peer relations have focused on the characteristics of children's or adolescents' friends, mainly in regard to deviant behavior. Two studies investigated the quality of adolescents' relationship with their best friend. Five studies examined youngsters' social experiences with the larger peer group (i.e., in regard to popularity and victimization). We now describe the findings with respect to each of these different types of peer experiences.

Friends' Characteristics

The earliest studies to examine potential genetic effects on friends' characteristics used the Sibling Inventory of Differential Experience (SIDE; Daniels & Plomin, 1985) as an index of the peer environment. This measure assesses to what extent participants perceive their friends to differ from those of their cosiblings with respect to three domains: college orientation, delinquency, and popularity. In one study based on a mixed twin and stepfamily (i.e., quasi-adoption) design with siblings ages 12–18 years, biological siblings reported having friends with more similar characteristics than did adoptive siblings, which suggests the presence of genetic effects (Nonshared Environment and Adolescent Development [NEAD] project; Daniels & Plomin, 1985). Another study using follow-up data from the same sample yielded similar results, although further analyses showed that genetic factors accounted only for friends' characteristics in the twin sample (Pike, Manke, Reiss, & Plomin, 2000). Yet another study using retrospective reports of friends' characteristics in adult twins also found that MZ twins had friends with more similar characteristics than did DZ twins, again suggesting a genetic contribution (Baker & Daniels, 1990).

The results from these studies thus suggest that the characteristics of a person's friends may partly be accounted for by that person's genetic disposition. However, the SIDE used a forced-comparison procedure between a child's own friends and those of the cotwin that may have artificially inflated the similarity among MZ twins, who may have a closer bond than (same-sex) DZ twins (Danby & Thorpe, 2006; Rose, 2002). In addition, because the SIDE scores reflect relative differences between siblings in regard to friends' characteristics, it is not possible to estimate the relative contribution of genes versus that of shared and nonshared environmental factors (Eaves & Carbonneau, 1998). Studies based on distinct peer relations measures for each individual are more useful in that regard. We now consider studies assessing the characteristics of the friendship group as a whole, before turning our attention to studies assessing the characteristics of specific, nominated friends.

Overall Friendship Group Characteristics

The first genetically informed study to use distinct measures of friends' characteristics was based on twin and nontwin siblings ages 10–18 years from the NEAD project (Manke, McGuire, Reiss, & Hetherington, 1995). Mothers' and fathers' perceptions of their children's friends' college orientation, delinquency, and popularity were examined. Genetic factors explained most of the variance in all measures, with estimated genetic effects ranging from 49 to 85%. Significant shared environmental factors also accounted for a significant part of the variance for most friendship group characteristics (from 13 to 35% of explained variance), with the remainder explained by nonshared environmental factors. The findings for parent reports may have been partly due to rater bias, however, because parents may not necessarily have known all of their adolescent children's friends. This may have prompted them to overestimate peer-related similarity among siblings in general and among MZ twins in particular, resulting in inflated estimates for genetic or shared environmental effects.

Three studies based on adolescents' self-reports indeed do not show consistently strong genetic effects on friends' characteristics. In the first study (Rose, 2002), 16-year-old MZ and DZ twins were asked to evaluate the overall level of their friends' substance use (drinking and smoking). The pattern of twin correlations showed only slightly larger similarity among the friends of MZ twins than among the friends of DZ twins. Effect sizes based on these correlations indicated 22% of variance accounted for by genes, with the residual variance explained mostly by shared environment (45%). A second study used a two-sample design: One sample comprised 13- to 21-year-old pairs of twins and nontwin siblings from the NEAD project; the other sample included nontwin sibling pairs from adoptive and nonadoptive families for whom repeated measures were available at 13–16 years of age (Iervolino et al., 2002). For both samples, self-reports were obtained about their friendship group's college orientation and delinquency. Aggregated across sex and age, the results showed substantial genetic contributions (between 42 and 47%) to friends' college orientation in both samples, but genetic factors played a negligible role (0%) for friends' delinquency when only same-sex siblings were considered. Instead, interindividual differences in friends' delinquency in the two samples were mostly explained by nonshared environmental factors (varying from 73 to 79%). In a third study, strong environmental effects—but no genetic effects—were also reported in 14-year-old twin pairs' reports about their friendship group's delinquency and substance use (Walden, McGue, Iacono, Burt, & Elkins, 2004). Teachers also rated the level of deviance of each participant's friendship group. Factor analysis showed that both the variance and the covariance of participants' and teachers' reports of friends' deviancy was completely accounted for by environmental factors. Specifically, shared environmental factors were responsible for the covariation among participants' own and their teachers' reports of friends' deviancy. The residual variance of participants' and teachers' reports of friends' deviancy was mainly explained by nonshared environmental factors.

Nominated Friends' Characteristics

Although adolescents may have greater insight than their parents into their friends' behavior, the reliance on individuals' accounts may be problematic due to the propensity to project one's own characteristics onto others (Bauman & Ennett, 1996). This often leads to an exaggerated correlation between individuals' own and their friends' behavioral characteristics (Berndt & Keefe, 1995), which, in the case of genetically sensitive designs, may translate into inflated heritability or shared environment estimates for friends' behavior. Potential halo effects might be increased further if the characteristics of the friendship group are evaluated as a whole instead of judging the behavior of specific, nominated friends.

To address this issue, we examined a sample of 6-year-old twin pairs drawn from the Quebec Newborn Twin Study (QNTS), for whom teacher and peer reports of aggressive behavior were obtained for each twin child and his or her nominated two best friends in the classroom (Van Lier et al., 2007). Teacher ratings were combined with the respective peer-rated scores. Interestingly, 73% of twins attended a different classroom than their cotwin, so that twins of those pairs were rated by different peers and teachers. As in previous studies (DiLalla, 2002), children's own aggression was found to be highly heritable, with 70% of the variance explained by genetic factors and the residual variance explained by nonshared environmental factors. However, friends' aggression was unrelated to children's genes. Instead, 74% of the variance of friends' aggression was accounted for by nonshared environmental effects, with the remaining variance explained by shared environmental factors.

Similar findings were obtained in a follow-up study where we examined the genetic and environmental contributions to friends' aggressive characteristics, but this time contrasting physical with indirect aggression (Brendgen, Boivin, Vitaro, Bukowski, et al., 2008). Using data from the QNTS, collected when the twins were 7 years of age, children's and their friends' characteristics were assessed according to the same procedure as that in the Van Lier et al. (2007) study. Children's own physical and social aggression were significantly accounted for by genetic factors (58 and 43%, respectively), with the remaining variance explained by nonshared environmental factors. In contrast, exposure to physically aggressive or to indirectly aggressive friends was unrelated to children's genetic disposition. Instead, friends' physical aggression was entirely accounted for by nonshared environmental factors, whereas friends' indirect aggression was explained by nonshared (87%) and by shared environmental factors (13%).

As in other studies, most genetically informed studies on peer relations have relied on questionnaire-based measures. A more direct observational assessment of friends' problem behavior was conducted with a sample of 7- to 13-year-old identical and fraternal twins (Leve, 2001). Each twin was asked to select a close, same-age friend to participate in the study and the twin-friend dyads were then observed in two 5-minute discussion sessions about a fun activity and about the next school year. Each twin's and his or her friend's negative behaviors (i.e., negative verbal content or negative affect) were rated separately by independent observers. In contrast to the twins' own behavior, which was significantly accounted for by genetic factors, friends' negative behavior was unrelated to the twins' genetic disposition. Rather, friends' negative behavior was almost entirely associated with nonshared environmental factors (100% when the twins' negative behavior was partialed out, and 85% when the twins' negative behavior was not controlled).

Few genetic effects on friends' characteristics were also found in a sample of 12-year-old identical and fraternal Finnish twins (Rose, 2002). Participants were asked to nominate their best friends in the classroom, and classroom-based peer nominations were then used to assess the best friends' behavior problems (hyperactivity–impulsiveness, aggression, inattention), emotional problems (anxiety and depression), and positive adjustment (constructiveness, sociability, compliance). Friends who were shared by both twins were excluded from the analyses. The pattern of MZ versus DZ correlations suggested no genetic contributions to friends' characteristics for boys. For girls, small genetic contributions were found for behavioral and emotional problems (about 26 and 14% of explained variance, respectively), but not for positive adjustment. However, all friends' characteristics mostly reflected nonshared environmental contributions, ranging from 64 to 91% of explained variance.

Overall, these findings suggest that exposure to antisocial friends is a—mainly nonshared—feature of the social environment, with very little, if any, relation to a child's genetic disposition when raters evaluate each friend's behavior individually. Genetic contributions seem to emerge when raters provide a more generalized assessment of a child's friendship group. A direct test of this hypothesis was conducted in a recent study examining MZ and DZ twin pairs, ages 7–14 years, and their close, same-age friend (Bullock, Deater-Deckard, & Leve, 2006). Each twin of a pair was instructed to select a different friend than that selected by his or her cotwin. Friends' deviant behavior was assessed with three different methods: (1) Coders rated the friend's observed antisocial behavior during an interaction task with the twin child; (2) teachers rated the deviant behavior of each twin's close friend; and (3) teachers assessed the overall level of deviancy of a child's peer group. The different raters also assessed the target children's own deviant behavior. Significant genetic effects were found for the twins' own deviant behavior. As in our studies, friends' deviant behavior was not significantly associated with genetic factors when the behavior of a friend was directly observed: 63% of the variance was explained by nonshared environmental effects, with shared environmental effects accounting for the remaining variance (37%). Nonshared environmental effects were even stronger for teachers' ratings of individual friends' deviant behavior (100% of the variance). However, when teachers rated the general level of deviance of a twin's larger peer group, a small but significant genetic contribution emerged: 18% of the variance was explained by genetic effects, and 82% was explained by nonshared environmental effects.

The Bullock et al. (2006) findings support the view that, compared to a global evaluation of the friendship group, the assessment of specific friends' characteristics may yield very small or no genetic effects. This conclusion, however, may apply only to younger children and early adolescents. Indeed, considerable genetic effects on nominated friends' characteristics were found in two reports from the National Longitudinal Study of Adolescent Health (Add Health; Harris et al., 2003), which includes a sample of twin and nontwin siblings in grades 7–9 (mean age = 16 years). The first study examined friends' tobacco and alcohol use (Cleveland, Wiebe, & Rowe, 2005). Participants were asked to nominate up to five male and five female school friends, who then reported on their own smoking and drinking. Genetic factors were found to explain 64% of the variance of a composite score of friends' averaged substance use, with nonshared environment accounting for the remaining variance. The second study focused specifically on the first nominated same-sex and opposite-sex friends, and examined the following characteristics: academic achievement, verbal intelligence, aggression, and depression (Guo, 2006). Although relative effects of genetic and environmental factors were not reported, the pattern of sibling correlations suggested strong genetic contributions on all examined features, at least for same-sex friends. Approximate effect size calculations (Falconer, 1989) based on the MZ and DZ correlations indicate that 62% of the variance of friends' academic achievement, 36% of the variance of friends' verbal intelligence, 100% of friends' aggression, and 40% of friends' depression was explained by adolescents' genetic disposition. The remaining variance seemed to be explained by nonshared environmental factors. For opposite-sex friends' characteristics, however, twin correlations were of the same magnitude for MZ and DZ twins, indicating no genetic effects but substantial shared environment contributions.

So what can we conclude from existing studies about the extent of genetic contributions to friends' characteristics? Overall, strong genetic effects seem to be found mostly when characteristics of the peer group are evaluated globally—especially by sources external to the friendship, such as parents—instead of assessing the characteristics of specific, nominated friends. Findings based on specific nominated friends' characteristics suggest a developmental pattern whereby friends' characteristics are unrelated to individuals' genetic disposition in younger children and preadolescents, but genetic effects appear to emerge in older adolescents, indicating a possible selection of friends based on heritable characteristics. Nevertheless, the bulk of the findings points toward a considerable—and mainly nonshared—environmental contribution to friends' characteristics, regardless of age group and methodology. If this is the case, then friends' influence could indeed make members of a family different from each other.

Friendship Quality

Compared with genetically informed research on friends' characteristics, behavioral-genetics studies on the quality of children's friendships are extremely scarce. One of the two exceptions is the previously mentioned study of same-sex twin and nontwin siblings, ages 10–18 years from the NEAD project (Manke et al., 1995). In addition to reports of friends' characteristics, adolescents also reported on positive aspects (warmth and support) and negative aspects (conflict and negativity) of their relationship with their best friend. The results showed that genetic factors explained 31% of the variance of positive friendship quality, with the remaining variance essentially explained by nonshared environmental factors. Negative friendship quality was unrelated to genetic factors; rather, it was explained by nonshared environmental factors. Similar findings were reported in a study with 12-year-old MZ and DZ twins (Pike & Atzaba-Poria, 2003). Participants were asked to describe their relationship with their best friend in regard to five positive dimensions (validation and caring, conflict resolution, help and guidance, companionship and recreation, and intimate exchange) and in regard to one negative dimension (conflict and betrayal). Although estimates did not always reach statistical significance due to the relatively small sample size, considerable genetic contributions were found for all positive dimensions of friendship quality, ranging from 29 to 56% of explained variance. The largest part of the variance was explained by nonshared environmental effects, however. In contrast, conflict and betrayal within friendships was completely unrelated to genes, and was instead accounted for by shared (39%) and nonshared (61%) environmental factors.

As an explanation for the disparity of genetic contributions to positive versus negative friendship quality, Manke et al. (1995) argued that negative interactions within enduring friendships may be of an ephemeral nature and may not necessarily reflect the partners' underlying (and presumably partly heritable) behavioral characteristics. In contrast, positive valuations of friendships may be based on repeated positive interactions over time, which may have a greater opportunity to be based on partners' underlying and genetically influenced characteristics. These explanations are highly speculative due to the dearth of genetically sensitive data on friendship quality. Nevertheless, the few existing findings suggest that some aspects of experiences with close friends may be shaped in part by adolescents' personal, heritable characteristics, although these experiences mainly constitute a nonshared environmental feature.

Popularity and Victimization in the Peer Group

So far, most genetically informed studies have examined various aspects of children's dyadic friendships. However, group-based peer experiences, such as those captured by peer-group popularity and victimization, have also been the object of attention. For example, in one study, teacher-rated popularity was examined in a sample of 12-year-old adoptive and biological siblings (O'Connor, Jenkins, Hewitt, DeFries, & Plomin, 2001). The results showed that the intraclass correlation (IC) among biological siblings was almost twice as high (IC = .45) as that between adoptive siblings (IC = .25), suggesting a genetic contribution to child popularity. Interestingly, these results also held when previous teacher-rated popularity at age 10 years was taken into account, which indicates that genetic factors were partly responsible for the change in popularity over time. However, for the most part, interindividual variance in popularity was associated with nonshared environmental factors, as indicated by the moderate level of overall similarity between sibling pairs, regardless of their level of genetic relatedness.

Genetic contributions to popularity among peers are also suggested by two studies using youngsters' self-reports. Specifically, using data from the NEAD project on 10- to 18-year-old adolescents, McGuire and colleagues (1999) examined the relative contribution of genetic and environmental effects on self-perceived social acceptance. These assessments were repeated twice over a 3-year interval. Significant genetic contributions were found for perceived social acceptance at both assessment times, with genetic factors accounting for between 49 and 51% of the variance. The remaining variance was explained entirely by nonshared environmental effects at both time points. Using, in part, data from the same sample but a different measure of peer acceptance, Iervolino and colleagues (2002) reached a similar conclusion. Specifically, examining adolescents' self-reports about their perceived popularity in the peer group, these authors found that genetic factors accounted for 38% of the variance of perceived popularity in the NEAD twin sample, with the remainder explained by nonshared environmental factors. Different findings were obtained for the nontwin sample, however, with perceived popularity entirely accounted for by nonshared environmental influences. Nevertheless, for the most part, the two studies using self-reports yielded relatively comparable findings. A potential limitation arises from the fact that self-perceived popularity measures show only modest overlap with actual peer-rated popularity (Brendgen, Vitaro, Turgeon, & Poulin, 2002), because they basically reflect a component of the self-system (Boivin & Hymel, 1997; Boivin, Vitaro, & Gagnon, 1992). Thus, the results could very well reflect biased estimates of genetic and environmental contributions to peer popularity.

We know of only one genetically informed study, the QNTS (see below) that used peer nomination or traditional rating procedures to assess popularity among peers. Classroomwide sociometric nominations were collected (in the spring session) when the MZ and DZ twins of QNTS were attending kindergarten and first grade. Liking and disliking nominations were gathered and combined into a peer preference score, a composite measure of peer popularity–rejection (Coie, Dodge, & Coppotelli, 1982). Peer victimization was also assessed through peer nominations. Peer-reported victimization is typically negatively correlated with popularity and reflects actual negative peer experiences in the peer group (Boivin, Hymel, & Hodges, 2001; McDougall, Hymel, Vaillancourt, & Mercer, 2001). We found no genetic contribution to peer preference or to peer victimization in kindergarten (Boivin et al., 2007; Brendgen, Boivin, Vitaro, Girard, et al., 2008). Rather, 75% of the variance in peer preference and 71% of the variance in peer victimization were accounted for by nonshared environmental factors, leaving 25 and 29% of the respective variances to shared environmental factors. However, a very different picture emerged in first grade, where significant genetic contributions were found for both dimensions: Genetic factors accounted for 55% of the variance in social preference and for 28% of the variance in peer victimization (Boivin et al., 2007). In both cases, familial aggregation was entirely explained by genetic factors, with no significant contribution of shared environmental factors. In other words, when twins of the same family were exposed to similar peer relations difficulties in first grade, this similar exposure was associated with their shared genes rather than with an environment they shared inside or outside the family. The unique environment component was more important in the case of peer victimization (72%) than in the case of social preference (45%), perhaps due to the contextual constraint associated with the expression of negative behaviors in the classroom.

This pattern of results, along with those reported by previous studies (McGuire et al., 1999), suggests a possible social-developmental dynamic underlying the emergence of peer relation difficulties in middle childhood. Specifically, acceptance–rejection and victimization may initially (i.e., at school entry) be determined by environmental conditions that foster positive or negative interactions in the group, because they are not yet fully influenced by individual behavioral tendencies and the ensuing social reputations. These environmental conditions may include teachers' awareness or responses to negative peer interactions (Fekkes, Pijpers, & Verloove-Vanhorick, 2005; Newman & Murray, 2005), or peer attitudes and reactions toward victimization in the classroom (Salmivalli, Kaukiainen, & Voeten, 2005). However, children's experiences with the peer group may become progressively more crystallized around their social reputation, partly founded on their behavioral tendencies as perceived by peers. This in turn is likely to elicit reactions such as prosocial behavior, aggression, or depression (Bukowski et al., 2007), which may in turn reinforce children's position among peers (Eisenberg et al., 1996; Hodges, Malone, & Perry, 1997; Lamarche et al., 2006). Such a sequence could then take the form of specific gene–environment processes—in particular gene–environment interactions and gene–environment correlations—linking child behavior and peer relations in a negative cycle that might manifest at different developmental stages. In the following sections, we describe in more detail such gene–environment processes in regard to peer relations, as well as existing empirical evidence in this context.

Central Issue: Gene–Environment Processes

The potential of behavioral genetics for theory testing extends beyond the question of heritability of phenotypes. Of particular interest to peer researchers are the etiological mechanisms that explain the link between peer relations and other aspects of child functioning. Within a genetically sensitive framework, at least three major hypotheses can be tested that may account for the association between peer experiences and child characteristics: the *gene–environment main effects versus gene–environment interaction* hypothesis, the *gene–environment correlation* hypothesis, and the *social homogamy* hypothesis. Although these hypotheses reflect different theoretical models linking peer experiences and child characteristics, they are not mutually exclusive. In the following sections, we explain each of these models in more detail.

Gene–Environment Main Effects versus the Interaction Model

Most existing genetically informative studies suggest that peer relations are a strongly environmentally driven feature that may play an important role in child development. However, environmental influences do not necessarily operate independently of genes. Indeed, the common view among scientists is that most developmental outcomes are the result of joint, rather than additive, effects of genetic (G) and environmental (E) factors (Rutter & Silberg, 2002). Accordingly, a first G–E process of interest in regard to peer relations and their association with child adjustment refers to a possible gene–environment interaction (G × E), which would be indicated if, for example, the effect of peer rejection on depressed mood were differentially manifested as a function of genetic risk for depression (Kendler & Eaves, 1986). Such a mechanism would be consistent with the diathesis–stress hypothesis, according to which an environmental stressor is more likely to lead to maladjustment among individuals with preexisting genetic vulnerabilities (Zuckerman, 1999).

Specific conditions facilitate the evaluation of G × E interaction. Genes do not have to be directly measured to test for a potential G × E interaction, but the putative environmental variable (e.g., peer rejection) has to be. Moreover, finding statistical evidence for a G × E interaction is most likely if the measured behavior is under strong genetic influence and if, in contrast, the measured putative "environmental" variable has little or no relation to genetic factors (Jaffee et al., 2005). In the absence of a G × E interaction, genes and exposure to a specific environment may, of course, independently affect child behavior and compound in an additive fashion, thus indicating general rather than conditional effects of the environment and of the genotype (i.e., a G & E main effect model).

To our knowledge, only three studies have examined a potential G × E interaction linking peer experiences and child behavior, and all of these studies have focused on child aggression as the behavioral outcome. One of these studies, described earlier, was conducted on a sample of 6-year-old twins (Van Lier et al., 2007). As mentioned, strong genetic effects were found to underlie individual differences in twins' aggression (i.e., a combined peer- and teacher-rated index of aggression), but genes were unrelated to their friends' level of aggression, which was instead entirely accounted for by nonshared environmental factors. We then tested whether exposure to aggressive friends moderated the contribution of genes to children's own aggression. This was indeed the case, but only for boys: Aggression was highest for genetically vulnerable boys who were exposed to highly aggressive friends. The contribution of genes to aggressive behavior was less pronounced, however, for boys who were exposed to friends with very low levels of aggression. For girls, the results revealed main effects of genes and of friends' aggression, suggesting that genetic vulnerability *and* exposure to aggressive friends operate as independent risk factors for aggressive behavior in girls.

It is possible that indirect rather than physical aggression may be more indicative of girls' disruptive behavior (Crick & Zahn-Waxler, 2003), and G × E processes may operate differently for these two types of aggressive behavior. Empirical evidence, again, from a previously described study, indeed suggests that the G × E interaction linking children's own and their friends' aggression operates for physical aggression but not for indirect aggression (Brendgen, Boivin, Vitaro, Bukowski, et al., 2008). Instead, genetic risk and exposure to indirectly aggressive friends showed additive (i.e., independent) contributions to children's own indirect aggression. We explain this finding by the different social consequences associated with indirect aggression compared to physical aggression: The lack of negative sanctions and the potential for positive consequences that are sometimes associated with indirect aggression (Cillessen & Mayeux, 2004; Leadbeater, Boone, Sangster, & Mathieson, 2006) may prompt children who are exposed to indirectly aggressive friends to use indirect aggression even in the absence of a predisposing genetic risk for this type of behavior.

Evidence was also found for a G × E interaction linking peer victimization and aggressive behavior (Brendgen, Boivin, Vitaro, Girard, et al., 2008). However, this interaction was only observed in girls, not in boys. Specifically, the association between peer victimization and girls' aggression gradually diminished with decreasing genetic risk for such behavior. Girls without a genetic disposition for aggressive behavior may be less inclined to display aggression when faced with abusive behavior from peers. In contrast, perhaps because aggressive responses to hostile peer provocations may be more acceptable for boys, victimized boys may be more likely generally to retort with aggression, regardless of whether they have a genetic disposition for such behavior.

Gene–Environment Correlation Model

As reviewed previously, children's experiences with peers are likely to be partly dependent on genetic factors. Indeed, some studies suggest a significant genetic contribution to various aspects of peer relations, including friends' characteristics, as well as peer popularity and peer victimization. One possible explanation for genes impinging on a purportedly "environmental" variable is that individuals evoke their environment as a function of heritable traits (Scarr & McCartney, 1983). Thus, children may become popular with peers due to heritable characteristics, such as good looks or superior athletic skills. Conversely, a child may suffer rejection and victimization because he or she behaves inappropriately in the eyes of the peer group, and these behaviors may be partly due to genetic vulnerabilities. This process, referred to as an "evocative gene–environment correlation" (rGE; Plomin, DeFries, & Loehlin, 1977), may be seen as a special case of "child effects" on his or her relations with peers. Another possible mechanism linking genes with environmental factors is that of an active selection of a peer environment according to one's genetic disposition (i.e., an "active gene–environment correlation"). For example, in the context of friendship affiliations, children may actively seek out friends with similar behavioral characteristics as a function of their own genetic disposition toward this behavior (e.g., aggression). Such an active G–E correlation corresponds to the notion of selection or "niche-picking," based on heritable characteristics, and may partly account for the similarity between children and their friends. Again, although genes do not have to be directly measured to test for a potential G–E correlation within a behavioral genetic framework, child characteristics and the putative environmental variable (e.g., friends' characteristics, peer victimization) have to be measured directly. When the measured child characteristic is significantly associated with the measured environmental feature, a twin design makes it possible to evaluate the extent to which this association is accounted by the child's genes, thus pointing to a G–E correlation phenomenon.

Most studies that found genetic effects on peer-related variables did not extend their investigations to potential links with child characteristics. To our knowledge, there are only two exceptions. In a previously mentioned study, positive, but not negative, friendship quality with the best friend among 12-year-old twins was explained to a considerable extent by genetic factors (Pike & Atzaba-Poria, 2003). Participants' temperamental features (i.e., activity, and sociability as assessed through the combined ratings of self- and parent reports) were also found to be associated with substantial genetic effects (with 56 and 43% of explained variance, respectively). Both activity and sociability were correlated with positive friendship quality. Bivariate genetic analyses revealed that these correlations were partly accounted for by an overlap in genetic factors, thus indicating a G–E correlation. Specifically, 27% of the phenotypic correlation between sociability and positive friendship quality, and 23% of the phenotypic correlation between activity and positive friendship quality were explained by shared genes.

In another previously reported study, we found significant genetic contributions for both first-grade social preference and peer victimization (Boivin et al., 2007). In that same study, the child's aggressive behavior in kindergarten (i.e., a combined score of peer and teacher ratings) was found significantly to predict these peer relation difficulties, and for both social preference and peer victimization, genetic factors in the child essentially accounted for that predictive association, which again signals a possible evocative G–E correlation. These findings provide an important first indication of a G–E correlation as a plausible mechanism linking child characteristics and peer experiences.

The Social Homogamy Model

In contrast to the previous models, the *social homogamy* model suggests that genetic factors do not play any role in the link between peer relations and child characteristics (Neale & Cardon, 1992). Instead, behavioral resemblance is explained by environmental conditions that simultaneously foster a specific behavior in all individuals who are exposed to these conditions (e.g., in the target child, his or her siblings, and his or her friends). For example, children may show similar levels of academic achievement simply because they are in the same academic track or because they attend the same afterschool academic counseling program, rather than because they share genes that lead them (or their parents) to select these features of the environment. Thus, a social homogamy process necessarily implies a significant contribution of shared environmental factors on the measured phenotype. Notably, these shared environmental influences are believed to operate outside of the family and are assumed to be shared by not only siblings and their friends but also all other children exposed to the same environmental conditions.

Social homogamy has rarely been tested as an explanation of similarity among friends. Preliminary empirical evidence for a possible social homogamy process in regard to friendships comes from a previously described study of 14-year-old twins (Walden et al., 2004). This study considered the participants' own deviancy (based on self-reports, cotwin reports, and mother reports), as well as their peer-group deviancy (based on self- and teacher reports). Both participants' and their peers' deviancy were entirely accounted for by shared and unique environmental factors. Most importantly, a series of bivariate analyses further revealed that the association between participants' deviancy and their peers' deviancy was essentially due to shared environmental influences operating on both phenotypes.

Although these findings hint at a possible social homogamy process, they do not necessarily imply that the link between peer deviancy and adolescents' substance use is entirely explained by shared environmental conditions external to the family. Indeed, shared environmental conditions within the family were not distinguished from those outside the family. A more stringent test of the social homogamy hypothesis with respect to deviancy was conducted with a school-based sample of full-sibling pairs in grades 7–12, drawn from the National Longitudinal Study of Adolescent Health (Gilson, Hunt, & Rowe, 2001). Participants completed a self-report delinquency questionnaire and a verbal intelligence test. They were also asked to nominate up to 10 friends from their school. Averaged delinquency and verbal IQ scores, respectively, was computed for the first male and the first female friend each participant had nominated within the school. Structural equation analyses were then performed to investigate different models: (1) a selection–socialization model characterized by direct effects between child and friend characteristics versus (2) a social homogamy model characterized by latent shared, nonfamilial environmental effects on child, sibling, and friend characteristics. Controlling for family-level effects (i.e., reflecting genes and shared familial environment), the results revealed that a social homogamy model best described the similarity between children and their friends in regard to verbal intelligence. In contrast, a combined social homogamy and selection–socialization process best explained the similarity between children and their friends in regard to delinquent behavior. These results suggest that although selection and socialization processes account for much of the behavioral similarity between friends, environmental influences external to the relationship also play an important part in making friends similar to each other.

Future Directions

As this review shows, behavioral-genetics studies can provide a more comprehensive understanding of the nature of peer experiences and their association with child adjustment. By disentangling genetic from environmental effects, important questions about selection versus socialization and about potential moderating factors of peer influence may be investigated. At this time, genetically sensitive research is only just beginning to explore peer relations, and many questions remain. We conclude this chapter by outlining specific methodological problems that limit the interpretation of findings, and that need to be considered in future research. We also discuss potential sex and age differences in the G–E processes linking peer relations and child adjustment, which have been largely ignored in current studies. Finally, we examine the possible role of molecular genetics in informing peer relations research beyond behavioral-genetics designs.

Many behavioral-genetics studies examining peer relations rely on self-, parent, or teacher reports to facilitate data collection and to increase the sample size to reach the power necessary to detect complex genetic and environmental effects. This approach, however, may produce biased results with respect to not only the nature of individuals' peer relations but also in terms of their underlying G–E etiology. For example, empirical evidence indicates that self-reports with respect to children's popularity or rejection in the peer group are only moderately correlated with the peer group's view in this regard (Brendgen et al., 2002). With respect to friendship relations, the reliance on individuals' accounts of their friends' behavior—instead of the use of the friends' self-reports—is problematic due to individuals' propensity to project their own characteristics onto others (Bauman & Ennett, 1996). Moreover, the vast majority of studies do not consider the potential overlap in siblings' friendship choices, despite evidence that identical twins tend to share the same friends more often than do fraternal twins (Pike & Atzaba-Poria, 2003; Rose, 2002; Thorpe & Gardner, 2006). Thus, including shared friends in the analyses can inflate genetic effects on friends' characteristics. The use of parent and teacher reports may also be problematic when the same person assesses both twins of the same family. In that case, the fact that the characteristics of the twins and the features of their environment are not assessed independently for each twin may yield biased estimates. Despite the associated costs and logistic challenges, behavioral-genetics studies might benefit from the use of multiple and independent evaluations when assessing children of the same family, including the use of peers as additional sources of information, especially when identifying and evaluating specific friends. It may also be useful to incorporate observational data that allow the investigation of microprocesses within peer relations—especially in regard to peer influence—within a genetically sensitive design.

An important problem with existing research concerns the fact that genetically informed studies rarely test for potential sex differences. The reason for this may be the limitations in statistical power when samples are broken down by sex. There is, however, some preliminary evidence that G–E processes may differ between girls and boys (Brendgen, Boivin, Vitaro, Girard, et al., 2008; Rose, 2002; Van Lier et al., 2007). Thus, combining the two sex groups without a specific test of sex differences may lead to potentially misleading conclusions about the role of genes in the link between peer relations and child adjustment. A related problem refers to the fact that many studies combined data across different age groups, thus obscuring possible age differences. This issue is important, because the pattern of results so far indicates that the relative contribution of genetic factors to peer experiences may change over the course of development, playing a stronger role for adolescents than for younger children. The large variability of effect sizes reported in the current studies makes it difficult to draw a definite conclusion in this respect, however. This variability is likely due to the vast differences in reporting sources, the targeted age range, the specific measures used, and the behavioral characteristics assessed. Indeed, developmental patterns may depend on the specific peer variable measured and may also differ for boys and girls. More longitudinal data are needed to assess developmental trends in regard to G–E processes within peer relations. Some studies (e.g., Boivin et al., 2007; Iervolino et al., 2002; O'Connor et al., 2001; Pike, Manke, Reiss,

& Plomin, 2000) already have repeated measures on peer relations that offer exciting possibilities for future longitudinal analyses.

Another exciting avenue for future research on G–E processes in regard to peer relations may be offered by molecular genetics (Eley, 2001). In contrast to behavioral genetics, which require the use of specific samples (e.g., twins or biological and adoptive siblings) to estimate the effect of latent genetic factors on a given phenotype, molecular genetics aims at identifying specific measured genes related to that phenotype. Once identified, measured genes can then be incorporated into regular studies and analyzed together with other measured variables. Collecting DNA has become simple and relatively inexpensive, and can now be obtained via mail using cheek swabs (Plomin & Rutter, 1998). Unlike single-gene disorders, such as cystic fibrosis or phenylketonuria, however, complex social behaviors are unlikely to be caused by a single gene; thus, measured genes would necessarily have relatively small effects (Eley, 2001). In fact, evidence so far points to a lack of main effects for measured genes and instead suggests that genes interact with each other or with specific environmental conditions in shaping individual behavior (Moffitt, Caspi, & Rutter, 2005). So far, the investigation of G × E interaction effects on social behavior involving measured genes has been limited to the family environment (e.g., Bakermans-Kranenburg & van IJzendoorn, 2006; Fox et al., 2005; Kim-Cohen et al., 2006). Nevertheless, given that these findings are in line with G × E interactions reported in recent behavioral-genetics studies on peer experiences (Brendgen, Boivin, Vitaro, Girard, 2008; Van Lier et al., 2007), the inclusion of measured genes, together with measured environmental variables, offers exciting possibilities for our understanding of G–E transactions in child development.

In conclusion, behavior-genetics research on peer relations is in its infancy. The initial reports reviewed here clearly show the potential of genetically informed designs to deepen our knowledge about the determinants and consequences of peer relations. Through the continuing study of potential interactions between genetic factors and peer environments, this line of research will likely help to clarify the unique contribution of peer experiences and relations to child development. The main challenge now lies in our capacity to use these powerful tools to understand the complex G–E interplay underlying the multifaceted aspects of peer relations and social development in a fully developmental perspective.

References

Baker, L. A., & Daniels, D. (1990). Nonshared environmental influences and personality differences in adult twins. *Journal of Personality and Social Psychology, 58*, 103–110.

Bakermans-Kranenburg, M. J. M., & van IJzendoorn, M. H. (2006). Gene–environment interaction of the dopamine D4 receptor (DRD4) and observed maternal insensitivity predicting externalizing behavior in preschoolers. *Developmental Psychobiology, 48*(5), 406–409.

Bauman, K. E., & Ennett, S. T. (1996). On the importance of peer influence for adolescent drug use: Commonly neglected considerations. *Addiction, 91*, 185–198.

Berndt, T. J., & Keefe, K. (1995). Friends' influence on adolescents' adjustment to school. *Child Development, 66*, 1312–1329.

Boivin, M., Brendgen, M., Dionne, G., Vitaro, F., Tremblay, R. E., & Pérusse, D. (2007, March). *Evidence of an emerging G–E correlation affecting peer rejection and victimization at school entry.* Presented at the Biennial Meeting of the Society for Research in Child Development, Boston, MA.

Boivin, M., & Hymel, S. (1997). Peer experiences and social self-perceptions: A sequential model. *Developmental Psychology, 33*(1), 135–145.

Boivin, M., Hymel, S., & Hodges, E. V. E. (2001). Toward a process view of peer rejection and harassment In J. Juvonen & S. Graham (Eds.), *Peer harassment in school: The plight of the vulnerable and victimized* (pp. 265–289). New York: Guilford Press.

Boivin, M., Vitaro, F., & Gagnon, C. (1992). A reassessment of the self-perception profile for children: Factor structure, reliability and convergent validity of a French version among second through sixth grade children. *International Journal of Behavioral Development, 15*, 275–290.

Boivin, M., Vitaro, F., & Poulin, F. (2005). Peer relationships and the development of aggressive behavior in early childhood. In R. E. Tremblay, W. W. Hartup, & J. Archer (Eds.), *Developmental origins of aggression* (pp. 376–397). New York: Guilford Press.

Brendgen, M., Boivin, M., Vitaro, F., Bukowski, W. M., Dionne, G., Tremblay, R. E., et al. (2008). Linkages between children's and their friends' social and physical aggression: Evidence for a gene–environment interaction? *Child Development, 79*, 13–29.

Brendgen, M., Boivin, M., Vitaro, F., Girard, A., Dionne, G., & Pérusse, D. (2008). Gene–environment interaction between peer victimization and child aggression. *Development and Psychopathology, 20*, 455–471.

Brendgen, M., Vitaro, F., Turgeon, L., & Poulin, F. (2002). Assessing aggressive and depressed children's social relations with classmates and friends: A matter of perspective. *Journal of Abnormal Child Psychology, 30*, 609–624.

Bukowski, W. M., Brendgen, M., & Vitaro, F. (2007). Peers and socialization: Effects on externalizing and internalizing problems. In J. E. Grusec & P. D. Hastings (Eds.), *Handbook of socialization* (pp. 355–381). New York: Guilford Press.

Bullock, B. M., Deater-Deckard, K., & Leve, L. D. (2006). Deviant peer affiliation and problem behavior: A test of genetic and environmental influences. *Journal of Abnormal Child Psychology, 34*(1), 29–41.

Cillessen, A. H. N., & Mayeux, L. (2004). From censure to reinforcement: Developmental changes in the association between aggression and social status. *Child Development, 75*(1), 147–163.

Cleveland, H. H., Wiebe, R. P., & Rowe, D. C. (2005). Sources of exposure to smoking and drinking friends among adolescents: A behavioral–genetic evaluation. *Journal of Genetic Psychology, 166*(2), 153–169.

Coie, J. D., Dodge, K. A., & Coppotelli, H. (1982). Dimensions and types of social status: A cross-age perspective. *Developmental Psychology, 18*, 557–570.

Conger, K. J., & Conger, R. D. (1994). Differential parenting and change in sibling differences in delinquency. *Journal of Family Psychology, 8*, 287–302.

Crick, N. R., & Zahn-Waxler, C. (2003). The development of psychopathology in females and males: Current progress and future challenges. *Development and Psychopathology, 15*(3), 719–742.

Danby, S., & Thorpe, K. (2006). Compatibility and conflict: Negotiation of relationships by dizygotic same-sex twin girls. *Twin Research and Human Genetics, 9*(1), 103–112.

Daniels, D., & Plomin, R. (1985). Differential experiences of siblings in the same family. *Developmental Psychology, 21*, 747–760.

DiLalla, L. F. (2002). Behavior genetics of aggression in children: Review and future directions. *Developmental Review, 22*, 593–622.

Dunn, J., & Plomin, R. (1990). *Separate lives: Why siblings are so different.* New York: Basic Books.

Dunn, J., Stocker, C., & Plomin, R. (1990). Nonshared experiences within the family: Correlates of behavior problems in middle childhood. *Development and Psychopathology, 2*, 113–126.

Eaves, L. J., & Carbonneau, R. (1998). Recovering components of variance from differential ratings of behavior in pairs of relatives. *Developmental Psychology, 34*, 125–129.

Eisenberg, N., Fabes, R. A., Karbon, M., Murphy, B. C., Wosinski, M., Polazzi, L., et al. (1996). The relations of children's dispositional prosocial behavior to emotionality, regulation, and social functioning. *Child Development, 67*, 974–992.

Eley, T. C. (2001). From behavioral genetics to molecular genetics: Direct tests of genetic hypotheses for behavioral phenotypes. In K. Deater-Deckard & S. A. Petrill (Eds.), *Gene–environment processes in social behaviors and relationships* (pp. 57–75). New York: Haworth Press.

Falconer, D. S. (1989). *Introduction to quantitative genetics.* Essex, UK: Longman.

Fekkes, M., Pijpers, F. I. M., & Verloove-Vanhorick, S. P. (2005). Bullying: Who does what, when and where?: Involvement of children, teachers and parents in bullying behavior. *Health Education Research, 20*(1), 81–91.

Fox, N. A., Nichols, K. E., Henderson, H. A., Rubin, K., Schmidt, L., Hamer, D., et al. (2005). Evidence for a gene–environment interaction in predicting behavioral inhibition in middle childhood. *Psychological Science, 16*(12), 921–926.

Gilson, M. S., Hunt, C. B., & Rowe, D. C. (2001). The friends of siblings: A test of social homogamy vs. peer selection and influence. In K. Deater-Deckard & S. A. Petrill (Eds.), *Gene–environment processes in social behaviors and relationships* (pp. 205–224). New York: Haworth Press.

Guo, G. (2006). Genetic similarity shared by best friends among adolescents. *Twin Research and Human Genetics, 9*(1), 113–121.

Harris, J. R. (1998). *The nurture assumption.* New York: Free Press.

Harris, K. M., Florey, F., Tabor, J., Bearman, P. S., Jones, J., & Udry, J. R. (2003). *The National Longitudinal Study of Adolescent Health: Research design. Technical report.* Carolina Population Center, University of North Carolina, Chapel Hill.

Hodges, E. V. E., Malone, M. J., & Perry, D. G. (1997). Individual risk and social risk as interacting determinants of victimization in the peer group. *Developmental Psychology, 33*(6), 1032–1039.

Iervolino, A. C., Pike, A., Manke, B., Reiss, D., Hetherington, E. M., & Plomin, R. (2002). Genetic and environmental influences in adolescent peer socialization: Evidence from two genetically sensitive designs. *Child Development, 73*(1), 162–174.

Jaffee, S. R., Caspi, A., Moffitt, T. E., Dodge, K. A., Rutter, M., Taylor, A., et al. (2005). Nature × nurture: Genetic vulnerabilities interact with physical maltreatment to promote conduct problems. *Development and Psychopathology, 17*(1), 67–84.

Kendler, K. S., & Eaves, L. J. (1986). Models for the joint effect of genotype and environment on liability to psychiatric illness. *American Journal of Psychiatry, 143*(3), 279–289.

Kim-Cohen, J., Caspi, A., Taylor, A., Williams, B., Newcombe, R., Craig, I. W., et al. (2006). MAOA, maltreatment, and gene–environment interaction predicting children's mental health: New evidence and a meta-analysis. *Molecular Psychiatry, 11*(10), 903–913.

Lamarche, V., Brendgen, M., Boivin, M., Vitaro, F., Pérusse, D., & Dionne, G. (2006). Do friendships and sibling relationships provide protection against peer victimization in a similar way? *Social Development, 15*(3), 373–393.

Leadbeater, B. J., Boone, E. M., Sangster, N. A., & Mathieson, L. C. (2006). Sex differences in the personal costs and benefits of relational and physical aggression in high school. *Aggressive Behavior, 32*, 409–419.

Leve, L. D. L. (2001). Observation of externalizing behavior during a twin–friend discussion task. *Marriage and Family Review, 33*(2), 225–250.

Manke, B., McGuire, S., Reiss, D., & Hetherington, E. M. (1995). Genetic contributions to adolescents' extrafamilial social interactions: Teachers, best friends, and peers. *Social Development, 4*(3), 238–256.

McDougall, P., Hymel, S., Vaillancourt, T., & Mercer, L. (2001). The consequences of childhood peer rejection. In M. Leary (Ed.), *Interpersonal rejection* (pp. 213–247). New York: Oxford University Press.

McGuire, S., Manke, B., Saudino, K. J., Reiss, D., Hetherington, E. M., & Plomin, R. (1999). Perceived competence and self-worth during adolescence: A longitudinal behavioral genetic study. *Child Development, 70*(6), 1283–1296.

McHale, S. M., Crouter, A. C., McGuire, S., & Updegraff, K. A. (1995). Congruence between mothers' and fathers' differential treatment of siblings: Links with family relations and children's well-being. *Child Development, 66*, 116–128.

Moffitt, T. E. (2005). The new look of behavioral genetics in developmental psychopathology: Gene–environment interplay in antisocial behaviors. *Psychological Bulletin, 131*(4), 533–554.

Moffitt, T. E., Caspi, A., & Rutter, M. (2005). Strategy for investigating interactions between measured genes and measured environments. *Archives of General Psychiatry, 62*, 473–481.

Neale, M. C., & Cardon, L. R. (1992). *Methodology for genetic studies of twins and families.* Dortrecht, the Netherlands: Kluwer Academic.

Newman, R. S., & Murray, B. J. (2005). How students and teachers view the seriousness of peer harassment: When is it appropriate to seek help? *Journal of Educational Psychology, 97*(3), 347–365.

O'Connor, T. G., Jenkins, J. M., Hewitt, J., DeFries, J. C., & Plomin, R. (2001). Longitudinal connections between parenting and peer relationships in adoptive and biological families. In K. Deater-Deckard & S. A. Petrill (Eds.), *Gene–environment processes in social behaviors and relationships* (pp. 251–271). New York: Haworth Press.

Petrill, S. A. (2002). Examining social behavior and relationships using genetically sensitive designs: An introduction. *Marriage and Family Review, 33*(1), 3–10.

Pike, A., & Atzaba-Poria, N. (2003). Do sibling and friend relationships share the same temperamental origins?: A twin study. *Journal of Child Psychology and Psychiatry and Allied Disciplines, 44*(4), 598–611.

Pike, A., Manke, B., Reiss, D., & Plomin, R. (2000). A genetic analysis of differential experiences of adolescent siblings across three years. *Social Development, 9*, 96–114.

Plomin, R., DeFries, J. C., & Loehlin, J. C. (1977). Genotype–environment interaction and correlation in the analysis of human behavior. *Psychological Bulletin, 84*, 309–322.

Plomin, R., & Rutter, M. (1998). Child development, molecular genetics, and what to do with the genes once they are found. *Child Development, 69*, 1223–1242.

Rose, R. J. (2002). How do adolescents select their friends?: A behavior–genetic perspective. In L. Pulkkinen & A. Caspi (Eds.), *Paths to successful development: Personality in the life course* (pp. 106–125). New York: Cambridge University Press.

Rutter, M., & Silberg, J. (2002). Gene–environment interplay in relation to emotional and behavioral disturbance. *Annual Review of Psychology, 53*(1), 463–490.

Salmivalli, C., Kaukiainen, A., & Voeten, M. (2005). Anti-bullying intervention: Implementation and outcome. *The British Journal of Educational Psychology, 75*(3), 465–487.

Scarr, S., & McCartney, K. (1983). How people make their own environments: A theory of genotype–environment effects. *Child Development, 54*(2), 424–435.

Thorpe, K., & Gardner, K. (2006). Twins and their friendships: Differences between monozygotic, dizygotic, same-sex, and dizygotic mixed-sex pairs. *Twin Research and Human Genetics, 9*(1), 155–164.

Van Lier, P., Boivin, M., Dionne, G., Vitaro, F., Brendgen, M., Koot, H., et al. (2007). Kindergarten children's genetic vulnerabilities interact with friends' aggression to promote children's own aggression. *Journal of the American Academy of Child and Adolescent Psychiatry, 46*, 1080–1087.

Vitaro, F., Brendgen, M., & Tremblay, R. E. (2001). Preventive intervention: Assessing its effects on the trajectories of delinquency and testing for mediational processes. *Applied Developmental Science, 5*, 201–213.

Walden, B., McGue, M., Iacono, W. G., Burt, S. A., & Elkins, I. (2004). Identifying shared environmental contributions to early substance use: The respective roles of peers and parents. *Journal of Abnormal Psychology, 113*(3), 440–450.

Zuckerman, M. (1999). *Vulnerability to psychopathology: A biosocial model.* Washington, DC: American Psychological Association.

CHAPTER 26

Temperament, Self-Regulation, and Peer Social Competence

NANCY EISENBERG
JULIE VAUGHAN
CLAIRE HOFER

The quality of children's peer interactions is undoubtedly affected by a variety of factors, including heredity, children's dispositional characteristics, and environmental influences, such as parenting and interactions with peers and teachers (Rubin, Bukowski, & Parker, 2006). In this chapter, we summarize the literature on the relations of children's temperament-based characteristics to children's peer acceptance, quality of peer interactions and related social skills, and friendships.

Relevant Theory

Temperament and Its Components

"Temperament" refers to individual differences in reactivity and self-regulation and is believed to be influenced by genetics, other constitutional factors, and environmental factors (Rothbart & Bates, 2006). It is widely believed to contribute to the development of personality, defined as "patterns of thoughts, emotion and behavior that show consistency across situations and stability over time" (Rothbart & Bates, 2006, p. 100). By childhood, temperament and personality are difficult to differentiate, although personality is believed to include a wider range of individual differences in feeling, thinking, and behaving than temperament (Caspi & Shiner, 2006). In this chapter, we use the term "temperament" when we refer to research involving measures of that construct and "personality" when researchers have used measures that typify that body of work (e.g., measures of the "Big Five" personality characteristics).

Although there are multiple models of temperament, that of Mary Rothbart is currently the most influential. In her model, *regulation* and *reactivity* are the two primary dimensions (e.g., Rothbart & Bates, 2006). The core of temperamental regulation is effortful control (EC), defined as "the efficiency of executive attention—including the ability to inhibit a dominant response and/or to activate a subdominant response, to plan, and to detect errors" (Rothbart & Bates, 2006, p. 129). EC includes skills such as the abilities to shift and focus attention as needed, to adapt and to activate and to inhibit behavior as needed, especially when one does not feel like doing so; these skills are involved in integrating information, planning, and modulating emotion and behavior. Reactivity "refers to the arousability of motor, affective, and sensory response systems" (Rothbart, Ahadi, Hershey, & Fisher, 2001, p. 1395), and includes "responsiveness to change in the external and internal environment" (Rothbart & Bates, 2006, p. 100). It includes emotions such as fear, anger, and sadness; positive affect; and behavioral tendencies such as impulsivity, shyness, and behavioral inhibition.

An aspect of temperament in some models is "adaptability," or the ability to adjust to new situations; a related construct, "soothability," is the ability to recover from emotional arousal (often with external assistance; Rothbart et al., 2001). Conceptually, soothability seems to tap both regulatory skills and emotionality, but in Rothbart et al.'s (2001) research, it loads more heavily (but inversely) with negative emotionality than with EC. "Sociability" and "shyness," or behavioral inhibition, are also assessed in some measures of temperament (e.g., Buss & Plomin, 1975), although only shyness and a positive approach to things (including people) are included in the Rothbart et al. (2001) measure of temperament, and behavioral inhibition is often measured observationally (e.g., Kagan & Fox, 2006).

The interrelations among components of temperament vary with the particular measurement scale, and with the age of the child and perhaps the type of culture (e.g., see Rothbart & Bates, 1998, 2006). Rothbart et al. (2001) found three factors: (1) negative affectivity, including emotions such as anger, fear, sadness, and discomfort, as well as low soothability; (2) extraversion/surgency, including high-intensity pleasure, positive anticipation, impulsivity, high activity level, and low shyness (and to some degree, high levels of smiling/laugher); and (3) EC, including attention focusing, inhibitory control, low-intensity pleasure, perceptual sensitivity, and often smiling/laughter.

In this chapter, we review the relations of temperament and closely related aspects of personality to indices of functioning with peers, including sociometric status, the quality of peer interactions and social skills, and the quality or quantity of friendships. We focus primarily on self-regulatory capacities (EC) and emotionality, although we review more briefly other aspects of temperament and sometimes personality, including sociability, shyness/behavioral inhibition, and activity level. First, we discuss reasons to expect relations of temperament–personality to children's and adolescents' peer relationships and interactions. Then we review relations of temperament and personality to EC/self-regulation, negative emotionality, positive emotionality, sociability or shyness/behavioral inhibition, and composite or less studied aspects of temperament. Our review is illustrative, and we focus primarily on measures of social status and observed or reported quality of peer/friend interactions, and less on global indices of children's social competence—often reported by parents or teachers—that probably tap more than competence with peers.

Central Issues and Relevant Research

Relations of Temperament–Personality to Peer Competence and Status

Because temperament and personality include characteristics of the child that are relatively stable over time, it is logical that they should relate to individual differences in social skills and social relationships (e.g., Asendorpf & van Aken, 2003a; see Figure 26.1). Children tend to want to be with others who express positive emotion (Halberstadt, Denham,

& Dunsmore, 2001; Lyubomirsky, King, & Diener, 2005; Sroufe, Schork, Motti, Lawroski, & LaFreniere, 1985) and to avoid those who characteristically express negative emotion (Furr & Funder, 1998). Positive emotionality broadens the scope of attention and cognitive flexibility (Fredrickson & Branigan, 2005), which is likely to result in more socially skilled behavior. In addition, people who are well-regulated generally act in more appropriate ways (see Eisenberg, Fabes, Guthrie, & Reiser, 2000) and are low in aggression (e.g., Dodge, Coie, & Lynam, 2006), which tends to foster relatively positive peer relationships (Rubin, Bukowski, et al., 2006). They are also more likely to behave in constructive rather than inappropriate ways when angered (Eisenberg, Fabes, Nyman, Bernzweig, & Pinuelas, 1994). Children who are not overly controlled (inhibited) and rigid in their behavior are viewed by adults as socially competent and socially appropriate (Eisenberg et al., 2000; Spinrad et al., 2006). In addition, children who are sociable rather than shy would be expected to have less trouble interacting with peers.

Personality characteristics predict getting along with peers. For example, children who are high in EC tend to be high in agreeableness (Cumberland-Li, Eisenberg, & Reiser, 2004), and more agreeable children are better liked by peers (Jensen-Campbell, Adams, et al., 2002; Jensen-Campbell & Malcolm, 2007) and deal more constructively with interpersonal conflict (Jensen-Campbell, Gleason, Adams, & Malcolm, 2003).

In summary, in general, we would expect temperament to feed into personality, and that both temperament and personality would predict children's status with peers, quality of their friendships, and the quality children's behaviors with peers and friends in social interactions (see Figure 26.1). Moreover, the quality of children's peer relationships is likely to affect aspects of children's functioning, such as loneliness and self-esteem, which Asendorpf and van Aken (2003a) labeled as surface rather than core (i.e., basic temperament–personality) characteristics. Nonetheless, over time, it is plausible that negative peer experiences increase children's feelings of anger, frustration, and sadness, which might affect their self-regulation and attempts to interact with new or known peers. If this is true, peer interactions might have an effect on aspects of functioning that are typically measured by indices of temperament or personality (although this relation is not depicted in Figure 26.1).

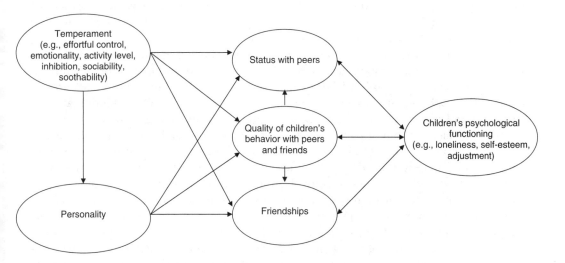

FIGURE 26.1. Conceptual model of the relations between temperament and peer relations.

Self-Regulation/Effortful Control and Impulsivity

Many researchers examining temperamental aspects of self-regulation have used questionnaire or behavioral indices believed to tap aspects of children's EC, including the abilities to manage attention, willfully inhibit or activate behavior as needed to be appropriate, delay gratification, and persist on frustrating tasks. These measures vary considerably based on when the study was conducted and the age of the children. Although impulsivity likely reflects behavioral reactivity rather than EC (Eisenberg et al., 2004), investigators often have not tried, or been able to, differentiate EC from impulsivity, and these constructs tend to be negatively correlated. Thus, we do not attempt to differentiate between the two constructs in this review.

Sociometric Status

Even during the preschool years, children who are viewed by adults as well regulated—for example, high in EC and behavioral self-control and/or low in task distractibility—generally are relatively well liked rather than rejected by peers (e.g., Gunnar, Sebanc, Tout, Donzella, & van Dulmen, 2003; Maszk, Eisenberg, & Guthrie, 1999; Walker, Berthelsen, & Irving, 2001). For example, Olson and Lifgren (1988) found that behavioral measures of low regulation and high impulsivity were correlated with concurrent negative nominations from preschool peers. In that study, high levels of positive peer nominations and/or low levels of negative nominations also predicted high self-regulation and low impulsivity on the tasks a year later—a finding that highlights the possibility that popular children have more opportunities to develop their self-regulation.

Often constructive coping has been viewed as indicative of self-regulation. Fabes and Eisenberg (1992) found that popular preschool girls were likely to cope with anger by expressing their disapproval of the provocateur and unlikely to cope with anger by venting emotion or seeking revenge. Popular boys were likely to cope with their anger by actively resisting (i.e., attempting physically or verbally to defend one's position, possessions, or self-esteem in nonaggressive ways) or expressing their disapproval of the provocateur, and were relatively unlikely to seek adult assistance when angered. Similarly, Eisenberg et al. (1994) found that preschoolers observed to use constructive methods of dealing with real-life anger were better liked by peers. Thus, preschoolers who are well liked by peers tend to use constructive means of coping.

Among elementary schoolers, similar findings have been obtained. For example, Wilson (2003) found that popular and prosocial kindergartners and first graders exhibited less difficulty shifting attention from negative to positive affect and were better able to regulate their behavior after experiencing social failure. In a study of Swiss kindergartners, children's and adults' (combined) reports of high impulsivity/inattention were related to sociometric rejection, but not acceptance (Perren, Von Wyl, Stadelmann, Burgin, & Von Klitzing, 2006). In a study of kindergartners to third graders, children rated as high in attentional EC were well liked by peers and perceived as popular by teachers; those who scored relatively high on reactive control rather than impulsivity were rated as socially appropriate/prosocial by both peers and adults (Eisenberg et al., 1997; also see Ollendick, Weist, Borden, & Greene [1992] for a focus on attentional problems and peer rejection, and Mostow, Izard, Fine, & Trentacosta [2002], who used a more inclusive measure of self-control). In a study of fourth graders, McDowell and Parke (2005) found that children who exhibited positive emotion when they received a disappointing gift scored high in positive peer nominations (an aggregate of being liked, having good sense of humor, and prosociality), whereas those who exhibited negative emotion scored relatively high in negative peer nominations (being disliked, sad, and spending time alone). Because inhibition of negative emotion and displays of positive emotion when one is disappointed are considered to be demonstrations of self-regulation, these findings support a connection between regulation and peer status (see also Graziano, Keane, & Calkins, 2007). This conclusion also applies to children in another culture. Thus, Eisenberg, Pidada, and Liew (2001) found that adult-reported, low EC was related to negative peer evaluations (being disliked, fighting) for Indonesian third graders, whereas high EC was related to positive peer nominations (being liked, prosociality). Findings were similar 3 years later, although significant effects held only for boys (Eisenberg et al., 2004).

Few researchers have examined the relation of EC to peer competence in adolescence. The personality trait of conscientiousness is believed partly to reflect self-regulation and to be linked to EC (Caspi & Shiner, 2006); indeed, measures of EC and conscientiousness are related (e.g., Jensen-Campbell, Rosselini, et al., 2002). Thus, it is not surprising that Jensen-Campbell and Malcolm (2007) found that a composite score of self-, teacher-, and parent-rated conscientiousness related positively to peers' ratings of liking in a sample of adolescents.

Quality of Peer Interactions

EC/self-regulation frequently has been associated with high-quality interactions with peers. For example, several researchers have reported a positive relation between teacher-reported self-regulation and social competence (Brody, Murray, Kim, & Brown, 2002; Eisenberg et al., 2000; Spinrad et al., 2006). Others have found a positive relation between teacher reports of self-regulation (e.g., emotion regulation) and children's peer interaction (e.g., high play interaction, low play disruption, and low play disconnection; Fantuzzo, Sekino, & Cohen, 2004; see also Fabes, Martin, Hanish, Anders, & Madden-Derdich, 2003; Izard et al., 2008).

Relatedly, ratings of observed self-regulation (using a Q-sort method) are positively related to adult-reported interactive peer play and negatively related to adult-reported disruptive and disconnected play behaviors (Fantuzzo, Perry, & McDermott, 2004). Eisenberg et al. (1993) reported that boys' attentional control was positively related to observers' ratings of boy's global social skills, whereas Zhou, Eisenberg, Wang, and Reiser (2004) found that EC was related to peers' ratings of sociability among Chinese children.

Other researchers have used observations to assess the quality of peer interactions. For example, Fabes et al. (1999) found a positive relation between EC and a composite of observed socially competent behaviors (e.g., helping others, being friendly). Similarly, David and Murphy (2007) found that EC predicted low levels of problematic peer behaviors (including observed hostility, negative affect, and provocative behavior during peer interactions and teacher-rated low social competence).

Sometimes contextual variables moderate relations of EC with measures of peer relationships. For example, Deynoot-Schaub and Riksen-Walraven (2006) noted no first-order relation between children's play behaviors (e.g., positive and negative initiatives, involved and uninvolved play) during free play with peers and parent-reported difficult temperament (low self-regulation combined with high negative emotionality). However, when the quality of day care was considered, they found a negative relation between difficult temperament and the initiation of play with peers within low-quality day care centers (there were no differences among children in high-quality child care centers). Analogously, Li-Grining, Votruba-Drzal, Bachman, and Chase-Lansdale (2006) found that preschoolers with high EC were rated as exhibiting greater social competence than children with lower EC if their mothers experienced job loss or entered the welfare system (but not when they left welfare or entered work). Thus, temperament may be more likely to be associated with peer competence in stressful contexts.

Social Solitude

In a study of the lack of peer interaction, Spinrad et al. (2004) found that EC was positively related to children's observed reticence (i.e., not playing or being involved in any activity) with peers and negatively related to a change in solitary play (i.e., engaging in some activity alone) from early to later in the school year. Other researchers have argued that some forms of solitary play are common for preschool-age children and therefore, even well-regulated children would be likely to engage in this type of play behavior (see Rubin, Coplan, Fox, & Calkins, 1995). Spinrad et al. (2004) suggested that solitary play might be less socially appropriate than the other types of play during outdoor play and might in turn be related to low levels of children's EC. In fact, Spinrad et al. found that children who engaged in reticent activity were relatively well liked by peers, whereas those who were high in solitary play were less well liked by their peers.

Aggression

Aggressive behavior that is sustained across childhood tends to be associated with problems in attention and impulsivity. For example, Wilson (2006) found that children who were labeled by their peers as aggressive–rejected were more impulsive (as rated by parents) than nonaggressive–popular children and made more inappropriate attempts at engaging in social interactions with their classmates (e.g., taking another's toy, making demands, exhibiting aggression) than nonaggressive–popular children. Similarly, victimization by peers is associated with youths' attentional problems (Jensen-Campbell & Malcolm, 2007). Thus, it is likely that EC affects children's aggression (see Eisenberg et al., 2000, 2004), which in turn influences the quality of their interactions and relationships with peers.

Quantity and Quality of Friendships

A distinction has been made between the general quality of peer relationships and friendships. Both the quantity and quality of friendships are considered important. When investigating friendship quality, researchers often focus on the dimensions of intimacy, companionship, and emotional and social support (Rubin, Wojslawowicz, Rose-Krasnor, Booth-LaForce, & Burgess, 2006).

Walden, Lemerise, and Smith (1999) found an inverse relation between emotion dysregulation (an aggregate of teachers' ratings of low regulation and high affective intensity and emotional expressivity) and number of reciprocated preschool friendships. In another study of young children (ages 3–5 years), Gleason, Gower, Hohmann, and Gleason (2005) found that the children who were most frequently nominated by peers as friends were also viewed by teachers as high on impulsivity and soothability. The finding with soothability is logical: Children who score high on soothability are well-regulated, a characteristic that favors positive social interactions and likely increases attractiveness as a friend. However, the finding regarding impulsivity was less expected. The researchers highlighted the fact that impulsivity is not always related to negative outcomes, and that children high on a nondisruptive type of impulsivity might be noticed by other kids and, therefore, likely to be picked as friends. Indeed, in preschool and early school-age children, impulsivity and resiliency tend to be positively related, and resilient children are viewed by teachers as popular (e.g., Cumberland-Li et al., 2004; Spinrad et al., 2006). However, when impulsivity is part of a pattern of hyperactivity, inattention, and conduct problems, it appears to be associated with a dearth of friends (Gresham, MacMillan, Bocian, Ward, & Forness, 1998). Finally, in a study of adolescents, Jensen-Campbell and Malcolm (2007) found a relation between adult-reported attentional problems and low number of reciprocated friendships and self-reports of low-quality friendships.

Negative Emotion

Children's dispositional negative emotionality and its intensity have been fairly consistently related to children's sociometric status. This may be because the ability to modulate strong emotions, such as anger within peer encounters, is likely to aid the child in conflict management and the maintenance of social activity (see Eisenberg et al., 1994). Expressions of anger are likely to elicit antagonism and rejection from peers. In addition, unsociable children who are poor emotion regulators appear to be more behaviorally anxious, wary, reticent, and prone to internalizing problems (Rubin et al., 1995), all of which may undermine children's social relationships and status with peers.

Sociometric Status and Rated Popularity

An inverse association between children's negative emotionality and peer acceptance has been found in studies of preschoolers (e.g., Eisenberg et al., 1993; for boys only) (Maszk et al., 1999; Stocker & Dunn, 1990) and adolescents (Dodge, Coie, Pettit, & Price, 1990; Fabes & Eisenberg, 1992). Moreover, in a meta-analysis, Newcomb, Bukowski, and Pattee (1993) reported that a combination of anger/hostility and negative behavior was related to social rejection across the years of childhood.

Whereas some researchers have found that internalizing behaviors, such as depression and anxiety, predict social status (Olson & Lifgren, 1988; Perren et al., 2006), others have not (e.g., Ollendick, Weist, Borden, & Greene, 1992). Nonetheless, in their meta-analysis, Newcomb et al. (1993) found that anxiety and depression were associated with peer rejection. Although anxiety, depression, and anger may reflect responses to the environment, including reactions to peer rejection, these emotions appear to have a temperamental and personality basis in negative emotionality (and the personality trait of neuroticism; Caspi & Shiner, 2006).

The aforementioned studies were conducted in Western cultures. However, similar findings have been obtained elsewhere. For example, parents' and teachers' reports of third-grade Indonesian children's negative emotional intensity were positively related to peers' negative nominations (disliked, fights) and negatively related to positive peer nominations (liked, prosocial). In addition, peer-rated child anger was substantially positively related to negative peer nominations (Eisenberg, Pidada, & Liew, 2001). Three years later, the findings were weaker, although teacher- and peer-rated negative emotionally were still related to peer rejection for boys (Eisenberg et al., 2004).

Quality of Peer Interactions

Negative emotionality also has been related to the *reported* quality of peer interaction. For example, in a study of older elementary school children, Murphy, Shepard, Eisenberg, and Fabes (2004) found a negative relation between negative emotionality and social competence; Zhou et al. (2004) found that anger/frustration was related to low levels of social competence and sociability/leadership among Chinese children. More recently, Jensen-Campbell and Malcolm (2007) reported that adolescents' emotional stability (low negative emotionality) and peer victimization were inversely related, even after they controlled for sex and age.

Other researchers have examined negative emotionality as a correlate or predictor of *observed* peer interaction. Fabes et al. (1999) found that children who displayed more negative emotion during the peer interactions also exhibited less socially competent behavior (e.g., helping others, being friendly) than children who were not as negatively expressive, and negative emotionality appeared to mediate the relation between teacher-reported regulation and children's observed social behavior. In another study, Fabes, Hanish, Martin, and Eisenberg (2002) reported that preschoolers who were high in teacher-rated dispositional negative emotionality engaged in more solitary play over time, which likely served to isolate them from peers. Similarly, Ladd and Profilet (1996) found that preschool children who were rated as anxious–fearful by their teachers were low in observed positive and aggressive interactions with peers and high in nonsocial behaviors.

Rubin et al. (1995) examined the relation of children's observed play behaviors (e.g., social wariness and disruptiveness) with same-sex peers and parent-reported emotional reactivity. They created groups based on children's social interaction styles (observed group play and peer conversation) and parent-reported negative emotionality/low soothability. Children in the low social engagement/emotion *dysregulation* group were higher in observed social wariness (and had more internalizing problems) than the low social engagement/emotion *regulation* and average groups.

Some researchers have assessed specific types of negative emotions. For example, Diener and Kim (2004) asked parents to rate preschoolers' anger proneness. They found that boys' (not girls') anger proneness was negatively related to their prosocial behaviors, positively related to their aggressive behaviors, and unrelated to social withdrawal. Similarly, in a study of elementary school children, observed anger and observed sadness were negatively related to teacher-reported social competence for boys, but not for girls. However, parent-reported negative emotional intensity was negatively related to teacher-reported social competence for both sexes, and both observed and teacher-reported affective balance (positive vs. negative emotionality) were positively related to social competence (Jones, Eisenberg, Fabes, & MacKinnon, 2002). In a study of preschoolers (Spinrad et al., 2004), a composite of observed and adult-reported anger was negatively related to observed reticence (onlooking, unoccupied play); parent-reported anxious–fearful emotionality was positively related to reticence early in the school year, whereas adult-reported (teacher and parent) anxious–fearful emotionality tended to be related to solitary play later in the school year.

Not all researchers have found significant negative relations between children's negative emotionality and quality of peer interactions. For example, Dunn and Cutting (1999) did not find a relation between negative emotionality and a number of children's observed play behaviors (i.e., connected conversation, conflict, and cooperative pretend play), but they found a positive relation between coordinated play and negative emotionality. Moreover, Eisenberg et al. (1993) found nonsignificant relations between adult-reported quantity and intensity of negative emotionality and observers' ratings of children's social skills. Blair, Denham, Kochanoff, and Whipple (2004) also reported that children's parent-reported irritability/soothability and sadness were unrelated to teacher-reported social competence (e.g., comforting and assisting peers in difficulty, taking the other child's viewpoint). Results probably vary not only as a consequence of sample size, but also based on the type of peer interaction assessed and the method of measurement.

Quality and Quantity of Friendships

In studies of young children, Dunn and colleagues reported that indices of negative emotionality were associated with negative markers of friendship. For example, Dunn and Cutting (1999) observed several aspects of the interactions between two close friends: joint pretense, frequency of play other than joint pretense, conflict, communication failure and success, and amity (the sharing of amusement and positive affect). They found that mother-reported negative emotionality related to communication failure (failed bids). Furthermore, negative emotionality related to less amity displayed in the children's interactions. Supporting these findings, Pellegrini, Galda, Flor, Bartini, and Charak (1997) found that children's high reactivity (including not only negative emotionality but also distractibility, persistence, and activity) was related to high levels of both observed conflict and resolution between friends while engaging in both a writing task and a play context. Children who were emotionally dysregulated appeared not only to have more conflicts but also tended to resolve conflicts more often, likely because they had more opportunities to do so. And similarly, Pike and Atzaba-Poria (2003) found that negative emotionality related positively to 12–15-year-old twins' reports of conflict and betrayal on a friendship quality questionnaire.

Positive Emotion

Although Denham et al. (2003) found that the ability to express an array of emotions during play predicted children's social competence 1 year later, it is children's positive emotionality that seems to be most often positively related to their social competence, especially across time. In several studies of children ranging widely in age, researchers have reported positive relations between the expression of positive affect and child and adolescent popularity, sociability, social competence, and dominance in the peer group (Izard et al., 2008; Jones et al., 2002; LaFreniere & Sroufe, 1985; Lengua, 2002). Moreover, children who are relatively low in observed positive affect at school tend to play alone or to be reticent to enter into play with peers (Spinrad et al., 2004).

It is likely that high-intensity positive emotion has mixed relations with peer competence. High levels of positive emotion in situations where it may reflect exuberance have been linked to low regulation (Kochanska, Murray, & Harlan, 2000). In addition, parent-reported exuberance has been linked to externalizing problems in the preschool and elementary school years, as well as low prosocial behavior in preschool (Rydell, Berlin, & Bohlin, 2003), whereas parent-reported high-intensity pleasure has been associated with externalizing problems in preadolescence (Oldehinkel, Hartman, de Winter, Veenstra, & Ormel, 2004). Children who are prone to high-intensity pleasure are also likely to be impulsive and to have high activity levels (Rothbart et al., 2001), so that they may often behave inappropriately with peers. Thus, it is important to consider the measure of positive emotionality and to examine whether positive affect is well-regulated.

Sociability and Behavioral Inhibition

Although sociability and behavioral inhibition/shyness are conceptually related, these constructs are not simply two sides of a coin. Caspi and Shiner (2006) suggested that sociability is a pure marker of extraversion, whereas social inhibition is a more complex blend of low extraversion and high fear or anxiety in the presence of novel situations. Moreover, others note the importance of differentiating among shyness, social disinterest, and social avoidance (e.g., Coplan & Armer, 2007; Rubin & Coplan, 2004). However, the two constructs are related. For example, Fox, Henderson, Rubin, Calkins, and Schmidt (2001) found that mothers rated as shy and socially fearful young children who scored high on measures of behavioral inhibition (to unfamiliar social and/or nonsocial stimuli) and were stable in their behavioral inhibition over the first years of life, whereas they rated continuously uninhibited children as sociable and low in shyness.

Sociability and inhibition/shyness have obvious implications for peer interactions: Sociable children are more likely than behaviorally inhibited or shy individuals to have interactions with peers. As would be expected, sociable children tend to be liked by peers (Skarpness & Carson, 1986) and to engage in positive interactions with them (Eisenberg, Cameron, Tryon, & Dodez, 1981), whereas shy, inhibited children are less popular, and often rejected, especially as they move through the elementary school years (see Rubin, Bowker, & Kennedy, Chapter 17, this volume).

Measures of sociability or extraversion, shyness, and behavioral inhibition also have been associated with observed or reported play behavior with peers, with many findings in the expected direction. Even at age 2, parent-rated approach versus avoidance tendencies (e.g., anger proneness vs. social fearfulness) have been associated with agonistic behaviors (e.g., grabbing, pushing) with peers (Rubin, Burgess, Dwyer, & Hastings, 2003). Asendorpf and van Aken (2003b) found that children rated as extraverted by their teachers at multiple aggregated assessments at ages 4–6 years exhibited less inhibited behavior when interacting with peers at preschool or kindergarten. Similarly, preschoolers reported by teachers to be withdrawn rather than approach-oriented have also been reported to display withdrawn and avoidant behavior during play (Coplan & Rubin, 1998; Mendez, Fantuzzo, & Cicchetti, 2002). Moreover, preschoolers observed to be asocial with peers are reported by teachers to be excluded by their peers (Ladd & Profilet, 1996). Also, elementary school children who scored high on a behavioral inhibition scale were less likely to ask an unknown peer to play and were rated by parents (but not teachers) as low in social competence (Van Brakel, Muris, & Bogels, 2004). Henderson, Marshall, Fox, and Rubin (2004) found that 4-year-old children who were reticent in their observed play with unfamiliar peers (i.e., in the company of unfamiliar peers, taking a long time to respond to others, remaining unoccupied, and carefully watching the activities of others) were viewed by their mothers as socially fearful at 2 years of age.

A few investigators have examined the relations of temperamental shyness, inhibition, and sociability to the quality of friendships. Dunn and Cutting (1999) found shyness to be related to a lack of responsiveness with friends. Pellegrini et al. (1997) found that inhibition was positively related to high conflict and high levels of resolution while children engaged in a writing task and in play with a friend; this relation was reversed for nonfriends. Finally, Rubin, Wojslawowicz, et al. (2006) reported that friendship quality of shy 10- and 11-year-old children was lower than that of their non-shy agemates.

In regard to sociability, Pike and Atzaba-Poria (2003) found that highly sociable children had high-quality friendships; moreover, their friendships were less conflicted. Stocker and Dunn (1990) found that children's sociability (as reported by mothers and, to some extent, teachers) was associated with closer, more positive, less hostile, and less negative relationships with best friends. Jensen-Campbell and Malcolm (2007) found that extraversion was positively related to adolescents' reports of the quality of their friendships, but not to either the number of friendships or general peer status (also see Jensen-Campbell, Adams, et al., 2002). Similarly, Asendorpf and van Aken (2003a) found that extraversion at age 12 was correlated with perceived support from school friends and nonschool friends at age 17; moreover, extraversion predicted nonschool friends' support at age 17 (but perceived peer support did not predict extraversion over time). Their analyses suggested that extraversion, which reflects temperamental sociability, predicts the quality of later friendships, but that friendships have a minimal effect on personality.

The relation of social inhibition/shyness and sociability with indices of peer relationships may vary as a function of culture and historical time and place (see Chen, Chung, & Hsiao, Chapter 24, this volume). Consistent with this argument, Chen and colleagues initially argued that in traditional Chinese culture, shy, sensitive, and restrained behavior traditionally has been considered indicative of social accomplishment and maturity; their initial findings indicated that shyness was associated with measures of social competence and peer acceptance (Chen, Rubin, & Sun, 1992; Chen, Rubin, & Li, 1995). However, other researchers found that, similar to children in Western cultures, socially withdrawn Chinese children were unpopular with peers (Chang et al., 2005; Hart et al., 2000; Schwartz, Chang, & Farver, 2001). In their most recent follow-up, Chen, Cen, Li, and He (2005) reported similar findings and suggested that Chinese culture has become Westernized in recent years, with the consequence that assertiveness is now valued, whereas inhibited behavior is not.

Activity Level, Adaptability, and Global Temperament

Some researchers have examined the relation of activity level and/or adaptability to children's social competence. For example, Mendez et al. (2002) found that African American Head Start children's activity level (i.e., motoric vigor) and low adaptability (ease and skill with which one adjusts to new situations) were positively related to teacher-reported aggressive and antisocial play behavior, and negatively related to creative, cooperative, and helpful play behavior. Moreover, adaptability was related to low levels of "play disconnection" (withdrawn and avoidant behavior during play). In addition, Pike and Atzaba-Poria (2003) found that activity level related to all positive aspects of friendship quality (validation and caring, conflict resolution, help and guidance, companionship and recreation, and intimate exchange). Gleason et al. (2005) suggested that these findings may differ for boys and girls. They found that boys chose friends with a higher activity level, whereas girls chose friends with a relatively lower activity level. This finding is consistent with the argument that girls and boys typically gravitate toward styles of play consistent with their "cultures" (calmer, inside play for girls; outside, high-activity play for boys; Fabes et al., 2003; Maccoby, 1998).

A number of researchers have constructed global measures of difficult temperament. Preschoolers with a difficult temperament are less well accepted by their peers

(Szewczyk-Sokolowski, Bost, & Wainwright, 2005). McCoy, Brody, and Stoneman (2002) found that difficult temperament (based on mothers' and fathers' ratings of children's activity, emotional intensity, and low persistence) in 4- to 11-year-old boys was related to discord with their best friends 5 years later. For girls, the relation between having a difficult temperament and low quality of best friendships was evident only if they had a relationship with their older sister that was low in warmth (for support in the friendship) or high in conflict (for discord in the friendship). In addition, Criss, Pettit, Bates, Dodge, and Lapp (2002) found a negative relation between mother-reported resistant temperament (e.g., ignoring directives, getting upset when removed from something in which he or she is interested but should not be getting into) and both sociometric status and the number of reciprocated friendships in 5-year-old children.

Finally, Rubin et al. (2003) constructed an index of emotion dysregulation that reflected global difficult temperament (i.e., social fearfulness; anger proneness; and reverse-coded pleasure expression, activity level, and interest–persistence). They found a positive relation between their measure of emotion dysregulation and children's observed conflict initiations and aggression during peer interactions.

Future Directions and Conclusions

In summary, from the literature reviewed herein, it may be concluded that dispositional self-regulation, including EC, is positively associated with peer acceptance, socially competent behavior, and friendship quality. In contrast, negative emotionality and global measures of difficult temperament tend to be negatively related to a variety of measures of peer competence. Positive emotionality generally is positively related to peer status and competence; however, high-intensity positive emotionality, including exuberance, is related to relatively high levels of maladaptive behavior (externalizing problems) and low levels of prosocial behavior with peers, likely because it reflects lack of regulation.

Whereas sociability generally has been positively associated with peer status and competence, behavioral inhibition and shyness often have been negatively related to peer acceptance and social competence. However, findings in regard to inhibition are less clear than for some other aspects of temperament because inhibition may increasingly become socially detrimental with age and may be less problematic for children in some cultures than others.

One question that merits examination is whether the potential effects of children's temperament on the quality of peer interactions and relationships are moderated by the temperaments of their social partners. It is possible that negative temperamental characteristics, such as low regulation and high negative emotionality, are viewed more favorably by children with similar characteristics, and that children similar in temperamental characteristics are more likely to be friends. Gleason et al. (2005) reported that the similarity in temperament between the two friends did not increase the likelihood of being nominated as friends, whereas Dunn and Cutting (1999) and Rubin, Wojslawowicz, et al. (2006) found similarities in friends' temperaments. Thus, it is important to examine the moderating influence of peers' dispositional characteristics in future work. Moreover, the temperament–personality of peer partners may contribute to the quality of their interactions (Jensen-Campbell, Gleason, Adams, & Malcolm, 2003).

In addition, moderating variables, such as sex and age, have not been explicitly examined. Fabes, Shepard, Guthrie, and Martin (1997) found that arousable boys, but not girls, who engaged in relatively high levels of same-sex play were likely to exhibit problem behaviors at preschool and were low in social status. Because desired qualities in friends change somewhat with age, and because there are probably gender differences in these and in preferred styles of peer interaction (Maccoby, 1998; Rubin, Bukowski, et al., 2006), it is important to examine the ways in which age and sex moderate associations between children's temperament–personality and peer competence.

Finally, researchers would do well to chart the mediating variables in the relations between temperament–personality characteristics and children's social competence. Often the quality of peer interaction may be predicted by children's dispositions and may in turn affect peer status (Fabes et al., 1997; see Figure 26.1).

Acknowledgment

Writing of this chapter was supported by grants from the National Institute of Mental Health and the National Institute of Child Health and Development to Nancy Eisenberg.

References

Asendorpf, J. B., & van Aken, M. A. G. (2003a). Personality–relationship transaction in adolescence: Core versus surface personality characteristics. *Journal of Personality, 71*, 629–666.

Asendorpf, J. B., & van Aken, M. A. G. (2003b). Validity of Big Five personality judgments in childhood: A 9 year longitudinal study. *European Journal of Personality, 17*, 1–17.

Blair, K. A., Denham, S. A., Kochanoff, A., & Whipple, B. (2004). Playing it cool: Temperament, emotion regulation, and social behavior in preschoolers. *Journal of School Psychology, 42*, 419–443.

Brody, G. H., Murray, V. M., Kim, S., & Brown, A. C. (2002). Longitudinal pathways to competence and psychological adjustment among African American children living in rural single-parent households. *Child Development, 73*, 1505–1516.

Buss, A. H., & Plomin, R. (1975). *A temperament theory of personality development.* New York: Wiley.

Caspi, A., & Shiner, R. L. (2006). Personality development. In N. Eisenberg (Vol. Ed.) & W. Damon & R. M. Lerner (Series Eds.), *Handbook of child psychology: Vol. 3. Social, emotional, and personality development* (6th ed., pp. 300–365). New York: Wiley.

Chang, L., Li, L., Li, K. K., Lui, H., Guo, B., Wang, Y., et al. (2005). Peer acceptance and self-perceptions of verbal and behavioral aggression and social withdrawal. *International Journal of Behavioral Development, 29*, 48–57.

Chen, X., Cen, G., Li, D., & He, Y. (2005). Social functioning and adjustment in Chinese children: The imprint of historical time. *Child Development, 76*, 182–195.

Chen, X., Rubin, K. H., & Li, Z. (1995). Social functioning and adjustment in Chinese children: A longitudinal study. *Developmental Psychology, 31*, 531–539.

Chen, X., Rubin, K. H., & Sun, Y. (1992). Social reputation and peer relationships in Chinese and Canadian children: A cross-cultural study. *Child Development, 63*, 1336–1343.

Coplan, R. J., & Armer, M. (2007). A multitude of "solitude": A closer look at social withdrawal and nonsocial play in early childhood. *Child Development Perspectives, 1*, 1–63.

Coplan, R. J., & Rubin, K. H. (1998). Exploring and assessing non-social play in the preschool: The development and validation of the Preschool Play Behavior Scale. *Social Development, 7*, 72–91.

Criss, M. M., Pettit, G. S., Bates, J. E., Dodge, K. A., & Lapp, A. L. (2002). Family adversity, positive peer relationships, and children's externalizing behavior: A longitudinal perspective on risk and resilience. *Child Development, 73*, 1220–1237.

Cumberland-Li, A., Eisenberg, N., & Reiser, M. (2004). Relations of young children's agreeableness and resiliency to effortful control and impulsivity. *Social Development, 13*, 191–212.

David, K. M., & Murphy, B. C. (2007). Interparental conflict and preschoolers' peer relations: The moderating roles of temperament and gender. *Social Development, 16*, 1–20.

Denham, S. A., Blair, K. A., DeMulder, E., Levitas, J., Sawyer, K., Auerbach-Major, S., et al. (2003). Preschool emotional competence: Pathway to social competence. *Child Development, 74,* 238–256.

Deynoot-Schaub, M. J., & Riksen-Walraven, J. M. (2006). Peer contacts of 15-month-olds in child-care: Links with child temperament, parent–child interaction, and quality of childcare. *Social Development, 15,* 709–729.

Diener, M. L., & Kim, D. (2004). Maternal and child predictors of preschool children's social competence. *Applied Developmental Psychology, 25,* 3–24.

Dodge, K. A., Coie, J. D., & Lynam, D. (2006). Aggression and antisocial behavior in youth. In W. Damon & R. M. Lerner (Series Eds.) & N. Eisenberg (Vol. Ed.), *Handbook of child psychology: Vol. 3. Social, emotional, and personality development* (6th ed., pp. 719–788). New York: Wiley.

Dodge, K. A., Coie, J. D., Pettit, G. S., & Price, J. M. (1990). Peer status and aggression in boys' groups: Developmental and contextual analyses. *Child Development, 61,* 1289–1309.

Dunn, J., & Cutting, A. L. (1999). Understanding others, and individual differences in friendship interactions in young children. *Social Development, 8,* 201–219.

Eisenberg, N., Cameron, E., Tryon, K., & Dodez, R. (1981). Socialization of prosocial behavior in the preschool classroom. *Developmental Psychology, 17,* 773–782.

Eisenberg, N., Fabes, R. A., Bernzweig, J., Karbon, M., Poulin, R., & Hanish, L. (1993). The relations of emotionality and regulation to preschoolers' social skills and sociometric status. *Child Development, 64,* 1418–1438.

Eisenberg, N., Fabes, R. A., Guthrie, I. K., & Reiser, M. (2000). Dispositional emotionality and regulation: Their role in predicting quality of social functioning. *Journal of Personality and Social Psychology, 78,* 136–157.

Eisenberg, N., Fabes, R. A., Nyman, M., Bernzweig, J., & Pinuelas, A. (1994). The relations of emotionality and regulation to children's anger-related reactions. *Child Development, 65,* 109–128.

Eisenberg, N., Fabes, R. A., Shepard, S. A., Murphy, B. C., Guthrie, I. K., Jones, S., et al. (1997). Contemporaneous and longitudinal prediction of children's social functioning from regulation and emotionality. *Child Development, 68,* 642–664.

Eisenberg, N., Pidada, S., & Liew, J. (2001). The relations of regulation and negative emotionality to Indonesian children's social functioning. *Child Development, 72,* 1747–1763.

Eisenberg, N., Spinrad, T. L., Fabes, R. A., Reiser, M., Cumberland, A., Shepard, S. A., et al. (2004). The relations of effortful control and impulsivity to children's resiliency and adjustment. *Child Development, 75,* 25–46.

Fabes, R. A., & Eisenberg, N. (1992). Young children's coping with interpersonal anger. *Child Development, 63,* 116–128.

Fabes, R. A., Eisenberg, N., Jones, S., Smith, M., Guthrie, I., Poulin, R., et al. (1999). Regulation, emotionality, and preschoolers' socially competent peer interactions. *Child Development, 70,* 432–442.

Fabes, R. A., Hanish, L. A., Martin, C. L., & Eisenberg, N. (2002). Young children's negative emotionality and social isolation: A latent growth curve analysis. *Merrill–Palmer Quarterly, 48,* 284–307.

Fabes, R. A., Martin, C. L., Hanish, L. D., Anders, M. C., & Madden-Derdich, D. A. (2003). Early school competence: The roles of sex-segregated play and effortful control. *Developmental Psychology, 39,* 848–858.

Fabes, R. A., Shepard, S. A., Guthrie, I. K., & Martin, C. L. (1997). Roles of temperamental arousal and gender-segregated play in young children's social adjustment. *Developmental Psychology, 33,* 693–702.

Fantuzzo, J., Perry, M. A., & McDermott, P. (2004). Preschool approaches to learning and their relationship to other relevant classroom competencies for low-income children. *School Psychology Quarterly, 19,* 212–230.

Fantuzzo, J., Sekino, Y., & Cohen, H. L. (2004). An examination of the contributions of interactive peer play to salient classroom competencies for urban Head Start children. *Psychology in the Schools, 41*, 323–336.

Fox, N. A., Henderson, H. A., Rubin, K. H., Calkins, S. D., & Schmidt, L. A. (2001). Continuity and discontinuity of behavioral inhibition and exuberance: Psychophysiological and behavioral influences across the first four years of life. *Child Development, 72*, 1–21.

Fredrickson, B. L., & Branigan, C. (2005). Positive emotions broaden the scope of attention and thought-action repertoires. *Cognition and Emotion, 19*, 313–332.

Furr, R. M., & Funder, D. C. (1998). A multimodal analysis of personal negativity. *Journal of Personality and Social Psychology, 74*, 1580–1591.

Gleason, T. R., Gower, A. M., Hohmann, L. M., & Gleason, T. C. (2005). Temperament and friendship in preschool-aged children. *International Journal of Behavioral Development, 29*, 336–344.

Graziano, P. A., Keane, S. P., & Calkins, S. D. (2007). Cardiac vagal regulation and early peer status. *Child Development, 78*, 264–278.

Gresham, F. M., MacMillan, D. L., Bocian, K. M., Ward, S. L., & Forness, S. R. (1998). Comorbidity of hyperactivity–impulsivity–inattention and conduct problems: Risk factors in social, affective, and academic domains. *Journal of Abnormal Child Psychology, 26*, 393–406.

Gunnar, M. R., Sebanc, A. M., Tout, K., Donzella, B., & van Dulmen, M. M. (2003). Peer rejection, temperament, and cortisol activity in preschoolers. *Developmental Psychobiology, 43*, 346–358.

Halberstadt, A. G., Denham, S. A., & Dunsmore, J. C. (2001). Affective social competence. *Social Development, 10*, 79–119.

Hart, C. H., Yang, C., Nelson, L. J., Robinson, C. C., Olsen, J. A., Nelson, D. A., et al. (2000). Peer acceptance in early childhood and subtypes of socially withdrawn behavior in China, Russia, and the United States. *International Journal of Behavioral Development, 24*, 73–81.

Henderson, H. A., Marshall, P. J., Fox, N. A., & Rubin, K. H. (2004). Psychophysiological and behavioral evidence for varying forms and functions of nonsocial behavior in preschoolers. *Child Development, 75*, 251–263.

Izard, C. E., King, K. A., Trentacosta, C. J., Morgan, J. K., Laurenceau, J.-P., Krauthamer-Ewing, E. S., et al. (2008). Accelerating the development of emotion competence in Head Start children: Effects on adaptive and maladaptive behavior. *Development and Psychopathology, 20*, 369–397.

Jensen-Campbell, L. A., Adams, R., Perry, D. G., Workman, K. A., Furdella, J. Q., & Egan, S. K. (2002). Agreeableness, extroversion, and peer relations in early adolescence: Winning friends and deflecting aggression. *Journal of Research in Personality, 36*, 224–251.

Jensen-Campbell, L. A., Gleason, K. A., Adams, R., & Malcolm, K. T. (2003). Interpersonal conflict, agreeableness, and personality development. *Journal of Personality, 71*, 1059–1085.

Jensen-Campbell, L. A., & Malcolm, K. T. (2007). The importance of conscientiousness in adolescent interpersonal relationships. *Personality and Social Psychology Bulletin, 33*, 368–383.

Jensen-Campbell, L. A., Rosselini, M., Workman, K. A., Santisi, M., Rios, J. D., & Bojan, D. (2002). Agreeableness, conscientiousness, and effortful control processes. *Journal of Research in Personality, 36*, 476–489.

Jones, S., Eisenberg, N., Fabes, R. A., & MacKinnon, D. P. (2002). Parents' reactions to elementary school children's negative emotions: Relations to social and emotional functioning at school. *Merrill–Palmer Quarterly, 48*, 133–159.

Kagan, J., & Fox, N. (2006). Biology, culture, and temperamental biases. In N. Eisenberg (Vol. Ed.) & W. Damon & R. M. Lerner (Series Eds.), *Handbook of child psychology: Vol. 3. Social, emotional, personality development* (pp. 167–225). New York: Wiley.

Kochanska, G., Murray, K. T., & Harlan, E. T. (2000). Effortful control in early childhood: Continuity and change, antecedents, and implications for social development. *Developmental Psychology, 36*, 220–232.

Ladd, G. W., & Profilet, S. M. (1996). The Child Behavior Scale: A teacher-report measure of young children's aggressive, withdrawn, and prosocial behaviors. *Developmental Psychology, 32*, 1008–1024.

LaFreniere, P. J., & Sroufe, L. A. (1985). Profiles of peer competence in preschool: Interrelations between measures, influence of social ecology, and relation to attachment history. *Developmental Psychology, 21,* 56–69.

Lengua, L. J. (2002). The contribution of emotionality and self-regulation to the understanding of children's multiple risk. *Child Development, 73,* 144–161.

Li-Grining, C. P., Votruba-Drzal, E., Bachman, H. J., & Chase-Lansdale, P. L. (2006). Are certain preschoolers at risk in the era of welfare reform?: The moderating role of children's temperament. *Children and Youth Social Services, 28,* 1102–1123.

Lyubomirsky, S., King, L., & Diener, E. (2005). The benefits of frequent positive affect: Does happiness lead to success? *Psychological Bulletin, 131,* 803–855.

Maccoby, E. E. (1998). *The two sexes: Growing up apart, coming together.* Cambridge, MA: Belknap.

Maszk, P., Eisenberg, N., & Guthrie, I. K. (1999). Relations of children's social status to their emotionality and regulation: A short-term longitudinal study. *Merrill–Palmer Quarterly, 45,* 468–492.

McCoy, J. K., Brody, G. H., & Stoneman, Z. (2002). Temperament and the quality of best friendships: Effect of same-sex sibling relationships. *Family Relations, 51,* 248–255.

McDowell, D. J., & Parke, R. D. (2005). Parental control and affect as predictors of children's display rule use and social competence with peers. *Social Development, 14,* 440–457.

Mendez, J. L., Fantuzzo, J., & Cicchetti, D. (2002). Profiles of social competence among low-income African American preschool children. *Child Development, 73,* 1085–1100.

Mostow, A. J., Izard, C. E., Fine, S., & Trentacosta, C. J. (2002). Modeling emotional, cognitive, and behavioral predictors of peer acceptance. *Child Development, 73,* 1775–1787.

Murphy, B. C., Shepard, S. A., Eisenberg, N., & Fabes, R. A. (2004). Concurrent and across time prediction of young adolescents' social functioning: The role of emotionality and regulation. *Social Development, 13,* 56–86.

Newcomb, A. F., Bukowski, W., & Pattee, L. (1993). Children's peer relations: A meta-analytic review of popular, rejected, neglected, controversial, and average sociometric status. *Psychological Bulletin, 113,* 99–128.

Oldehinkel, A. J., Hartman, C. A., de Winter, A. F., Veenstra, R., & Ormel, J. (2004). Temperament profiles associated with internalizing and externalizing problems in preadolescence. *Development and Psychopathology, 16,* 421–440.

Ollendick, T. H., Weist, M. D., Borden, M. C., & Greene, R. W. (1992). Sociometric status and academic, behavioral, and psychological adjustment: A five-year longitudinal study. *Journal of Consulting and Clinical Psychology, 60,* 80–87.

Olson, S. L., & Lifgren, K. (1988). Concurrent and longitudinal correlates of preschool peer sociometrics: Comparing rating scale and nomination measures. *Journal of Applied Developmental Psychology, 9,* 409–420.

Pellegrini, A. D., Galda, L., Flor, D., Bartini, M., & Charak, D. (1997). Close relationships, individual differences, and early literacy learning. *Journal of Experimental Child Psychology, 67,* 409–422.

Perren, S., Von Wyl, A., Stadelmann, S., Burgin, D., & Von Klitzing, K. (2006). Associations between behavioral/emotional difficulties in kindergarten children and the quality of their peer relationships. *Journal of American Child Adolescent Psychiatry, 45,* 867–876.

Pike, A., & Atzaba-Poria, N. (2003). Do sibling and friend relationships share the same temperamental origins?: A twin study. *Journal of Child Psychology and Psychiatry and Allied Disciplines, 44,* 598–611.

Rothbart, M. K., Ahadi, S. A., Hershey, K. L., & Fisher, P. (2001). Investigations of temperament at three to seven years: The children's behavior questionnaire. *Child Development, 72,* 1394–1408.

Rothbart, M. K., & Bates, J. E. (1998). Temperament. In N. Eisenberg (Vol. Ed.) & W. Damon & R. M. Lerner (Series Eds.), *Handbook of child psychology: Vol. 3. Social, emotional, and personality development* (6th ed., pp. 105–176). New York: Wiley.

Rothbart, M. K., & Bates, J. E. (2006). Temperament. In N. Eisenberg (Vol. Ed.) & W. Damon & R.

M. Lerner (Series Eds.), *Handbook of child psychology: Vol. 3. Social, emotional, and personality development* (6th ed., pp. 99–166). New York: Wiley.

Rubin, K., Bukowski, W. M., & Parker, J. G. (2006). Peer interactions, relationships, and groups. In N. Eisenberg (Vol. Ed.) & W. Damon & R. M. Lerner (Series Eds.), *Handbook of child psychology: Vol. 3. Social, emotional, and personality development* (6th ed., pp. 571–645). New York: Wiley.

Rubin, K. H., Burgess, K. B., Dwyer, K. M., & Hastings, P. D. (2003). Predicting preschoolers' externalizing behaviors from toddler temperament, conflict, and maternal negativity. *Developmental Psychology, 39,* 164–176.

Rubin, K. H., & Coplan, R. J. (2004). Paying attention to and not neglecting social withdrawal and social isolation. *Merrill–Palmer Quarterly, 50,* 506–534.

Rubin, K. H., Coplan, R. J., Fox, N. A., & Calkins, S. (1995). Emotionality, emotion regulation, and preschoolers' social adaptation. *Development and Psychopathology, 7,* 49–62.

Rubin, K. H., Wojslawowicz, J. C., Rose-Krasnor, L., Booth-LaForce, C. L., & Burgess, K. B. (2006). The best friendships of shy/withdrawn children: Prevalence, stability, and relationship quality. *Journal of Abnormal Child Psychology, 34,* 139–153.

Rydell, A., Berlin, L., & Bohlin, G. (2003). Emotionality, emotion regulation, and adaptation among 5- to 8-year-old children. *Emotion, 3,* 30–47.

Schwartz, D., Chang, L., & Farver, J. M. (2001). Correlates of victimization in Chinese children's peer groups. *Developmental Psychology, 37,* 520–532.

Skarpness, L. R., & Carson, D. K. (1987). Correlates of kindergarten adjustment: Temperament and communicative competence. *Early Childhood Research Quarterly, 2,* 367–376.

Spinrad, T. L., Eisenberg, N., Cumberland, A., Fabes, R. A., Valiente, C., Shepard, S. A., et al. (2006). The relations of temperamentally based control processes to children's social competence: A longitudinal study. *Emotion, 6,* 498–510.

Spinrad, T., Eisenberg, N., Harris, E., Hanish, L., Fabes, R. A., Kupanoff, K., et al. (2004). The relation of children's everyday nonsocial peer play behavior to their emotionality, regulation, and social functioning. *Developmental Psychology, 40,* 67–80.

Sroufe, A., Schork, E., Motti, E., Lawroski, N., & LaFreniere, P. (1985). The role of affect in social competence. In C. E. Izard, J. Kagan, & R. B. Zajonc (Eds.), *Emotion, cognition, and behavior* (pp. 289–319). New York: Cambridge Press.

Stocker, C., & Dunn, J. (1990). Sibling relationships in childhood: Links with friendships and peer relationships. *British Journal of Developmental Psychology, 8,* 227–244.

Szewczyk-Sokolowski, M., Bost, K. K., & Wainwright, A. B. (2005). Attachment, temperament, and preschool children's peer acceptance. *Social Development, 14,* 379–397.

Van Brakel, A. M., Muris, P., & Bogels, S. M. (2004). Relations between parent- and teacher-reported behavioral inhibition and behavioral observations of this temperamental trait. *Journal of Clinical Child and Adolescent Psychology, 33,* 579–589.

Walden, T., Lemerise, E., & Smith, M. C. (1999). Friendship and popularity in preschool classrooms. *Early Education and Development, 10,* 351–371.

Walker, S., Berthelsen, D., & Irving, K. (2001). Temperament and peer acceptance in early childhood: Sex and social status differences. *Child Study Journal, 31,* 177–192.

Wilson, B. J. (2003). The role of attentional processes in children's prosocial behavior with peers: Attention shifting and emotion. *Development and Psychopathology, 15,* 313–329.

Wilson, B. J. (2006). The entry behavior of aggressive/rejected children: The contributions of status and temperament. *Social Development, 15,* 463–479.

Zhou, Q., Eisenberg, N., Wang, Y., & Reiser, M. (2004). Chinese children's effortful control and dispositional anger/frustration: Relations to parenting styles and children's social functioning. *Developmental Psychology, 40,* 352–366.

CHAPTER 27

Child–Parent Attachment Relationships, Peer Relationships, and Peer-Group Functioning

CATHRYN BOOTH–LaFORCE
KATHRYN A. KERNS

Links between children's experiences in the family and their interactions and relationships with peers have been the subject of much theoretical and empirical work in the last 15 years. In 1992, Parke and Ladd's edited volume focused attention on the topic and provided several relevant theoretical perspectives that sparked subsequent research. Debate on how family and peer relationships are interlinked has continued, offering diverse opinions: Whereas Harris (1995) has argued that parents' socialization efforts have little impact on children's relationships with peers, Sroufe, Egeland, and Carlson (1999) have referred to families and peers as one integrated social world. We believe that there are strong theoretical reasons and extensive empirical evidence to suggest that children's experiences in the family are connected in important ways to the quality of their relationships and interactions with peers. In this chapter we explore one of these links, namely, the relation between children's security of attachment to their parents, and their experiences and relationships with peers.

Attachment theory has provided one of the most well-developed and -validated theoretical perspectives for understanding individual differences in children's social–emotional development. It is well known that the quality of early parenting, specifically, the history of the primary caregiver's sensitivity and responsiveness to the infant, forms the basis for the development of the child's security or insecurity of attachment to the primary caregiver (Ainsworth, Blehar, Waters, & Wall, 1978; De Wolff & van IJzendoorn, 1997). The child's quality of attachment to the primary caregiver(s) is significant for understanding the ongoing nature of their relationship, but a great deal of the import accorded to attachment theory derives from the notion that the child's early attachment-related experiences set the stage for his or her subsequent social–emotional functioning beyond the family. In particular, the influence of individual differences in attachment security on children's peer relationships and peer-group functioning has been the subject of much empirical work.

This work is the focus of this chapter. Our aims are (1) to provide a framework for understanding and studying the relations between child–parent attachment security, and children's functioning and relationships with peers; (2) to summarize broadly the key studies and extant literature in this area; (3) to discuss significant issues and emerging trends in attachment–peer research; and (4) to identify gaps and future directions. Note that we have limited our review of the literature to studies of infancy through middle childhood, although our thinking is informed by theory and research across the lifespan. Also note that we distinguish children's *relationships* with peers (i.e., friendships) from their *general functioning* within the peer group—including their social competence, acceptance by the peer group, and problematic behaviors in relation to their peers.

Central Issues

Conceptualizing Attachment–Peer Links

The links between attachment security and children's relationships and functioning with peers have been conceptualized in a number of ways. Foremost among these is the notion that through the history of attachment-related interactions with the primary caregiver, the child develops a set of "internal working models" (IWMs; i.e., internal representations about the world; Bowlby, 1973, 1980; Bretherton, 2005; Bretherton & Munholland, 1999; Sroufe & Fleeson, 1986). These representations encompass views of the self, the "other," and the nature of relationships, and lead to "interpretive filters" that guide subsequent beliefs and expectations about how to behave and what to expect from the social world. As such, these IWMs are said to form the bridge between experiences in the parent–child relationship and the quality of relationships with others (Bretherton & Munholland, 1999), including peers. For example, an internal representation of the self as unworthy and ineffective, arising from a history of insensitive parental care, might be expressed as dependent, immature behavior with others (Bowlby, 1973), thereby leading to avoidance or rejection by peers, as well as confirmation of the IWM, and a continuation of maladaptive behavior with peers (Rubin & Lollis, 1988).

The IWM is an appealing construct that has been used extensively in the literature as an explanation for links between attachment security and a wide variety of other child attributes. Because this construct is very broad in terms of delineating a basis for how children think and feel about themselves and others, and what they expect from relationships, it is possible to invoke IWMs as an explanation for most *any* aspect of social–emotional development. Indeed, the explanatory power of IWMs has been questioned by a number of developmentalists (Belsky & Cassidy, 1994; Hinde, 1988; Thompson & Raikes, 2003; Thompson, 2005), who cite lack of both specificity and theoretical development for this "conceptual metaphor" (Thompson & Raikes, 2003).

A more nuanced framework for examining and explaining attachment–peer links has been developed by Sroufe and colleagues (Sroufe et al., 1999; Sroufe, Egeland, Carlson, & Collins, 2005), who have conceptualized the following ways in which attachment security may promote the development of peer relationships:

(1) A motivational base, involving expectations of connectedness; (2) an attitudinal base, involving expectations of responsiveness; (3) an instrumental base centered on exploratory

and play capacities; (4) an emotional base, including entrained capacities for arousal and emotional regulation; and (5) a relational base, involving empathy and expectations of mutuality. (Sroufe et al., 2005, p. 57)

According to this view of attachment–peer links, part of the legacy of attachment security is a set of specific expectations about relationships and interactions with others, as well as the interactive skills and emotion-regulation abilities to engage successfully with peers. By delineating these distinct aspects of child functioning, Sroufe et al. have provided a useful framework for evaluating the *processes* whereby attachment security is linked with peer relationships and peer-group functioning, without resorting to a more general IWM explanation. In a subsequent section, we review the literature on such mediating processes.

A Developmental Framework and Developmental Issues

In addition to conceptualizing the processes linking attachment security with peer relationships and functioning, it is also important to consider the child's interface with the peer world from the perspective of relevant developmental tasks. There is general agreement that peers are important social partners by the preschool years, but many different ideas have been proposed regarding the ways in which the central issues in peer relationships may change across childhood. For example, Howes (1988) suggested that, within the early childhood years, the focus shifts from communicating shared meaning during play with peers to developing social knowledge of the peer group. Gottman and Mettetal (1986) indicated that whereas the key issue in peer relationships in early childhood is coordinated interaction with peers, in middle childhood it is inclusion in the peer group. Sroufe et al. (1999, 2005) suggested that during the preschool period, the primary peer-related task is positive engagement (e.g., selecting peer partners, participating in groups, and learning to maintain interaction), whereas the primary task in middle childhood is greater investment in the peer world (e.g., development and maintenance of close friendships and functioning in stable groups of peers). Similarly, Sullivan (1953) proposed that children develop the need for peers in middle childhood, with friendships taking on special significance by the end of middle childhood. Despite these different perspectives, a common thread among them is the focus on the development of coordinated and sustained interactions with peers in early childhood, with greater concern for friendship and one's standing in the peer group emerging in middle childhood.

Changing manifestations of attachment security with age are important to consider as well. By the end of the first year, infants' attachment behaviors have become organized around the goal of using the parent as a secure base (i.e., seeking contact when distressed, yet using the parent as a secure base from which to explore in the absence of threat). The attachment behaviors that are readily observable in infancy evolve into the "goal-corrected partnership" (Bowlby, 1969/1982), with the child increasingly able to take into consideration the caregiver's needs and preferences. By middle childhood, the attachment system has evolved from the goal of physical proximity to a focus on the availability of caregivers (Ainsworth, 1990), with children becoming more able to spend increasing amounts of time away from them (for additional discussion, see Kerns, 2008). Obviously, these changes have implications for methods of assessing attachment security, and some methods have a greater body of evidence supporting their validity than do others (Dwyer, 2005). For example, the decline in the frequency and intensity of observable attachment behaviors with age has necessitated the development of methods to assess children's representations of attachment relationships (Kerns & Richardson, 2005; Solomon & George, 1999).

These developmental changes in attachment and peer relationships have implications for the ways in which their linkages are studied; that is, in addition to the specific measures of each construct varying with the age of the child, the hypothesized links between the two constructs may change across childhood, with effects being the strongest when the most developmentally salient aspects of peer relationships are targeted (Kerns, 1994; Sroufe et al., 1999). Thus, studies linking attachment with friendship quality, for example, may be more relevant in middle childhood than in earlier years. By contrast, studies of attachment and peer social interaction skills (e.g., coordinated interaction) may be most relevant during early childhood, when peer interaction skills are emerging (Kerns, 1994).

Research Evidence

Early/Classic Studies

The earliest reports linking child–mother attachment with peer interactions and relationships came from the Minnesota Studies (Sroufe et al., 2005; Waters, Wippman, & Sroufe, 1979). One goal of these longitudinal projects was to understand how individual differences in infant–mother attachment forecast a child's subsequent social and emotional development. Sroufe (1979) had suggested that secure attachment might be an indicator of social competence in infancy, and peer competence, an indicator of social competence in the preschool years. Furthermore, he suggested a degree of continuity in development, with children who were securely attached as infants being more likely to show greater competence with peers as preschoolers. This hypothesis was tested in a series of studies in which child–mother attachment was shown to predict children's later competence with peers in both low-income and middle-class samples. For example, children who were securely attached as infants, compared with those who were insecure, were later rated by teachers as more socially competent with peers (e.g., ego resilient, leaders; Sroufe, 1983; Waters et al., 1979), were less hostile and more empathic (Sroufe, 1983), and displayed more positive affect with playmates (Sroufe, Schork, Motti, Lawroski, & LaFreniere, 1984). In subsequent follow-up studies with the Minnesota low-income sample, Sroufe et al. (2005) showed that early attachment continued to predict peer relationships in middle childhood and adolescence. For example, children who had been securely attached in infancy, compared with those who had been insecure, were later rated by teachers and camp counselors to be more competent with peers and more likely to develop higher-quality friendships, and they showed greater maintenance of gender boundaries (Shulman, Elicker, & Sroufe, 1994; Sroufe, Bennett, Englund, Urban, & Shulman, 1993; Sroufe, Egeland, & Kreutzer, 1990; Sroufe et al., 1999). In the following years, several other investigators replicated or extended these findings (e.g., Suess, Grossmann, & Sroufe, 1992).

A number of other studies indicated a relation between attachment and peer relationships when the two were assessed concurrently. In these studies, several different aspects of peer relationships were investigated. For example, child–mother attachment security was found to be related to peer acceptance (e.g., Cohn, 1990), friendship quality (e.g., Park & Waters, 1989), and positive social engagement with an unfamiliar peer (but not the quality of observed interpersonal problem-solving skills with the peer; Rose-Krasnor, Rubin, Booth, & Coplan, 1996).

It should be noted that in the later articles from this period, the conceptual rationale for a link between attachment and peer relationships was elaborated beyond an expectation for continuity in children's social competence. In a classic article, Sroufe and Fleeson (1986) proposed that part of what children internalize through participation in attachment relationships with caregivers is a broader understanding of the dynamics of close relationships, and that this understanding guides children in their new relationships. Additionally, Belsky and Cassidy (1994) suggested that attachment should be most highly related to children's *close* relationships with peers. These ideas led researchers to focus on more specific ways in which attachment might be linked to the quality of children's peer relationships (e.g., Park & Waters, 1989; Troy & Sroufe, 1987), including a differentiation of attachment in relation to close friendships and to more general functioning within the peer group.

By the end of the century, the literature on attachment–peer links had increased a great deal, to the extent that a meta-analysis was warranted. To that end, Schneider, Atkinson, and Tardif (2001) performed such an analysis to evaluate the strength of the association between child–parent attachment and children's peer relationships. The authors included 63 studies involving 3,510 children and found an overall effect size of 0.20 in these studies, which differed significantly from zero. Additionally, they randomly matched studies involving attachment–friendship relations with studies pertaining to unfamiliar peers, and the mean effect size for the friendship studies (0.24) was significantly larger than the mean for the unfamiliar peer studies (0.14). There were no gender differences in effect sizes. However, effect sizes were larger in studies involving maternal ratings of their children's peer competencies rather than measures from other informants and sources; in studies investigating sociability/leadership rather than aggression or withdrawal; and in studies of children in middle childhood and adolescence (age 8 years and older) rather than earlier in life. Regarding the latter point, it is interesting that the time between attachment and peer assessments did not affect the strength of the association between variables (i.e., effect sizes were similar for cross-sectional and longitudinal studies). Finally, studies involving child–father attachment were too few in number to be meaningfully evaluated, and studies of non–North American samples yielded effect sizes that were similar to those in North America—but this result is also qualified by the relatively small number of such studies conducted in other cultures.

Recent Research

In our review of the current literature, we limited our detailed search to publications in the last 10 years, because the Schneider et al. (2001) meta-analysis included most of the relevant earlier research. (In a few sections we have included earlier references due to a paucity of research in particular areas.) In separate sections we consider the literature on attachment and social competence, behavior problems, peer acceptance, and friendship.

Social Competence

Several studies in the preschool and early school period have continued to support the link between attachment security and children's social competence with peers. Belsky and Fearon (2002) demonstrated that 15-month security, as assessed in the Strange Situation (Ainsworth et al., 1978), was related to mother-reported social competence at 36 months, especially when high-sensitive mothering also was observed at 24 months. From the same set of data (the NICHD Study of Early Child Care and Youth Development), the NICHD Early Child Care Research Network (ECCRN; 2006) found that children who had been securely attached at 15 months, compared with those who were insecure–avoidant, had higher social competence scores from 54 months to 6 years. Using the Waters Attachment Q-Sort procedure (Waters, Vaughn, Posada, & Kondo-Ikemura, 1995) at 3–4 years of age, Bost, Vaughn, Washington, Cielinski, and Bradbard (1998) found that security was related to a composite measure of social competence that included observed competence and sociometric data. Finally, Stams, Juffer, and van IJzendoorn (2002) found that attachment security at 12 months of age from the Strange Situation predicted a composite measure of social competence at age 7, derived from mother and teacher reports, as well as from sociometric data.

In middle childhood, there is also evidence for an association between secure attachment and peer competence, with most studies using a cross-sectional rather than a longitudinal design. In these studies, peer competence has been measured with either global ratings or observational assessments of peer interactions, with children who are securely attached to their mothers demonstrating more competent behavior with peers (Bohlin, Hagekull, & Rydell, 2000; Contreras, Kerns, Weimer, Gentzler, & Tomich, 2000; Yunger, Corby, & Perry, 2005; but for an exception, see Easterbrooks & Abeles, 2000). Additionally, using evaluations by mothers, teachers, and peers, Booth-LaForce, Oh, Kim, Rubin, Rose-Krasnor, and Burgess (2006) found that attachment security in relation to mothers *and* fathers was related to children's social competence.

Taken together, the most recent studies continue to support the links between attachment security and peer social competence, evaluated predictively or contemporaneously. However, what is missing from these reports is a more fine-grained analysis of *types* of insecurity (most used secure–insecure or continuous security scores) and the ways these different types may vary in their social competence.

Behavior Problems

Although this chapter is focused primarily on links between child–parent attachment security and children's peer interactions and relationships, it is worthwhile to consider the literature on attachment and behavior problems. Many of the attributes of children with internalizing and externalizing problems affect interactions and relationships with peers.

One approach to the study of attachment and behavior problems has been to link general security–insecurity, or a continuous security score, with behavior-problem levels. In these studies, secure attachment, compared with insecure or less-secure attachment, has been associated with relatively lower levels of internalizing problems (Bohlin et al., 2000; Davies, Harold, Goeke-Morey, & Cummings, 2002; Easterbrooks & Abeles, 2000; Graham & Easterbrooks, 2000; Granot & Mayseless, 2001; Harold, Shelton, Goeke-Morey, & Cummings, 2004; Muris, Mayer, & Meesters, 2000) and externalizing problems (Belsky & Fearon, 2002; Booth-LaForce et al., 2006; Davies, Cummings, & Winter, 2004; DeMulder, Denham, Schmidt, & Mitchell, 2000; El-Sheikh & Buckhalt, 2003; Harold et al., 2004; Stams et al., 2002).

Another approach has been to link specific *types* of insecurity to either internalizing or externalizing problems. According to the "specific linkage hypothesis" (see Finnegan, Hodges, & Perry, 1996), children who are insecure–avoidant are more likely to have externalizing problems, and those who are insecure–resistant (or preoccupied, in older children) are more likely to have internalizing problems. The link between insecure–avoidant attachment and aggression/externalizing behavior problems has been found in some studies (Booth-LaForce et al., 2006; Burgess, Marshall, Rubin, & Fox, 2003; Easterbrooks & Abeles, 2000; Granot & Mayseless, 2001; Hodges, Finnegan, & Perry, 1999; Keller, Spieker, & Gilchrist, 2005; McElwain, Cox, Burchinal, & Macfie, 2003; NICHD ECCRN, 2006; Yunger et al., 2005). Alternatively, Lyons-Ruth (1996) has proposed that *disorganized* attachment might be most strongly related to externalizing problems. Although there is some evidence to support this idea (Granot & Mayseless, 2001; Moss, Cyr, & Dubois-Comtois, 2004), disorganized attachment also has been associated with elevated internalizing problems (Carlson, 1998; Granot & Mayseless, 2001).

In other studies, researchers have examined how internalizing problems are related to specific forms of insecurity. Although there has been speculation that internalizing problems are most likely to be related to ambivalent or preoccupied attachment (Finnegan et al., 1996; Renken, Egeland, Marvinney, Mangelsdorf, & Sroufe, 1989), extant studies have yielded a mixture of results. Specifically, internalizing problems have been linked with avoidance (Moss, Rousseau, Parent, St. Laurent, & Saintonge, 1998; NICHD ECCRN, 2006; Pierrehumbert, Miljkovitch, Plancherel, Halfon, & Ansermet, 2000; Yunger et al., 2005), ambivalent/preoccupied attachment (Hodges et al., 1999; Yunger et al., 2005), and attachment disorganization (Graham & Easterbrooks, 2000; Moss et al., 2004; NICHD ECCRN, 2006). The lack of specificity in the associations with different insecure patterns is difficult to evaluate, given that in the few available studies, researchers have used different measures of internalizing problems (e.g., depression, anxiety, social withdrawal, aggregated internalizing symptom measures) and different measures of attachment (observations and questionnaires).

In general, researchers' attempts to link attachment security with problematic behavior have yielded a negative connection between the two, but evidence for the specific linkage hypothesis is mixed, and stronger for externalizing than internalizing problems. Also, it is important to note that in most of these studies, teacher or mother reports of externalizing and internalizing problems were used, or these indices were combined with peer sociometric or observational data to form a composite variable. Consequently, it is more challenging to tease apart the links between attachment security and problems with peers *specifically* (e.g., aggression, social withdrawal in relation to peers) than that between attachment and more general behavior problems.

Friendship

In accordance with the increasing developmental salience of friendship during the middle childhood years, most of the studies of links between attachment security and friendship have been conducted in middle childhood or later. Studies attempting to link attachment and prevalence of friendship (i.e., having or not having a close friend) or number of friends have yielded mixed results: In some studies, positive associations have been reported (Kerns, Klepac, & Cole, 1996, Study 1); in others, results have not supported the posited link between attachment and friendship prevalence (Booth, Rubin, & Rose-Krasnor, 1998; Lieberman, Doyle, & Markiewicz, 1999). This inconsistent evidence may be due to the fact that most children in middle childhood have at least one friend (Epstein, 1986). In contrast to the mixed findings regarding friendship prevalence, researchers have found consistently that attachment is related to the *quality* of children's friendships, as indexed by child reports of support, companionship, responsiveness, and (low) conflict, and by observers' ratings of friends' interactions (Howes & Tonyan, 1999; Kerns et al., 1996, Study 2; Lieberman et al., 1999; McElwain & Volling, 2004; Rubin et al., 2004).

An area of attachment–friendship research that has received almost no attention in the middle childhood period is friendship "homophilies"; that is, the extent to which children form friendships with peers who are similar to them in terms of attachment security. The extant evidence comes from two studies, one with preschoolers (Park & Waters, 1989) and the other with preadolescents (Kerns et al., 1996), in which researchers recruited friend pairs and gathered attachment information for each child. These studies indicated that the number of secure–secure, secure–insecure, and insecure–insecure pairs did not differ from what would be expected by chance, suggesting that attachment security may not be a dimension on which friends match. It is still important to consider the developmental consequences for children whose closest friends share, or do not share, their attachment characteristics. For example, although attachment matching did not predict friendship stability (Kerns et al., 1996), the interactions of secure–secure and secure–insecure friend pairs differed (Kerns, 2000; Kerns et al., 1996). Thus, it is possible that the impact of friendship on development might vary in relation to the degree of attachment homophily.

Peer Acceptance

In another group of studies, researchers tested the hypothesis that children who form secure versus insecure attachments to caregivers are more likely to experience high acceptance by their peers. Typically, this research has focused on children between the ages of 8 and 11 years, with sociometric nominations or ratings of acceptance–rejection obtained from the peers of the study children. These studies have yielded mixed evidence for an association between attachment and peer acceptance: In three studies, investigators reported a positive association between security and peer acceptance (Bohlin et al., 2000; Granot & Mayseless, 2001; Kerns et al., 1996, Study 1); in two studies, an association was found between secure attachment and peer popularity for child–father but not child–mother attachment (Verschueren & Marcoen, 2002, 2005); and in one study, neither child–mother nor child–father attachment security was associated with peer popularity (Lieberman et al., 1999).

The substantial literature on the correlates of peer acceptance (Rubin, Bukowski, & Parker, 2006) might inform future studies investigating links between attachment and peer acceptance. It may be the case that securely attached children typically possess only some of the characteristics that are associated with peer acceptance (e.g., securely attached children may develop adaptive emotion-regulation strategies but may not necessarily possess other characteristics associated with peer popularity such as physical attractiveness). Additional theorizing on *why* attachment might foster greater liking from peers would advance research in this area. Recent studies also are limited in that most have examined how variations in attachment security are related to peer liking, and therefore have not considered how particular types of insecurity (i.e., avoidance, ambivalence, disorganization) are related to specific peer sociometric categories (e.g., neglected status; but for an exception see Granot & Mayseless, 2001).

Emerging Trends

In this section we introduce and discuss a variety of issues and emerging trends in research investigating attachment–peer links, specifically, mediating processes, the role of fathers, and early versus ongoing and changing experiences.

Mediating Processes

As researchers have become more attuned to the need to understand the *processes* whereby attachment security and peer relations are linked, they have focused more attention on identifying and testing additional variables that may mediate the relation between the existence of a secure base and consequent social competence with peers. One such candidate is children's self-esteem, which is an idea derived from Bowlby's (1973) suggestion that attachment influences working models that children develop for the self and for others. In fact, a number of researchers have found that security is related to children's self-esteem (Booth-LaForce et al., 2006; Simons, Paternite, & Shore, 2001; Verschueren & Marcoen, 2002, 2005). Other researchers have linked insecure attachment with children's negative perceptions and attributions about peer intentions in hypothetical situations that could be interpreted as accidental or deliberately aggressive (Cassidy, Kirsch, Scolton, & Parke, 1996; McElwain, Booth-LaForce, & Lansford, 2007; Suess et al., 1992; Wartner, Grossmann, Fremmer-Bombik, & Suess, 1994). Also, attachment is purported to provide a base from which to develop emotion regulation capacities (Contreras & Kerns, 2000; Sroufe et al., 1999); researchers have found support for this suggestion (Contreras et al., 2000; Kerns, Abraham, Schlegelmilch, & Morgan, 2007; Sroufe, 1983).

As a group, these studies show that attachment is related to several possible mediating mechanisms. Yet mediational models with appropriate statistical tests have been included in very few studies (Booth-LaForce et al., 2006; Cassidy et al., 1996; Contreras et al., 2000). As researchers move beyond the basic demonstration of links between attachment and peer variables, the "why" of these connections has gained increasing importance, both theoretically and empirically. Thus, the development and testing of more elaborated models of mediating mechanisms are important directions for future research.

The Role of Fathers

Bowlby (1969/1982) proposed that children tend to form their first attachments to their mother or to a mother figure, but by 18 months of age, the norm is for most infants to have formed multiple attachment relationships, usually with both fathers and mothers. Furthermore, Bowlby suggested that children often have one primary figure to whom they turn when in need of comforting, and that mothers play this role in most societies. The theory's emphasis on children's attachments to their mothers was later captured by the "mother primacy hypothesis" (Suess et al., 1992), which states that the child's attachment relationship with the mother is more predictive of child social–emotional outcomes than is the child's attachment relationship with father. In fact, some studies have found that child–mother attachment predicted children's social and emotional development more strongly than did child–father attachment (e.g., Main, Kaplan, & Cassidy, 1985; Suess et al., 1992).

Other research has not supported the mother primacy hypothesis (e.g., Youngblade, Park, & Belsky, 1993). Verschueren and Marcoen (1999) have proposed an alternative hypothesis, in which they suggest that child–mother and child–father attachment may influence different domains of development. They found that child–mother attachment is more strongly related to children's self-esteem, whereas child–father attachment is more strongly related to children's anxious or withdrawn behavior. These findings suggest that child–father attachment may be particularly relevant in the realm of children's relationships with peers.

Although fathers are deemed important, there has been very little research on the child–father relationship and how it is linked with children's functioning and relationships with peers; consequently, neither of these hypotheses has been tested adequately. Nevertheless, studies in early childhood have shown that child–father attachment is related to several aspects of peer relationships, including preschool teacher ratings of friendly–cooperative behavior (Kerns & Barth, 1995) or anxious–withdrawn behavior (Verschueren & Marcoen, 1999), observer ratings of children's behavior with peers (Suess et al., 1992), and the quality of interactions with a best friend (Youngblade et al., 1993). The child–father attachment relationship may become even more salient and predictive of outcomes in middle childhood (Cohn, Patterson, & Christopoulos, 1991) and beyond. A few studies in middle childhood have included both child–father and child–mother attachment measures. For example, Lieberman et al. (1999) found that child–father security was related to lower conflict in best-friend relationships, but not to peer popularity; among 10- and 11-year-olds, Rubin and colleagues (2004) found a positive association between attachment to fathers and the quality of the child's best friendship. Verschueren and Marcoen (2002) found that popular children had higher child–father security scores than did rejected–nonaggressive children, and that child–father security was related to peer acceptance at ages 8 and 11 (Verschueren & Marcoen, 2005).

Booth-LaForce et al. (2006) found that children's security with both parents was related to social competence, but security with the father (and not the mother) was related to lower aggression with peers. This latter result is interesting in relation to evidence in the literature that fathers tend to interact with their children in more playful ways, and mothers, in more nurturing ways (see Lamb, 1997; Parke, 2002). In fact, the work of Grossmann et al. (2002) indicates that fathers foster secure attachment via "sensitive and challenging interactive play" (p. 315), and serve as supportive guides in the context of children's exploratory behavior. If we extrapolate this exploratory behavior to the world of peers, then it is possible to imagine that supportive fathers encourage more adaptive, less aggressive solutions to peer conflicts. It is also possible that within the context of father–child play, these fathers may help their securely attached children to learn the boundaries between play and aggression.

Early versus Ongoing and Changing Experiences

An issue discussed in the attachment literature is the extent to which the *early* experience of attachment security or insecurity is a primary determinant of subsequent behavior, or whether correlations between attachment and later social adjustment are a function of ongoing stability in the nature and quality of relationships and experiences with parents and other social partners. These differing views are sometimes referred to as the prototype versus revisionist perspectives (Fraley, 2002). The "prototype" perspective (e.g., Sroufe et al., 1990) maintains that early attachment experiences give rise to a stable prototype that guides the selection of later attachment experiences. Some have incorrectly assumed that this view implies absolute (or high) stability of individual differences; instead, it argues for the enduring significance of early experiences (Roisman, Collins, Sroufe, & Egeland, 2005) and the recognition that the development of a secure or insecure attachment does not solely determine later events but may make certain developmental pathways and outcomes more or less likely (Bowlby, 1988; Sroufe et al., 2005). In contrast, the "revisionist" perspective holds that any observed stability in security is due to continuity in ongoing social experiences.

It is important to note that both approaches suggest that IWMs can be changed beyond infancy, and that current levels of security influence the selection of subsequent experiences (e.g., the nature of the peers with whom the child forms close friendships). These perspectives differ, however, in terms of what they posit regarding the malleability of IWMs established in infancy.

In relation to attachment–peer links, the Minnesota Study has provided the most extensive data to test a pathways perspective. In general, some peer outcomes are predicted better by early attachment security, and others by intervening variables (e.g., middle childhood social competence); such intervening variables are predicted by early attachment security, but they are stronger predictors of outcomes than are early attachment variables (Sroufe et al., 2005). These varying predictive patterns remind us of the importance of staying open to different ways in which early attachment security may be related to subsequent peer outcomes, as well as the significance of developmental pathways, and highlight the advantages of long-term longitudinal studies.

Summary and Future Directions

We began this chapter by presenting alternative frameworks for thinking about the links between attachment security with the primary caregiver and the child's relationships/ functioning with peers. The framework proposed by Sroufe and his colleagues (1999, 2005) outlines several specific ways in which attachment security may promote the development of peer relationships. According to this view, from the attachment relationship with the primary caregiver, the child gains a set of specific expectations about relationships and interactions with others, as well as the interactive skills and emotion regulation abilities to engage successfully with peers. Although elements of this framework are not especially unique, the advantage of such a framework is that it provides guidance about specific areas in which we might expect attachment–peer links, as well as some specific mediating variables that are likely to be important. In addition, the more recent emphasis on linking attachment-focused IWMs with other cognitive processes (e.g., memory, development of event schemas) holds promise for a greater understanding of IWMs and how they operate (see Bretherton & Munholland, 1999; Crittenden, 1990); such research will inform the attachment–peer literature as well. That said, there is still much theoretical and empirical work to be done in terms of offering differential predictions from attachment security to varying aspects of peer relationships and functioning in the peer group. Regardless of the conceptual framework employed, it is clear that we must continue to address the nonproductive issue of attachment being related to "everything," and the uninformative notion that "all good things go together" (Belsky & Cassidy, 1994; Thompson, 2005). As we noted earlier, considering the developmental context of peer relationships may lead to more precise hypotheses regarding the ways in which attachment and peer relationships are likely to be associated at different developmental periods.

The literature on attachment and peer relationships has focused primarily on establishing associations between the two. It is important to consider that some of the relations between attachment security and relationships/functioning with peers may be due to unmeasured "third variables," which might include other aspects of parent–child relationships. Ladd (1992) proposed a distinction between direct and indirect parent–child relationship influences on peer relationships. "Indirect influences" (including attachment) are aspects of parent–child relationships that may influence peer relationships, even though parents are not developing these relationship patterns for the specific purpose of promoting their child's functioning with peers. For example, it is doubtful that a parent's primary motivation for fostering a secure relationship with the child is to facilitate the child's relationships with peers. Ladd noted that parents do engage in some direct actions specifically to enhance their children's peer relationships (e.g., setting up playdates). Also, it may be that attachment is related to children's peer relationships, in part because parents of securely attached children value relationships and take actions to enhance directly their children's relationships with peers (Kerns, Cole, & Andrews, 1998). For example, a primary caregiver who is sensitive and responsive in terms of meeting the child's emotional needs might also be good at teaching appropriate social behaviors to be used in the company of peers. Therefore, the child's social competence might relate more directly to the parent's teaching efforts than to the child's attachment security (Contreras & Kerns, 2000; see also Rose-Krasnor et al., 1996). We know very little about how attachment is associated with parents' direct efforts to foster peer relationships (for an exception, see Kerns et al., 1998).

In fact, it is important that we do not lose sight of the bigger developmental picture as we focus in on attachment–peer links. Attachment is just one component of the parent–child relationship, which, in turn, is embedded within a broader context. There are multiple aspects of the parent–child relationship to consider, and multiple aspects of peer relationships and peer-group functioning. We know, for example, that the relative effects of early attachment security and maternal style may differ depending on the social outcomes studied (e.g., Booth, Rose-Krasnor, McKinnon, & Rubin, 1994; Rose-Krasnor et al., 1996). It is likely that any consideration of long-term links between early attachment security and subsequent peer variables would benefit from consideration of these other sources of variance (Sroufe et al., 2005).

As well, it is important to consider that a variety of life changes and stressors may impact the nature and quality of both parenting and peer relationships, which challenges us to think about, and to measure, potential sources of change in predicted links between attachment security and peer variables that may alter children's developmental trajectories. Although it is beyond the scope of this chapter to delve into the literature on "lawful discontinuity" (Belsky & Fearon, 2002; Belsky, Fish, & Isabella, 1991; Lewis, Feiring, & Rosenthal, 2000; NICHD ECCRN, 2006; Sameroff, Bartko, Baldwin, Baldwin, & Seifer, 1998)—the idea that continuity, as well as change, can be predictable—it is worth mentioning in the context of strategies for studying longitudinal attachment–peer relations. Most studies of attachment and peer relationships have been cross-sectional rather than longitudinal, and most of the longitudinal studies have examined how attachment is related to subsequent peer relationships, without considering intervening experiences with attachment figures and peers. Longitudinal studies that focus on identifying pathways to peer competence, with careful consideration of both parent–child and peer relationship influences across development, are needed (for an excellent example, see Sroufe et al., 1999, 2005).

In addition to the need for larger, longer-term studies, we have highlighted a number of future directions for research. Primary among these is a continuing emphasis on identifying mediating variables that link attachment security with children's peer relationships/functioning. Such studies promise to provide greater understanding of the processes whereby the quality of the attachment relationship with the primary caregiver provides the foundation for children's developing social competence and relationship quality with peers and friends. A second area in need of greater attention is the role of fathers, particularly in the middle childhood period. A few recent studies (not surprisingly) have emphasized that mothers and fathers play different roles in children's lives in the areas of both attachment security and engagement with peers. However, there is still much to discover.

In conclusion, we agree with Schneider et al. (2001), who on the basis of their meta-analysis suggest that "relatively little will be gained with new correlational studies linking mother–child attachment with the mainstays of peer-relations assessment" (p. 96). Though necessary as a first step, future studies should advance our understanding of *why* and in *what specific ways* attachment security is connected with child outcomes in relation to peers.

References

Ainsworth, M. D. S. (1990). Epilogue: Some considerations regarding theory and assessment relevant to attachments beyond infancy. In M. T. Greenberg, D. Cicchetti, & E. M. Cummings (Eds.), *Attachment in the preschool years* (pp. 463–488). Chicago: University of Chicago Press.

Ainsworth, M. D. S., Blehar, M. C., Waters, E., & Wall, S. (1978). *Patterns of attachment: A psychological study of the strange situation*. Hillsdale, NJ: Erlbaum.

Belsky, J., & Cassidy, J. (1994). Attachment: Theory and evidence. In M. Rutter & D. Hay (Eds.), *Developmental principles and clinical issues in psychology and psychiatry* (pp. 373–402). London: Blackwell.

Belsky, J., & Fearon, R. M. (2002). Early attachment security, subsequent maternal sensitivity, and later child development: Does continuity in development depend upon continuity of caregiving? *Attachment and Human Development, 4*, 361–387.

Belsky, J., Fish, M., & Isabella, R. (1991). Continuity and discontinuity in infant negative and positive emotionality: Family antecedents and attachment consequences. *Developmental Psychology, 27*, 421–431.

Bohlin, G., Hagekull, B., & Rydell, A. M. (2000). Attachment and social functioning: A longitudinal study from infancy to middle childhood. *Social Development, 9*, 24–39.

Booth, C. L., Rose-Krasnor, L., McKinnon, J., & Rubin, K. H. (1994). Predicting social adjustment in middle childhood: The role of preschool attachment security and maternal style. *Social Development, 3*, 189–204.

Booth, C. L., Rubin, K. H., & Rose-Krasnor, L. (1998). Perceptions of emotional support from mother and friend in middle childhood: Links with social–emotional adaptation and preschool attachment security. *Child Development, 69*, 427–442.

Booth-LaForce, C., Oh, W., Kim, A. H., Rubin, K. H., Rose-Krasnor, L., & Burgess, K. (2006). Attachment, self-worth, and peer-group functioning in middle childhood. *Attachment and Human Development, 8*, 309–325.

Bost, K. K., Vaughn, B. E., Washington, W. N., Cielinski, K. L., & Bradbard, M. R. (1998). Social competence, social support, and attachment: Demarcation of construct domains, measurement, and paths of influence for preschool children attending Head Start. *Child Development, 69*, 192–218.

Bowlby, J. (1973). *Attachment and loss: Vol. 2. Separation.* New York: Basic Books.

Bowlby, J. (1980). *Attachment and loss: Vol. 3. Loss, sadness and depression.* New York: Basic Books.

Bowlby, J. (1982). *Attachment and loss: Vol. 1. Attachment.* New York: Basic Books. (Original work published 1969)

Bowlby, J. (1988). Developmental psychiatry comes of age. *American Journal of Psychiatry, 145,* 1–10.

Bretherton, I. (2005). In pursuit of the internal working model construct and its relevance to attachment relationships. In K. E. Grossmann, K. Grossmann, & E. Waters (Eds.), *Attachment from infancy to adulthood* (pp. 13–47). New York: Guilford Press.

Bretherton, I., & Munholland, K. A. (1999). Internal working models in attachment relationships: A construct revisited. In J. Cassidy & P. R. Shaver (Eds.), *Handbook of attachment: Theory, research, and clinical applications* (pp. 89–111). New York: Guilford Press.

Burgess, K. B., Marshall, P. J., Rubin, K. H., & Fox, N. A. (2003). Infant attachment and temperament as predictors of subsequent externalizing problems and cardiac physiology. *Journal of Child Psychology and Psychiatry, 44,* 819–831.

Carlson, E. A. (1998). A prospective longitudinal study of attachment disorganization/disorientation. *Child Development, 69,* 1107–1128.

Cassidy, J., Kirsh, S. J., Scolton, K. L., & Parke, R. D. (1996). Attachment and representations of peer relationships. *Developmental Psychology, 32,* 892–904.

Cohn, D. A. (1990). Child–mother attachment of six-year-olds and social competence at school. *Child Development, 61,* 152–162.

Cohn, D. A., Patterson, C. J., & Christopoulos, C. (1991). The family and children's peer relations. *Journal of Social and Personal Relationships, 8,* 315–346.

Contreras, J. M., & Kerns, K. A. (2000). Emotion regulation processes: Explaining links between parent–child attachment and peer relationships. In K. A. Kerns, J. M. Contreras, & A. M. Neal-Barnett (Eds.), *Family and peers: Linking two social worlds* (pp. 1–25). Westport, CT: Praeger.

Contreras, J. M., Kerns, K. A., Weimer, B. L., Gentzler, A. L., & Tomich, P. L. (2000). Emotion regulation as a mediator of associations between mother–child attachment and peer relationships in middle childhood. *Journal of Family Psychology, 14,* 111–124.

Crittenden, P. M. (1990). Internal representational models of attachment relationships. *Infant Mental Health Journal, 11,* 259–277.

Davies, P. T., Cummings, E., & Winter, M. A. (2004). Pathways between profiles of family functioning, child security in the interparental subsystem, and child psychological problems. *Development and Psychopathology, 16,* 525–550.

Davies, P. T., Harold, G. T., Goeke-Morey, M. C., & Cummings, E. (2002). Child emotional security and interparental conflict. *Monographs of the Society for Research in Child Development, 67*(3), vii–viii.

DeMulder, E. K., Denham, S., Schmidt, M., & Mitchell, J. (2000). *Q*-sort assessment of attachment security during the preschool years: Links from home to school. *Developmental Psychology, 36,* 274–282.

De Wolff, M. S., & van IJzendoorn, M. H. (1997). Sensitivity and attachment: A meta-analysis on parental antecedents of infant attachment. *Child Development, 68,* 571–591.

Dwyer, K. M. (2005). The meaning and measurement of attachment in middle and late childhood. *Human Development, 48,* 155–182.

Easterbrooks, M., & Abeles, R. (2000). Windows to the self in 8-year-olds: Bridges to attachment representation and behavioral adjustment. *Attachment and Human Development, 2,* 85–106.

El-Sheikh, M., & Buckhalt, J. A. (2003). Parental problem drinking and children's adjustment: Attachment and family functioning as moderators and mediators of risk. *Journal of Family Psychology, 17,* 510–520.

Epstein, J. L. (1986). Friendship selection: Developmental and environmental influences. In E. C. Mueller & C. R. Cooper (Eds.), *Process and outcome in peer relationships* (pp. 129–160). Orlando, FL: Academic Press.

Finnegan, R. A., Hodges, E. V., & Perry, D. G. (1996). Preoccupied and avoidant coping during middle childhood. *Child Development, 67*, 1318–1328.

Fraley, R. C. (2002). Attachment stability from infancy to adulthood: Meta-analysis and dynamic modeling of developmental mechanisms. *Personality and Social Psychology Review, 6*, 123–151.

Gottman, J., & Mettetal, G. (1986). Speculations about social and affective development: Friendship and acquaintanceship through adolescence. In J. M . Gottman & J. G. Parker (Eds.), *Conversations of friends* (pp. 192–237). New York: Cambridge University Press.

Graham, C. A., & Easterbrooks, M. (2000). School-aged children's vulnerability to depressive symptomatology: The role of attachment security, maternal depressive symptomatology, and economic risk. *Development and Psychopathology, 12*, 201–213.

Granot, D., & Mayseless, O. (2001). Attachment security and adjustment to school in middle childhood. *International Journal of Behavioral Development, 25*, 530–541.

Grossmann, K., Grossmann, K. E., Fremmer-Bombik, E., Kindler, H., Scheuerer-Englisch, H., & Zimmermann, P. (2002). The uniqueness of the child–father attachment relationship: Father's sensitive and challenging play as a pivotal variable in a 16-year longitudinal study. *Social Development, 11*, 307–331.

Harold, G. T., Shelton, K. H., Goeke-Morey, M. C., & Cummings, E. (2004). Marital conflict, child emotional security about family relationships and child adjustment. *Social Development, 13*, 350–376.

Harris, J. R. (1995). Where is the child's environment?: A group socialization theory of development. *Psychological Review, 102*, 458–489.

Hinde, R. A. (1988). Continuities and discontinuities: Conceptual issues and methodological considerations. In M. Rutter (Ed.), *Studies of psychosocial risk: The power of longitudinal data* (pp. 367–383). Cambridge, UK: Cambridge University Press.

Hodges, E. V., Finnegan, R. A., & Perry, D. G. (1999). Skewed autonomy-relatedness in preadolescents' conceptions of their relationships with mother, father, and best friend. *Developmental Psychology, 35*, 737–748.

Howes, C. (1988). Peer interaction of young children. *Monographs of the Society for Research in Child Development, 53*(Serial No. 217).

Howes, C., & Tonyan, H. (1999). Peer relations. In L. Balter & C. S. Tamis-LeMonda (Eds.), *Child psychology: A handbook of contemporary issues* (pp. 143–157). New York: Psychology Press.

Keller, T. E., Spieker, S. J., & Gilchrist, L. (2005). Patterns of risk and trajectories of preschool problem behaviors: A person-oriented analysis of attachment in context. *Development and Psychopathology, 17*, 349–384.

Kerns, K. A. (1994). A developmental model of the relations between mother–child attachment and friendship. In R. Erber & R. Gilmour (Eds.), *Theoretical frameworks for personal relationships* (pp. 129–156). Hillsdale, NJ: Erlbaum.

Kerns, K. A. (2000). Types of preschool friendships. *Personal Relationships, 7*, 311–324.

Kerns, K. A. (2008). Attachment in middle childhood. In J. Cassidy & P. R. Shaver (Eds.), *Handbook of attachment* (2nd ed., pp. 366–382). New York: Guilford Press.

Kerns, K. A., Abraham, M. M., Schlegelmilch, A., & Morgan, T. A. (2007). Mother–child attachment in later middle childhood: Assessment approaches and associations with mood and emotion regulation. *Attachment and Human Development, 9*, 33–53.

Kerns, K. A., & Barth, J. (1995). Attachment and play: Convergence across components of parent–child relationships and their relations to peer competence. *Journal of Social and Personal Relationships, 12*, 243–260.

Kerns, K. A., Cole, A., & Andrews, P. B. (1998). Attachment security, peer management practices, and peer relationships in preschoolers. *Merrill–Palmer Quarterly, 44*, 504–522.

Kerns, K. A., Klepac, L., & Cole, A. (1996). Peer relationships and preadolescents' perceptions of security in the child–mother relationship. *Developmental Psychology, 32*, 457–466.

Kerns, K. A., & Richardson, R. A. (Eds.). (2005). *Attachment in middle childhood*. New York: Guilford Press.

Ladd, G. W. (1992). Themes and theories: Perspectives on processes in family-peer relationships. In R. D. Parke & G. W. Ladd (Eds.), *Family–peer relationships: Modes of linkage* (pp. 1–34). Hillsdale, NJ: Erlbaum.

Lamb, M. E. (1997). Fathers and child development: An introductory overview and guide. In M. E. Lamb (Ed.), *The role of the father in child development* (3rd ed., pp. 1–18). New York: Wiley.

Lewis, M., Feiring, C., & Rosenthal, S. (2000). Attachment over time. *Child Development, 71*, 707–720.

Lieberman, M., Doyle, A. B., & Markiewicz, D. (1999). Developmental patterns in security of attachment to mother and father in late childhood and early adolescence: Associations with peer relations. *Child Development, 70*, 202–213.

Lyons-Ruth, K. (1996). Attachment relationships among children with aggressive behavior problems: The role of disorganized early attachment patterns. *Journal of Consulting and Clinical Psychology, 64*, 64–73.

Main, M., Kaplan, N., & Cassidy, J. (1985). Security in infancy, childhood, and adulthood: A move to the level of representation. *Monographs of the Society for Research in Child Development, 50*(Serial No. 209), 66–104.

McElwain, N. L., Booth-LaForce, C., & Lansford, J. E. (2007). *Social information processing and language relations with early child–mother attachment and later social–emotional functioning during the transition to school.* Manuscript submitted for publication.

McElwain, N. L., Cox, M. J., Burchinal, M. R., & Macfie, J. (2003). Differentiating among insecure mother–infant attachment classifications: A focus on child–friend interaction and exploration during solitary play at 36 months. *Attachment and Human Development, 5*, 136–164.

McElwain, N. L., & Volling, B. L. (2004). Attachment security and parental sensitivity during infancy: Associations with friendship quality and false-belief understanding at age 4. *Journal of Social and Personal Relationships, 21*, 639–667.

Moss, E., Cyr, C., & Dubois-Comtois, K. (2004). Attachment at early school age and developmental risk: Examining family contexts and behavior problems of controlling–caregiving, controlling–punitive, and behaviorally disorganized children. *Developmental Psychology, 40*, 519–532.

Moss, E., Rousseau, D., Parent, S., St. Laurent, D., & Saintonge, J. (1998). Correlates of attachment at school age: Maternal reported stress, mother–child interaction, and behavior problems. *Child Development, 69*, 1390–1405.

Muris, P., Mayer, B., & Meesters, C. (2000). Self-reported attachment style, anxiety, and depression in children. *Social Behavior and Personality, 28*, 157–162.

NICHD Early Child Care Research Network. (2006). Infant–mother attachment classification: Risk and protection in relation to changing maternal caregiving quality. *Developmental Psychology, 42*, 38–58.

Park, K. A., & Waters, E. (1989). Security of attachment and preschool friendships. *Child Development, 60*, 1076–1081.

Parke, R. D. (2002). Fathers and families. In M. H. Bornstien (Ed.), *Handbook of parenting: Vol. 3. Being and becoming a parent* (2nd ed., pp. 27–74). Mahwah, NJ: Erlbaum.

Parke, R. D., & Ladd, G. W. (1992). *Family–peer relationships: Modes of linkage*. Hillsdale, NJ: Erlbaum.

Pierrehumbert, B., Miljkovitch, R., Plancherel, B., Halfon, O., & Ansermet, F. (2000). Attachment and temperament in early childhood; Implications for later behavior problems. *Infant and Child Development, 9*, 17–32.

Renken, B., Egeland, B., Marvinney, D., Mangelsdorf, S., & Sroufe, L. A. (1989). Early childhood antecedents of aggression and passive-withdrawal in early elementary school. *Journal of Personality, 57*, 257–281.

Roisman, G. I., Collins, W. A., Sroufe, L. A., & Egeland, B. (2005). Predictors of young adults' representations of and behavior in their current romantic relationship: Prospective tests of the prototype hypothesis. *Attachment and Human Development, 7*, 105–121.

Rose-Krasnor, L., Rubin, K. H., Booth, C. L., & Coplan, R. J. (1996). Maternal directiveness and child attachment security as predictors of social competence in preschoolers. *International Journal of Behavioral Development, 19*, 309–325.

Rubin, K. H., Bukowski, W., & Parker, J. (2006). Peer interactions, relationships, and groups. In N. Eisenberg (Ed.), *Handbook of child psychology: Social, emotional, and personality development* (6th ed., pp. 571–645). New York: Wiley.

Rubin, K. H., Dwyer, K. M., Booth-LaForce, C. L., Kim, A. H., Burgess, K. B., & Rose-Krasnor, L. (2004). Attachment, friendship, and psychosocial functioning in early adolescence. *Journal of Early Adolescence, 24*, 326–356.

Rubin, K. H., & Lollis, S. (1988). Origins and consequences of social withdrawal. In J. Belsky & T. Nezworski (Eds.), *Clinical implications of attachment* (pp. 219–252). Hillsdale, NJ: Erlbaum.

Sameroff, A. J., Bartko, W. T., Baldwin, A., Baldwin, C., & Seifer, R. (1998). Family and social influences on the development of child competence. In M. Lewis & C. Feiring (Eds.), *Families, risk, and competence* (pp. 161–185). Hillsdale, NJ: Erlbaum.

Schneider, B. H., Atkinson, L., & Tardif, C. (2001). Child–parent attachment and children's peer relations: A quantitative review. *Developmental Psychology, 37*, 86–100.

Shulman, S., Elicker, J., & Sroufe, L. A. (1994). Stages of friendship growth in preadolescence as related to attachment history. *Journal of Social and Personal Relationships, 11*, 341–361.

Simons, K. J., Paternite, C. E., & Shore, C. (2001). Quality of parent/adolescent attachment and aggression in young adolescents. *Journal of Early Adolescence, 21*, 182–203.

Solomon, J., & George, C. (1999). The measurement of attachment security in infancy and childhood. In J. Cassidy & P. R. Shaver (Eds.), *Handbook of attachment* (pp. 287–316). New York: Guilford Press.

Sroufe, L. A. (1979). The coherence of individual development. *American Psychologist, 34*, 834–841.

Sroufe, L. A. (1983). Infant–caregiver attachment and patterns of adaptation in preschool: The roots of maladaptation and competence. In M. Perlmutter (Ed.), *Minnesota Symposia on Child Psychology: Vol. 16. Development and policy concerning children with special needs* (pp. 41–81). Hillsdale, NJ: Erlbaum.

Sroufe, L. A., Bennett, C., Englund, M., Urban, J., & Shulman, S. (1993). The significance of gender boundaries in preadolescence: Contemporary correlates and antecedents of boundary violation and maintenance. *Child Development, 64*, 455–466.

Sroufe, L. A., Egeland, B., & Carlson, E. A. (1999). One social world: The integrated development of parent–child and peer relationships. In W. A. Collins & B. Laursen (Eds.), *Minnesota Symposia on Child Psychology: Vol. 30. Relationships as developmental contexts: Festschrift in honor of Willard W. Hartup* (pp. 241–261). Mahwah, NJ: Erlbaum.

Sroufe, L. A., Egeland, B., Carlson, E., & Collins, W. A. (2005). Placing early attachment experiences in developmental context. In K. E. Grossmann, K. Grossmann, & E. Waters (Eds.), *Attachment from infancy to adulthood* (pp. 48–70). New York: Guilford Press.

Sroufe, L. A., Egeland, B., & Kreutzer, T. (1990). The fate of early experience following developmental change: Longitudinal approaches to individual adaptation in childhood. *Child Development, 61*, 1363–1373.

Sroufe, L. A., & Fleeson, J. (1986). Attachment and the construction of relationships. In W. Hartup & Z. Rubin (Eds.), *Relationships and development* (pp. 51–71). Hillsdale, NJ: Erlbaum.

Sroufe, L. A., Schork, E., Motti, E., Lawroski, N., & LaFreniere, P. (1984). The role of affect in social competence. In C. Izard, J. Kagan, & R. Zajonc (Eds.), *Emotion, cognition, and behavior* (pp. 289–319). New York: Plenum Press.

Stams, G. J., Juffer, F., & van IJzendoorn, M. H. (2002). Maternal sensitivity, infant attachment, and temperament in early childhood predict adjustment in middle childhood: The case of adopted children and their biologically unrelated parents. *Developmental Psychology, 38*, 806–821.

Suess, G., Grossmann, K., & Sroufe, L. A. (1992). Effects of infant attachment to mother and father on quality of adaptation in preschool: From dyadic to individual organization of the self. *International Journal of Behavioral Development, 15*, 43–66.

Sullivan, H. S. (1953). *The interpersonal theory of psychiatry.* New York: Norton.

Thompson, R. A. (2005). Multiple relationships multiply considered. *Human Development, 48*, 102–107.

Thompson, R. A., & Raikes, H. A. (2003). Toward the next quarter-century: Conceptual and methodological challenges for attachment theory. *Development and Psychopathology, 15*, 691–718.

Troy, M., & Sroufe, L. A. (1987). Victimization of pre-schoolers: Role of attachment relationship history. *Journal of the American Academy of Child and Adolescent Psychiatry, 26*, 166–172.

Verschueren, K., & Marcoen, A. (1999). Representation of self and socioemotional competence in kindergartners: Differential and combined effects of attachment to mother and to father. *Child Development, 70*, 183–201.

Verschueren, K., & Marcoen, A. (2002). Perceptions of self and relationship with parents in aggressive and nonaggressive rejected children. *Journal of School Psychology, 40*, 501–522.

Verschueren, K., & Marcoen, A. (2005). Perceived security of attachment to mother and father: Developmental differences and relations to self-worth and peer relationships at school. In K. A. Kerns & R. A. Richardson (Eds.), *Attachment in middle childhood* (pp. 212–230). New York: Guilford Press.

Wartner, U. G., Grossmann, K., Fremmer-Bombik, E., & Suess, G. (1994). Attachment patterns at age six in south Germany: Predictability from infancy and implications for preschool behavior. *Child Development, 65*, 1014–1027.

Waters, E., Vaughn, B. E., Posada, G., & Kondo-Ikemura, K. (Eds.). (1995). Caregiving, cultural and cognitive perspectives on secure-base behavior and working models: New growing points of attachment theory and research. *Monographs of the Society for Research in Child Development, 60*(2–3, Serial No. 244).

Waters, E., Wippman, J., & Sroufe, L. A. (1979). Attachment, positive affect, and competence in the peer group: Two studies in construct validation. *Child Development, 50*, 821–829.

Youngblade, L. M., Park, K. A., & Belsky, J. (1993). Measurement of young children's close friendship: A comparison of two independent assessment systems and their associations with attachment security. *International Journal of Behavioral Development, 16*, 563–587.

Yunger, J. L., Corby, B. C., & Perry, D. G. (2005). Dimensions of attachment in middle childhood. In K. A. Kerns & R. A. Richardson (Eds.), *Attachment in middle childhood* (pp. 89–114). New York: Guilford Press.

CHAPTER 28

Family Influences
on Children's Peer Relationships

HILDY ROSS
NINA HOWE

Central Issues

For many reasons, what happens in the family should affect children's peer interactions and relationships. First, family life is ubiquitous, multifaceted, and complex. Some of the complexity arises because families entail a set of interacting relationships, any of which can influence the development of children and, through that, their relationships beyond the family. Second, diverse socialization processes no doubt operate from within the family; families provide models of interpersonal relationships that can be adopted or adapted to suit peer situations, offer direct guidance as to how children should treat one another, and set atmospheres of harmony and cooperation or competition and conflict. Families also select neighborhoods, and with these, school and peer-group characteristics; they set the conditions for and supervise peer experiences, especially early in life. Third, there are many indirect pathways through which family life may interact with and affect the attributions, beliefs, emotional security, and the confidence or reticence of each family member. Genetic similarities among family members complicate the developmental story, and reciprocal influences can often mean that children are affecting their own developmental pathways both within the family and in their wider social networks. The psychologists' search for the "direction of causality" is often frustrated by both the ethical and practical limitations of much of the existing research. Thus, our goals are limited: We seek a comprehensive appraisal of the links that exist between children's development within their families and their experiences of peer interaction and relationships. We take an eclectic approach to the theoretical models of family influence and pay special attention to research that disambiguates processes through which family and peer relationships might exert their influence on one another. We limit our coverage to young children and focus on the role of relationships within the immediate family—those between parents and children, siblings, and marital partners.

We emphasize sibling relationships, as well as those between parents and children. Sibling relationships are important for two reasons: First, sibling relationships are more similar to relationships that children will develop with their peers, because these relationships involve greater equality of status and ability than those with parents, and because play and companionship are central to sibling relationships, as they are to relationships with peers (Dunn, 1983). Moreover, sibling relationships provide models of relationship characteristics that are far more akin to those that develop with peers than are parent–child relationships. Second, parents socialize children within families that normatively contain more than one child. If they are to influence how children treat their peers and what children are to expect from their peers, then they do so often in the context of sibling relationships and may relate those socializing efforts not directly to children's peer relationships but to their ongoing relations with sisters and brothers (Ross, Filyer, Lollis, Perlman, & Martin, 1994). Moral issues arise in families most often when siblings violate one another's rights or welfare, so parents deal with children's developing moral standards in the context of sibling relationships. Children expect their parents to treat them equally, or that when inequality arises, the reasons for it will be understandable (Kramer & Kowal, 2005); thus, differential treatment becomes an important debilitating factor in children's sibling relationships that may carry forward into children's views of how the world treats them.

Key Classical and Modern Research Studies

An influential collection of papers edited by Ross Parke and Gary Ladd (1992) did much to set the agenda for the study of parents' influences on children's peer relationships. Importantly, two types of parent influences were distinguished: "Direct influences" are those parenting practices aimed at fostering children's relationships with peers. These include parents' efforts to arrange and supervise peer encounters, to intervene directly when difficulties arise with children's agemates, or to coach their children in anticipation of peer-group involvement (Lollis, Tate, & Ross, 1992). Underlying these direct pathways of influence are parental beliefs regarding the importance of promoting their children's positive interactions with siblings and peers (Rubin, Bukowski, & Parker, 2006). We begin our review of the existing literature by considering direct influences on children's peer relationships.

"Indirect influences" occur as a result of parenting practices leading to the children's development of the positive and negative characteristics that influence their abilities to interact with peers and to form friendships (Parke & Ladd, 1992). Parenting behavior and sibling relationships that foster social competence, interpersonal confidence, or aggression might be particularly relevant to the development of children's peer relationships. Social imitation, expectations concerning relationship processes, and abilities to regulate negative emotions are processes hypothesized to develop within family relationships and to link family and peer relationships. Family members might also be expected to react differently to children who are eager to make friends and to play with others, who are confident or insecure in peer situations, or who behave aggressively in the playground or the preschool.

Direct Family Influences on Children's Peer Relationships

Parents Supervise and Provide Opportunities
for the Development of Peer Competence

Parents often act in a management capacity, providing various opportunities and activities for children to interact with peers (Ladd & Pettit, 2002; Lollis et al., 1992), although the degree of direct involvement varies according to the child's age. The overriding parental goal is to facilitate opportunities for children to develop skills to initiate and maintain prosocial peer interactions. Whereas parents may take a proactive role in the early years, school-age children begin to manage their own social interactions to a greater degree. Parental management strategies include social planning, participation in activities, monitoring, and the integration of adult and child social networks. We discuss each strategy in turn.

One arena in which parents take an early role in facilitating their children's peer relations is social planning, by providing informal interaction opportunities (e.g., playdates). During the toddler and preschool years, parents are frequently proactive and concerned with the "who," "where," "what," and "when" of arranging peer contact (Ladd, Le-Sieur, & Profilet, 1993). Thus, parents act as social directors by orchestrating opportunities for informal peer contacts, although often there are also more formal opportunities (e.g., child care, preschool, community activities). These opportunities allow children (and parents) to build social networks and to develop important social skills for getting along with individual playmates and groups of children.

Toddlers develop distinctive styles of interacting together and enduring positive relationships as a result of frequent informal opportunities to play together (Ross & Lollis, 1989). Preschoolers whose parents are more active in initiating opportunities have more playmates and exhibit more prosocial behaviors compared to children of less active parents (Kerns, Cole, & Andrews, 1998). Furthermore, kindergarten boys whose parents are moderately active (vs. over- or underinvolved) in the preschool years are better liked by their classmates and engage in more prosocial behavior (Ladd & Hart, 1992). Also, school-age children become more active in arranging their own peer contacts, especially if their parents have been proactive in the earlier years. Thus, during the preschool years, parents may have modeled or supported behaviors required to arrange peer contact, so that by school age, children are able to initiate peer contact on their own.

Parents' strategies for promoting children's positive peer relations also include participation, often in the form of interacting, coaching, or supervising play with peers. When parents become active play partners, they may scaffold positive interactions between children, a strategy that is most appropriate with very young children (Lollis et al., 1992). Parental guidance during toddlers' peer interactions is associated with more frequent child–child interactions (e.g., turn taking, sharing), suggesting that parents may guide their children in learning the dynamics of social interaction. Older preschoolers require less parental involvement to maintain positive peer interactions (Ladd & Golter, 1988). Children have higher peer status when their mothers employ effective supervision and coaching strategies (regarding group entry, conflicts, or cooperation) during peer interactions compared to children whose mothers are less effective coaches (Finnie & Russell, 1988, 1990).

Parents are also most active in intervening in children's conflicts with agemates (Lollis et al., 1992; Ross, Tesla, Kenyon, & Lollis, 1990). When children fight over property, mothers consistently urge their own children to consider the rights and welfare of their companions, and to acquiesce to their peers' demands. Interestingly, this often produces inconsistencies in parents' reasoning, because they sometimes ask children to yield to the demands of owners ("because it's his") or to nonowners ("because she doesn't have one of these to play with at home"). Parents rarely address or discipline their children's play-mates, but leave this task to the peer's mother. Thus, mothers emphasize the well-being of others rather than children's property rights as they attempt to resolve peer conflicts.

As children become more proficient in their peer relations during middle childhood and are less likely to want direct parental involvement, they may instead turn to parents for advice or guidance in managing social interactions (Cohen, 1989). Thus, parents' involvement becomes more distal, but they may take advantage of informal opportunities to discuss the state of their children's peer relations. These decontextualized discussions may include opportunities to "teach" children how to deal with difficult situations or to encourage more prosocial interaction, or they may be times to provide advice and sup-port (Lollis et al., 1992). The school-age children of supportive, noninterfering mothers who provide timely advice exhibited more positive peer relations (Cohen, 1989). Thus, distal forms of discussion versus direct involvement may be normative in this period.

As children move into middle childhood, when the importance of peers increases in their lives, parental monitoring becomes increasingly distal. Monitoring is concep-tualized as parents' awareness, knowledge, and supervision regarding their children's whereabouts, activities, and choice of friends (Ladd & Pettit, 2002). Lack of parental monitoring has been associated with less optimal social and academic outcomes (Kilg-ore, Snyder, & Lentz, 2000), suggesting that more active monitoring by parents sends a positive message to children regarding their extrafamilial experiences. Interestingly, parents' perceptions of neighborhood safety influence the degree of parental supervi-sion; in less desirable neighborhoods, increased parental supervision is associated with greater social competence (O'Neil, Parke, & McDowell, 2001). Even as early as pre-school, parents who seem unconcerned about their children's whereabouts or exposure to violence and other potentially negative peer and adult influences have children who display more severe conduct problems both in preschool and kindergarten (Kilgore et al., 2000). Such parents are unlikely to be very discerning in selecting schools, and poor school selection is a critical link in the pathway from the early lack of parental moni-toring to young children's aggressiveness on the playground and behavior problems in kindergarten classrooms.

As all parents of young children know, their own social networks and those of their children become intertwined. Initially parents may seek out playmates for their very young children from among the families in their adult networks, thus maintaining some control over their children's peer relations. Yet, as children's networks expand through informal (e.g., neighbors) or more formal contacts (e.g., child care, preschool, school, extracurricular activities), these networks often mesh with the parents' networks. This intermeshing of parent and child networks may be beneficial for children's peer rela-tions, because it provides wider social support for families; parents can rely on appro-priate supervision and encouragement of prosocial interaction by the parents of their children's friends, and they are likely to share common values (Parke et al., 2002). The outcome of these intertwined social networks may be beneficial for children's social com-petence, although there appear to be few direct tests of this notion in early and middle childhood.

Do Siblings Directly Influence Children's Peer Relationships?

The answer to this question is that we do not know. Very little evidence exists concerning the direct influence of siblings on children's peer relationships. Siblings could potentially impact peer relationships by including one another in play with friends in the neighborhood or at school, by offering protection from bullies, by excluding or instigating aggression themselves, or by monitoring and coaching siblings' peer relationships. The one recent study that addresses direct sibling influences suggests that prosocial twin siblings, even those who do not share classrooms, provide protection against peer-group victimization, although the means by which they do so is not clear (Lamarche et al., 2006). Older siblings, in particular, are likely to have more expertise with peer culture than parents, and to be present or nearby when monitoring or intervention is needed. The role of siblings in directly supporting children's peer relationships is clearly a topic of some merit for future research.

Indirect Family Influences on Children's Peer Relationships

If children derive models of relationships from those they experience in the family, then marital discord, harsh or punitive parenting, and aggressive siblings may dispose them to consider aggression as normative and potentially effective in reaching their goals. If coercive interaction pays off in the family, then similar negative patterns might be carried forward to the peer domain. If parents and siblings are companionable and enjoyable interactive partners, then social competence should develop and influence children's peer relationships. Both harmonious and acrimonious family interactions influence children's emotional resources, and the security and confidence with which they approach peer relationships (Davies, Harold, Goeke-Morey, & Cummings, 2002; Katz, Kramer, & Gottman, 1992; Rubin, Hastings, Chen, Stewart, & McNichol, 1998). On the other hand, children's competence or hostility with peers could also be the cause of similar dispositions at home, reversing the direction of effects advanced by most theories linking family to peer processes (Kramer & Kowal, 2005; Jenkins, Simpson, Dunn, Rasbash, & O'Connor, 2005; Snyder, Cramer, Afrank, & Patterson, 2005). The theoretical literature provides not so much competing as compatible propositions for how mutual influences link family and peer domains, nor is the empirical literature generally directed to differentiate among alternative explanations. It asks, more simply, whether there are associations between family processes and children's interaction with peers, and seeks to uncover the pathways through which mutual influences might exert themselves. How strong is the empirical evidence for links between families and peers?

Parenting and Children's Social Competence

Social competence is the ability to initiate and maintain positive interactions, to develop affiliative ties (i.e., make friends, be accepted by peers), and to avoid negative roles (e.g., rejection, victimization) and outcomes (e.g., loneliness, anxiety) (Ladd & Pettit, 2002). Promoting social competence requires parents to be sensitive and responsive to the children's characteristics (e.g., temperament, attachment), while taking into account their developmental stage, history of familial and extrafamilial experiences (e.g., child care, school, neighborhood), interests (e.g., sports, arts), and preferences for social interaction. Accordingly, knowledgeable, responsive, and sensitive parents may be well-placed to promote children's positive peer interactions.

The quality of the children's primary attachments to their parents is believed to be the basis for their later social interactions (Sroufe & Fleeson, 1988). Thus, sensitive and responsive parents facilitate the development of secure, warm parent–child attachments that allow children to learn autonomy and skills important for other relationships, such as those with peers. During this process, children also develop internal working models about the nature of relationships and apply these internalized notions to their interactions with playmates. Specifically, securely attached children enter play situations with the expectation that their partners will be responsive, warm, engaged, and nurturant. In fact, secure parent–child attachments enhance the likelihood that children will have more positive, friendly, and prosocial peer interactions, as well as their acceptance by preschool and school-age peers (Booth, Rose-Krasnor, & Rubin, 1991). Secure attachments also have an impact on the quality of children's friendships and social acceptance in middle childhood (see Booth-LaForce & Kerns, Chapter 27, this volume), indicating the long-term importance of early parent–child attachments. Thus, secure parent–child attachments may lay the foundation for children to generalize their social–emotional behaviors and skills to prosocial peer exchanges and positive friendships in middle childhood. Interestingly, in a meta-analysis, Schneider, Atkinson, and Tardif (2001) reported stronger associations between attachment and friendship than between attachment and peer-group acceptance, suggesting that the intimate, intense quality of the attachment relationship is more likely to influence other close and reciprocated relationships, such as friendships, than are group perceptions or acceptance. Although children are attached to their siblings (Stewart, 1983), the contribution of sibling attachment to children's peer relationships has not been examined.

One aspect of parenting that has garnered attention is the influence of childrearing styles on children's development. Maccoby and Martin (1983) outlined two constructs (warmth, control) to develop a typology of four styles of childrearing that combined low and high levels of these two constructs (i.e., authoritative, authoritarian, permissive, uninvolved). In particular, authoritative childrearing may promote positive peer interactions, because parents who are high on acceptance and responsivity not only employ high yet flexible control, use inductive reasoning, have high but realistic expectations, and encourage autonomy and joint decision making, but also monitor their children's activities and peer relations. Authoritative childrearing is positively associated with more optimal social outcomes for children, including peer relations, than the other parental styles (Rubin & Burgess, 2002). Furthermore, parental warmth and praise are also positively linked to prosocial behavior and peer-group acceptance (for a recent review, see Eisenberg, Fabes, & Spinrad, 2006). Pettit, Bates, and Dodge (1997) assessed the influence of authoritative or supportive parenting practices (warmth, inductive discipline, interest/involvement in peer relations, and teaching social skills) in a longitudinal study of children's adjustment from before school entry to grade 6. Supportive parenting predicted adjustment (including peer relations) in grade 6, even after researchers controlled for adjustment in kindergarten and authoritarian parenting. Parental techniques of calm discussion regarding problems, proactive teaching of social skills, and maternal involvement at an early age were predictive of later positive peer relations. Apparently, authoritative parents model caring, supportive approaches to relationships, encourage children to think about and solve social problems, and encourage positive social interactions in the family and in the wider world. This approach may be influential in charting the course of children's relationships with others (e.g., siblings, peers).

In recent years there has been a shift from studying global styles of childrearing to examining the influence of specific parent–child behaviors on children's peer relations (Ladd & Pettit, 2002). Parent–child play is an early context for learning to engage in positive social interactions and may provide a training ground for later prosocial peer interactions (Tamis-LeMonda, Uzgiris, & Bornstein, 2002). Why is parent–child play so important in facilitating young children's interpersonal interaction? First, play is one context for learning about appropriate emotional expression and, particularly, pretense is a safe venue for experimenting with positive and negative emotions. Dunn and colleagues (Brown, Donelan-McCall, & Dunn, 1996; Dunn, 2006) have demonstrated that some mothers and children employ frequent references to internal states (thoughts, feelings, desires) during play that are related to children's later affective perspective taking and friendly sibling and peer interaction. Second, play serves communicative functions that allow youngsters to construct knowledge about turn taking; reciprocity of exchanges; initiating, maintaining, and ending interactions; and co-construction and negotiation of play scenarios. Third, play provides a social context for learning about the "rules and boundaries of social contact" (Tamis-LeMonda et al., 2002, p. 227). Finally, pretend play is a context for learning about cultural and conventional norms practiced in the family (Farver & Howes, 1993).

In fact, the evidence supports the view that early parent–child play contributes to children's ability to generalize and to apply the skills learned during this context to their social interactions with peers. Parke and colleagues (MacDonald & Parke, 1984; Parke et al., 1989) conducted several studies on preschooler–parent play and concluded that this context facilitates important aspects of children's social and emotional competence with peers: Parental directiveness, engagement, and ability to elicit positive affect in the child were key factors. Parental directiveness may allow children to learn to regulate interactions and emotions during play, which become the foundation for peer interactions. The ability to sustain play with parents, in particular, maternal engagement with sons, was also related to children's subsequent peer popularity. Gerrits, Goudena, and van Aken (2005) found that 7-year-olds with high social status engaged in mutually responsive interactions and more simultaneous, coordinated play with parents and peers than did low-status children. In summary, the ability to sustain and co-construct play scenarios and to develop reciprocal interactions (reflecting a balance between partners' initiations, ideas, and responses) are key features of high-quality sibling and peer interactions (Howe, Petrakos, Rinaldi, & LeFebvre, 2005; Lindsey, Mize, & Pettit, 1997).

Positive behaviors, affect, and contingent interactions during parent–child play are related to social competence in young children (LaFreniere & Dumas, 1992). Putallaz (1987) argued that mothers may evoke positive child responses, and children may in turn influence maternal behavior, making the direction of effects unclear. Perhaps mothers were responding positively to their children's agreeable behavior, which increased the likelihood that their children would reciprocate. In any case, children may use skills learned with parents during peer interactions. Furthermore, children's abilities to express positive affect mediate the relation between parental positive affect during play and peer acceptance (Isley, O'Neil, Clatfelter, & Parke, 1999). Finally, father–child play is positively associated with youngsters' ability to form higher-quality friendships (Youngblade & Belsky, 1992).

So several mechanisms may account for the associations between parental behavior and children's friendly peer relations (Parke et al., 2002). Parents spend considerable time, especially with very young children, teaching emotion regulation skills that include appropriate emotional displays, emotional understanding, and encoding and decoding skills. These affective management skills are critical for ensuring appropriate and positive interactions in familial and extrafamilial contexts (Cassidy, Parke, Butovsky, & Braungart, 1992). For example, in families in which mothers and siblings discuss internal states (i.e., thoughts, feelings, desires, or beliefs), children are more likely to employ internal state language in their interactions with siblings (Howe & Rinaldi, 2004; Jenkins, Turrell, Takei, Lollis, & Ross, 2003). A second mechanism is attentional regulatory processes; parents actively teach young children to pay attention to relevant cues, to employ cognitive strategies for emotional regulation, and to engage in behaviors that promote social competence and important relationship skills. Finally, Parke et al. (2002) highlight the importance of cognitive representation models, namely, internal working models, as discussed earlier, which play a role in children's interpersonal interactions.

Siblings as Contributors to Children's Positive Peer Relations

The sibling relationship is a natural laboratory for children to develop their social understanding and interaction skills (Dunn, 2002). A small literature on parenting of siblings (for a review, see Furman & Lanthier, 2002) demonstrates associations between warm and affectionate parenting and prosocial sibling-directed behavior (Volling, 2003). For example, when mothers and older siblings talk about a newborn younger sibling as a person with feelings and thoughts, the two children are likely to develop a friendly relationship over time (Dunn, 2002; Howe & Ross, 1990). As well, family discussions about internal states are positively associated with sibling play and caretaking (Howe & Rinaldi, 2004). Young children with a secure mother–child attachment are more likely to have a friendly sibling relationship (Volling & Belsky, 1992). Siblings in early and middle childhood are more likely to engage in prosocial behavior when their mothers have been generally positive and responsive (Volling, 2003).

Clearly, the sibling relationship is an important part of most children's social world, and given the frequently intense nature of the relationship, an extended history of shared experiences, and the concern that parents have for promoting positive exchanges, it is an important context for children to develop their prosocial skills and understanding of relationship dynamics (Dunn, 2002). Nevertheless, only a limited literature has examined how children may generalize to other relationships the skills learned during sibling interactions. In fact, support for associations in early childhood between the quality of sibling and peer relationships is rather mixed, with some studies showing no (e.g., Cutting & Dunn, 2006) or limited associations (Volling, Youngblade, & Belsky, 1997).

Furthermore, the question of whether parenting of siblings and the nature of sibling relations may mediate the links between parenting and children's positive peer relations during early childhood remains largely unexplored, although it has been investigated in relation to sibling aggression in older, school-age children (MacKinnon-Lewis, Starnes, Volling, & Johnson, 1997). McCoy, Brody, and Stoneman (1994) reported that positive parent–child relationship quality is associated with children's friendly sibling relationships between 9 and 16 years of age, which in turn is positively related to the quality of children's friendships. Thus, the quality of sibling relations appears to mediate the association between parenting and children's friendships.

How Do Parents Influence Children's Conflict and Aggression?

Conflict occurs within virtually all close relationships. It has the potential to be highly destructive to relationships and to the well-being of individuals as aggression and hostility build, as bullies impact others' lives, and as aggressive conduct disorders develop. However, experience with conflict is also potentially beneficial, because it may teach children to recognize their connections with others. As children come to respect others' goals and to tailor their own desires to the necessity of compromise and conciliation, they begin to master a central challenge of social life. Despite the possibility that families may be the source of positive responses to conflict, most attention is focused on links between family hostility and peer aggression.

The empirical research supports the association of hostile parenting and children's aggression; however, the correlations tend to be modest at best. Putallaz (1987), in a groundbreaking study, found that mothers' demanding and disagreeable behavior was associated with children's demanding, self-focused squabbling and lack of agreement when playing with their peers. Furthermore, mothers' use of threats, reprimands, and hostile affect with toddlers or preschoolers is positively associated with children's later aggression in school (Booth, Rose-Krasnor, McKinnon, & Rubin, 1994; Kochanska, 1992), and fathers' authoritarian parenting style is associated with teacher ratings of children's physical aggression with peers in preschool (Russell, Hart, Robinson, & Olsen, 2003). Similarly, Dishion, Duncan, Eddy, Fagot, and Fetrow (1994) found only weak correlations between children's coercive behavior with their parents and with peers on the playground. Moreover, investigation of parents' psychological coercion, withdrawal of love, lack of responsiveness, and use of hostile control have not indicated clear links with children's relational aggression with peers (e.g., Hart, Nelson, Robinson, Olsen, & McNeilly-Choque, 1998; Russell et al., 2003).

Perhaps the most intensive work on the link between family hostility and children's peer aggression has been that of Dodge, Bates, Pettit, and their coworkers. In their large-scale, multisite study, parenting was measured with interviews and observations before children entered school, and behavior with peers was assessed with both teacher and peer nominations. Emphasis was placed on mothers' harsh discipline practices, described, at the extreme, as "severe, strict, often physical" discipline (e.g., Dodge, Pettit & Bates, 1994; Pettit et al., 1997; Nix et al., 1999). Positive, but generally modest, relations were found between harsh parenting and children's externalizing problems according to both teacher and peer assessments from kindergarten through grade 6.

Thus, the search for simple pathways from parent hostility to peer aggression has yielded consistent but very modest effects. These findings are reinforced by a unique study that controlled for genetic influences in antisocial behavior in a sample of monozygotic (MZ) twins:

> Correlating MZ twin differences in experience with MZ-twin differences in outcome is a strong, unambiguous test of environmental experiences independent of genetics; it rules out the two possibilities (a) that a genetically transmitted liability explains both the parenting of the mother and the behavior of the child and (b) that genetically influenced differences between the children evoke different material treatments. (Caspi et al., 2004, p. 151)

Interviewer ratings of mothers' criticism or warmth in describing or interacting with their twin children were related to children's antisocial behavior (teacher ratings) when children were 5 and 7 years of age. Children's antisocial behavior was associated with differences in maternal expressed emotion, contemporaneously and longitudinally, and also predicted teacher-rated outcomes at age 7. Controls for genetic differences and earlier child behavior provide a substantially stronger case for maternal influence than is found in most studies.

Mutual Influences

More robust associations between parenting and children's peer aggression are found in studies that include rather than control for children's behavior, because they recognize explicitly the contribution of children to continuities in family and peer behavior. Parenting behavior is not independent of the influences that children bring to parent–child interaction. When mothers are disagreeable and hostile in their interactions with their children, children are disagreeable and squabble with their mothers, and these children are also both aggressive and likely to receive aggression from their peers (Kochanska, 1992; Hinde, Tamplin, & Barrett, 1993). Additionally, when mothers are harsh and punitive in the face of child misbehavior prior to their children's school entry, children are aggressive according to both their teachers and their peers in kindergarten and, for boys at least, up to third grade (McFadyen-Ketchum, Bates, Dodge, & Pettit, 1996). Both children's own aggressiveness and mothers' reactions to it played a role in this association. Parenting also acts to moderate relationships between children's negativity and peer outcomes. For example, Rubin et al. (1998) found that angry, resistant toddler boys were aggressive with their peers, but only if their mothers were also negative and dominant.

Snyder et al. (2005), looking at relations between children's aggression at home and at school, combined observations in the home and on the playground with parents' or teachers' reports of child behavior problems in each setting in a longitudinal study of children from low socioeconomic status neighborhoods. Their focus was on effects of observed ineffective and irritable discipline, and hostile attributions for children's misbehavior as mothers described their children and talked about how they would deal with common challenging behaviors. Mothers' hostile attributions were those suggesting that their children's misbehavior was due to child selfishness, purposeful defiance, or the like. The findings support a complex, multiprocess model that includes reciprocal influences between parents' ineffective discipline and children's conduct problems at home, and that generalize to increasing school conduct problems largely through the mediation of conduct problems at home. Discipline and conduct problems at home are co-constructed over time by both parent and child, and the joint contributions of ineffective parenting and hostile attributions accelerate the transfer of aggression from home to school. These findings remind us that parents' discipline is interactive; parents are reactive to children's behavior and misbehavior, and to children's own responses to parental control. Models that take children's behavior into account provide a stronger basis for predicting peer outcomes than do those that focus on parenting alone.

Sibling Contributions to Children's Peer Aggression

What of sibling relationships? Are negativity and aggression found with siblings rather than with parents more closely associated with peer interaction? There are reasons to suppose that they might be. Sibling interaction more strongly resembles relationships with peers on many dimensions. Sibling conflict, even with asymmetries in age, provides experience in both the resolution of disagreements and the management of aggression and hostility that can be similar to that experienced with peers. Consistent with this, children without siblings tend to be more aggressive, more likely to receive aggression, and less popular with preschool classmates (Kitzman, Cohen, & Lockwood, 2002). However, marked individual differences exist in both the warmth and hostility of sibling relationships. To what extent are such differences manifested in relationships with peers?

Early evidence provided contradictory findings. Abramovitch, Corter, Pepler, and Stanhope (1986) observed 5- and 7-year-old siblings and friends playing, finding no differences in either physical or verbal aggression between siblings and friends, and considerable reciprocity in agonistic behavior within each pair. However, these researchers failed to find any evidence of associations between children's interactions with siblings and with friends. Berndt and Bulleit (1985) observed preschool-age children at home and at preschool, and also found few correlations between the children's behavior in these two setting. The important exception to these null results was that aggression observed at home was closely related to that at school. Hinde et al. (1993) also found that children whose sibling interactions lacked warmth and cooperation tended to be aggressive with peers, and that the girls tended to receive aggression from peers. More recently, McElwain and Volling (2005) observed 4-year-olds with their next-oldest siblings and their friends in parallel play sessions. Like other researchers, they found few correlations between children's behavior in the two settings; the two exceptions related to the sophistication of play and the intensity of conflict when the siblings shared a single attractive toy. Both sibling and friendship quality were independently related to children's disruptive behavior, and positive relationships with either siblings or with friends tended to buffer the negative effects of negative relationships within the other relationship.

Thus, peer and sibling relationships appear to be linked more through children's tendencies to manage or mismanage conflict and aggression than through more positive forms of interaction. Importantly, links might not always take the form of direct associations, but compensatory and amplifying effects of hostility in each relationship on the other and on children's well-being, may be the more promising direction for understanding the links between sibling and peer domains.

Additionally, sibling factors do not work in isolation from other family influences on children's peer aggression. Models that take into account multiple sources of family negativity fare far better than those focused on hostility in one relationship or another in predicting children's negativity with peers. MacKinnon-Lewis et al. (1997) reported that the combination of mothers' rejection and aggression in the sibling relationship predicted patterns of school-age boys' aggression and social acceptance by peers; interestingly, the association between mothers' rejection and their sons' peer aggression was nearly fully mediated by sibling aggression. In another study, both parental rejection and destructive sibling conflict were related to teacher-reported aggression and to increases in aggression for 5-year-old boys from low-income families (Garcia, Shaw, Winslow, & Yaggi, 2000). Sibling physical aggression, angry yelling and swearing, and denigration predicted increases in the boys' aggression at school when accompanied by rejecting parenting; rejecting parenting in turn predicted increased aggression when sibling conflict was intense.

More constructive forms of conflict engagement with peers are also better predicted by considering the combined influence of mother and sibling strategies (Dunn & Herrera, 1997; Herrera & Dunn, 1997). Mothers', siblings', and children's own use of other-oriented arguments strongly predicted children's later abilities to resolve differences with friends; children who earlier experienced conflicts in which they and their mothers made self-centered arguments were later less likely to resolve differences with their friends.

Taking Bidirectional Causal Processes Seriously

Much of the developmental research seeks links between earlier family processes and later interaction with peers. Researchers make a strong case for family processes being the causes of later behavior with peers when children's family relationships are measured before they enter a new peer group (e.g., Dodge et al., 1994). Reversals of this design are not possible with parent–child relationships; however, firstborn children often establish friendships before the arrival of a sibling, and early friendships may prepare children for resolving difficulties they might encounter with their younger siblings. Using this strategic natural design, Kramer and Gottman (1992) established that the positive quality of play with peers prior to the siblings' birth and the relative absence of unmanaged conflict were associated with harmonious sibling interaction up to a year and a half later. Indeed, in follow-up observations during adolescence, children who had positive relationships with friends prior to their siblings' births were less competitive, agonistic, and controlling as they discussed interpersonal problems (Kramer & Kowal, 2005).

Peer mediation training studies also suggest that bidirectional causal processes should be taken seriously. Peer mediation programs facilitate positive conflict resolution in the context of disputes between children at school by emphasizing the clear articulation of conflict issues, respect in discussing differences, and mutual understanding of disputants' respective emotions and interests. In light of this understanding, and under the control of a mediator, conflicting parties are often able to resolve differences in constructive ways (Smith & Ross, 2007). Peer mediation programs introduced at school are reported to benefit conflict resolution at home (Gentry & Benenson, 1992; Johnson, Johnson, Dudley, Ward, & Magnusson, 1995). Johnson et al., for example, trained third- and fourth-grade children in mediation and rotated the role of mediator (as well as a T-shirt designating this role) among the students. Prior to training, the mediation group did not differ from randomly selected control children, often reporting the use of force, withdrawing from the situation, or reaching compromises without negotiating. The use of force declined and negotiation increased dramatically after mediation training. Mediation children resolved conflict issues and negotiated new solutions that integrated both parties' interests. Adult-brokered resolutions declined in frequency. Most important for our purposes, the training that children received at school generalized fully to their disputes with siblings at home. No differences were found between conflicts resolved at school and those that occurred in the family.

How Does Marital Conflict Influence Children's Peer Relationships?

An additional source of stress and further models of negativity are experienced when children see their parents fight. Effects of marital conflict are seldom studied on their own, largely because negativity in the marital relationship often spills over to negative parenting. Repeated experience with parental conflict sensitizes children to the negative emotional effects associated with family conflict (Davies et al., 2002). In an early study, Katz et al. (1992) found that a pattern of cool, uninvolved marital conflict discussions was related to cold, unresponsive parenting and to anger and noncompliance by children.

Over time, a mutually hostile conflict resolution style between parents, and especially the wife's icy superiority and moralistic disapproval, was associated with later teacher ratings of children's externalizing.

There is some dispute about whether hostility between spouses has a direct effect on children's well-being, or whether those effects are largely associated with negative parenting. For example, Stocker and Youngblade (1999) found that marital conflict was related to both sibling conflict and problematic peer relationships, but that paternal hostility fully mediated those relationships. In contrast, others have found that marital conflict contributes to children's aggression, over and above the influences of parents' hostility or unresponsiveness to their children (Hart et al., 1998). One of the most potent sources of influence is parental conflicts concerning their children. Jenkins et al. (2005) used a powerful, within-family design that included multiple siblings (ages 4–17 years) and modeled individual- and family-level influences on children's aggression across a 2-year time span. Marital conflict about children predicted changes in teachers' ratings of children's externalizing after researchers controlled for earlier behavior. Importantly, reversals of this causal direction were also explored. Earlier child externalizing predicted increases in marital conflict. The effect of children's externalizing on marital arguments about children was particularly strong when all the children in the family scored high in externalizing. These patterns were not mediated by mother–child relationships; associations remained significant when mothers' negativity was added to the model. Parents, like their children, react to the stress created by dealing with aggressive children, especially when more than one child exhibits behavior problems, and when children are disruptive at school. Thus, research generally supports both direct and mediated pathways from marital conflict to children's peer aggression, as well as influences of children's misbehavior on marital processes.

Adding destructive sibling conflict to that found in parent–child and marital relationships illustrates the cumulative effects of hostility in the home (Ingoldsby, Shaw, & Garcia, 2001). These three relatively independent sources of family conflict were each related to children's aggression with peers on school entry. Together, these sources of family conflict accounted for 24% of the variance in children's aggression, compared with less than 10% of variance for any single predictor. When all three sources of family conflict were high, children displayed the highest levels of destructive peer conflict, demonstrating a synergistic effect of family conflict. Children who experience extremes of negativity with parents and siblings are not passive but are full participants in destructive family interaction, and those who watch parents fight are involved witnesses in the same processes.

Relationships with Peers Moderate the Influence of Family Members on Children's Aggressiveness

Although various sources of family hostility are linked to children's peer aggression, and more so if these are cumulative, one would expect that children's peer aggressiveness is more powerfully and directly determined by the more immediate influences of their peers. Additionally, there is growing evidence that the potential impact of families on peer relationships depends upon processes found in the peer group. Of particular relevance, peers moderate the influence of families on children's aggressiveness. Criss, Pettit, Bates, Dodge, and Lapp (2002) found associations between ecological disadvantage, violent marital conflict, and harsh discipline in mothers of 5-year-old boys, and first-grade teachers' ratings of externalizing. Although each family variable was associated with children's problem behavior at school, both children's friendships and their popularity with peers moderated the impact of adverse family characteristics on teachers' perceptions of externalizing; family variables were strongly related to externalizing in children who were not well accepted in the peer group, and the influence of harsh maternal discipline was also moderated by the number of children's reciprocated friendships. Similarly, links between mother–son aggression and children's peer aggression were mediated by peer dislike (MacKinnon-Lewis & Lofquist, 1996). Thus, pathways between children's family life and peer aggression involved a causal chain of events that included relationships within the peer group itself. If family experiences serve as the origins of negative trajectories, peer processes can weaken or accelerate the development of problems within the group.

Family Precursors of Peer-Group Victimization

Children's aggressiveness also has its victims, and often the same children are selected repeatedly as targets of others' harassment and abuse. Being repeatedly victimized can often have dire consequences for children's development and well-being, and they are likely to be anxious and withdrawn, mistrustful, insecure, and lonely (Ladd & Ladd, 1998; Rubin, Wojslawowicz, Rose-Krasnor, Booth-LaForce, & Burgess, 2006). Given the serious consequences of peer victimization, researchers have been moved to ask whether patterns of family interaction are associated with young children being selectively victimized by peers.

Ladd and Ladd (1998) observed aspects of parent–child relationships in kindergarten children that they reasoned were likely to be linked to a passive, withdrawn profile of child behavior. Measures of parental intrusive demands (interrupting, overriding initiatives, demanding conformity) and responsiveness, as well as judgments of intense closeness, were all related to children's victimization. Other research has focused attention on children who are both aggressive and victimized within the peer group—children identified both as bullies and as victims (Schwartz, Dodge, Pettit, & Bates, 1997). These authors classified 10-year-old boys into aggressive, victimized, aggressive victims, and children who were neither victims nor aggressors, and compared these groups based on the patterns of family life observed prior to kindergarten entry. Aggressive victims differed most dramatically from all other children: They were more likely to have experienced maternal hostility, restrictive discipline, parental aggression, and marital aggression. Family interviewers estimated that 38% of these boys were likely to have experienced physical harm at the hands of their parents, as compared to half as many of the aggressive boys and 6% in the two nonaggressive groups. Passive, nonaggressive victims did not differ from the normative group on any prekindergarten measures. Thus, the family socialization variables are consistent with a profile of aggressive victims as angry, overreactive, and poorly controlled. Links between victimization and later problems at home were also examined (Schwartz, McFadyen-Ketchum, Dodge, Pettit, & Bates, 1998). Victimization at age 8 was associated with increases in both immature, dependent behavior and with externalizing, as rated by the children's mothers 2 years later. Thus, associations between early family interaction and later victimization are accompanied by associations between victimization and later problems in the family, forming a cycle of mutual and detrimental influences on children's adjustment at home and at school.

At the same time, positive relationships with agemates can protect children from bullying. Friendship has been found to be a moderator of the effects of harsh parenting on peer-group victimization (Schwartz, Dodge, Pettit, & Bates, 2000). Harsh, punitive parenting and hostile family environments predicted victimization over the early school years for children with few friends; however, for those with many friends, no such relationship was found. Similarly, highly prosocial twin siblings and friends moderate the influence of children's own reactive aggression on peer-group victimization (Lamarche et al., 2006). Having friends per se did not offer protection from bullying. However, prosocial friends—those who often invite others to play or who can stop quarrels between their peers—did make a difference. For children whose reciprocal friends showed low levels of prosocial behavior, children's own aggression was strongly related to the likelihood that they would be victimized by peers, but for children whose friends were highly prosocial, no such relationship was evident. Prosocial siblings, even those who did not share classrooms, provided similar protection against victimization. Together, these findings emphasize that interaction and relationships within the peer group are central to understanding the limited impact of family processes on children's behavior with peers. What happens within the peer group can outweigh deleterious home conditions and children's own hostility with respect to their vulnerability to others' aggression. These findings of moderating influences of peer relationships are in addition to any "main effects" of the peer culture or of the particular composition of the peer group. Friends and siblings may offer direct protection or reduce the impression that others might have of a child's vulnerability. Prosocial friends or siblings might also model prosocial behavior that allows potential victims to acquire the skills that could help them to regulate their emotions and to control their own aggressive responses to peer provocation.

Conclusions and Future Directions

Clearly, the empirical research provides support for the existence of links between family and peer relationships. Both parents and siblings exert their own influences; however, the effects of any single relationship are relatively modest. It is only when one deals with multiple influences in the family that pathways leading to peer competence and aggression become more robust. Genetic similarities do not seem to account fully for the links between family and peer domains (Caspi et al., 2004), and it would be important to replicate this type of design in studies of other processes. Additionally, those few studies that have taken bidirectional processes seriously and tested models of transmission from peer to family relationships appear to show that social influences are mutual and reciprocal, and suggest that future research will need to follow these examples.

Despite all this, the development of peer relationships occurs within a complex context of interacting agemates, each with an individual family background and entering into peer associations that are multifaceted and diverse. With development, children establish relationships and networks of relationships with peers that occur within settings that typically are far removed from the direct supervision of family members. Each of these varied peer contexts has its own culture of activities, norms, patterns of inclusiveness, and valued characteristics. Each includes its own mix of individuals who themselves are attracted to particular characteristics of others. Physical environment, supervision, and group size each play a role in determining how children's peer relationships will develop. For these reasons, family influences on children's peer relationships are subtle and have proven to be more influential in some peer contexts than in others. Family relationships may be supportive or may undermine children's abilities to interact peaceably and productively with their peers, but processes within the peer group itself may ultimately exert more powerful influences on children's relationships with one another.

References

Abramovitch, R., Corter, C., Pepler, D. J., & Stanhope, L. (1986). Sibling and peer interaction: A final follow-up and comparison. *Child Development, 57,* 217–229.

Berndt, T., & Bulleit, T. N. (1985). Effects of sibling relationships on preschoolers behavior at home and at school. *Developmental Psychology, 21,* 761–767.

Booth, C. L., Rose-Krasnor, L., McKinnon, J., & Rubin, K. H. (1994). Predicting social adjustment in middle childhood: The role of preschool attachment security and maternal style. *Social Development, 3,* 189–204.

Booth, C. L., Rose-Krasnor, L., & Rubin, K. H. (1991). Relating preschoolers' social competence and their mothers' parenting behaviors to early attachment security and high risk status. *Journal of Social and Personal Relationships, 8,* 363–382.

Brown, J., Donelan-McCall, N., & Dunn, J. (1996). Why talk about mental states?: The significance of children's conversations with friends, siblings, and mothers. *Child Development, 67,* 836–849.

Caspi, A., Moffitt, T. E., Morgan, J., Ruter, M., Taylor, A., Arsenault, L., et al. (2004). Paternal expressed emotion predicts children's antisocial behavior problems: Using monozygotic-twin differences to identify environmental effects on behavioral development. *Developmental Psychology, 40,* 149–161.

Cassidy, J., Parke, R., Butkovsky, L., & Braungart, J. M. (1992). Family-peer connections: The roles of emotional expressiveness within the family and children's understanding of emotions. *Child Development, 63,* 603–618.

Cohen, J. S. (1989). *Maternal involvement in children's peer relationships during middle childhood.* Unpublished doctoral dissertation, University of Waterloo, Waterloo, Ontario, Canada.

Criss, M. M., Pettit, G. S., Bates, J. E., Dodge, K. A., & Lapp, A. L. (2002). Family adversity, positive peer relationship, and children's externalizing behavior: A longitudinal perspective on risk and resilience. *Child Development, 73,* 1220–1237.

Cutting, A. L., & Dunn, J. (2006). Conversations with siblings and with friends: Links between relationship quality and social understanding. *British Journal of Developmental Psychology, 24,* 73–87.

Davies, P. T., Harold, G. T., Goeke-Morey, M. C., & Cummings, E. M. (2002). Child emotional security and interparental conflict. *Monographs of the Society for Research in Child Development, 67*(3, Serial No. 270), 1–29.

Dishion, T. J., Duncan, T. E., Eddy, J. M., Fagot, B. I., & Fetrow, R. (1994). The world of parents and peers: Coercive exchanges and children's social adaptation. *Social Development, 3,* 255–268.

Dodge, K. A., Pettit, G. S., & Bates, J. E. (1994). Socialization mediators of the relation between socioeconomic status and child conduct problems. *Child Development, 65,* 649–665.

Dunn, J. (1983). Sibling relationships in early childhood. *Child Development, 54,* 787–811.

Dunn, J. (2002). Sibling relationships. In P. K. Smith & C. H. Hart (Eds.), *Blackwell handbook of childhood social development* (pp. 223–237). Oxford, UK: Blackwell.

Dunn, J. (2006). Parent–child discourse and the early development of understanding. *Merrill–Palmer Quarterly, 52,* 151–157.

Dunn, J., & Herrera, C. (1997). Conflict resolution with friends, siblings, and mothers: A developmental perspective. *Aggressive Behavior, 23,* 343–357.

Eisenberg, N., Fabes, R. A., & Spinrad, T. L. (2006). Prosocial behavior. In N. Eisenberg (Vol. Ed.), & W. Damon, & R. M. Lerner (Series Eds.), *Handbook of child psychology: Vol. 3. Social, emotional, and personality development* (6th ed., pp. 646–718). New York: Wiley.

Farver, J. M., & Howes, C. (1993). Cultural differences in American and Mexican mother–child pretend play. *Merrill–Palmer Quarterly, 39,* 344–358.

Finnie, V., & Russell, A. (1988). Preschool children's social status and their mothers' behaviors and knowledge in the supervisory role. *Developmental Psychology, 24,* 789–801.

Finnie, V., & Russell, A. (1990). Preschool children's social status and maternal instructions to assist group entry. *Developmental Psychology, 26,* 603–611.

Furman, W., & Lanthier, R. (2002). Parenting siblings. In M. Bornstein (Ed.), *Handbook of parenting* (pp. 165–188). Mahwah, NJ: Erlbaum.

Garcia, M. M., Shaw, D. S., Winslow, E. B., & Yaggi, K. E. (2000). Destructive sibling conflict and the development of conduct problems in young boys. *Developmental Psychology, 36,* 44–53.

Gentry, D., & Benenson, W. (1992). School-age peer mediators transfer knowledge and skills to home setting. *Mediation Quarterly, 10,* 101–109.

Gerrits, M. H., Goudena, P. P., & van Aken, M. A. G. (2005). Child–parent and child–peer interaction: Observational similarities and differences at age seven. *Infant and Child Development, 14,* 229–241.

Hart, C. H., Nelson, D. A., Robinson, C. C., Olsen, S. F., & McNeilly-Choque, M. K. (1998). Overt and relational aggression in Russian nursery-school-age children: Parenting style and marital linkages. *Developmental Psychology, 34,* 687–697.

Herrera, C., & Dunn, J. (1997). Early experiences with family conflict: Implications for arguments with a close friend. *Developmental Psychology, 33,* 869–881.

Hinde, R. A., Tamplin, A., & Barrett, J. (1993). Home correlates of aggression in preschool. *Aggressive Behavior, 19,* 85–105.

Howe, N., Petrakos, H., Rinaldi, C., & LeFebvre, R. (2005). "This is a bad dog, you know … ": Constructing shared meanings during sibling pretend play. *Child Development, 76,* 783–794.

Howe, N., & Rinaldi, C. (2004). "You be the big sister": Maternal–preschooler internal state discourse, perspective-taking, and sibling caretaking. *Infant and Child Development, 13,* 217–234.

Howe, N., & Ross, H. S. (1990). Socialization, perspective-taking and the sibling relationship. *Developmental Psychology, 26,* 160–165.

Ingoldsby, E. M., Shaw, D. S., & Garcia, M. M. (2001). Intrafamily conflict in relation to boys' adjustment at school. *Development and Psychopathology, 13,* 35–52.

Isley, S. L., O'Neil, R., Clatfelter, D., & Parke, R. D. (1999). Parent and child expressed affect and children's social competence: Modeling direct and indirect pathways. *Developmental Psychology, 35,* 547–560.

Jenkins, J., Simpson, A., Dunn, J., Rasbash, J., & O'Connor, T. G. (2005). Mutual influence of marital conflict and children's behavior problems: Shared and nonshared family risks. *Child Development, 76,* 24–39.

Jenkins, J. M., Turrell, S., Takei, Y., Lollis, S., & Ross, H. (2003). The dynamics of mental state talk in families. *Child Development, 74,* 905–920.

Johnson, D. W., Johnson, R., Dudley, B., Ward, M., & Magnusson, D. (1995). The impact of peer mediation training on the management of school and home conflicts. *American Educational Research Journal, 32,* 829–844.

Katz, L. F., Kramer, L., & Gottman, J. M. (1992). Conflict and emotions in marital, sibling, and relationships. In C. U. Shantz & W. W. Hartup (Eds.), *Conflict in child and adolescent development* (pp. 122–149). New York: Cambridge University Press.

Kerns, K. A., Cole, A. K., & Andrews, P. B. (1998). Attachment security, parent peer management practices, and peer relationships in preschoolers. *Merrill–Palmer Quarterly, 44*(4), 504–522.

Kilgore, K., Snyder, J., & Lentz, C. (2000). The contribution of parental discipline, parental monitoring, and school risk to early-onset conduct problems in African American boys and girls. *Developmental Psychology, 36,* 835–845.

Kitzman, K. M., Cohen, R., & Lockwood, R. L. (2002). Are only children missing out?: Comparison of the peer-related social competence of only children and siblings. *Journal of Social and Personal Relationships, 19,* 299–316.

Kochanska, G. (1992). Children's interpersonal influence with mothers and peers. *Developmental Psychology, 28,* 491–499.

Kramer, L., & Gottman, J. M. (1992). Becoming a sibling: "With a little help from my friends." *Developmental Psychology, 28*, 685–699.

Kramer, L., & Kowal, A. K. (2005). Sibling relationship quality from birth to adolescence: The enduring contribution of friends. *Journal of Family Psychology, 19*, 503–511.

Ladd, G. W., & Golter, B. (1988). Parents' management of preschoolers' peer relations: Is it related to children's social competence? *Developmental Psychology, 24*, 109–117.

Ladd, G. W., & Hart, C. H. (1992). Creating informal play opportunities: Are parents' and preschoolers' initiations related to children's competence with peers? *Developmental Psychology, 28*, 1179–1187.

Ladd, G. W., & Ladd, B. K. (1998). Parenting behaviors and parent–child relationships: Correlates of peer victimization in kindergarten? *Developmental Psychology, 34*, 1450–1458.

Ladd, G. W., Le Sieur, K. D., & Profilet, S. M. (1993). Direct parental influences of young children's peer relations. In S. Duck (Ed.), *Learning about relationships* (pp. 152–183). London: Sage.

Ladd, G. W., & Pettit, G. S. (2002). Parenting and the development of children's peer relationships. In M. Bornstein (Ed.), *Handbook in parenting* (Vol. 5, pp. 269–309). Mahwah, NJ: Erlbaum.

LaFreniere, P. J., & Dumas, J. E. (1992). A transactional analysis of early childhood anxiety and social withdrawal. *Development and Psychopathology, 5*, 385–402.

Lamarche, V., Brengden, M., Boivin, M., Vitaro, F., Pérusse, D., & Dionne, G. (2006). Do friendships and sibling relationships provide protection against peer victimization in a similar way? *Social Development, 15*, 373–393.

Lindsey, E. W., Mize, J., & Pettit, G. S. (1997). Differential play patterns of mothers and fathers of sons and daughters: Implications for children's gender role development. *Sex Roles, 37*, 643–661.

Lollis, S. P., Tate, E., & Ross, H. S. (1992). Parents' regulation of their children's peer interactions: Direct influences. In R. Parke & G. Ladd (Eds.), *The family and peer relationships* (pp. 255–281). Hillsdale, NJ: Erlbaum.

Maccoby, E. E., & Martin, J. A. (1983). Socialization in the context of the family: Parent–child interaction. In P. H. Mussen (Series Ed.) & E. M. Hetherington (Vol. Ed.), *Handbook of child psychology: Vol. 4. Socialization, personality, and social development* (4th ed., pp. 1–101). New York: Wiley.

MacDonald, K. B., & Parke, R. D. (1984). Bridging the gap: Parent–child play interaction and interactive competence. *Child Development, 55*, 1265–1277.

MacKinnon-Lewis, C., & Lofquist, A. (1996). Antecedents and consequences of boys' depression and aggression: Family and school linkages. *Journal of Family Psychology, 10*, 490–500.

MacKinnon-Lewis, C., Starnes, R., Volling, B., & Johnson, S. (1997). Perceptions of parenting as predictors of boys' sibling and peer relations. *Developmental Psychology, 33*, 1024–1031.

McCoy, J. K., Brody, G. H., & Stoneman, Z. (1994). Longitudinal analysis of sibling relationships as mediators of the link between family processes and youths' best friendships. *Family Relationships, 43*, 400–408.

McElwain, N. L., & Volling, B. L. (2005). Preschool children's interactions with friends and older siblings: Relationship specificity and joint contributions to problem behavior. *Journal of Family Psychology, 19*, 486–496.

McFadyen-Ketchum, S. A., Bates, J. E., Dodge, K. A., & Pettit, G. S. (1996). Patterns of change in early childhood aggressive–disruptive behavior: Gender differences in predictions from early coercive and affectionate mother–child interactions. *Child Development, 67*, 2417–2433.

Nix, R. L., Pinderhughes, E. E., Dodge, K. A., Bates, J. E., Pettit, G. S., & McFadyen-Ketchum, S. A. (1999). The relation between mothers' hostile attribution tendencies and children' externalizing problems: The mediating role of mothers' harsh discipline practices. *Child Development, 70*, 896–909.

O'Neil, R., Parke, R. D., & McDowell, D. J. (2001). Objective and subjective features of children's neighborhoods: Relations to parental regulatory strategies and children's social competence. *Applied Developmental Psychology, 22*, 135–155.

Parke, R. D., & Ladd, G. W. (Eds.). (1992). *Family–peer relationships: Modes of linkage.* Hillside, NJ: Erlbaum.

Parke, R. D., MacDonald, K. V. M., Carson, J., Bhavnagri, N., Barth, J. M., & Beitel, A. (1989). Family and peer linkages: In search of linkages. In K. Kreppner & R. M. Lerner (Eds.), *Family systems and life span development* (pp. 65–92). Hillside, NJ: Erlbaum.

Parke, R. D., Simpkins, S. D., McDowell, D. J., Kim, M., Killian, C., Dennis, J., et al. (2002). Relative contributions of families and peers to children's social development. In P. K. Smith & C. H. Hart (Eds.), *Blackwell handbook of childhood social development* (pp. 156–177). Oxford, UK: Blackwell.

Pettit, G. S., Bates, J. E., & Dodge, K. A. (1997). Supportive parenting, ecological context, and children's adjustment: A seven-year longitudinal study. *Child Development, 68,* 908–923.

Putallaz, M. (1987). Maternal behavior and children's sociometric status. *Child Development, 58,* 324–340.

Ross, H. S., Filyer, R. E., Lollis, S. P., Perlman, M., & Martin, J. L. (1994). Administering justice in the family. *Journal of Family Psychology, 18,* 254–273.

Ross, H. S., & Lollis, S. P. (1989). A social relations analysis of toddler peer relationships. *Child Development, 60,* 1082–1091.

Ross, H. S., Tesla, C., Kenyon, B., & Lollis, S. P. (1990). Maternal intervention in toddler peer conflict: The socialization of principles of justice. *Developmental Psychology, 26,* 994–1003.

Rubin, K. H., Bukowski, W., & Parker, J. (2006). Peer interactions, relationships, and groups. In N. Eisenberg (Ed.), *Handbook of child: Social, emotional, and personality development* (6th ed., pp. 571–645). New York: Wiley.

Rubin, K. H., & Burgess, K. (2002). Parents of aggressive and withdrawn children. In M. Bornstein (Ed.), *Handbook of parenting* (Vol. 1, pp. 383–418). Hillsdale, NJ: Erlbaum.

Rubin, K. H., Hastings, P., Chen, X., Stewart, S., & McNichol, K. (1998). Intrapersonal and maternal correlates of aggression, conflict and externalizing problems in toddlers. *Child Development, 69,* 1614–1629.

Rubin, K. H., Wojslawowicz, J. C., Rose-Krasnor, L., Booth-LaForce, C. L., & Burgess, K. B. (2006). The best friendships of shy/withdrawn children: Prevalence, stability, and relationship quality. *Journal of Abnormal Child Psychology, 34,* 139–153.

Russell, A., Hart, C. H., Robinson, C. C., & Olsen, S. F. (2003). Children' sociable and aggressive behaviour with peers: A comparison of the U.S. and Australia, and contributions of temperament and parenting styles. *International Journal of Behavioral Development, 27,* 74–86.

Schneider, B. H., Atkinson, L., & Tardif, C. (2001). Child–parent attachment and children's peer relations: A quantitative review. *Developmental Psychology, 37,* 86–100.

Schwartz, D., Dodge, K. A., Pettit, G. S., & Bates, J. E. (1997). The early socialization of aggressive victims of bullying. *Child Development, 68,* 665–675.

Schwartz, D., Dodge, K. A., Pettit, G. S., & Bates, J. E. (2000). Friendship as a moderating factor in the pathway between early harsh home environment and later victimization in the peer group. *Developmental Psychology, 36,* 646–662.

Schwartz, D., McFadyen-Ketchum, S. A., Dodge, K. A., Pettit, G. S., & Bates, J. E. (1998). Peer victimization as a predictor of behavior problems at home and at school. *Development and Psychopathology, 10,* 87–100.

Smith, J., & Ross, H. (2007). Training parents to mediate siblings disputes affects children's negotiation and conflict understanding. *Child Development, 78,* 790–805.

Snyder, J., Cramer, A., Afrank, J., & Patterson, G. R. (2005). The contribution of ineffective discipline and parent hostile attributions of child misbehavior to the development of conduct problems at home and at school. *Developmental Psychology, 41,* 30–41.

Sroufe, L. A., & Fleeson, J. (1988). The coherence of family relationships. In R. A. Hinde & J. Stevenson-Hinde (Eds.), *Relationships within families: Mutual influences* (pp. 27–47). Oxford, UK: Oxford University Press.

Stewart, R. B. (1983). Sibling attachment relationships: Child–infant interactions in the Strange Situation. *Developmental Psychology, 19*, 192–199.

Stocker, C. M., & Youngblade, L. (1999). Marital conflict and parental hostility: Links with children's sibling and peer relationships. *Journal of Family Psychology, 13*, 589–609.

Tamis-LeMonda, C. S., Uzgiris, I. C., & Bornstein, M. H. (2002). Play in parent–child interactions. In M. Bornstein (Ed.), *Handbook of parenting* (Vol. 5, pp. 221–241). Mahwah, NJ: Erlbaum.

Volling, B. (2003). Sibling relationships. In M. H. Bornstein, L. Davidson, C. L. M. Keyes, & K. A. Moore (Eds.), *Well-being: Positive development across the life course* (pp. 205–220). Mahwah, NJ: Erlbaum.

Volling, B. L., & Belsky, J. (1992). The contribution of mother–child and father–child relationships to the quality of sibling interaction: A longitudinal study. *Child Development, 63*, 1209–1222.

Volling, B., Youngblade, L. M., & Belsky, J. (1997). Young children's social relationships with siblings and friends. *American Journal of Orthopsychiatry, 6*, 102–111.

Youngblade, L. M., & Belsky, J. (1992). Parent–child antecedents of 5-year-olds' close friendships: A longitudinal analysis. *Developmental Psychology, 28*, 700–713.

PART VII

Childhood Peer Experiences and Later Adjustment

CHAPTER 29

Peers and Academic Functioning at School

KATHRYN R. WENTZEL

Peers are of central importance to children throughout childhood and adolescence. They provide companionship and entertainment, help in solving problems, personal validation and emotional support, and a foundation for identity development. In turn, children who engage in positive activities with peers also tend to experience levels of emotional well-being, beliefs about the self, and values for prosocial forms of behavior and social interaction that are stronger and more adaptive than levels of children who do not (see Rubin, Bukowski, & Parker, 2006). In addition, children who enjoy positive interactions and relationships with their peers also tend to be more engaged in and even to excel at academic tasks than those who experience problems with peers (see Wentzel, 2003). In light of this evidence that links children's adaptive functioning across social and academic domains, a central question addressed in this chapter is how students' social competence with peers might be related to academic motivation and accomplishments. Toward this end, peer-related activities are discussed in terms of children's interactions and their interpersonal relationships with classmates as they occur within the broader social structures of school settings.

Although many researchers use the terms "interactions" and "relationships" interchangeably when referring to contexts of peer influence, this practice masks the distinct contribution that various aspects of the peer system can make to academically related outcomes. As described herein, certain types of peer interactions, in and of themselves, can be influential in advancing the development of discrete cognitive skills, whereas interactions within the context of dyadic or group-level relationships can provide the added incentives and interpersonal resources to support competent academic functioning at school. School-level social systems also can influence the nature and quality of peer interactions and relationships, and moderate their impact on academic outcomes. These multiple levels of peer activities require qualitatively different models and approaches to the study of peer influence on academic functioning. The historical progression of work in this area is marked by initial interest in peer interactions as causal determinants of cognitive development, followed by increased recognition that relationships and even schools can serve as contextual affordances that provide essential resources to support children's academic functioning. In this chapter, each of these approaches is discussed in turn. In conclusion, thoughts and provocations for future research are offered.

Central Issues and Theories

Peer Interactions and Cognitive Development

Conceptual approaches to the study of peer activities and cognitive outcomes have focused on various aspects of peer relations, ranging from the nature of interactions involved in intellectual problem solving to group pressures to adopt norms and values associated with academic performance. Early work on peer activities and cognitive functioning was concerned almost exclusively with the role of peer interactions in motivating cognitive change and development. Theoretical explanations were based on the broad notion that positive interactions with peers contribute directly to intellectual functioning. For example, Piaget (e.g., 1932/1965) proposed that mutual discussion, perspective taking, and conflict resolution with peers can motivate the accommodation of new and more sophisticated approaches to intellectual problem solving. For Piaget, development was contingent on the relatively symmetrical nature of same-age peer interactions that allowed conflict resolution within the context of mutual reciprocity. Vygotsky (1978) suggested that peers can contribute directly to the development of academic skills when competent students teach specific learning strategies and standards for performance to peers who are less skilled. In this case, asymmetrical interactions were believed to contribute to cognitive gains primarily by way of cooperative and collaborative exchange.

Experimental research has supported both positions in that active discussion, problem solving, and elaborative feedback among peers are associated with advances in a range of cognitive competencies, including problem-solving skills, conceptual understanding, and metacognitive reasoning in samples ranging from preschool to high school (see Gauvain & Perez, 2007; Rogoff et al., 2007). However, of central importance for understanding the relevance of this work for academic functioning is that most theoretically based research on peer interactions has focused on specific cognitive capacities with identified developmental trajectories, such as those measured with performance on Piagetian-type tasks (e.g., Azmitia, 1988; Tudge, 1992). These outcomes typically are assessed in experimental settings that are relatively free of normative and contextual cues for performance. With regard to applications to school learning, a core assumption is that these cognitive skills have a fairly strong link to academic performance. In fact, this link is fairly tenuous, especially as students enter into the secondary school years (Snow & Yalow, 1982). In large part, this disconnect can be attributed to individual differences in students' social and emotional functioning, and the nature of social norms that define learning.

The potentially confounding influence of these social and contextual factors is evidenced in classroom intervention studies indicating that dyadic peer interactions contribute most (albeit modestly) to learning outcomes for minority, urban-dwelling, and young children, and when dyads are homogeneous with respect to gender (Rohrbeck, Ginsburg-Block, Fantuzzo, & Miller, 2003). In addition, interactions with friends rather than acquaintances tend to yield more predictable cognitive advances, presumably because friends have well-established interaction patterns and are sensitive to each others' interests and needs (e.g., Fonzi, Schneider, Tani, & Tomada, 1997).

Similarly, as predicted by co-constructivist models, the effects of cooperative learning on achievement are generally positive when students engage in cognitive elaboration, are required to work together toward common goals, and when the learning tasks require equal status for all group members (Cohen, 1986; Slavin, Hurley, & Chamberlain, 2003). However, cooperative learning structures tend to work differentially for girls and boys. In mixed-gender groups, girls perform less well than boys (see Slavin et al., 2003). Working with friends rather than acquaintances tends to result in more positive outcomes for girls than for boys (Kutnick & Kington, 2005). Pressures to display gender-stereotypical characteristics also can result in some girls downplaying their intellectual abilities and in boys displaying reluctance to engage in academic pursuits altogether (Maccoby, 2002). Group learning with children also tends to be largely unsuccessful in producing cognitive gains when group members differ as a function of ability, race, ethnicity, and socioeconomic status (SES) (Cohen, 1986).

Finally, engagement in cooperative learning activities has been associated consistently with social, motivational, and behavioral outcomes. For example, cooperative learning can lead to increased peer acceptance and enhanced cross-group relations, increased intrinsic motivation, positive attitudes toward school, a heightened sense of efficacy, and increased prosocial interactions (Slavin et al., 2003). As described in the following section, these varied social–emotional outcomes also have been related to academic functioning. Therefore, it is not clear whether positive learning outcomes are the result of intellectual gains emanating from peer interactions or from motivational, social, and behavioral benefits. In fact, direct pathways from collaborative and cooperative forms of learning to cognitive gains rarely have been established when accounting for the complex social and motivational aspects of peer interactions in groups.

Given the added complexities that social and motivational functioning bring to the task of learning in school settings, it stands to reason that the nature and level of peer contributions to school-based academic performance might be quite different from their contribution to the development of cognitive capacities and skills. Because academic performance requires not only cognitive skills but also specific motivational and social orientations toward learning, peer-related activities can influence academic outcomes by way of their impact on students' social and emotional adjustment to school. In this regard, dyadic and group-level relationships have the potential to provide the added incentives and interpersonal resources to support competent academic functioning. This perspective is discussed in the following section.

Peer Relationships as Contextual Affordances

More recent advances to the understanding of how and why peers might contribute to each other's academic functioning have adopted contextual approaches that focus on the nature of competence in social settings. These approaches recognize peer interactions as taking place within ongoing relationships and established groups. Moreover, they view academic performance partly as an aspect of social competence, because it takes place within, and is shaped by, the social affordances and constraints of the school setting (see Wentzel, 2005). The development and expression of discrete intellectual skills also can be understood as a function of social–cultural contexts (Greenfield, 1997). However, it is clear that school-based indicators of cognitive functioning are far more reflective of social-cognitive skills, such as detection and interpretation of social cues, in coordination with self-regulatory skills, such as goal setting, evaluating levels of efficacy and self-determination, and emotion regulation.

In support of this approach, Bronfenbrenner (1989) argued that competence can only be understood in terms of context-specific effectiveness, being a product of personal attributes such as social-cognitive and self-regulatory skills, and ways in which these attributes contribute to meeting situational requirements and demands. He further suggested that competence is facilitated by contextual supports that provide opportunities for the growth and development of these personal attributes, as well as for learning what is expected by the social group. Based on this perspective, being a competent and successful student requires not only demonstrations of skills and behaviors that meet with social approval and acceptance but also provisions of social supports and resources that motivate and enable such demonstrations (see also Ford, 1992; Wentzel, 2005). It follows that understanding peer contributions to academic achievement necessitates a consideration of academic outcomes that are related to peer approval and acceptance, and of ways in which peer relationships and contexts might support their development.

In the following section, the literature that links peer relationships to motivational and academic outcomes is reviewed, followed by a description of ways in which peer relationships provide students with resources and opportunities to excel academically. Next, social behaviors that are the hallmark of peer, as well as school-related, competence are discussed as additional student outcomes that might mediate between peer relationships and academic functioning. Finally, research on school-level structures that can influence the nature of peer relationships at school and their impact on academic outcomes are described. Peer relationships are construed broadly to include dyadic friendships, peer groups, and networks, and as a central source of social acceptance and approval at school.

Key Research Studies

Peer Relationships, Academic Motivation, and Achievement

An extensive body of work supports the notion that various aspects of peer relationships are related to children's motivational and academic functioning at school (for a review, see Wentzel, 2005). Research indicates that sociometrically rejected children experience academic difficulties, whereas sociometrically popular children are academically proficient; social preference scores on a continuum ranging from well accepted to rejected yield highly similar findings. Results are most consistent with respect to classroom grades, although peer acceptance has been related positively to standardized test scores, as well as to IQ. These findings are robust for elementary-age children, as well as adolescents, and longitudinal studies document the stability of relations between peer acceptance and academic accomplishments over time. Sociometric status and peer acceptance also has been related to motivation, including satisfaction with school, pursuit of goals to learn, interest in school, and perceived academic competence.

Studies of peer-group membership also have focused on academic and motivational outcomes. For example, ethnographic studies describe adolescents as characterizing certain peer crowds in terms of academic standing (Brown, 1989; Brown, Mounts, Lamborn, & Steinberg, 1993; Stone & Brown, 1999). "Brains," or students who get high grades, typically enjoy average status in crowd hierarchies, although the social status of this group appears to have a developmental trajectory, with "Brain" crowd status being highest during middle school and the end of high school, and lowest at the beginning of high school (see Stone & Brown, 1999). Crowd affiliation at the beginning of high school also is related to different levels of achievement as students progress through high school (Steinberg, Brown, & Dornbusch, 1996). In addition, students tend to self-select into groups of peers that have motivational orientations to school similar to their own; over the course of the school year, these orientations appear to become stronger and more similar within groups (e.g., Kindermann, 1993; Kindermann, McCollam, & Gibson, 1996).

Finally, having friends has been related positively to grades and test scores in elementary school and middle school (Berndt & Keefe, 1995; Wentzel, Barry, & Caldwell, 2004; Wentzel & Caldwell, 1997), although these relations tend to be weaker than those between other aspects of peer relationships and achievement (Wentzel & Caldwell, 1997). Friendship-based groups in middle school have been related to changes over the course of the school year in the degree to which students perform academically (A. Ryan, 2001; Wentzel & Caldwell, 1997). In addition, having friends at school has been related to positive aspects of motivation and classroom engagement in school-related activities (e.g., Berndt & Keefe, 1995; Ladd, 1990; Wentzel et al., 2004; Wentzel & Caldwell, 1997).

Peer Relationships as Socializers of Academic Competence

How might peer relationships promote these positive academic and motivational outcomes? Although rarely used to study peer influence, models that describe how adults socialize children suggest at least three general mechanisms whereby social relationships might influence competence development (see Grusec & Hastings, 2007; Wentzel & Looney, 2007). First, ongoing social interactions within relationships teach children what they need to do to become accepted and competent members of their social worlds. Second, relationships that are supportive and nurturing are likely to motivate children to adopt and internalize these goals and standards as their own. Finally, adults provide children with direct instruction and training in desired skills and outcomes. Similarly, within the context of peer relationships, children are likely to provide each other with valued goals and related standards for behavior, the affective support and approval to motivate the adoption of these goals and standards, and opportunities to develop the requisite skills to achieve them. Applied to classroom settings, this implies that students will engage in academic activities, in part, when their peers communicate positive expectations and standards for academic performance; provide direct assistance and help on academic tasks; and create a climate of emotional support that facilitates positive engagement in classroom activities, including protection from physical threats and harm. Findings that support this perspective on perceived academic competence are described next.

Communicating Goals and Expectations for Performance

Academically oriented goals and standards for performance are strong and consistent predictors of academic engagement and achievement (Wentzel & Wigfield, 1998). Teachers and parents are obvious socializers of these goals and values. Although not well documented, it also is reasonable to assume that students communicate to each other specific academic values and expectations for performance (e.g., Altermatt, Pomerantz, Ruble, Frey, & Greulich, 2002). During early adolescence, students report that their classmates expect them to perform well academically at school; for example, approximately 80% of students from three predominantly middle-class middle schools reported that their peers strongly valued academic learning (Wentzel, Looney, & Battle, 2003). However, as students advance through their middle school and high school years, the degree to which their goals and values support positive academic accomplishments can become fairly attenuated. In samples of high school students, only 40% of adolescents report similar levels of peer academic expectations (Wentzel, Monzo, Williams, & Tomback, 2007).

In addition to general expectations concerning academic achievement, peers also provide proximal input concerning reasons for engaging in academic tasks. In support of this notion, students who perceive relatively high expectations for academic learning and engagement from their peers also report that they pursue goals to learn for internalized reasons (e.g., because it is important or fun) significantly more often than for more extrinsic reasons (e.g., because they believe they will get in trouble or lose social approval if they do not; Wentzel, 2004; for similar findings in the social domain, see Wentzel, Filisitti, & Looney, 2007). Therefore, peers who convey expectations that others are likely to experience a sense of importance or enjoyment with regard to academic engagement are likely to lead others to form similar, intrinsically oriented attitudes toward learning (Bandura, 1986).

Although children articulate sets of goals that they would like and expect each other to achieve, specific aspects of peer contexts that lead children to adopt these academic goals and values are not well understood. However, the larger peer group can be a source of behavioral standards, and group pressures can provide a mechanism whereby adherence to group standards and expectations is monitored and enforced. For example, adolescent peer groups differ in the degree to which they pressure members to become involved in academic activities, with "Jocks" and "Popular" groups providing significantly more pressure for academic involvement than other groups (Clasen & Brown, 1985). Students also have been observed to monitor each other by ignoring noninstructional behavior and responses during group instruction, and by the private sanctioning of inappropriate conduct (Eder & Felmlee, 1984). It should be noted that peer monitoring of behavior will contribute to positive motivational orientations only insofar as the peer group has adopted adult standards for achievement and norms for conduct. As children enter middle school and establishing independence from adult influence becomes a developmental task, they are less likely to acknowledge the legitimacy of adult-imposed norms (Smetana & Bitz, 1996) or to enforce classroom rules automatically (Eccles & Midgley, 1989).

Another way that peers contribute to students' expectations and values for performance is by way of influence on perceptions of ability; students' beliefs about their academic efficacy are powerful predictors of academic performance (Schunk & Pajares, 2005). Children utilize their peers for comparative purposes as early as 4 years of age (for a review, see Butler, 2005). As children work on academic tasks that require fairly specific skills, and that are evaluated with respect to clearly defined standards, they use each other to monitor and to evaluate their own abilities. Experimental work also has shown that peers serve as powerful models that influence the development of academic self-efficacy (see Schunk & Pajares, 2005), especially when children observe similar peers who demonstrate successful ways to cope with failure. These modeling effects are especially likely to occur when students are friends (Crockett, Losoff, & Petersen, 1984), although students who have higher-achieving friends tend to have lower levels of self-efficacy than those with lower-achieving friends (Altermatt & Pomerantz, 2005).

Providing Help and Assistance

Perhaps the most explicit and obvious way in which peers can have a direct influence on students' academic competence is by way of help giving. Indeed, students who enjoy supportive relationships with their peers will also have greater access to resources and information that can help them accomplish academic tasks than those who do not. These resources can take the form of information and advice, modeled behavior, or specific experiences that facilitate learning (e.g., Cooper, Ayers-Lopez, & Marquis, 1982; Schunk, 1987). Teachers play the central pedagogical function of transmitting knowledge and training students in academic subject areas. However, at least during adolescence, students report that their peers are as, or more, important sources of instrumental aid than are their teachers (Lempers & Clark-Lempers, 1992). Developmental research on peer help giving is rare. However, findings on middle school students making the transition into high school suggest that receiving academic help from familiar peers tends to increase over the course of the transition (Wentzel, Filisetti, et al., 2007). One reason for this growing dependence on peers is that when adolescents enter new high school structures, the relative uncertainty and ambiguity of having multiple teachers and different sets of classmates for each class, new instructional styles, and more complex class schedules necessitates that students turn to each other for social support, ways to cope, and academic help.

Providing Emotional Support and Security

Feelings of emotional security and being socially connected are believed to facilitate the adoption of goals and interests valued by others, and desires to contribute in positive ways to the overall functioning of the social group (e.g., Ryan & Deci, 2000). Therefore, differences in the degree to which students believe that their peers accept and care about them might also account for significant relations between the nature of peer relationships at school and academic functioning. In support of this notion is an extensive literature relating positive academic outcomes to perceived emotional support from peers. Students who perceive that their peers support and care about them tend to be interested and engaged in positive aspects of classroom life, whereas students who do not perceive their relationships with peers as positive and supportive tend to be at risk for motivational academic problems (e.g., Goodenow, 1993; Wentzel, 1998; Wentzel et al., 2003).

One reason for these findings is that exclusion from supportive peer relationships can result in negative outcomes in the form of emotional distress. Children who are without friends or are socially rejected often report feeling lonely, emotionally distressed, and depressed (Wentzel & Caldwell, 1997; Wentzel et al., 2003). Moreover, researchers have established significant relations between psychological distress and depression and a range of achievement-related outcomes, including interest in school (Wentzel, Weinberger, Ford, & Feldman, 1990), negative attitudes toward academic achievement, performance (Dubow & Tisak, 1989; Wentzel et al., 1990), and ineffective cognitive functioning (Jacobsen, Edelstein, & Hoffmann, 1994). Therefore, students' affective functioning is likely to be an important outcome that links peer-related activity to academic outcomes (e.g., Juvonen, Nishina, & Graham, 2000; Wentzel, 1998).

Of related interest is that students who are accepted by their peers and who have established friendships with classmates also are more likely to enjoy a relatively safe school environment and less likely to be the targets of peer-directed violence and harassment than their peers who do not have friends (Hodges, Boivin, Vitaro, & Bukowski, 1999; Pellegrini, Bartini, & Brooks, 1999; Schwartz, Dodge, Pettit, Bates, & the Conduct Problems Prevention Research Group, 2000). The general effects of peer harassment on student motivation and academic competence have not been studied frequently. However, threats to physical safety at school can have a significant impact on students' academic self-concept and emotional functioning (Buhs, 2005; Buhs & Ladd, 2001). Students who are frequently victimized also tend to report higher levels of distress and depression than those who are not routinely victimized (e.g., Boivin & Hymel, 1997; Kochenderfer-Ladd & Waldrop, 2001; Olweus, 1993). Few studies have identified pathways whereby peer victimization and harassment affects academic outcomes. However, as with perceived support, peer abuse and exclusion are likely to be associated with academic achievement by way of emotional distress (Buhs, 2005; Flook, Repetti, & Ullman, 2005).

Social Behavior as a Mediator of Peer and Academic Competence

In addition to providing specific, academically related supports in the form of expectations, help, and emotional nurturance, peers might also have an impact on academic outcomes because they promote displays of competent forms of social behavior. Indeed, positive social outcomes, such as cooperation, following rules, and getting along with others, have been central goals for students throughout the history of U.S. education (Wentzel, 2003). Therefore, adopting a competence perspective to understand peer relationship–academic achievement connections highlights the fact that being a competent student requires not only the demonstration of intellectual proficiency but also the display of prosocial and socially responsible behavior. Researchers have reported that positive forms of social behavior are related to peer acceptance and friendships, as well as to academic performance. Displays of prosocial and socially responsible behavior and restraint from disruptive and antisocial forms of behavior have been related consistently and positively to peer acceptance, whereas aggressive and negative forms of social interactions have been related to peer rejection (Crick, Murray-Close, Marks, & Mohajeri-Nelson, Chapter 16, this volume). These same aspects of social behavior also are strongly related to intellectual accomplishments, including grades, test scores, and IQ. Tendencies to be prosocial and empathic, prosocial interactions with peers, appropriate classroom conduct, and compliance are related positively to classroom grades and standardized test scores throughout the school years, even when taking into account factors such as IQ, sex, grade level, and other demographic variables, and when following students over time (for a review, see Wentzel, 2003).

Additional evidence indicates that prosocial and responsible behavior might provide a pathway by which peer relationships support academic achievement. For example, helping, cooperating, and sharing have been shown to mediate relations between sociometric status and academic accomplishments in early childhood and early adolescence (Buhs & Ladd, 2001; Wentzel, 1991); when these positive forms of behavior are taken into account, significant relations between peer acceptance and academic outcomes tend to decrease in strength or become nonsignificant. Positive relations between having friends and academic outcomes also tend to be explained, at least in part, by these prosocial forms of behavior (e.g., Wentzel & Caldwell, 1997).

One explanation for these mediational effects is that socially competent behavior provides a necessary foundation for learning, such that a basic ability to engage in and benefit from social interactions is necessary for children to benefit from classroom instruction. Interventions that teach children appropriate social responses to instruction, such as paying attention and volunteering answers, have led to significant and stable gains in academic achievement (Cobb & Hops, 1973; Hops & Cobb, 1974). Similarly, boys with attention-deficit/hyperactivity disorder (ADHD) can learn effective intellectual problem-solving strategies in collaborative situations when first trained to engage in positive social skills that support ongoing interactions with their peer partners (Wentzel & Watkins, 2002). An unanswered question concerns the degree to which peer relationships at school also promote these positive forms of social behavior. However, causal relations between behavioral and peer-related competence are likely reciprocal; it is clear that experiences with peers can teach children valuable social skills, and that demonstrations of valued social skills are a strong determinant of peer acceptance and approval.

Social Structures, Academic Functioning, and Peer Activities

Of final importance for understanding associations between peer activities and academic outcomes is a consideration of the broader social context of school. There are several ways in which social structures of schools can influence students' academic and peer-related competencies, including the nature of peer support at the school level, school-wide norms for peer interaction, the organizational structure of classrooms, and teachers' interactions with groups of children. Few researchers have documented ways in which peer influence, aggregated at the level of the school, might be related to the development and quality of academic functioning. However, the cumulative effects of having positive relationships with many classmates over time, and in multiple classroom and school settings, contribute to a student's sense of school community and belongingness (see Goodenow, 1993; Roeser & Eccles, 1998). The power of these broad levels of support is evidenced by positive relations of school belongingness to students' academic and behavioral outcomes, with effects often being moderated by students' sex, race, and school size (see Wentzel, in press).

Institutional rules and norms also can influence the nature of peer interactions and academic functioning. For instance, reform efforts designed to instill schools and classrooms with a sense of community and opportunities for social and moral development have resulted in schools within which students engage in positive and prosocial interactions with peers, perceive strong levels of emotional support and caring, and hold positive motivational orientations toward both social and academic outcomes (e.g., Watson, Solomon, Battistich, Schaps, & Solomon, 1989). School-level norms also can have a negative impact on academic motivation and achievement by influencing ways in which students interact with each other. This occurs most often when schools establish competitive academic standards and norm-referenced evaluations of achievement that in turn heighten social comparison among students. Such practices tend to result in students adopting orientations toward learning that focus on performance rather than mastery of subject matter, and in lowered levels of academic efficacy and aspirations for achievement especially among low-ability students (Butler, 2005).

Organizational aspects of classrooms also can have fairly powerful effects on the nature of peer relationships and interactions. For instance, middle and high school students in classrooms where frequent interactions with classmates are condoned, that is, where students are encouraged to talk to each other about class assignments, to work in small groups, and to move about while working on activities, also are less likely to be socially isolated or rejected by their classmates, enjoy greater numbers of friends, and experience more diversity and stability in their friendships (Epstein, 1983). The degree to which middle schools and high schools are ethnically diverse, as opposed to having clear majority and minority groupings, also can influence the nature and stability of friendships and group membership (Urberg, Degirmencioglu, Tolson, & Halliday-Scher, 1995).

Although the literature implies that peers might be the primary source of threats to students' physical safety and well-being, of central importance to understanding this process is that teachers and school administrators can play a central role in creating schools that are free of peer harassment and in alleviating the negative effects of harassment once it has occurred (Olweus, 1993). Interventions designed to offset the often negative influence of peer groups and gangs are especially successful if students have access to adults who provide them with warmth and strong guidance (Heath & McLaughlin, 1993). Teachers' verbal and nonverbal behavior toward certain children, especially when critical, also has been related to how these children are treated by their peers (Harper & McCluskey, 2003; White & Kistner, 1992). Teachers also can contribute to the formation of social norms that can impact the nature of peer interactions and academic accomplishments (Craig, Pepler, & Atlas, 2000; Smith, 2007).

The quality of students' relationships with teachers also is relevant for understanding school- and classroom-level effects on peer relationships and achievement. Research indicates that preschool children who enjoy emotionally secure relationships with their teachers are more likely to demonstrate prosocial, gregarious, and complex play, and less likely to show hostile aggression and withdrawn behavior toward their peers (e.g., Howes & Hamilton, 1993). Moreover, the affective quality of teacher–student relationships predicts peer-related and behavioral competence up to 8 years later (Hamre & Pianta, 2001). Although the nature of causal connections between teacher–student and peer relationships is unclear (see Wentzel, in press), it is reasonable to assume that the development of positive relationships with peers might be due in large part to systematic regulation of student behavior and the establishment of positive adult–child relationships in formal school settings.

Emerging Trends and Future Directions

Why might social competence with peers influence or even be related to academic outcomes? The research described in this chapter has established clear and often strong associations between the nature and quality of peer interactions and relationships, and students' academic motivation and performance. These findings appear to be robust for students of all ages. For the most part, the focus of this chapter has been on mechanisms and pathways of influence by which peers might influence academic functioning at school. The proposed models are those that have been studied most extensively in the literature. For example, social interactions with peers lead to academic accomplishments, because they motivate cognitive change and development (Piaget, 1932/1965; Vygotsky, 1978). Models of indirect influence in which peers serve as motivational contexts also were proposed. In these cases, positive relationships with peers serve as contextual affordances that support the development of positive motivational orientations toward achievement or result directly in academic assistance (Wentzel, 2005).

However, other pathways are feasible. At the simplest level, competence with peers and academic outcomes might simply be correlated but not causally related domains of functioning. In this case, social-behavioral outcomes might explain both positive peer relationships and academic accomplishments; students can be rewarded by teachers for their positive behavior with high grades or high-quality instruction and help (e.g., Brophy & Good, 1974) just as they are rewarded for positive behavior with social approval and acceptance by peers. Positive correlations between achievement and peer relationships also could reflect reputational biases rather than causal influence. To illustrate, some middle school students attribute positive academic characteristics to sociometrically popular peers, but not to sociometrically neglected students who also are high achievers but not as well-liked (Wentzel & Asher, 1995). Therefore, when classmates inform assessments of both social and academic competence, significant relations between peer acceptance and academic accomplishments might simply reflect a halo effect that leads students to evaluate well-liked classmates positively in both academic and social domains. However, peer reputational biases might also lead to real change in student outcomes over time as academic reputations become self-fulfilling prophecies (e.g., Gest, Domitrovich, & Welsh, 2005).

Additional causal mechanisms also might be operative. Significant relations between peer relationships and academic accomplishments, at least for some students, might reflect how excelling at academic tasks results in peer approval and acceptance. In other words, academic excellence would be one criterion for establishing positive relationships with peers. Interactions with peers have been viewed most often as having a potentially negative motivational impact on the pursuit and achievement of educational goals (Berndt, 1999). However, this negative influence is not universal across all peer groups and, as illustrated earlier, peer expectations can have a positive impact on students' academic functioning. Another relatively unexplored possibility is that improvements in cognitive abilities can lead to more skilled peer interactions. However, interventions to increase academic skills do not necessarily lead to decreases in types of antisocial behavior associated with peer rejection (Patterson, Bank, & Stoolmiller, 1990), nor do they enhance social skills typically associated with peer acceptance (Hops & Cobb, 1974). Therefore, a strong causal connection between academic skills and social competence is unlikely.

The role of specific, school-level factors in facilitating or negating the effects of peers on academic outcomes also requires additional examination. The fact that teachers have the potential to influence peer-related activities in powerful ways raises two important issues with respect to the role of peers in children's academic functioning. First, few studies on the quality of students' peer relationships and supports have also included assessments of teacher–student relationships. Available evidence yields mixed results. On the one hand, the quality of students' relationships with teachers tends to predict academic outcomes over and above the nature and quality of relationships with peers and parents (Furrer & Skinner, 2003; Ladd & Burgess, 2001). A study of middle school students further supports this finding; students who had few friends and were neither well-liked nor disliked by their peers (sociometrically neglected children), were the most well-liked by their teachers, the most highly motivated students, and were equally self-confident when compared to their average status peers (Wentzel & Asher, 1995). These findings might reflect the fact that not all students are motivated to interact with their peers when pursuing academic goals. This is especially true for high-achieving students in cooperative learning settings, who tend to view less able peers as not contributing to group efforts, and who believe their performance will suffer because of accountability to their peers (Ames, 1984). These students are likely to look to teachers rather than to peers for information and guidance.

On the other hand, aspects of peer rather than teacher relationships have been related to behavioral competence at school, especially prosocial forms of behavior (Wentzel, 1998; Wentzel & McNamara, 1999). Recent work suggests that peer, but not teacher, expectations predict middle school students' prosocial behavior (Wentzel, Filisetti, et al., 2007). In this latter study, peer expectations also predicted students' internalized reasons (e.g., "It's important") for behaving prosocially. Therefore, although findings indicate that students' relationships with teachers might have a more proximal influence on their academic achievement than their peer relationships, the relatively unique influence of peer relationships on students' prosocial behavior should not be discounted. Learning to cooperate with peers is a central requirement of educational institutions, and prosocial behavior is a powerful predictor of academic outcomes that tend to mediate relations between peer activities and academic competencies (Wentzel, 2003).

The relative contribution of different types of peer activities to academic outcomes also remains a relatively unexplored area of research. When children are with friends, they engage in more positive interactions, resolve more conflicts, and accomplish tasks with greater proficiency than when they are with nonfriends (Newcomb & Bagwell, 1995); not having a friend predicts less than optimal levels of emotional well-being (e.g., Brendgen, Vitaro, & Bukowski, 2000; Parker & Asher, 1993). In contrast, friends are believed to play a relatively minor role in socializing each other with respect to larger group norms and expectations (Hartup & Stevens, 1997). Therefore, the role of friendships in supporting academic competence should be most positive when students are collaborating with friends on academic activities, and when friends are available to provide emotional support when needed. Peer groups and crowds are likely to provide students with performance standards and behavioral norms that are commonly expected and sanctioned; peer values are communicated and modeled frequently, so that they can be easily learned and adopted by group members (Brown, Mory, & Kinney, 1994). Ecological perspectives (Bronfenbrenner, 1989; Cairns, Xie, & Leung, 1998) also call attention to the role of peer groups and crowds as intermediaries between the individual and broader peer and adult communities. For these reasons, it is likely that peer groups and crowds play a more central role than dyadic relationships in contributing to students' academic values and overall competencies (see Brown & Dietz, Chapter 20, and Kindermann & Gest, Chapter 6, this volume).

An additional issue with respect to peer activities and academic adjustment is that little is understood about peer cultures and what students themselves value and expect of each other to gain approval. The complexity of this undertaking is reflected in findings that personal attributes and behavior valued by students tend to differ as a function of gender, as well as race (e.g., Benenson, Apostoleris, & Parnass, 1998; Graham, Taylor, & Hudley, 1998). Similarly, ways in which characteristics of families, neighborhoods, and schools interact with peer relationships to influence children's academic functioning must be considered (e.g., Ge, Brody, Conger, Simmons, & Murray, 2002; Pettit, Bates, Dodge, & Meece, 1999). Therefore, conceptual models that take into account the diversity of student backgrounds need to be developed (see Chen, Chung, & Hsiao, Chapter 24, and Graham, Taylor, & Ho, Chapter 22, this volume). In this regard, researchers also need to identify ways in which students learn to coordinate their own social and academic goals with those prompted by others.

Finally, more studies in this area must take into account the age-related interests and capabilities of the child. From a developmental perspective, the role of peers in motivating academic accomplishments is likely to be especially critical during the middle and high school years. Although children are interested in and even emotionally attached to their peers at all ages, they exhibit increased interest in their peers, spend more time with them, and exhibit a growing psychological and emotional dependence on them for support and guidance as they make the transition into adolescence (Youniss & Smollar, 1989). Moreover, whereas friendships are enduring aspects of children's peer relationships at all ages, peer groups and crowds emerge primarily in the middle school years, peak at the beginning of high school, then diminish in prevalence, as well as influence, by the end of high school (Brown, 1989). Therefore, efforts to understand the influence of peer relationships on academic motivation and achievement must be sensitive to the qualities and types of relationships that students form with each other at different points in their educational careers.

References

Altermatt, E. R., & Pomerantz, E. M. (2005). The implications of having high-achieving versus low-achieving friends: A longitudinal analysis. *Social Development, 14*, 61–81.

Altermatt, E. R., Pomerantz, E. M., Ruble, D. N., Frey, K. S., & Greulich, F. K. (2002). Predicting changes in children's self-perceptions of academic competence: A naturalistic examination of evaluative discourse among classmates. *Developmental Psychology, 38*, 903–917.

Ames, C. (1984). Competitive, cooperative, and individualistic goal structures: A cognitive–motivational analysis. In R. Ames & C. Ames (Eds.), *Research in motivation in education* (pp. 177–208). New York: Academic Press.

Azmitia, M. (1988). Peer interaction and problem solving: When are two heads better than one? *Child Development, 59*, 87–96.

Bandura, A. (1986). *Social foundations of thought and action: A social cognitive theory*. Englewood Cliffs, NJ: Prentice-Hall.

Benenson, J., Apostoleris, N., & Parnass, J. (1998). The organization of children's same-sex peer relationships. *New Directions for Child Development, 80*, 5–23.

Berndt, T. J. (1999). Friends' influence on students' adjustment to school. *Educational Psychologist, 34*, 15–28.

Berndt, T. J., & Keefe, K. (1995). Friends' influence on adolescents' adjustment to school. *Child Development, 66*, 1312–1329.

Boivin, M., & Hymel, S. (1997). Peer experiences and social self-perceptions: A sequential model. *Developmental Psychology, 33*, 135–145.

Brendgen, M., Vitaro, F., Bukowski, W. M. (2000). Deviant friends and early adolescents' emotional and behavioral adjustment. *Journal of Research on Adolescence, 10*, 173–189.

Bronfenbrenner, U. (1989). Ecological systems theory. In R. Vasta (Ed.), *Annals of child development* (Vol. 6, pp. 187–250). Greenwich, CT: JAI.

Brophy, J. E., & Good, T. L. (1974). *Teacher–student relationships: Causes and consequences*. New York: Holt, Rinehart & Winston.

Brown, B. B. (1989). The role of peer groups in adolescents' adjustment to secondary school. In T. J. Berndt & G. W. Ladd (Eds.), *Peer relationships in child development* (pp. 188–215). New York: Wiley.

Brown, B. B., Mory, M. S., & Kinney, D. (1994). Casting adolescent crowds in a relational perspective: Caricature, channel, and context. In R. Montemayor, G. R. Adams, & T. P. Gullotta (Eds.), *Personal relationships during adolescence* (pp. 123–167). Newbury Park, CA: Sage.

Brown, B. B., Mounts, N., Lamborn, D. D., & Steinberg, L. (1993). Parenting practices and peer group affiliation in adolescence. *Child Development, 64*, 467–482.

Buhs, E. S. (2005). Peer rejection, negative peer treatment, and school adjustment: Self-concept and classroom engagement as mediating processes. *Journal of School Psychology, 43*, 407–424.

Buhs, E. S., & Ladd, G. W. (2001). Peer rejection as an antecedent of young children's school adjustment: An examination of mediating processes. *Developmental Psychology, 37*, 550–560.

Butler, R. (2005). Competence assessment, competence, and motivation between early and middle childhood. In A. Elliot & C. Dweck (Eds.), *Handbook of competence and motivation* (pp. 202–221). New York: Guilford Press.

Cairns, R., Xie, H., & Leung, M. (1998). The popularity of friendship and the neglect of social networks: Toward a new balance. *New Directions for Child Development, 80*, 25–53.

Clasen, D. R., & Brown, B. B. (1985). The multidimensionality of peer pressure in adolescence. *Journal of Youth and Adolescence, 14*, 451–468.

Cobb, J. A., & Hops, H. (1973). Effects of academic survival skills training on low achieving first graders. *Journal of Educational Research, 67*, 108–113.

Cohen, E. G. (1986). *Designing group work: Strategies for the heterogeneous classroom.* New York: Teachers College Press.

Cooper, C. R., Ayers-Lopez, S., & Marquis, A. (1982). Children's discourse during peer learning in experimental and naturalistic situations. *Discourse Processes, 5*, 177–191.

Craig, W. M., Pepler, D., & Atlas, R. (2000). Observations of bullying in the playground and in the classroom. *School Psychology International, 21*, 22–36.

Crockett, L., Losoff, M., & Petersen, A. C. (1984). Perceptions of the peer group and friendship in early adolescence. *Journal of Early Adolescence, 4*, 155–181.

Dubow, E. F., & Tisak, J. (1989). The relation between stressful life events and adjustment in elementary school children: The role of social support and social problem-solving skills. *Child Development, 60*, 1412–1423.

Eccles, J. S., & Midgley, C. (1989). Stage–environment fit: Developmentally appropriate classrooms for young adolescents. In C. Ames & R. Ames (Eds.), *Research on motivation in education* (Vol. 3, pp. 139–186). New York: Academic Press.

Eder, D. E., & Felmlee, D. (1984). The development of attention norms in ability groups. In P. L. Peterson, L. C. Wilkinson, & M. Hallinan (Eds.), *The social context of instruction: Group organization and group processes* (pp. 189–225). New York: Academic Press.

Epstein, J. L. (1983). The influence of friends on achievement and affective outcomes. In J. L. Epstein & N. Karweit (Eds.), *Friends in school* (pp. 177–200). New York: Academic Press.

Flook, L., Repetti, R. L., & Ullman, J. B. (2005). Classroom social experiences as predictors of academic performance. *Developmental Psychology, 41*, 319–327.

Fonzi, A., Schneider, B. H., Tani, F., & Tomada, G. (1997). Predicting children's friendship status from their dyadic interaction in structured situations of potential conflict. *Child Development, 68*, 496–506.

Ford, M. E. (1992). *Motivating humans: Goals, emotions, and personal agency beliefs.* Newbury Park, CA: Sage.

Furrer, C., & Skinner, E. (2003). Sense of relatedness as a factor in children's academic engagement and performance. *Journal of Educational Psychology, 95*, 148–162.

Gauvain, M., & Perez, S. M. (2007). The socialization of cognition. In J. E. Grusec & P. D. Hastings (Eds.), *Handbook of socialization: Theory and research* (pp. 588–613). New York: Guilford Press.

Ge, A., Brody, G. H., Conger, R. D., Simons, R. L., & Murray, V. M. (2002). Contextual amplification of pubertal transition effects on deviant peer affiliation and externalizing behavior among African-American children. *Developmental Psychology, 38*, 42–54.

Gest, S. D., Domitrovich, C. E., & Welsh, J. A. (2005). Peer academic reputation in elementary school: Associations with changes in self-concept and academic skills. *Journal of Educational Psychology, 97*, 337–346.

Goodenow, C. (1993). Classroom belonging among early adolescent students: Relationships to motivation and achievement. *Journal of Early Adolescence, 13*, 21–43.

Graham, S., Taylor, A., & Hudley, C. (1998). Exploring achievement values among ethnic minority early adolescents. *Journal of Educational Psychology, 90*, 606–620.

Greenfield, P. M. (1997). You can't take it with you: Why ability assessments don't cross cultures. *American Psychologist, 52*, 1115–1124.

Grusec, J. E., & Hastings, P. D. (Eds.). (2007). *Handbook of socialization: Theory and research.* New York: Guilford Press.

Hamre, B. K., & Pianta, R. C. (2001). Early teacher–child relationships and the trajectory of children's school outcomes through eighth grade. *Child Development, 72*, 625–638.

Harper, L. V., & McCluskey, K. S. (2003). Teacher–child and child–child interactions in inclusive preschool settings: Do adults inhibit peer interactions? *Early Childhood Research Quarterly, 18*, 163–184.

Hartup, W. W., & Stevens, N. (1997). Friendships and adaptation in the life course. *Psychological Bulletin, 121*, 355–370.

Heath, S. B., & McLaughlin, M. W. (1993). *Identity and inner-city youth.* New York: Teachers College Press.

Hodges, E. V., Boivin, M., Vitaro, F., & Bukowski, W. M. (1999). The power of friendship: Protection against an escalating cycle of peer victimization. *Developmental Psychology, 35*, 94–101.

Hops, H., & Cobb, J. A. (1974). Initial investigations into academic survival-skill training, direct instruction, and first-grade achievement. *Journal of Educational Psychology, 66*, 548–553.

Howes, C., & Hamilton, C. E. (1993). The changing experience of child care: Changes in teachers and in teacher–child relationships and children's social competence with peers. *Early Childhood Research Quarterly, 8*, 15–32.

Jacobsen, T., Edelstein, W., & Hofmann, V. (1994). A longitudinal study of the relation between representations of attachment in childhood and cognitive functioning in childhood and adolescence. *Developmental Psychology, 30*, 112–124.

Juvonen, J., Nishina, A., & Graham, S. (2000). Peer harassment, psychological adjustment, and school functioning in early adolescence. *Journal of Educational Psychology, 92*, 349–359.

Kindermann, T. A. (1993). Natural peer groups as contexts for individual development: The case of children's motivation in school. *Developmental Psychology, 29*, 970–977.

Kindermann, T. A., McCollam, T. L., & Gibson, E. (1996). Peer networks and students' classroom engagement during childhood and adolescence. In J. Juvonen & K. R. Wentzel (Eds.), *Social motivation: Understanding children's school adjustment* (pp. 279–312). New York: Cambridge University Press.

Kochenderfer-Ladd, B., & Waldrop, J. L. (2001). Chronicity and instability of children's peer victimization experiences as predictors of loneliness and social satisfaction trajectories. *Child Development, 72*, 134–151.

Kutnick, P., & Kington, A. (2005). Children's friendships and learning in school: Cognitive enhancement through social interaction? *British Journal of Educational Psychology, 75*, 521–538.

Ladd, G. W. (1990). Having friends, keeping friends, making friends, and being liked by peers in the classroom: Predictors of children's early school adjustment. *Child Development, 61*, 1081–1100.

Ladd, G. W., & Burgess, K. B. (2001). Do relational risks and protective factors moderate the linkages between childhood aggression and early psychological and school adjustment? *Child Development, 72*, 1579–1601.

Lempers, J. D., & Clark-Lempers, D. S. (1992). Young, middle, and late adolescents' comparisons of the functional importance of five significant relationships. *Journal of Youth and Adolescence, 21*, 53–96.

Maccoby, E. E. (2002). Gender and group process: A developmental perspective. *Current Directions in Psychological Science, 11*, 54–58.

Newcomb, A. F., & Bagwell, C. L. (1995). Children's friendship relations: A meta-analytic review. *Psychological Bulletin, 117*, 306–347.

Olweus, D. (1993). Victimization by peers: Antecedents and long-term outcomes. In K. Rubin & J. B. Asendorf (Eds.), *Social withdrawal, inhibition, and shyness in childhood* (pp. 315–341). Chicago: University of Chicago Press.

Parker, J. G., & Asher, S. R. (1993). Friendship and friendship quality in middle childhood: Links with peer group acceptance and feelings of loneliness and social dissatisfaction. *Developmental Psychology, 29*, 611–621.

Patterson, G. R., Bank, C. L., & Stoolmiller, M. (1990). The preadolescent's contributions to disrupted family process. In R. Montemayor, G. R. Adams, & T. P. Gullota (Eds.), *From childhood to adolescence: A transitional period?* (Vol. 2, pp. 107–133). Newbury Park, CA: Sage.

Pellegrini, A. D., Bartini, M., & Brooks, F. (1999). School bullies, victims, and aggressive victims: Factors relating to group affiliation and victimization in early adolescence. *Journal of Educational Psychology, 91*, 216–224.

Pettit, G. S., Bates, J. E., Dodge, K. A., & Meece, D. W. (1999). The impact of after-school peer contact on early adolescent externalizing problems is moderated by parental monitoring, perceived neighborhood safety, and prior adjustment. *Child Development, 70*, 768–778.

Piaget, J. (1965). *The moral judgment of the child.* New York: Free Press. (Original work published 1932)

Roeser, R. W., & Eccles, J. S. (1998). Adolescents' perceptions of middle school: Relation to longitudinal changes in academic and psychological adjustment. *Journal of Research on Adolescence, 8*, 123–158.

Rogoff, B., Moore, L., Najafi, B., Dexter, A., Correa-Chavez, M., & Solis, J. (2007). Children's development of cultural repertoires through participation in everyday routines and practices. In J. E. Grusec & P. D. Hastings (Eds.), *Handbook of socialization: Theory and research* (pp. 490–515). New York: Guilford Press.

Rohrbeck, C. A., Ginsburg-Block, M. D., Fantuzzo, J. W., & Miller, T. R. (2003). Peer-assisted learning interventions with elementary school students: A meta-analytic review. *Journal of Educational Psychology, 95*, 240–257.

Rubin, K. H., Bukowski, W., & Parker, J. (2006). Peer interactions, relationships, and groups. In N. Eisenberg (Ed.), *Handbook of child psychology: Social, emotional, and personality development* (6th ed., pp. 571–645). New York: Wiley.

Ryan, A. (2001). The peer group as a context for the development of young adolescent motivation and achievement. *Child Development, 72*, 1135–1150.

Ryan, R. M., & Deci, E. L. (2000). Self-determination theory and the facilitation of intrinsic motivation, social development, and well-being. *American Psychologist, 55*, 68–78.

Schunk, D. H. (1987). Peer models and children's behavioral change. *Review of Educational Research, 57*, 149–174.

Schunk, D. H., & Pajares, F. (2005). Competence perceptions and academic functioning. In A. Elliot & C. Dweck (Eds.), *Handbook of competence and motivation* (pp. 85–104). New York: Guilford Press.

Schwartz, D., Dodge, K. A., Pettit, G. S., Bates, J. E., & the Conduct Problems Prevention Research Group. (2000). Friendship as a moderating factor in the pathway between early harsh home environment and later victimization in the peer group. *Developmental Psychology, 36*, 646–662.

Slavin, R. E., Hurley, E. A., & Chamberlain, A. (2003). Cooperative learning and achievement: Theory and research. In W. Reynolds & G. Miller (Eds.), *Handbook of psychology: Vol. 7. Educational psychology* (pp. 177–198). New York: Wiley.

Smetana, J., & Bitz, B. (1996). Adolescents' conceptions of teachers' authority and their relations to rule violations in school. *Child Development, 67*, 1153–1172.

Smith, J. (2007). "Ye've got to 'ave balls to play this game sir!": Boys, peers and fears: The negative influence of school-based "cultural accomplices" in constructing hegemonic masculinities. *Gender and Education, 19*, 179–198.

Snow, R. E., & Yalow, E. (1982). Education and intelligence. In R. Sternberg (Ed.), *Handbook of human intelligence* (pp. 493–585). New York: Cambridge University Press.

Steinberg, L., Brown, B. B., & Dornbusch, S. M. (1996). Beyond the classroom: Why school reform has failed and what parents need to do. New York: Simon & Schuster.

Stone, M. R., & Brown, B. B. (1999). Identity claims and projections: Descriptions of self and crowds in secondary school. *New Directions for Child and Adolescent Development, 84*, 7–20.

Tudge, J. R. H. (1992). Processes and consequences of peer collaboration: A Vygotskian analysis. *Child Development, 63*, 1364–1379.

Urberg, K. A., Degirmencioglu, S. M., Tolson, J. M., & Halliday-Scher, K. (1995). The structure of adolescent peer networks. *Developmental Psychology, 31*, 540–547.

Vygotsky, L. S. (1978). *Mind in society: The development of higher psychological processes.* Cambridge, MA: Harvard University Press.

Watson, M., Solomon, D., Battistich, V., Schaps, E., & Solomon, J. (1989). The Child Development Project: Combining traditional and developmental approaches to values education. In L. Nucci (Ed.), *Moral development and character education: A dialogue* (pp. 51–92). Berkeley: McCutchan.

Wentzel, K. R. (1991). Relations between social competence and academic achievement in early adolescence. *Child Development, 62,* 1066–1078.

Wentzel, K. R. (1998). Social support and adjustment in middle school: The role of parents, teachers, and peers. *Journal of Educational Psychology, 90,* 202–209.

Wentzel, K. R. (2003). School adjustment. In W. Reynolds & G. Miller (Eds.), *Handbook of psychology, Vol. 7: Educational psychology* (pp. 235–258). New York: Wiley.

Wentzel, K. R. (2004). Understanding classroom competence: The role of social-motivational and self-processes. In R. Kail (Ed.), *Advances in child development and behavior* (Vol. 32, pp. 213–241). New York: Elsevier.

Wentzel, K. R. (2005). Peer relationships, motivation, and academic performance at school. In A. Elliot & C. Dweck (Eds.), *Handbook of competence and motivation* (pp. 279–296). New York: Guilford Press.

Wentzel, K. R. (in press). Students' relationships with teachers. In J. Meece & J. Eccles (Eds.), *Handbook of research on schools, schooling, and human development.* New York: Erlbaum.

Wentzel, K. R., & Asher, S. R. (1995). Academic lives of neglected, rejected, popular, and controversial children. *Child Development, 66,* 754–763.

Wentzel, K. R., Barry, C., & Caldwell, K. (2004). Friendships in middle school: Influences on motivation and school adjustment. *Journal of Educational Psychology, 96,* 195–203.

Wentzel, K. R., & Caldwell, K. (1997). Friendships, peer acceptance, and group membership: Relations to academic achievement in middle school. *Child Development, 68,* 1198–1209.

Wentzel, K. R., Filisetti, L., & Looney, L. (2007). Adolescent prosocial behavior: The role of self-processes and contextual cues. *Child Development, 78,* 895–910.

Wentzel, K. R., & Looney, L. (2007). Socialization in school settings. In J. E. Grusec & P. D. Hastings (Eds.), *Handbook of socialization: Theory and research* (pp. 382–403). New York: Guilford Press.

Wentzel, K., Looney, L., & Battle, A. (2003). *Social and academic motivation in adolescence.* Unpublished manuscript, University of Maryland, College Park.

Wentzel, K. R., & McNamara, C. (1999). Interpersonal relationships, emotional distress, and prosocial behavior in middle school. *Journal of Early Adolescence, 19,* 114–125.

Wentzel, K. R., Monzo, J., Williams, A. Y., & Tomback, R. M. (2007, April). *Teacher and peer influence on academic motivation in adolescence: A cross-sectional study.* Paper presented at the biennial meeting of the Society for Research in Child Development, Boston, MA.

Wentzel, K. R., & Watkins, D. (2002). Peer relationships and collaborative learning as contexts for academic enablers. *School Psychology Review, 31,* 366–377.

Wentzel, K. R., Weinberger, D. A., Ford, M. E., & Feldman, S. S. (1990). Academic achievement in preadolescence: The role of motivational, affective, and self-regulatory processes. *Journal of Applied Developmental Psychology, 11,* 179–193.

Wentzel, K. R., & Wigfield, A. (1998). Academic and social motivational influences on students' academic performance. *Educational Psychology Review, 10,* 155–175.

White, K. J., & Kistner, J. (1992). The influence of teacher feedback on young children's peer preferences and perceptions. *Developmental Psychology, 28,* 933–940.

Youniss, J., & Smollar, J. (1989). Adolescents' interpersonal relationships in social context. In T. J. Berndt & G. Ladd (Eds.), *Peer relationships in child development* (pp. 300–316). New York: Wiley.

CHAPTER 30

Peer Reputations
and Psychological Adjustment

MITCHELL J. PRINSTEIN
DIANA RANCOURT
JOHN D. GUERRY
CAROLINE B. BROWNE

Children begin to develop remarkably stable peer reputations early in their lives. Research has demonstrated that children's likability among peers can be measured reliably within just the first few years of life (e.g., ages 3–5 years; Ladd & Troop-Gordon, 2003). These reputations appear to be stable across contexts; indeed, children's reputations of likability among familiar peers are very quickly replicated within groups of unfamiliar peers (Coie & Kupersmidt, 1983; Dodge, 1983). Moreover, there is good evidence to suggest that children's peer reputations endure over multiple developmental transitions, with moderate stability coefficients over at least 5 years (Coie & Dodge, 1983). Given the extraordinary consistency in children's experiences among peers, it is not surprising that investigators frequently have examined whether these peer reputations may have consequences for later adjustment outcomes. This chapter focuses specifically on research that has explored childhood peer reputations as predictors of later psychological symptoms.

There is substantial research to suggest that peer reputations are associated longitudinally with a variety of important developmental outcomes. For instance, prior work has suggested that children who are strongly disliked among peers are less likely to complete secondary education (e.g., Coie, Lochman, Terry, & Hyman, 1992; Ollendick, Weist, Borden, & Greene, 1992), to develop long-term romantic relationships (Connolly & Johnson, 1996), or to demonstrate vocational competence as adults (e.g., Bagwell, Newcomb, & Bukowski, 1998; Nelson & Dishion, 2004). Research regarding normative developmental outcomes has been reviewed in other chapters within this volume. Our review is focused on the prediction of three domains of psychopathology: (1) externalizing symptoms; (2) health-risk behaviors; and (3) internalizing symptoms. "Externalizing symptoms" include disruptive, oppositional, and/or aggressive behaviors. Externalizing symptoms can include DSM-IV diagnoses of oppositional defiant disorder, conduct disorder, or attention-deficit/hyperactivity disorder (predominantly hyperactive/impulsive or combined subtypes) (American Psychiatric Association, 2000) but frequently are examined by assessing related outcomes or constructs. For instance, many studies within the peer relations literature have examined measures of delinquency; teacher-, child-, or parent-reported aggressive/oppositional symptoms; or illegal behaviors as markers of externalizing symptoms.

"Health-risk behaviors" include several types of serious behaviors associated with short- or long-term health morbidity or mortality. Substance use, sexual-risk behaviors, eating-related behaviors, and self-harm behaviors are included within the domain of health-risk outcomes. Although many health-risk behaviors co-occur with either internalizing or externalizing symptoms, these behaviors are distinct and not merely indicative of the presence of other psychopathology. Health-risk behaviors therefore represent important, discrete clinical outcomes.

"Internalizing symptoms" most frequently include difficulties with mood or anxiety. Internalizing diagnoses include major depressive disorder, dysthymia, bipolar disorder, and several anxiety disorders (e.g., generalized anxiety, posttraumatic stress disorder, social phobia, specific phobia, obsessive–compulsive disorder). However, the vast majority of studies examining internalizing outcomes have focused specifically on depressive symptoms, generalized anxiety, or social anxiety symptoms, as well as other markers of potential internalizing distress, such as loneliness.

It is essential to examine associations between peer reputations and psychological symptoms from a developmental psychopathology perspective (Parker, Rubin, Erath, Wojslawowicz, & Buskirk, 2006). Developmental psychopathology theory emphasizes a multidisciplinary approach toward understanding typical and atypical development. The study of normative developmental processes, and the identification of aberrations in normative development that may confer adjustment risk, can help inform an understanding of psychopathology. Examining atypical development often can elucidate normative processes by highlighting perturbations in normal developmental competencies. Developmental psychopathology research on peer relations to date has been somewhat skewed toward the study of normative processes only. In other words, most prior research examining peer reputations as predictors of adjustment outcomes have involved normative samples, and the prediction of elevations on screening measures of psychological symptoms. Rarer are studies that have examined peer relationships within a clinical sample of youth experiencing severe psychopathology. These latter data may be especially helpful for understanding reciprocal transactions between peer reputations and adjustment that likely occur over time. We review the normative and clinical sample literature below.

Central Issues

The association between peer reputation and psychological symptoms is dependent upon youth development. Specifically, it is essential to consider developmental variation in both (1) the construct of peer reputation, and (2) the presentation and assessment of psychological symptoms. A brief overview of each issue is offered below. Until recently, there has been remarkable consistency in operationalizing the construct of "peer reputations." Specifically, for over 30 years there has been a strong consensus regarding the reliance on both positive and negative peer nominations of peer acceptance and rejection as a basis for understanding children's reputations among peers. The emphasis on peer nominations is consistent with the notion that peers are optimal informants for understanding and reporting peers' attitudes toward other youth. The use of both positive and negative nominations allows for the identification of children who are likable and/or dislikable among peers (see Cillessen, Chapter 5, this volume). From such nomination data, youth can be identified as sociometrically "popular" (strongly liked, rarely disliked), "rejected" (strongly disliked, rarely liked), "neglected" (rarely nominated), and "controversial" (strongly liked, strongly disliked). The vast majority of research on peer reputations has examined this preference-based measure of status (i.e., sometimes referred to as "sociometric popularity") as a predictor of later adjustment outcomes.

Relatively recently, the assessment of peer reputations among adolescents has led to the development of a second construct of peer status. Investigations of peer reputations in middle childhood and adolescence have revealed that youth are increasingly capable of distinguishing between their own personal *preferences* and their peers' global reputations of popularity among others. With increasing age, youth are able to provide reports of two distinct constructs of peer status (see Cillessen, Chapter 5, and Asher & McDonald, Chapter 13, this volume). Thus, youth are capable of directly reporting their peers' reputations of popularity. This reputation-based construct has been referred to as "peer-perceived popularity" (e.g., LaFontana & Cillessen, 2002; Parkhurst & Hopmeyer 1998), and often is assessed by asking youth to nominate peers who are "most popular" and "least popular." These nominations reflect youths' perceptions of their peers' reputations of popularity rather than assess their preferences toward peers. Preference- and reputation-based measures of peer status are moderately intercorrelated (Cillessen, Chapter 5, and Asher & McDonald, Chapter 13, this volume). However, youth with high levels of reputation-based popularity include those who are sociometrically both popular and controversial (Parkhurst & Hopmeyer, 1998). Furthermore, the association between each type of peer status (i.e., sociometric popularity and peer-perceived popularity) and later psychological adjustment outcomes is quite distinct.

Development

It is important to consider the developmental period during which psychological symptoms are assessed as an outcome. Substantial literature suggests that the prevalence of specific psychological symptoms varies considerably over development. For example, the prevalence of depressive symptoms increases dramatically during the transition to adolescence, especially for girls (Hankin & Abramson, 2001). Among boys, the adolescent transition is associated with a marked increase in the prevalence of externalizing symptoms, including severe oppositional defiant and conduct disorder symptoms. However, there appear to be substantial differences in the antecedents, course, and prognosis of symptoms among youth who exhibit externalizing behaviors in childhood or adolescence (Moffitt, 1993). Given these developmental differences in the prevalence and correlates of psychological symptoms, some rationale is needed for the investigation of peer reputations as predictors of psychological symptoms at a particular age. Heteroscedasticity in psychological symptoms across different developmental periods also may result in spurious associations between peer reputations and psychological symptoms.

In addition to developmental variation in diagnoses, there also is considerable developmental heterogeneity in the symptoms that comprise a specific diagnosis. For instance, within the diagnosis of depression, there is some evidence to suggest that hopelessness and somatic symptoms may be rarer in childhood than in adolescence (e.g., Weiss & Garber, 2003). Studies assessing a single symptom as a marker for a clinical diagnosis may yield misleading findings, if developmental variation in the presentation of clinical syndromes is not considered.

It is important to consider a developmental rationale in the assessment of behaviors over time. Most studies examining the consequences of negative peer reputations assess peer experiences at an initial time point and psychological symptoms at a later time point. Although this design offers an important advantage in the ability to reveal prospective associations, it is unfortunate that many studies have not allowed for an examination of potential reciprocal, transactional associations. Developmental psychopathology theories emphasize substantial heterogeneity in the timing and course of psychological symptoms across individuals. Unless the initial time point in which predictors are assessed marks a uniform stressor or transition experience that is hypothesized to exert a homogeneous effect on all study participants, it is likely that the assessment window captures a period of substantial change in psychological functioning for only a minority of participants. In other words, the effect of pervasive peer reputations may be immediate or delayed, or may have been most evident on outcomes that occurred prior to study onset.

Last, developmental psychopathology theory suggests continuous transactions among different domains of development. For example, changes in social development are dependent upon and influence changes in behavioral development. Atypical developmental experiences (e.g., rejection by peers) are intertwined with altered trajectories of development in other domains of functioning (e.g., emotional competencies). Interpersonal experiences within the peer context may be both a cause and consequence of behavioral difficulties. Unfortunately, few investigations have examined such bidirectional associations between peer experiences and psychological adjustment.

Relevant Theory

Studies examining the effects of peer reputations generally have addressed one of two fundamental questions:

1. *Do* children's peer reputations predict later adjustment outcomes?
2. *Why* do children's peer reputations predict later adjustment outcomes?

Theoretical issues relevant to each research program are discussed below.

Examinations to determine the importance of childhood peer reputations as predictors of later psychological symptoms typically utilize one of two longitudinal designs. Follow-back designs identify youth or adults who have experienced a clinical outcome of interest (e.g., a specific diagnosis, the receipt of psychological treatment). Archival data from this identified group then may be analyzed, or sometimes evaluated with respect to a comparison group, to determine unique antecedent childhood predictors. Several of the most influential early studies of peer relations utilized follow-back longitudinal design, yielding provocative results (see Roff, 1961). For example, Cowen, Pedersen, Bagigian, Izzo, and Trost (1973) examined archival childhood data within a sample of adults who had received psychological treatment at a community mental health clinic. Prior school records from this sample included results from a peer nomination assessment (i.e., class play; Bower, 1969) conducted 11–13 years earlier. Results indicated that negative peer nominations (suggesting peer rejection) were significantly associated with mental health status in adulthood. Moreover, negative peer nominations were stronger predictors of adult outcomes than were teacher ratings of childhood psychological adjustment, physical health, intellectual potential, academic performance, self-esteem, and anxiety (Cowen et al., 1973). Results from these follow-back studies offered the first evidence to suggest that peer-reported peer rejection may confer unique risks for later psychological symptoms that are not explained by more general adult-rated indices of social-psychological predictors.

Although results from prior follow-back investigations have yielded intriguing results and have offered rare opportunities to study individuals experiencing clinically significant outcomes, the vast majority of research in this area has utilized a follow-forward design. This type of study typically involves comparatively large samples of youth recruited from a normative, community context, and repeated follow-up data collection over several months or even years. Notably, this approach more easily allows for the examination of prospective associations, tests of theoretically derived hypotheses, the assessment of processes at precise developmental periods or transition points, and the use of sophisticated analyses to understand longitudinal effects. Limitations of this approach have included a low prevalence of severe clinical outcomes at follow-up.

Due to the correlational nature of both follow-back and follow-forward investigations, it is especially difficult to determine whether peer reputations exert a unique and perhaps causal impact on later adjustment outcomes. This often has been discussed in the context of three heuristic models of peer reputations (Parker et al., 2006; Rubin, Bukowski, & Parker, 2006). One of these, the "incidental model," suggests that the apparent association between peer reputations and later adjustment outcomes may be due to a "third variable" that predicts each. For example, attachment theories suggest that an insecure attachment in early childhood, and the resulting biases in one's internal working model of relationships, may cause both difficulties with peers and later psychological symptoms (e.g., Sroufe, 1997). "Third variables" also may include early manifestations of psychological disorders. For example, aggressive behavior in childhood may be an earlier expression of the same disturbance that produces severe oppositional or conduct disorder symptoms in adolescence (i.e., heterotypic continuity). Because childhood aggressive behavior also is associated strongly with peer rejection, the apparent role of peer rejection as a predictor of later externalizing symptoms perhaps could be more accurately explained by the heterotypic continuity of aggressive behavior. The incidental model therefore suggests that once the effects of a third variable are accounted for, peer reputations may not have a direct effect on the development of psychopathology.

A second model, often referred to as a "causal model," hypothesizes a direct effect of peer experiences on psychological symptoms. Studies offering data consistent with a causal model control for relevant "third variables" and examine unique longitudinal effects of peer reputations over time. Although data from correlational studies are not able to offer causal conclusions, researchers have attempted to offer evidence that is most consistent with a direct and unique contribution of peer reputations on later psychological symptoms.

Developmental psychopathology theories more specifically suggest that development is guided by transactions between various aspects of adaptation, as well as between individuals and their environment. A "transactional model" therefore suggests bidirectional and mutually reinforcing associations between predisposing characteristics (e.g., behavioral inhibition, working models of relationships) and peer reputations (e.g.,

Rubin, Burgess, Kennedy, & Stewart, 2003). The continuous interaction and mutual rein-forcement between experiences of youth with peers and their development competence (e.g., emotional, behavioral, moral competencies) conjointly leads to the development of later psychological symptoms. Notably, the transactional model suggests that neither peer reputations nor behavioral/social-cognitive correlates are solely responsible for the development of psychopathology. Rather, psychological symptoms are best predicted by the dynamic interplay of these experiences and competencies over time.

One specific example of a transactional model is a moderator hypothesis, in which peer reputations change the nature of the association between early behavioral difficul-ties, or social-cognitive deficits, and later psychopathology. For example, many investiga-tions have suggested that peer rejection may actuate the longitudinal effects of social-cognitive deficits (e.g., cognitive biases) on psychological symptoms. Additionally, peer rejection may exacerbate the effects of early behavioral difficulties (e.g., aggression) on later symptoms of a disorder. In many cases, explorations of peer rejection as a potential moderator have been examined by considering subtypes of peer-rejected youth (e.g., rejected–aggressive; rejected–withdrawn/submissive; Cillessen, van IJzendoorn, van Lie-shout, & Hartup, 1992). Studies investigating such moderator hypotheses have been espe-cially fruitful and are reviewed in detail below.

In addition to research examining whether peer reputations may be associated with later psychological symptoms, a large literature has focused on the examination of pos-sible theoretical models that may help to explain the important role of peer experiences. Perhaps the most consistent and fruitful line of inquiry uses a social-cognitive framework for understanding links between peer reputations and adjustment. In particular, much work has focused on the manner in which children's peer experiences may be associated with how social information processing may mediate or moderate longitudinal associa-tions with later psychological symptoms. For example, Crick and Dodge's (1994) social information-processing model indicates that individuals' responses within interpersonal interactions (i.e., to a specific social stimulus) are mediated by several specific cognitive steps; intra, and interindividual variability at each of these steps is associated with interper-sonal schemas, scripts, and data from past experiences. The presence of cognitive biases at any of these steps alters the trajectory of subsequent processes, leading to aberrant or maladaptive behavior. Specifically, this model suggests that individuals first encode social stimuli, then generate an interpretation (i.e., causal and intent attributions) of encoded information. Behavioral strategies that are generated, selected, and enacted follow from cue interpretations.

Researchers have identified a unique cognitive bias, suggesting that a tendency to interpret ambiguous or benign social stimuli is due to hostile intent (i.e., a hostile attribu-tion bias; e.g., Crick & Dodge, 1996; Dodge, Bates, & Pettit, 1990; Dodge & Coie, 1987). This cognitive interpretation leads to the development and clarification of specific social goals (e.g., to maintain dominance, to avoid conflict), followed by the generation, selec-tion, and enactment of specific behavioral responses that are perceived to help achieve these goals (Crick & Dodge, 1994). Research suggests that individuals with a hostile attri-bution bias may be especially likely to generate, select, and enact aggressive behaviors (Dodge et al., 1990). Individuals who interpret ambiguous social stimuli as being due to perceived self-deficits are likely to generate passive or submissive behavioral responses (e.g., withdrawal; Prinstein, Cheah, & Guyer, 2005; Rubin & Rose-Krasnor, 1992). A dis-cussion of social information-processing theories that pertain to the links between peer reputations and psychological symptoms is offered below.

Key Classical and Modern Research Studies

Prediction of Externalizing Symptoms

At least 30 follow-forward longitudinal studies examined peer reputation as a predictor of externalizing symptoms. The results of these investigations have offered overwhelming evidence that children's status among peers is associated prospectively with later aggressive, delinquent, oppositional, and illegal behavior (e.g., Bagwell et al., 1998; Coie et al., 1992; Coie, Terry, Lenox, Lochman, & Hyman, 1995; Kupersmidt & Coie, 1990). However, findings have suggested that the nature of this association is highly dependent on the specific types of peer reputations and externalizing symptoms that are measured. Moreover, findings have offered conflicting results regarding the specific model that best explains the nature of this association.

Results consistently demonstrate that children who are disliked by their peers are more likely to exhibit externalizing symptoms later in development. Peer rejection appears to be a powerful predictor, with several studies suggesting the prediction of long-term outcomes 7 (e.g., Coie et al., 1995; Lewin, Davis, & Hops, 1999) or even over 10 years later (e.g., Laird, Pettit, Dodge, & Bates, 2005; Nelson & Dishion, 2004; Rabiner, Coie, Miller-Johnson, Boykin, & Lochman, 2005). This effect remains consistent for studies that have assessed peer rejection using peer-reported sociometric measures (e.g., Coie et al., 1995) or teacher-reported assessments of children's peer likability (Fergusson, Woodward, & Horwood, 1999). Additionally, the effect of peer rejection appears to be similar across different stages of development. Studies examining peer rejection in early childhood (e.g., kindergarten and first grade; Dodge et al., 2003), middle childhood (e.g., Coie et al., 1995; Kupersmidt & Coie, 1990; Ollendick et al., 1992), and adolescence (e.g., grades 8–10; French, Conrad, & Turner, 1995; Prinstein & Cillessen, 2003) have revealed both short- and long-term effects on later externalizing symptoms. Results also remain consistent for studies of peer rejection predicting elevations on symptom checklists (Coie et al., 1995; Kupersmidt & Patterson, 1991; Prinstein & La Greca, 2004), the presence of externalizing diagnoses, and public records of criminal offenses (Nelson & Dishion, 2004; Ollendick et al., 1992). It appears that these findings are similar for predominantly European American samples (Lewin et al., 1999), exclusively African American samples (Rabiner et al., 2005), and ethnically heterogeneous samples (Laird et al., 2005; Prinstein & La Greca, 2004).

Data from investigations attempting to explain better the longitudinal association between peer rejection and externalizing symptoms seem to fit a transactional model best; however, these data are still emerging. Compared to the number of studies examining the effects of peer rejection, few have simultaneously considered peer rejection as a competing or interacting predictor of externalizing symptoms. This has been a notable issue given the importance of peer aggression as a possible "third variable" that should be considered to determine the potential unique effects of peer rejection. Notably, most studies that do so have examined peer aggression using sociometric assessments, thus yielding a measure of youths' *reputations* of peer aggression.

Early studies assessing both peer rejection and aggression examined only incidental or causal models of externalizing symptoms; these investigations initially offered mixed results. Kupersmidt and Coie (1990) revealed that peer-reported aggressive behavior, but not peer rejection, was associated significantly with adolescent-reported externalizing outcomes 7 years later. Kupersmidt and Patterson (1991) revealed a similar pattern of results in a different sample of younger children assessed over 2 years (see also Coie et al., 1992, 1995). However, several contrasting studies suggest that peer rejection remains uniquely associated with externalizing symptoms after researchers controlled for peer aggression as a competing predictor (e.g., Dodge et al., 2003). The unique effects of peer rejection may be particularly evident when externalizing symptoms are assessed with the use of external reporters (i.e., parents, teachers; Coie et al., 1992, 1995).

Transactional theories propose that the nature of associations among peer rejection, peer aggression, and later externalizing symptoms may not be as simplistic as suggested in either the incidental or causal models (Rubin et al., 2006). Support for a transactional model is provided by findings that indicate reciprocal associations between peer rejection and peer aggression. Youth aggression may be triggered by social experiences (e.g., victimization or exclusion by others); simultaneously, aggressive behavior can alter subsequent social experiences by eliciting aversive responses or distorted expectations from others (Dodge et al., 2003). Thus, peer rejection and aggression are mutually reinforced and may subsequently delay developmental competencies more pervasively than either of these characteristics alone (Cillessen et al., 1992). Perhaps for this reason the stability of peer rejection is greater among aggressive than among nonaggressive youth (Cillessen et al., 1992). Researchers have suggested that the combination of peer rejection and aggression may be especially predictive of global social dysfunction, distorted cognitive biases, or inappropriate emotional expression and regulation, thus conferring unique and potent risks for psychopathology (Bierman & Wargo, 1995).

Past studies of a transactional model have considered the conjoint effects of peer rejection and peer aggression on later externalizing symptoms in one of two ways. Some researchers have examined this hypothesis by identifying subgroups of rejected youth who also are nominated as aggressive by their peers. Other investigations have statistically tested peer rejection as a moderator of the longitudinal association between peer aggression and later externalizing symptoms. With a few exceptions, many studies using both approaches have revealed that the conjoint effects of peer rejection and peer aggression are especially potent predictors of later externalizing symptoms (Bierman & Wargo, 1995; Dodge et al., 2003; French et al., 1995; Lochman & Wayland, 1994; Prinstein & La Greca, 2004). For example, Bierman and Wargo (1995) revealed that compared to rejected–nonaggressive or nonrejected–aggressive youth, rejected–aggressive boys exhibited the highest risks for later externalizing symptoms. Coie and colleagues (1995) demonstrated that, compared to others, rejected–aggressive boys had the steepest increasing trajectories of self-reported externalizing problems beginning in the third grade, and consistent levels of elevated parent-reported behavior problems beginning in the sixth grade for over 4 years. Additionally, Lochman and Wayland (1994) revealed that peer rejection moderated the association between aggressive behavior and externalizing symptoms 4 years later.

Another issue regarding the prediction of externalizing symptoms from peer reputations pertains to a predominant focus in past research on *boys'* development. Given substantial gender differences in the prevalence of many externalizing symptoms, this past research emphasis has offered an important opportunity to examine predictors of behaviors that are of high public health priority. However, recent data regarding sharply increasing levels of externalizing behaviors among young females have prompted greater attention to gender diversity.

Two types of studies have been conducted on girls' peer reputations and externalizing symptoms. First, some investigations have examined the prediction of externalizing symptoms using similar measures to those described earlier in investigations of boys' outcomes. Results have been somewhat consistent with work on boys' peer reputations. Findings have supported peer rejection as a unique longitudinal predictor of parent-reported externalizing symptoms (Coie et al., 1995) and self-reported externalizing symptoms (Kupersmidt & Patterson, 1991). Other findings have suggested that peer rejection is an incidental predictor of externalizing symptoms, with peer aggression more strongly predicting girls' outcomes (Miller-Johnson, Coie, et al., 1999). There also is significant support for peer rejection as a moderator of the longitudinal association between girls' peer aggression and parent-reported externalizing symptoms 6 years later (Prinstein & La Greca, 2004).

Second, recent work has revealed a set of aggressive behaviors that may be more common among girls than the types of overt and physically violent behaviors assessed in prior work on boys (Crick & Grotpeter, 1995; Galen & Underwood, 1997; Lagerspetz, Bjorkqvist, & Peltonen, 1988). Studies of peer reputations and later externalizing behaviors sometimes have focused specifically on the prediction of "social aggression" or "relational aggression." Unlike physical forms of aggression, social and relational forms of aggression utilize one's social reputation or an interpersonal relationship as a target for harm (through gossip, social exclusion, withdrawal of friendship support, etc.). As with the prediction of overt and physical externalizing symptoms among boys, emerging evidence suggests that peer rejection is a significant predictor of social and relational aggression. Werner and Crick (2004) revealed that peer rejection among children was associated with higher levels of girls' relational aggression 1 year later. Among adolescents, Prinstein and Cillessen (2003) revealed that peer rejection predicted increases in both girls' and boys' social and relational forms of aggression 17 months later (see also Sandstrom & Cillessen, 2006). Interestingly, no known studies have examined transactional models of the association between peer rejection and social/relational forms of aggression among girls.

Thus, there is substantial evidence to indicate that youth who are disliked by their peers may be at increased risk for later externalizing behaviors, including either overt/physical aggression, illegal behavior, delinquency, and disruptive behavior disorder diagnoses (among boys) or social and relational forms of aggression (among young girls and adolescents). The evidence suggests that peer rejection may change the nature of the association between early aggressive behavior among peers and later symptoms of externalizing psychopathology. The experience of being disliked by ones' peers appears to present unique risks, perhaps by exacerbating the cognitive, emotional, and/or social deficits that accompany aggressive behavior. As discussed below, the effects of peer rejection may be especially relevant for predicting later externalizing symptoms; other peer status reputations are not associated with adjustment in a similar manner.

Indeed, yet another issue regarding peer reputation as a predictor of externalizing symptoms pertains to recent research suggesting a different pattern of results for the adjustment correlates of peer-perceived popularity. As previously noted, although preference-based sociometric popularity and reputation-based peer-perceived popularity are moderately correlated, substantial evidence suggests that aggressive youth may be regarded as highly popular among their peers. Much of the work suggesting this association has been cross-sectional. For example, Rodkin, Farmer, Pearl, and Van Acker (2000) revealed a group of aggressive youth who were nominated by teachers as popular among peers. Moderate, positive associations between aggressive behavior and peer-perceived popularity also have been reported in studies using other methodologies, including peer-reported measures (Prinstein & Cillessen, 2003; Rose, Swenson, & Waller, 2004). Peer-perceived popularity has been conceived of as a measure of youths' positions of dominance, social influence, and access to resources; thus, consistent with studies in human and animal ethology, this measure of status should be associated with aggressive behavior.

Of particular note are findings from longitudinal studies that explore whether peer-perceived popularity may be associated with increases in aggressive behavior over time, after accounting for previous levels of aggression. Several studies now support this longitudinal effect. Higher levels of peer-perceived popularity are associated with increases in both overt/physical and social/relational aggressive behavior. This effect appears to be consistent for youth in middle childhood (Cillessen & Mayeux, 2004; Sandstrom & Cillessen, 2006), as well as adolescents (Prinstein & Cillessen, 2003; Rose et al., 2004). There is some evidence for a more complex association between peer-perceived popularity and externalizing outcomes, however. Considering the heterogeneity of different forms and functions of aggressive behavior, Prinstein and Cillessen (2003) hypothesized that adolescents at risk for aggressive behavior may include those with either low or high levels of reputation-based popularity. Analysis of curvilinear effects supported this idea. Results suggested that adolescents who were either perceived by peers as unpopular or as highly popular were more relationally aggressive than others. Additional results suggested that unpopular adolescents who act aggressively may do so impulsively, in response to frustration or anger (i.e., "reactive aggression"; Dollard et al., 1939), whereas popular adolescents may be more likely to engage in aggression as a strategic, planful, and goal-oriented strategy (i.e., "proactive aggression"; Dodge & Coie, 1987).

In addition to studies that have examined whether peer reputations may be associated with later externalizing symptoms, a body of research has examined possible mechanisms that may explain this association. Two theories have received substantial support. First, as noted earlier, social-cognitive theories have suggested that peer rejection may confer risks for various social information-processing biases that ultimately contribute to the development of externalizing diagnoses. Investigations of rejected and rejected–aggressive children's cue interpretations have offered good support for this hypothesis. Rejected and aggressive children appear to be especially likely to interpret ambiguous cues as hostile in nature (i.e., a hostile attribution bias; Dodge et al., 2003). This hostile attribution bias is significantly associated with a tendency to generate aggressive solutions to hypothetical provocation dilemmas and to behave aggressively toward peers (Dodge et al., 1990). Moreover, a hostile attribution bias is associated with a greater risk for continued and persistent aggressive behavior across development (Dodge, Pettit, Bates, & Valente, 1995). A longitudinal study offers compelling evidence that these social information-processing mechanisms appear to mediate the longitudinal association between peer rejection and later aggressive behavior (Dodge et al., 2003).

A second theory suggests that deviant peer-group affiliation may mediate the association between peer rejection and later externalizing behaviors. It has been suggested that peer rejection deprives children of an opportunity to participate in normative social activities that are essential for adaptive social development. Rejected children develop inadequate social skills, which, in combination with school failure and poor parental management, may be especially predictive of affiliation with deviant peers (e.g., Dishion, Patterson, & Griesler, 1994). Substantial research suggests that affiliation with deviant peers is strongly associated with the onset, maintenance, and exacerbation of antisocial behavior (for a review, see Prinstein & Dodge, 2008).

Although research with clinical populations of diagnosed youth are relatively rare, several findings support these theoretical mechanisms of the association between peer rejection and externalizing symptoms. For instance, children with disruptive behavior disorders, such as conduct disorder or attention-deficit/hyperactivity disorder (ADHD), often display large deficits in social functioning; indeed, social difficulties are often considered integral to the psychopathology of these disorders (e.g., Whalen & Henker, 1992). Children with ADHD are particularly likely to be rejected by peers. Given that many of the behavioral symptoms most associated with ADHD (talking and fidgeting excessively, impulse control problems, inattention, etc.) are socially aversive, and that children with ADHD tend to be aggressive, links with peer rejection are not entirely surprising. Erhardt and Hinshaw (1994) found that after only 3 days of interacting with previously unfamiliar peers at summer camp, children with ADHD earned lower liking ratings and were overwhelmingly more rejected than campers without ADHD. Aggression and disruptiveness, two major behavioral features of ADHD, were the strongest predictors of negative peer status across both groups. In another study utilizing peer sociometric methods, Hoza and colleagues (2005) found that a disproportionate number of boys and girls with ADHD were rejected by age- and sex-matched peers.

Children with ADHD also demonstrate certain social-cognitive deficits, including both cue encoding and cue interpretation biases. Indeed, despite their low sociometric status and probable experience of peer rejection, children with ADHD tend to perceive their own social acceptance as no worse than that of controls (Hoza, Pelham, Milich, Pillow, & McBridge, 1993), or even see their social performance as more favorable (Hoza, Waschbusch, Pelham, Molina, & Milich, 2000).

In summary, substantial research suggests that peer rejection is a particularly potent and potentially long-term predictor of externalizing symptoms, especially when combined with the effects of peer aggression. This finding has been remarkably consistent across studies using a variety of methodological designs, participant populations, and measures to assess externalizing outcomes. Studies largely support a transactional model, suggesting that reciprocal, longitudinal associations between peer rejection and aggression contribute to externalizing symptoms. The effects of these transactions on psychopathology likely are mediated by the conjoint effects of peer rejection and reputations of aggression in youth on both the development of specific social-cognitive skills (i.e., social information processing) and social environments (i.e., deviant peer-group affiliation).

Prediction of Health Risk Behaviors

As with the prediction of externalizing symptoms, studies from follow-forward longitudinal investigations indicate that childhood peer rejection is associated with later substance use. Again, this effect appears to be consistent regardless of when peer rejection is measured in the developmental process. Research by Dishion and colleagues suggests that peer rejection at age 9 years is longitudinally associated with adolescent boys' use of nicotine, alcohol, and marijuana (Dishion, Capaldi, Spracklen, & Li, 1995; Dishion, Capaldi, & Yoerger, 1999). Aloise-Young and Kaeppner (2005) revealed that rejected youth are at increased risk for the onset of cigarette use during the transition to adolescence, though not for the lifetime progression of cigarette use. Zettergren, Bergman, and Wangby (2006) have offered evidence to suggest that children rejected at ages 10–13 years are eight times more likely than sociometrically average children to abuse alcohol as young adults, up to 10 years later. However, whereas some studies have failed to find significant associations between peer rejection and later substance use (e.g., Lochman & Wayland, 1994), others have suggested that high levels of social preference may be associated with increased risk for minor delinquency, and alcohol and substance abuse (Allen, Porter, McFarland, Marsh, & McElhaney, 2005).

Consistent with a transactional model, there also is evidence to suggest that the conjoint effects of rejection and aggression may be especially strongly associated with later substance use. French and colleagues (1995) revealed that "rejected–antisocial" eighth-grade students were more likely to use tobacco and alcohol 2 years later compared to rejected–nonantisocial or peer-accepted students. Prinstein and La Greca (2004) revealed that peer rejection in grades 4–6 moderated the association of peer aggression and girls' substance use 6 years later. Among girls with low social preference scores (i.e., peer rejection), peer aggression was significantly associated with heavy episodic drinking, marijuana, and "hard" drug use; however, among girls with high social preference scores, peer aggression was not a significant predictor of later substance use.

Notably, the examination of substance use outcomes has offered several findings to suggest that youth with somewhat favorable peer reputations also may be at risk for future substance use. This finding has been demonstrated in two ways. Studies of sociometric popularity have suggested that in addition to the risk of peer rejection, sociometric controversial status predicts cigarette use (Aloise-Young & Kaeppner, 2005). Feldman and colleagues revealed that, independent of the effect of peer rejection, peer acceptance in sixth grade was longitudinally associated with boys' alcohol use 4 years later (Feldman, Rosenthal, Brown, & Canning, 1995). The effects of positive peer reputations on substance use outcomes also have been suggested by recent work on peer-perceived popularity. Although longitudinal studies of peer-perceived popularity are rare, results have suggested strong concurrent associations between reputation-based popularity and substance use (e.g., Engels, Scholte, van Lieshout, de Kemp, & Overbeek, 2006).

Both peer rejection and high peer status may be relevant as predictors of sexual risk behaviors. Underwood, Kupersmidt, and Coie (1996) reported that sociometrically controversial girls and aggressive girls were more likely to give birth in adolescence, had experienced more births than other adolescent mothers, and had given birth to their first child at earlier ages compared to other adolescent mothers. Examining peer status and aggression separately, Miller-Johnson and colleagues replicated these results only for childhood aggression; no significant effects were revealed for peer status (Miller-Johnson, Winn, et al., 1999; see also Feldman et al., 1995; Prinstein & La Greca, 2004). The associations of peer reputations and sexual behaviors may depend greatly on the extent of adolescents' engagement in behaviors perceived as risky. For instance, Prinstein, Meade, and Cohen (2003) found that, compared to sexually inactive adolescents, adolescents who report engagement in oral sex or sexual intercourse received far more nominations of peer-perceived popularity. However, among adolescents who engaged in sexual behavior, peer-perceived popularity was negatively associated with the number of adolescents' sexual partners.

Given the potentially important role of peer socialization in the development of health-risk behaviors, it is unfortunate that so few studies have examined peer reputations as predictors of other health-related outcomes. Some research suggests that this may indeed be a fruitful line of inquiry. For example, strong concurrent effects have been revealed for the association between peer reputation and weight-related behaviors. Lieberman, Gauvin, Bukowski, and White (2001) found that higher levels of girls' friendships nominations from peers (i.e., a possible proxy for peer acceptance) were associated with lower levels of body self-esteem and higher levels of dieting and bulimic behavior. Recently, Wang, Houshyar, and Prinstein (2006) found that lower levels of peer-perceived popularity were associated with boys' self-reports of thin and heavy body shapes, whereas higher levels of popularity were associated with boys' self-reports of muscular body shapes. Lower levels of peer-perceived popularity also were associated with girls' reports of both heavy body shapes and lower levels of dieting behavior.

A possible explanation for this association between peer status and later health-risk behaviors (i.e., substance abuse, risky sexual behavior, weight-related behaviors) is the impact of deviant peer affiliation. Research suggests that people generally choose to be friends with those who are like themselves (e.g., Rubin et al., 2006). As previously noted, peer status is predictive of later engagement in health-risk behaviors. Moreover, adolescents select friends of not only similar peer status (e.g., Drewry & Clark, 1985) but also similar risky behaviors (e.g., Hamm, 2000). Illustrating this progression is a longitudinal study by Patterson, Dishion, and Yoerger (2000) demonstrating that early involvement with deviant peers at age 10 was associated with increases in new forms of risk behavior at age 14. Thus, although peer status may contribute uniquely to participation in later health-risk behaviors, these behaviors are likely maintained through deviant peer selection and affiliation (see Dishion & Piehler, Chapter 32, this volume).

Prediction of Internalizing Symptoms

Studies examining associations between peer reputations and internalizing symptoms have offered decidedly mixed results, perhaps due to marked variability in the types of outcomes assessed and the method used to measure internalizing symptoms. Most studies in this area have examined sociometric peer status as a predictor of internalizing outcomes; few data are available to understand the possible role of peer-perceived popularity as a predictor of internalizing symptoms. Also, relatively few studies in this area have examined incidental, causal, or transactional models for predicting internalizing symptoms. In research that has examined possible moderators of the association between peer rejection and internalizing symptoms, there has been some exploration of other subtypes of rejected children. For example, it has been hypothesized that peer rejection may moderate the association between withdrawal/submissiveness and later internalizing symptoms.

Studies that have examined the prediction of internalizing symptoms as a broad domain of psychopathology (e.g., from an overall symptom checklist) generally have found that peer rejection is associated with later internalizing psychological symptoms (e.g., Hoza, Molina, Bukowski, & Sippola, 1995; Lochman & Wayland, 1994). In some instances, a combination of peer rejection and aggression (e.g., Coie et al., 1992), or a combination of peer rejection and reputations of withdrawal (Bell-Dolan, Foster, & Christopher, 1995) was associated with increases in internalizing symptoms over time. There also has been evidence to suggest that chronically rejected boys may be especially susceptible to internalizing difficulties (Burks, Dodge, & Price, 1995). Although this research offers an excellent opportunity to determine potential risk, a lack of specificity in the outcomes assessed presents some difficulty in contributing to theoretical models of specific psychological symptoms or the development of symptom-tailored psychosocial treatments.

In studies examining specific outcomes, the most robust findings have pertained to the prediction of loneliness. Although loneliness is not specifically an internalizing disorder in itself, it is a symptom of mood disorders and an especially important predictor of suicidality, particularly in adolescence (American Psychiatric Association, 2000). Peer rejection in early childhood (Ladd & Burgess, 1999), school-age years (Hymel, Rubin, Rowden, & LeMare, 1990) and at the adolescent transition (Boivin, Hymel, & Bukowski, 1995) is associated with loneliness up to 3 years later.

Results are somewhat mixed when other specific types of internalizing symptoms are examined. This is especially true for the prediction of depressive symptoms. Several studies have revealed that peer rejection is associated longitudinally with increasing levels of depressive symptoms (e.g., Kistner, Balthazor, Risi, & Burton, 1999; Panak & Garber, 1992; Vernberg, 1990), or that the combination of peer rejection and a reputation for aggression is associated with depression (Haselager, Cillessen, van Lieshout, Riksen-Walraven, & Hartup, 2002; French et al., 1995). Research has suggested that peer exclusion (i.e., a close correlate of peer rejection) also may moderate the association between anxious solitude and later depressive symptoms (e.g., Gazelle & Ladd, 2003).

More recent research suggests that the link between peer rejection and depressive symptoms may be best understood through the integration of work on cognitive theories of depression. For instance, consistent with a social information-processing model, encoding of peer rejection experiences by youth may be critical to internalizing outcomes. Several studies have suggested that youth perceptions of rejection by peers are more proximal longitudinal predictors of depression (e.g., Kistner et al., 1999) and may mediate the association between actual peer rejection and later depressive symptoms (Panak & Garber, 1992).

This model offers an interesting contrast to the association between peer rejection and externalizing symptoms. Findings have suggested that when compared with peer reports, aggressive children, as well as those with ADHD, overestimate their levels of peer acceptance and social competence, and underestimate their level of peer rejection (e.g., De Los Reyes & Prinstein, 2004; Hoza et al., 1993). Overestimation of their peer status contributes to misinterpretations of social events by youth and inappropriate behavioral responses that further exacerbate peer rejection and increase risk for future externalizing symptoms. In contrast, some youth appear to underestimate their peer status, perceiving far greater levels of rejection than measures of actual status suggest (Cillessen & Bellmore, 1999; Kistner et al., 1999). The discrepancy between actual and perceived youth peer status may be longitudinally predictive of increases in depression over time (Cillessen & Bellmore, 1999).

A second cognitive model relevant for understanding the link between peer rejection and depression in youth pertains to interpretations of stressful experiences. Cognitive vulnerability models of depression suggest that a tendency to interpret negative life events as due to internal, global, and stable causes (and positive events to external, unstable, and specific causes) may be associated with depression risk when combined with a stressful experience (Abramson, Metalsky, & Alloy, 1989). Peer rejection may be a relevant stressful experience that elicits variable cognitive interpretations. The interaction between a depressogenic attributional style and peer-nominated rejection is longitudinally associated with increases in depressive symptoms among both children (Panak & Garber, 1992) and adolescents (Prinstein & Aikins, 2004).

Social goals of youth within the peer context also may be relevant for understanding the risk for depressive symptoms. It may be that one buffer against the deleterious effects of peer rejection is a low level of importance ascribed to peer popularity. Thus, it may be that a youth's actual level of peer status is relevant for understanding depression, but especially if actual status is discrepant from an ideal or desired level of peer status (Kupersmidt, Buchele, Voegler, & Sedikides, 1996). For example, in a longitudinal study, Prinstein and

Aikins (2004) found that adolescents who were both rejected by peers and placed a high level of importance on their level of peer status (i.e., a condition that would produce cognitive dissonance) were at greatest risk for increases in depressive symptoms.

Interpersonal theories of depression propose reciprocal associations between problematic social experiences and depressive symptoms. Substantial evidence suggests that depressive symptoms in youth also are associated with increases in problematic peer relations. Although much of this work has pertained to the effects of depression on dyadic peer friendships (e.g., Borelli & Prinstein, 2006; Prinstein, Borelli, Cheah, Simon, & Aikins, 2005), some evidence indicates that depression also is associated with decreases in peer status. Kennedy, Spence, and Hensley (1989) reported that depressed primary school-age children received lower ratings of peer popularity, were more likely to receive negative sociometric nominations, and were less likely to receive positive sociometric nominations compared to nondepressed children. Evidence that peer rejection may occur in reaction to child depressive symptoms is provided by a video-based study conducted by Peterson, Mullins, and Ridley-Johnson (1985), in which children in grades 3–6 rated seemingly depressed peers as less attractive and less likable than nondepressed children.

A bidirectional model for understanding the association between peer status and psychological symptoms also is relevant for the study of anxiety symptom outcomes. Some research suggests that peer rejection may be associated with later anxiety or social anxiety symptoms (Vernberg, Abwender, Ewell, & Beery, 1992). However, the majority of research in this area has offered evidence for specific transactions between youth behavior, peer reputations, and psychological symptoms. Socially withdrawn youth appear to be at risk for later internalizing symptoms, such as loneliness, low self-worth, and anxiety (Rubin, Chen, McDougall, Bowker, & McKinnon, 1995; Rubin, Bowker, & Kennedy, Chapter 17, this volume). However, it may be that peer rejection contributes to this association, because peer rejection is both a predictor and a consequence of social withdrawal (Hymel et al., 1990). A combination of peer rejection and submissiveness or withdrawal appears to be particularly associated with later anxiety symptoms.

Future Directions

Much research suggests that peer rejection may exert a direct effect on later psychological adjustment, or may transact with other behavioral difficulties (e.g., aggression, withdrawal) to produce risk for psychopathology. Future research more fully examining the nature of these transactions, and possible theoretical mechanisms (e.g., social-cognitive skills), will be especially important to develop long-term preventions and interventions. Moreover, greater attention to developmental issues, including age, gender, ethnicity, and the specific context in which peer interactions occur, will be important to fully understand the processes that render peer experiences so important for adjustment. Last, emerging work on unique peer reputations (e.g., peer-perceived popularity) suggests that untapped dimensions of peer experiences may more fully elucidate the important role of peer relationships. Recent research suggests that such investigations will offer a much needed opportunity to integrate developmental and clinical psychology theories and methods with those from other psychological subdisciplines and other social sciences to examine best the manner in which relationships with contemporaries has a profound effect on the development of mental health.

References

Abramson, L. Y., Metalsky, G. I., & Alloy, L. B. (1989). Hopelessness depression: A theory-based subtype of depression. *Psychological Review, 96*, 358–372.

Allen, J. P., Porter, M. R., McFarland, F. C., Marsh, P., & McElhaney, K. B. (2005). The two faces of adolescents' success with peers: Adolescent popularity, social adaptation, and deviant behavior. *Child Development, 3*, 747–760.

Aloise-Young, P. A., & Kaeppner, C. J. (2005). Sociometric status as a predictor of onset and progression in adolescent cigarette smoking. *Nicotine and Tobacco Research, 7*, 199–206.

American Psychiatric Association. (2000). *Diagnostic and statistical manual of mental disorders* (4th ed., text rev.). Washington, DC: Author.

Bagwell, C. L., Newcomb, A. F., & Bukowski, W. M. (1998). Preadolescent friendship and peer rejection as predictors of adult adjustment. *Child Development, 69*, 140–153.

Bell-Dolan, D. J., Foster, S. L., & Christopher, J. S. (1995). Girls' peer relations and internalizing problems: Are socially neglected, rejected, and withdrawn girls at risk? *Journal of Clinical Child Psychology, 24*, 463–473.

Bierman, K. L., & Wargo, J. B. (1995). Predicting the longitudinal course associated with aggressive-rejected, aggressive (nonrejected), and rejected (nonaggressive) status. *Development and Psychopathology, 7*, 669–682.

Boivin, M., Hymel, S., & Bukowski, W. M. (1995). The roles of social withdrawal, peer rejection, and victimization by peers in predicting loneliness and depressed mood in children. *Development and Psychopathology, 7*, 765–785.

Borelli, J. L., & Prinstein, M. J. (2006). Reciprocal, longitudinal associations among adolescents' negative feedback-seeking, depressive symptoms, and peer relations. *Journal of Abnormal Child Psychology, 34*, 159–169.

Bower, E. M. (1969). *Early identification of emotionally handicapped children in school* (2nd ed.). Springfield, IL: Thomas.

Burks, V. S., Dodge, K. A., & Price, J. M. (1995). Models of internalizing outcomes of early rejection. *Development and Psychopathology, 7*, 683–695.

Cillessen, A. H. N., & Bellmore, A. D. (1999). Accuracy of social self-perceptions and peer competence in middle childhood. *Merrill–Palmer Quarterly, 45*, 650–676.

Cillessen, A. H. N., & Mayeux, L. (2004). From censure to reinforcement: Developmental changes in the association between aggression and social status. *Child Development, 75*, 147–163.

Cillessen, A. H. N., van IJzendoorn, H. W., van Lieshout, C. F., & Hartup, W. W. (1992). Heterogeneity among peer-rejected boys: Subtypes stabilities. *Child Development, 63*, 893–905.

Coie, J. D., & Dodge, K. A. (1983). Continuities and changes in children's social status: A five-year longitudinal study. *Merrill–Palmer Quarterly, 29*, 261–282.

Coie, J. D., & Kupersmidt, J. B. (1983). A behavioral analysis of emerging social status in boys' groups. *Child Development, 54*, 1400–1416.

Coie, J. D., Lochman, J. E., Terry, R., & Hyman, C. (1992). Predicting early adolescent disorder from childhood aggression and peer rejection. *Journal of Consulting and Clinical Psychology, 60*, 783–792.

Coie, J. D., Terry, R., Lenox, K., Lochman, J., & Hyman, C. (1995). Childhood peer rejection and aggression as predictors of stable patterns of adolescent disorder. *Development and Psychopathology, 7*, 697–714.

Connolly, J. A., & Johnson, A. M. (1996). Adolescents' romantic relationships and the structure and quality of their close interpersonal ties. *Personal Relationships, 3*, 185–195.

Cowen, E. L., Pedersen, A., Bagigian, H., Izzo, L. D., & Trost, M. A. (1973). Long-term follow-up of early vulnerable children. *Journal of Consulting and Clinical Psychology, 41*, 438–446.

Crick, N. R., & Dodge, K. A. (1994). A review and reformulation of social information-processing mechanisms in children's social adjustment. *Psychological Bulletin, 115*, 74–101.

Crick, N. R., & Dodge, K. A. (1996). Social information-processing mechanisms on reactive and proactive aggression. *Child Development, 67*, 993–1002.

Crick, N. R., & Grotpeter, J. K. (1995). Relational aggression, gender, and social-psychological adjustment. *Child Development, 66*, 710–722.

De Los Reyes, A., & Prinstein, M. J. (2004). Applying depression–distortion hypotheses to the assessment of peer victimization in adolescents. *Journal of Clinical Child and Adolescent Psychology, 33*, 325–335.

Dishion, T. J., Capaldi, D., Spracklen, K. M., & Li, F. (1995). Peer ecology of male adolescent drug use. *Development and Psychopathology, 7*, 803–824.

Dishion, T. J., Capaldi, D. M., & Yoerger, K. (1999). Middle childhood antecedents to progressions in male adolescent substance use: An ecological analysis of risk and protection. *Journal of Adolescent Research, 14*, 175–205.

Dishion, T. J., Patterson, G. R., & Griesler, P. C. (1994). Peer adaptations in the development of antisocial behavior: A confluence model. In L. R. Huesmann (Ed.), *Aggressive behavior: Current perspectives* (pp. 61–95). New York: Plenum Press.

Dodge, K. A. (1983). Behavioral antecedents of peer social status. *Child Development, 54*, 1386–1399.

Dodge, K. A., Bates, J. E., & Pettit, G. S. (1990). Mechanisms in the cycle of violence. *Science, 250*, 1678–1683.

Dodge, K. A., & Coie, J. D. (1987). Social information-processing factors in reactive and proactive aggression in children's peer groups. *Journal of Personality and Social Psychology, 53*, 1146–1158.

Dodge, K. A., Lansford, J. E., Burks, V. S., Bates, J. E., Pettit, G. S., Fontaine, R., et al. (2003). Peer rejection and social information-processing factors in the development of aggressive behavior problems in children. *Child Development, 74*, 374–393.

Dodge, K. A., Pettit, G. S., Bates, J. E., & Valente, E. (1995). Social information-processing patterns partially mediate the effect of early physical abuse on later conduct problems. *Journal of Abnormal Psychology, 104*, 632–643.

Dollard, J., Doob, L. W., Miller, N. E., Mowrer, O. H., Sears, R. R., Ford, C. S., et al. (1939). *Frustration and aggression*. Oxford: Yale University Press.

Drewry, D. L., & Clark, M. L. (1985). Factors important in the formation of preschoolers' friendships. *Journal of Genetic Psychology, 146*, 37–44.

Engels, R. C. M. E., Scholte, R. H. J., van Lieshout, C. F. M., de Kemp, R., & Overbeek, G. (2006). Peer group reputation and smoking and alcohol consumption in early adolescence. *Addictive Behaviors, 31*, 440–449.

Erhardt, D., & Hinshaw, S. P. (1994). Initial sociometric impressions of attention-deficit hyperactivity disorder and comparison boys: Predictors from social behaviors and from nonverbal variables. *Journal of Consulting and Clinical Psychology, 62*, 833–842.

Feldman, S. S., Rosenthal, D. R., Brown, N. L., & Canning, R. D. (1995). Predicting sexual experience in adolescent boys from peer rejection and acceptance during childhood. *Journal of Research on Adolescence, 5*, 387–411.

Fergusson, D. M., Woodward, L. J., & Horwood, L. J. (1999). Childhood peer relationship problems and young people's involvement with deviant peers in adolescence. *Journal of Abnormal Child Psychology, 27*(5), 357–369.

French, D. C., Conrad, J., & Turner, T. M. (1995). Adjustment of antisocial and nonantisocial rejected adolescents. *Development and Psychopathology, 7*, 857–874.

Galen, B. R., & Underwood, M. K. (1997). A developmental investigation of social aggression among children. *Developmental Psychology, 33*, 589–600.

Gazelle, H., & Ladd, G. W. (2003). Anxious solitude and peer exclusion: A diathesis–stress model of internalizing trajectories in childhood. *Child Development, 74*, 257–278.

Hamm, J. V. (2000). Do birds of a feather flock together?: The variation bases for African American,

Asian American, and European American adolescents' selection of similar friends. *Developmental Psychology, 36*, 209–219.

Hankin, B. L., & Abramson, L. Y. (2001). Development of gender differences in depression: An elaborated cognitive vulnerability–transactional theory. *Psychological Bulletin, 127*, 773–796.

Haselager, G. J. T., Cillessen, A. H. N., van Lieshout, C. F. M., Riksen-Walraven, J. M. A, & Hartup, W. W. (2002). Heterogeneity among peer-rejected boys across middle childhood: Developmental pathways of social behavior. *Developmental Psychology, 38*, 446–456.

Hoza, B., Molina, B., Bukowski, W. M., & Sippola, L. K. (1995). Aggression, withdrawal and measures of popularity and friendship as predictors of internalizing and externalizing problems during early adolescence. *Development and Psychopathology, 7*, 787–802.

Hoza, B., Mrug, S., Gerdes, A. C., Hinshaw, S. P., Bukowski, W. M., Gold, J. A., et al. (2005). What aspects of peer relationships are impaired in children with attention-deficit/hyperactivity disorder? *Journal of Consulting and Clinical Psychology, 73*(3), 411–423.

Hoza, B., Pelham, W. E., Milich, R., Pillow, D., & McBride, K. (1993). The self-perceptions and attributions of attention deficit hyperactivity disordered and nonreferred boys. *Journal of Abnormal Child Psychology, 21*, 271–286.

Hoza, B., Waschbusch, D. A., Pelham, W. E., Molina, B. S. G., & Milich, R. (2000). Attention-deficit/ hyperactivity disordered and control boys' responses to social success and failure. *Child Development, 72*(2), 432–446.

Hymel, S., Rubin, K. H., Rowden, L., & LeMare, L. (1990). Children's peer relationships: Longitudinal prediction of internalizing and externalizing problems from middle to late childhood. *Child Development, 61*, 2004–2021.

Kennedy, E., Spence, S. H., & Hensley, R. (1989). An examination of the relationship between childhood depression and social competence amongst primary school children. *Journal of Child Psychology and Psychiatry, 30*, 561–573.

Kistner, J., Balthazor, M., Risi, S., & Burton, C. (1999). Predicting dysphoria in adolescence actual and perceived peer acceptance in childhood. *Journal of Clinical Child Psychology, 28*, 94–104.

Kupersmidt, J. B., Buchele, K. S., Voegler, M. E., & Sedikides, C. (1996). Social self-discrepancy: A theory relating peer relations problems and school maladjustment. In J. Juvonen & K. R. Wentzel (Eds.), *Social motivation: Understanding children's school adjustment* (pp. 66–97). New York: Cambridge University Press.

Kupersmidt, J. B., & Coie, J. D. (1990). Preadolescent peer status, aggression, and school adjustment as predictors of externalizing problems in adolescence. *Child Development, 61*, 1350–1362.

Kupersmidt, J. B., & Patterson, C. J. (1991). Childhood peer rejection, aggression, withdrawal, and perceived competence as predictors of self-reported behavior problems in preadolescence. *Journal of Abnormal Child Psychology, 19*, 427–449.

Ladd, G. W., & Burgess, K. B. (1999). Charting the relationship trajectories of aggressive, withdrawn, and aggressive/withdrawn children during early grade school. *Child Development, 70*, 910–929.

Ladd, G. W., & Troop-Gordon, W. (2003). The role of chronic peer difficulties in the development of children's psychological adjustment problems. *Child Development, 74*, 1344–1367.

LaFontana, K. M., & Cillessen, A. H. N. (2002). Children's perceptions of popular and unpopular peers: A multimethod assessment. *Developmental Psychology, 38*, 635–647.

Lagerspetz, K. M., Bjorkqvist, K., & Peltonen, T. (1988). Is indirect aggression typical of females?: Gender differences in aggressiveness in 11- to 12-year-old children. *Aggressive Behavior, 14*, 403–414.

Laird, R. D., Pettit, G. S., Dodge, K. A., & Bates, J. E. (2005). Peer relationship antecedents of delinquent behavior in late adolescence: Is there evidence of demographic group differences in developmental processes? *Development and Psychopathology, 17*, 127–144.

Lewin, L. M., Davis, B., & Hops, H. (1999). Childhood social predictors of adolescent antisocial behavior: Gender differences in predictive accuracy and efficacy. *Journal of Abnormal Child Psychology, 27*, 277–292.

Lieberman, M., Gauvin, L., Bukowski, W. M., & White, D. R. (2001). Interpersonal influence and disordered eating behaviors in adolescent girls: The role of peer modeling, social reinforcement, and body-related teasing. *Eating Behaviors, 2*, 215–236.

Lochman, J. E., & Wayland, K. K. (1994). Aggression, social acceptance, and race as predictors of negative adolescent outcomes. *Journal of the American Academy of Child and Adolescent Psychiatry, 33*, 1026–1035.

Miller-Johnson, S., Coie, J. D., Maumary-Gremaud, A., Lochman, J., & Terry, R. (1999). Relationship between childhood peer rejection and aggression and adolescent delinquency severity and type among African-American youth. *Journal of Emotional and Behavioral Disorders, 7*, 137–146.

Miller-Johnson, S., Winn, D., Coie, J., Maumary-Gremaud, A., Hyman, C., Terry, R., et al. (1999). Motherhood during the teen years: A developmental perspective on risk factors for childbearing. *Development and Psychopathology, 11*, 85–100.

Moffitt, T. E. (1993). Adolescence-limited and life-course-persistent antisocial behavior: A developmental taxonomy. *Psychological Review, 100*(4), 674–701.

Nelson, S. E., & Dishion, T. J. (2004). From boys to men: Predicting adult adaptation from middle childhood sociometric status. *Development and Psychopathology, 16*(2), 441–459.

Ollendick, T. H., Weist, M. D., Borden, M. C., & Greene, R. W. (1992). Sociometric status and academic, behavioral, and psychological adjustment: A five-year longitudinal study. *Journal of Consulting and Clinical Psychology, 60*, 80–87.

Panak, W. F., & Garber, J. (1992). Role of aggression, rejection, and attributions in the prediction of depression in children. *Development and Psychopathology, 4*, 145–165.

Parker, J., Rubin, K. H., Erath, S., Wojslawowicz, J. C., & Buskirk, A. A. (2006). Peer relationships and developmental psychopathology. In D. Cicchetti & D. Cohen (Eds.), *Developmental psychopathology: Risk, disorder, and adaptation* (2nd ed., Vol. 2, pp. 419–493). New York: Wiley.

Parkhurst, J. T., & Hopmeyer, A. (1998). Sociometric popularity and peer-perceived popularity: Two distinct dimensions of peer status. *Journal of Early Adolescence, 18*(2), 125–144.

Patterson, G. R., Dishion, T. J., & Yoerger, K. (2000). Adolescent growth in new forms of problem behavior: Macro- and micro-peer dynamics. *Prevention Science, 1*, 3–13.

Peterson, L., Mullins, L. L., & Ridley-Johnson, R. (1985). Childhood depression: Peer reactions to depression and life stress. *Journal of Abnormal Child Psychology, 13*(4), 597–609.

Prinstein, M. J., & Aikins, J. W. (2004). Cognitive moderators of the longitudinal association between peer rejection and adolescent depressive symptoms. *Journal of Abnormal Child Psychology, 32*, 147–158.

Prinstein, M. J., Borelli, J. L., Cheah, C. S. L., Simon, V. A., & Aikins, J. W. (2005). Adolescent girls' interpersonal vulnerability to depressive symptoms: A longitudinal examination of reassurance-seeking and peer relationships. *Journal of Abnormal Psychology, 114*, 676–688.

Prinstein, M. J., Cheah, C. S. L., & Guyer, A. E. (2005). Peer victimization, cue interpretation, and internalizing symptoms: Concurrent and longitudinal findings for children and adolescents. *Journal of Clinical Child and Adolescent Psychology, 34*, 11–24.

Prinstein, M. J., & Cillessen, A. H. N. (2003). Forms and functions of adolescent peer aggression associated with high levels of peer status. *Merrill–Palmer Quarterly, 49*, 310–342.

Prinstein, M. J., & Dodge, K. A. (Eds.). (2008). *Understanding peer influence in children and adolescents.* New York: Guilford Press.

Prinstein, M. J., & La Greca, A. M. (2004). Childhood peer rejection and aggression as predictors of adolescent girls' externalizing and health risk behaviors: A six year longitudinal study. *Journal of Consulting and Clinical Psychology, 72*, 103–112.

Prinstein, M. J., Meade, C. S., & Cohen, G. L. (2003). Adolescent oral sex, peer popularity, and perceptions of best friend's sexual behavior. *Journal of Pediatric Psychology, 28*, 243–249.

Rabiner, D. L., Coie, J. D., Miller-Johnson, S., Boykin, A. M., & Lochman, J. E. (2005). Predicting the persistence of aggressive offending of African American males from adolescence into young adulthood: The importance of peer relations, aggressive behavior, and ADHD symptoms. *Journal of Emotional and Behavioral Disorders, 13*, 131–140.

Rodkin, P. C., Farmer, T. W., Pearl, R., & Van Acker, R. (2000). Heterogeneity of popular boys: Antisocial and prosocial configurations. *Developmental Psychology, 36*, 14–24.

Roff, M. (1961). Childhood social interactions and young adult bad conduct. *Journal of Abnormal Social Psychology, 63*, 333–337.

Rose, A. J., Swenson, L. P., & Waller, E. M. (2004). Overt and relational aggression and perceived popularity: Developmental differences in concurrent and prospective relations. *Developmental Psychology, 40*, 378–387.

Rubin, K. H., Bukowski, W. M., & Parker, J. G. (2006). Peer interactions, relationships, and groups. In N. Eisenberg, W. Damon, & R. M. Lerner (Eds.), *Handbook of child psychology: Vol. 3. Social, emotional, and personality development* (6th ed., pp. 571–645). Hoboken, NJ: Wiley.

Rubin, K. H., Burgess, K., Kennedy, A. E., & Stewart, S. (2003). Social withdrawal and inhibition in childhood. In E. Mash & R. Barkley (Eds.), *Child psychopathology* (2nd ed., pp. 372–406). New York: Guilford Press.

Rubin, K. H., Chen, X., McDougall, P., Bowker, A., & McKinnon, J. (1995). The Waterloo Longitudinal Project: Predicting internalizing and externalizing problems in adolescence. *Developmental Psychology, 7*, 751–764.

Rubin, K. H., & Rose-Krasnor, L. (1992). Interpersonal problem solving and social competence in children. In V. B. Van Hasselt & M. Hersen (Eds.), *Handbook of social development: A lifespan perspective* (pp. 283–323). New York: Plenum Press.

Sandstrom, M. J., & Cillessen, A. H. (2006). Likeable versus popular: Distinct implications for adolescent adjustment. *International Journal of Behavioral Development, 30*, 305–314.

Sroufe, L. A. (1997). Psychopathology as an outcome of development. *Development and Psychopathology, 9*, 251–268.

Underwood, M. K., Kupersmidt, J. B., & Coie, J. D. (1996). Childhood peer sociometric status and aggression as predictors of adolescent childbearing. *Journal of Research on Adolescence, 6*, 201–223.

Vernberg, E. M. (1990). Psychological adjustment and experiences with peers during early adolescence: Reciprocal, incidental, or unidirectional relationships? *Journal of Abnormal Child Psychology, 18*, 187–198.

Vernberg, E. M., Abwender, D. A., Ewell, K. K., & Beery, S. H. (1992). Social anxiety and peer relationships in early adolescence: A prospective analysis. *Journal of Clinical Child Psychology, 21*, 189–196.

Wang, S. S., Houshyar, S., & Prinstein, M. J. (2006). Adolescent girls' and boys' weight-related health behaviors and cognitions: Associations with reputation- and preference-based peer status. *Health Psychology, 25*, 658–663.

Weiss, B., & Garber, J. (2003). Developmental differences in the phenomenology of depression. *Development and Psychopathology, 15*, 403–430.

Werner, N. E., & Crick, N. R. (2004). Maladaptive peer relationships and the development of relational and physical aggression during middle childhood. *Social Development, 13*, 495–514.

Whalen, C. K., & Henker, B. (1992). The social profile of attention-deficit/hyperactivity disorder: Five fundamental facets. *Child and Adolescent Psychiatric Clinics of North America, 1*, 395–410.

Zettergren, P., Bergman, L. R., & Wangby, M. (2006). Girls' stable peer status and their adulthood adjustment: A longitudinal study from age 10 to age 43. *International Journal of Behavioral Development, 30*, 315–325.

CHAPTER 31

The Role of Friendship
in Child and Adolescent
Psychosocial Development

FRANK VITARO
MICHEL BOIVIN
WILLIAM M. BUKOWSKI

The role played by friendship in child and adolescent psychosocial development has been examined from two contrasting perspectives: the social bonding perspective and the social interaction perspective. The social bonding perspective emphasizes the bright side of friendships and stresses that friends—mostly conventional friends—contribute positively to children's emotional, cognitive, academic, and behavioral functioning. Guided by the ideas of Sullivan and Piaget, researchers who share this social-developmental view mainly examine *friendship participation* and *features of friendship* to understand how and when friendships play a positive role, or fail to do so.

In contrast, the social interaction perspective focuses on friends' characteristics—especially their negative characteristics—to investigate the putative dark side of friendships, particularly with regard to risk taking, antisocial behavior, or internalizing problems. Guided by a social learning framework, this approach examines *friends' behavior styles* and *friends' interactions* to explain how and when friends (especially when they are antisocial or depressed) have a negative impact on children's and adolescents' adjustment.

Throughout this chapter, we attempt to synthesize these two perspectives to form a comprehensive view of the processes through which friendships affect youth development. The fundamental premise of this endeavor is that friendships are generally beneficial for children's psychosocial development, except when friends have adjustment problems or support deviant behaviors, or when friendships are conflictual or of low quality. Under these conditions, friendships may be detrimental to development. The dual role of friendship is examined with respect to its operating mode (i.e., as main effect or as moderator) and its positive or negative impact on children's and adolescents' psychological (i.e., emotional, social-cognitive) and behavioral (i.e., externalizing, internalizing, and prosocial behaviors) adjustment. Finally, three aspects of friendships are examined to understand more fully how and when friendships make a positive or a negative contribution to psychosocial development: friendship participation, friends' characteristics, and features of friendships (see Hartup, 1996, 2005). Accordingly, this chapter is divided into three sections. The first section examines whether friendship participation contributes to psychosocial development directly (i.e., as a main effect), conditionally (i.e., as a moderator), or as part of an indirect pathway (i.e., as a mediator of other factors). The second section centers on friends' characteristics and aims to clarify the conditions under which friendship participation is beneficial or detrimental, as well as the processes that may account for these positive or negative effects. In the third section of the chapter, we turn our attention to the features of friendship that may explain how and when friendships foster positive or negative adjustment, as well as the processes that could account for these effects. Whenever possible, we focus on the results of studies that used a longitudinal or an experimental design (rather than cross-sectional studies), because of their added value with respect to causal inferences.

The Bright and the Dark Side of Friendship Participation

The first step in examining child and adolescent friendships is to establish *whether* the experience of friendship (i.e., friendship participation) does indeed play a role in development. "Friendship participation" is typically defined as having at least one mutual friendship with another child (Bukowski & Hoza, 1989; Parker & Asher, 1993). This dichotomous view of friendship participation was derived from the finding that the number of friends is not linearly related to individual adjustment (e.g., children with no mutual friends report more internalizing symptoms than those with one or more mutual friends, whereas those with more than one mutual friend do not differ from those with one mutual friend on this outcome; Parker & Seal, 1996).

Friendship Participation as a Main Effect

Several studies have shown that the presence of at least one friend is significantly related to later adjustment. However, studies have not always included the appropriate controls to ensure that the role of friendship participation was not spurious. A first set of variables to control is children's initial social-cognitive, behavioral, or emotional characteristics or states, because children who have friends tend to differ from children without friends on these characteristics (Newcomb & Bagwell, 1995). Specifically, controlling for these initial child characteristics ensures that friendship participation is not *incidentally* (or *spuriously*) associated with emotional, social-cognitive, or behavioral outcomes.

A second set of variables to control comprises correlated social experiences: Compared to children lacking friends, friended children may also be exposed to a variety of other experiences due to their personal characteristics. Hence, a third set of variables that is partially correlated with friendship participation and adjustment may account for the association between these two dimensions. One such potentially confounding experience is the degree of social acceptance by the peer group, because low-accepted children are less likely to have friends than average and high-accepted children (Parker & Asher,

1993). Another potentially confounding experience is the degree of embeddedness in a clique or a social network (Cairns, Leung, Buchanan, & Cairns, 1995), given that a majority of children who have friends are also part of larger peer groups (Ennett et al., 2006). Hence, any difference in children's or adolescents' social-cognitive, behavioral, or emotional development could be accounted for by peer status or group membership rather than by friendship per se.

Finally, family and school-related processes that are correlated both with friendship participation and children's or adolescents' development may also operate as a third set of variables (see Doyle & Markiewicz, 1996). Thus, controlling for selection (e.g., children's personal characteristics at the time of friendship formation) and correlated experiences (e.g., peer acceptance at the group level) is mandatory to demonstrate plausibly that friendship participation contributes to adjustment.

Only a few studies have included these controls in examining the main contribution of friendship participation to child and adolescent development. For example, fifth graders who had a stable best friend were found to view themselves more positively and to report fewer depressive feelings in early adulthood than those who were friendless (Bagwell, Newcomb, & Bukowski, 1998). These analyses took into account initial peer acceptance and perceptions of general competence. Interestingly, the benefits of having a friend were found to be specific to emotional well-being, because peer acceptance, but not friendship status, predicted school performance, professional aspiration level, and job performance. A recent longitudinal follow-up of a sample of children ages 6–13 revealed a similar pattern of results (Pedersen, Vitaro, Barker, & Borge, 2007): The number of years without at least one reciprocal friendship predicted loneliness and depressed feelings during early adolescence, even after accounting for personality factors, such as disruptiveness and anxiety, and peer rejection. The number of years without a friend was not, however, predictive of delinquent behaviors.

This general pattern of findings seems to hold over various age ranges. For instance, one study found that a lack of close friends at age 16 predicted depression symptoms at age 22, over and above previous levels of depressed mood (Pelkonen, Marttunen, & Aro, 2003). Another found that the lack of a close friend from grades 1 through 3 predicted feelings of loneliness and anxious–depressed behaviors 1 year later, above and beyond initial levels of these internalizing problems, peer rejection, and peer victimization (Ladd & Troop-Gordon, 2003).

Other data suggest that friendlessness may mediate the association between low popularity and feelings of loneliness and depression (Nangle, Erdley, Newman, Mason, & Carpenter, 2003). In other words, low popularity could create the conditions under which a child lacks friends, an experience that could then impact the child's emotional well-being. Support for this proposition, however, was based on a cross-sectional study, leaving open the question of the direction of association among these variables. The validity of these findings are also challenged by results showing that friendlessness does not mediate the link between peer relation difficulties (i.e., peer rejection and peer victimization) and later internalizing problems (Ladd & Troop-Gordon, 2003). It is more likely that friendlessness and general peer experiences each contribute uniquely (i.e., additively), and perhaps interactively (in a nonlinear fashion), to internalizing difficulties.

In summary, a number of methodologically sound studies have documented a predictive association between friendship participation and emotional well-being across childhood and adolescence. However, this association was not found for externalizing problems, nor for prosocial behavior, although very few studies have examined the latter.

In one such study, the presence of a friend in sixth grade did not predict prosocial behavior (or academic achievement) 2 years later (Wentzel, Barry, & Caldwell, 2004). However, friendlessness was related to emotional distress across the same time interval.

Most of these studies did not examine sex differences with respect to the predictive association between friendship participation and emotional well-being. However, the few studies that did test for sex differences found a stronger association for girls than for boys (e.g., Oldenburg & Kerns, 1997), which may reflect a greater orientation toward, and dependence upon, social relationships in females than in males (Archer & Lloyd, 2002). However, this last finding should be qualified by age, because such sex differences were not found among young school-age children (e.g., Ladd & Troop-Gordon, 2003).

Many processes may underlie the longitudinal association between participation in friendship and later emotional well-being. For instance, it has been suggested that friendlessness could deprive children of the "secure base" that is necessary to create comfort and willingness to explore new environments and to get involved in new social situations (Birch & Ladd, 1996). The lack of such a secure base could in turn generate anxiety and low self-confidence. Friendlessness may also negatively affect children's self-perceptions, which are central to emotional well-being and self-confidence (Ladd & Troop-Gordon, 2003). Finally, friendlessness may also deprive children of the protection against negative social experiences, and the instrumental and emotional support needed to cope with these adverse social circumstances that friends provide. Such support cannot be compensated for completely by relationships with adults (Boivin, Hymel, & Hodges, 2001). It should be noted that these processes are currently mostly speculative and clearly in need of empirical support. Furthermore, it is unclear whether they are generally true or conditional (i.e., applying only under specific circumstances through a moderation process).

Friendship Participation as Moderator

Having at least one close friend is not only beneficial to an individual's well-being but it may also protect against the negative emotional consequences of aversive social experiences. For example, unlike classmates who are rejected by the peer group and have no friends, rejected schoolchildren who have at least one reciprocated friendship do not differ from their more accepted peers in terms of their reported levels of loneliness and depression (Parker & Asher, 1993). The protective effect of friendship participation with respect to the psychological and behavioral problems associated with peer rejection has been observed in very young schoolchildren (Laursen, Bukowski, Aunola, & Nurmi, 2007). In this study, rejected first graders without friends reported an increase in internalizing problems and feelings of isolation over a 1-year period but no change in externalizing problems. In contrast, children with at least one reciprocated friendship experienced a decrease in both internalizing *and* externalizing problems. However, the power of friendship participation to mitigate the long-term consequences of peer rejection on internalizing problems may be limited (Lansford et al., 2007).

Friends may not only protect children against the negative effects of being rejected and excluded from the peer group, but also against actual peer victimization and its negative consequences (Boivin et al., 2001). For example, a study of fourth and fifth graders revealed that having a reciprocal best friend significantly reduced the likelihood of being victimized over a 1-year period (Hodges, Boivin, Vitaro, & Bukowski, 1999). For children with a best friend, the degree of protection afforded by this friend moderated the link between internalizing problems (a risk factor for victimization) and actual victimization experiences. Moreover, children with a best friend who were victimized did not show the increase in internalizing problems experienced by victimized children without a best friend.

Friends may protect against the negative consequences of peer victimization by providing companionship, emotional support, intimacy, and self-validation. Provision of this support could also account for the protective effect of friendship participation with respect to the psychological consequences usually associated with peer rejection or negative experiences within the family (Bolger, Patterson, & Kupersmidt, 1998; Criss, Pettit, Bates, Dodge, & Lapp, 2002; Gauze, Bukowski, Aquan-Assee, & Sippola, 1996).

Overall, available studies suggest that the presence of a friend is an important resource for emotional well-being, at least in the short term. This seems to be true in general (i.e., as main effect), as well as in more specific cases (i.e., as a moderator). However, the role of friendship is likely to vary depending on the children's and friends' characteristics, and the type of outcome considered. For example, disruptive children without friends were found to report less delinquency than disruptive children with disruptive friends (Vitaro, Brendgen, & Wanner, 2005; Vitaro, Tremblay, Kerr, Pagani, & Bukowski, 1997). These findings suggest that *not* having friends may be "protective" for disruptive children, perhaps because not affiliating with other disruptive children would keep them from becoming increasingly involved in delinquent acts. Similarly, rejected children without friends were not only less aggressive but also less likely to increase their aggressive behaviors over time than rejected children who had friends, probably because these friends were aggressive or supportive of aggressive behaviors (Boivin & Vitaro, 1995; Kupersmidt, Burchinal, & Patterson, 1995). Moreover, children and adolescents with disruptive–aggressive friends were found to report elevated levels of depression compared to children and adolescents with conventional friends (Brendgen, Vitaro, & Bukowski, 2000a; Mrug, Hoza, & Bukowski, 2004). Given that having deviant friends was also associated with more delinquent or aggressive behaviors, early adolescents involved in such friendships exhibited, on average, poorer outcomes than their friendless peers. Interestingly, however, children with friends seemed to be buffered from feelings of loneliness regardless of the friends' characteristics.

In summary, two conclusions can be derived from this first section. First, many of the studies that reported a positive "effect" of friendship participation on children's and adolescents' emotional well-being included primarily children with well-adjusted friends. Second, it is not possible to grasp the full contribution of friendship participation without considering the friends' characteristics.

Friends' Characteristics: For Better and Worse

Friends and Externalizing Problems

There is strong empirical evidence to suggest that friends' externalizing problems (e.g., delinquency, drug use, aggression) put children at risk for the acquisition, maintenance, and escalation of similar externalizing behavior problems (Elliott, Huizinga, & Ageton, 1985; Engels, Knibbe, De Vries, Drop, & Van Breukelen, 1999; Patterson, Dishion, & Yoerger, 2000; Scaramella, Conger, Spoth, & Simons, 2002). For example, early involvement with deviant peers (i.e., by age 10 years) predicts growth in antisocial behavior during adolescence (Patterson et al., 2000). Involvement with disruptive friends has also been found to mediate the predictive associations between early disruptiveness and rejection by normative peers, and later violent delinquency (Vitaro, Pedersen, & Brendgen, 2007). There is also evidence that friends can influence children's and adolescents' aggression-related social cognitions and attitudes (Brendgen, Bowen, Rondeau, & Vitaro, 1999).

Results from a limited number of short-term studies suggest that the negative consequences of exposure to deviant friends may already be apparent by early childhood (see Boivin, Vitaro, & Poulin, 2005). To illustrate, one study showed that the amount of time preschoolers spent with aggressive peers predicted an increase in observed and teacher-rated aggressive behavior over a 3-month interval (Snyder, Horsch, & Childs, 1997). Conversely, children who spent minimal time (less than 15%) with aggressive peers showed a decrease in aggression over the subsequent 3-month period. More recently, association with deviant peers in kindergarten was found to predict growth in overt conduct problems (e.g., aggressiveness), as well as covert conduct problems (e.g., lying aznd stealing), on the playground and in the classroom during the following 2 years (Snyder et al., 2005). However, the "influence" of friends' externalizing problems at this young age may be very specific. To illustrate, Lamarche et al. (2007) found that friends' reactive aggression specifically predicted increases in children's reactive aggression, whereas friends' proactive aggression specifically predicted increases in children's proactive aggression from kindergarten to grade 1. No such predictive associations were observed across dimensions.

Correlational versus Experimental Studies

In spite of the abundance of research on the developmental role of friendships, the available evidence is primarily correlational, albeit longitudinal, which limits our ability to draw causal inferences from these findings. Prevention/intervention studies using experimental designs can help to overcome this limitation. For example, affiliation with conventional friends has been found to explain partly the impact of multimodal prevention programs on later violent and delinquent behaviors (Eddy & Chamberlain, 2000; Vitaro, Brendgen, Pagani, Tremblay, & McDuff, 1999). Taken together, these results support the view that friends play a causal role in the development of problem behaviors. However, they do not provide direct proof, because the nature of friendships has not been experimentally manipulated in most prevention programs.

There are, however, some experimental studies that provide better evidence for the causal role of friendships in child development. The most notable example is a prevention study that actually produced iatrogenic effects (Dishion & Andrews, 1995). In this study, 158 high-risk early adolescents were randomly assigned to one of four groups: a peer-group intervention, a parent-group intervention, a group receiving both interventions, and a group receiving neither intervention (i.e., the control group). The peer-group intervention targeted social and self-regulatory skills, and aggregated six or seven at-risk youth together with an adult trainer. The parent group included parent training in monitoring and behavior management (but no direct intervention with the adolescents). The participants in the control condition actually received the same training as those in the peer-group condition, but through a self-administered procedure. At posttest, participants in both peer groups and the parent-only group manifested better skills and less conflict with parents than their counterparts in the control group. However, 1 and 3 years after the intervention, teachers' reports of behavior problems and participants' reports of tobacco use were higher for participants in the two peer-group conditions than for participants in either the parent-only or the control conditions (Poulin, Dishion, & Burraston, 2001). Given the high internal validity of the experimental design used in this study, it is likely that the iatrogenic effects resulted from a negative peer effect during or after the intervention sessions. Post hoc analyses of these sessions showed that the iatrogenic effects were accounted for by specific interpersonal interactions among the participants. This pattern of interactions was later termed "deviancy training." Other experimental studies that identified similar iatrogenic effects of deviant peers on specific behaviors were reported by Dodge, Dishion, and Lansford (2006). These studies have proved very informative about the role of deviant peers in influencing youth behaviors, especially when actual interactions among peers can be examined.

Friends and Prosocial Behavior

In contrast to the abundant studies linking friends' antisocial behavior to changes in children's or adolescents' externalizing problems, the evidence for the contribution of friends' prosocial behavior to changes in children's and adolescents' prosocial behavior is scarce. A few studies, however, warrant particular attention. For example, friends' prosocial behavior in sixth grade was found to predict adolescents' prosocial behavior in eighth grade through positive changes in personal motivation to behave prosocially (Wentzel et al., 2004). The presumed "influence" of friends' prosocial behavior seemed to depend on the difference between adolescents and friends in grade 6. Prosocial behavior increased for students with friends who were more prosocial than themselves, whereas it decreased for those with friends who were less prosocial. A follow-up study showed that a similar process was operative between grades 9 and 10 (Barry & Wentzel, 2006). In this study, reciprocal friends' self-reported prosocial behavior in ninth grade predicted changes in the participants' prosocial behavior over the 1-year interval. Interestingly, the links between friends' prosocial and participants' prosocial behavior were moderated by the perceived quality of the friendships (i.e., closeness and importance), the frequency of the interactions with the friends, and the stability of the friendships over the period of study.

Explanatory Mechanisms

In conformity with the social bonding perspective, Barry and Wentzel (2006) proposed that friends' prosocial behavior fostered changes in participants' prosocial behavior by increasing their motivation to behave prosocially. This explanatory hypothesis implicitly refers to internal psychological processes that might be triggered by friends' behaviors. However, these psychological processes may not be the only mediators involved in the association between friends' behaviors and changes in participants' behaviors. According to the social interaction perspective, changes in internal psychological processes may actually follow a series of microsocial processes at the interpersonal level. Evidence for these microsocial processes has been mainly collected through direct observations of interactions between friends.

A first microsocial process that can potentially impact youth behavior is positive verbal reinforcement by peers of the child's behaviors. This process, labeled "deviancy training" (Dishion, Spracklen, Andrews, & Patterson, 1996) because it often emerges in a context involving disruptive adolescents and their friends, has received substantial empirical support. Specifically, deviant friends tend to reinforce, through laughter or positive nonverbal feedback, rule-breaking talk or deviant acts and to ignore or punish normative behaviors (Buehler, Patterson, & Furniss, 1966). This differential reinforcement of deviant behaviors has been found to result in an increase in youngsters' subsequent delinquent behavior and substance use (Dishion, Poulin, & Burraston, 2001; Poulin et al., 2001). Deviancy training has also been found to mediate the predictive association between exposure to deviant peers at age 10 and increases in arrests, substance use, and sexual intercourse during adolescence (Patterson et al., 2000).

Deviancy training may occur among kindergarten children. Engaging in deviant talk and imitative play of deviant behaviors with same-gender peers predicted an increase in overt and covert conduct problems over a 1-year interval (Snyder et al., 2005) and of covert conduct problems over a 3-year interval (Snyder et al., 2008). These effects were positive even after researchers accounted for deviant peer involvement or peer coercion.

On the other side of the spectrum, "conformity training" (i.e., the opposite of deviancy training) may help explain the apparent positive influence of friends' prosocial behavior on children's and adolescents' prosocial behavior (Wentzel et al., 2004; Wentzel, Filisetti, & Looney, 2007). In conformity training, friends approve of each other's prosocial behaviors and disapprove of each other's antisocial behaviors. However, to our knowledge, the microsocial processes reflecting conformity training have not yet been documented.

A third microprocess that may serve as an indicator of deviancy (and conformity) training in the context of friendships is "norm-disobedience behaviors," that is, the pressure exerted within the relationship to conform to norm-breaking behaviors. For example, 10-year-old aggressive boys and their friends have been found to provide more enticement for rule violations in situations that provided opportunities for rule-breaking behavior than nonaggressive boys and their friends (Bagwell & Coie, 2004). As expected, aggressive boys and their friends engaged in more rule-breaking behavior than nonaggressive boys and their friends. Interestingly, nonaggressive dyads also engaged in what was referred to as "temptation talk" (i.e., exploration of potential rule violations), but they seldom escalated from temptation talk to actual norm-breaking behaviors (Bagwell & Coie, 2004).

Demonstration–imitation through observational learning of rule-breaking, aggressive, or prosocial behaviors is a fourth microprocess that may also explain how friends support the acquisition, maintenance, or escalation of aggressive–antisocial or prosocial acts (Berndt, 1999; Hartup & Stevens, 1997). Clear imitation effects have been reported through an experiment in which adolescents were randomly exposed to high- or low-status (virtual) peers in a laboratory setting (Cohen & Prinstein, 2006). When peers were ostensibly high in status, adolescents conformed more to these peers' aggressive/risky behaviors than when peers were low in status. This study clearly demonstrates that modeling effects do occur and peer social status (in addition to participants' levels of social anxiety) plays a moderating role in the relation between peer and adolescent behavior. However, this study involved peers rather than friends. Given that friends' characteristics cannot be manipulated directly, their modeling effects can only be inferred.

Antisocial children and adolescents have been found to be bossier with their friends and more frequently involved in coercive and conflictual exchanges than conventional children (Deptula & Cohen, 2004; Dishion, Andrews, & Crosby, 1995; Windle, 1994). These conflictual-negative interactions could set in motion a "coercive interactional process" (Patterson, Reid, & Dishion, 1992; Boivin & Vitaro, 1995) whereby coercing or threatening one's friend for some personal benefit, if successful, can increase the likelihood of similar coercive behaviors in the future through negative reinforcement. Consistent with this notion, conflict with a best friend predicted delinquency beyond peer rejection and best friend aggressiveness (Kupersmidt et al., 1995). In contrast, the diplomatic and empathic skills manifested by prosocial friends, or the use of adaptive reconciliation strategies after occasional conflicts, may enhance children's negotiation skills and tolerance, two important ingredients for prosocial development.

These processes may not always be involved in every instance of participant–friend interactions. Moreover, different processes may be related to different outcomes. As recently shown by Snyder, Schrepferman, Brooker, and Stoolmiller (2007), deviancy training and modeling may foster conduct problems of the covert type (i.e., stealing, cheating), whereas coercion may be involved with aggression-type outcomes.

Friends may foster internalizing outcomes in addition to externalizing behavior problems and prosocial development. Conflict with a best friend, for example, may foster internalizing problems, such as depressive feelings (Brendgen, Vitaro, & Bukowski, 2000b), especially if the friendship is valued by the child and the conflict results in the termination of the friendship. There are also ways that friends' deviancy can lead to depressed mood. For example, affiliation with deviant friends may lead to increases in externalizing behavior, such as delinquency and alcohol problems, which could then lead to interpersonal problems with parents and teachers—and an ensuing negative effect on mood (Fergusson, Wanner, Vitaro, Horwood, & Swain-Campbell, 2003). Subsequently, deviant friends may then share and further promote each other's negative feelings through co-rumination (Rose, 2002). "Co-rumination" refers to an excessive discussion of personal problems within a dyadic relationship, a focus on negative feelings generated by the personal problems, and a mutual encouragement of the ruminating behavior. Thus, co-rumination rests on a series of interpersonal interactions that are reminiscent of the microsocial processes underlying deviancy or conformity training described earlier. Co-rumination may, however, have a paradoxical effect: It may strengthen the friendship bond through mutual self-disclosure, while increasing depressive feelings through excessively dwelling on personal problems, and the negative feelings associated with those problems.

Thus, co-rumination may explain how friends' depressive feelings predict increases in adolescents' depressive feelings (Prinstein, 2007; Stevens & Prinstein, 2005). Also important are the factors that may aggravate or attenuate the linkages between friends' and adolescents' feelings. For example, in Prinstein's (2007) study, girls were found to be particularly vulnerable to friends' depressive feelings. High levels of social anxiety and lack of reciprocity in the friendship further exacerbated girls' vulnerability. For boys, higher levels of friends' peer-perceived popularity and lower levels of positive friendship quality were both associated with greater susceptibility to depressive symptom contagion. These results suggest that emulation of higher-status friends or social comparison may play an important role in this context (as intrapersonal motivational or emotional mechanisms following co-rumination).

An imbalance in friendship reciprocity and low friendship quality seem to exacerbate these processes. As mentioned above, low friendship quality exacerbates the risk associated with exposure to depressed friends (Prinstein, 2007). Low-quality friendships also strengthen the predictive linkages between friends' deviancy and increases in participants' delinquent behaviors (Poulin, Dishion, & Haas, 1999) as well as between friends' shyness/social withdrawal and participants' increases in shyness and social withdrawal (Berndt, Hawkins, & Jiao, 1999).

In contrast, at least three studies show that high—not low—friendship quality amplifies deviant friends' influence on externalizing behaviors, such as serious delinquency and drug use (Agnew, 1991; Piehler & Dishion, 2007; Urberg, Luo, Pilgrim, & Degirmencioglu, 2003). One way to reconcile these opposing results concerning the role of friendship quality is to link the moderating role of friendship quality to the nature of the interaction processes among friends. If the process is consensual and positive (as in deviancy or conformity training), then the link between friendship and either well-being or behavior might be enhanced more by high-quality friendships than by low-quality friendships. However, if the interactions between friends abound with conflict and are mutually coercive, then it is low quality friendships that might exacerbate the impact of interactions on mood and behavior. These empirical and theoretical points emphasize the need to consider friendship features as an additional and important dimension of friendship.

Friendship Features: The Bright and Dark Sides

As discussed by Berndt (1996; Berndt & McCandless, Chapter 4, this volume), the "features" of a friendship are its attributes or characteristics. The features can be either positive (e.g., intimacy, companionship) or negative (i.e., rivalry, conflict). Together, the positive and negative features of friendship define friendship quality.

Friendship quality may not only moderate the impact of friends' behaviors but also have a main effect of its own. However, the social bonding and the social interaction perspectives lead to different expectations regarding the role of friendship quality. According to the social interaction view, the quality of the relationship is a by-product of the exchange pattern among friends (Patterson et al., 1992; Poulin et al., 1999): When the microsocial processes between friends are accounted for, the quality of the relationship plays no additional, unique role with respect to the child's adjustment. However, the proponents of the social interaction perspective acknowledge that positive features of friendships may reinforce the deviancy training process, whereas low-quality friendships may exacerbate the coercive process. In other words, friendship quality can moderate the impact of friends' characteristics. In contrast, the social bonding tradition emphasizes friendship features and considers them to be at the heart of friends' contribution to child development. Authors who adhere to this perspective assume that friendships (usually) create contexts characterized by intimate conversations, provision of emotional security, intimacy and affection, as well as mutual assistance. Provided that they are positive, these features in turn are likely to increase children's well-being and interpersonal competence, irrespective of children's characteristics (e.g., Buhrmester, 1996; Hartup & Stevens, 1999; Parker, Rubin, Erath, Wojslawowicz, & Buskirk, 2006). To summarize, the social bonding view emphasizes the quality of the transactions between friends, whereas the social interaction view emphasizes the content of the transactions between friends.

There is evidence that friendships improve children's positive mood and feelings of well-being through the provision of companionship and social support (Birch & Ladd, 1996; Ladd, Kochenderfer, & Coleman, 1996), and of instrumental assistance and feelings of security (Wentzel, 1996). There is also evidence that early adolescents involved in high-quality friendships become more socially visible and gain in social reputation (Berndt, 2002). In contrast, virtually all published longitudinal studies failed to find any unique or mediating contribution of friendship quality to externalizing behaviors (i.e., delinquency) once researchers accounted for children's own and friends' characteristics (Haynie & Osgood, 2005; McElhany, Immele, Smith, & Allen, 2006; Poulin et al., 1999; Selfhout, Branje, & Meeus, 2008; Windle, 1994; Zimmerman, Ramirez-Valles, Zapert, & Maton, 2000). Short-term longitudinal studies also failed to find a main effect of friendship quality on depressive symptoms (Prinstein, 2007; Windle, 1994) or self-esteem (Berndt, 1996; Berndt et al., 1999).

Several reasons may explain this failure to detect a main effect of friendship quality. First, most studies relied on self-reports to assess friendship quality. This may have resulted in skewed ratings and limited variance (although similar findings are obtained when external raters are used to assess friendship quality, as in Poulin et al., 1999). Second, many studies have focused on the positive features of friendship or have combined the positive and negative features of the friendship through the use of a difference score (which favors the positive features, because most items in current friendship quality questionnaires tap these positive features). As shown in some cross-sectional studies, negative friendship features predict behavioral and academic outcomes better than the positive features (Berndt & Keefe, 1995; Burk & Laursen, 2005; Ladd et al., 1996), suggesting that the positive and negative features should be measured separately or be given equal importance in combined measures.

Third, the duration of the study is too short for the behavior or self-perception to change, or too long for the friendship to remain stable and of high quality (Berndt, 1996). Fourth, most studies considered only the participants' point of view about the quality of the relationship with the friend. However, the friend's view is essential to ascertain the nature of the relationship. Accordingly, the association between friendship quality and a series of outcomes is strongest when both friends strongly agree or strongly disagree about the nature of the friendship, especially with respect to negative features (Burk & Laursen, 2005).

Fifth, the way friendship quality is conceptualized and measured can also account for the mixed findings about the contribution of friendship quality. To illustrate, when friendship quality refers to personal feelings about the relationship or features such as attachment to the friend, feelings of security, or time spent together, there is little information conveyed about interaction and learning processes. Thus, it is unlikely that a specific contribution to behavioral adjustment will be identified. We argue that these specific contributions are more likely when features of friendship quality approximate some of the microsocial processes reviewed earlier. Finally, most studies do not examine the contribution of friendship quality separately for boys and girls. It is possible that friendship quality could play a stronger role for girls given their greater emphasis on dyadic relationships (as opposed to boys).

In conclusion, current empirical evidence supports a main effect of friendship quality on psychoemotional well-being but a moderating role with respect to behavioral adjustment. This tentative conclusion aims to reconcile the social interaction and the social bonding perspectives in an integrated way. Figure 31.1 illustrates the putative role of friends' characteristics and of intra- or interindividual processes, such as deviancy training, conformity training, coercion, and support in changing behaviors. Figure 31.1 also illustrates the role of intrapersonal affective and motivational processes in explaining how features of friendship are linked to emotional well-being. The absence of a direct link between the microsocial interindividual processes and changes in emotional well-being results from lack of research on this issue (with the exception of that on the co-rumination process) rather than on conceptual grounds. In turn, the absence of a direct link between features of friendship and changes in externalizing behaviors, and the illustration of a moderating role for features of friendship should be conceived not as definitive conclusions but as propositions based on current knowledge.

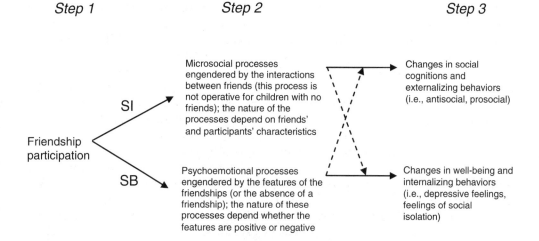

FIGURE 31.1. Integrated model illustrating how friendship participation can be linked to children's psychosocial development according both the social interaction (SI) and the social bonding (SB) perspectives. A host of moderating variables may be involved at every step of the process depicted here; some of these moderators refer to participants' characteristics, friends' characteristics, or contextual factors. They are not illustrated for the sake of clarity.

Conclusions

Friendships may have both positive and negative consequences for children's and adolescents' psychosocial development depending on (1) whether the friendships are present or absent; (2) whether the friends' behaviors are prosocial, antisocial, or depressogenic; (3) whether the friendships' features are positive or negative; and (4) whether friends' reactions are supportive of adaptive or maladaptive behaviors. A host of moderating variables may also be involved. Two theoretical perspectives were used to examine the roles played by these different friendship-related variables in affecting youth development. These two perspectives focus on different aspects of the friendship experience that might impact children's psychosocial development.

Although theoretically distinct, both the social bonding and the social interaction perspectives may be used to explain empirical research findings; thus, they are sometimes difficult to tease apart. For example, friends involved in deviancy or conformity training may also experience pleasure and feelings of validation through their friendships. In turn, many features of friendship that are so central to the social bonding perspective also involve microsocial transactions between friends similar to those suggested by the social interaction perspective.

In addition, a host of moderating factors may affect the full expression of either theoretical perspective. For example, reciprocity, a defining feature of friendship, does not always operate in the expected direction. Contrary to what may be predicted on the basis of the social bonding perspective, adolescents may adopt their friends' behaviors if the friendship nominations are unilateral, but not if they are reciprocated (Adams, Bukowski, & Bagwell, 2005; Aloise-Young, Graham, & Hansen, 1994; Bot, Engels, Knibbe,

& Meeus, 2005). Given that most mutual friends are initially more similar than desired unilateral friends, it is not totally surprising that unilateral friends have more "influence" than reciprocal friends, especially for behaviors that are popular among adolescents. Nevertheless, these results are important, because they indicate that it is not necessary for children or adolescents to interact closely with peers for influence or contagion to occur. In this case, the desired friends are most influential even though they are not as accessible as actual friends. These results also force us to consider reciprocity as another feature of friendship that could moderate the link between friends' behaviors and changes in participants' behaviors, instead of simply selecting only participants with mutual friends.

Another important set of potential moderators comprises children's personal, social, or sociofamilial characteristics. These factors may explain why not all children are equally "influenced" by their friends' behaviors (Caprara & Zimbardo, 1996; Prinstein, 2007; Van Lier, Wanner, & Vitaro, 2007; Vitaro et al., 1997; Vitaro, Brendgen, & Tremblay, 2000).

The issues raised in this chapter have implications for intervention strategies that attempt to improve children's adjustment by capitalizing on the power of friendships. Unfortunately, these strategies do not always ensure that friends possess prosocial skills, that friendships are of high quality, and that the friends interact in a socially acceptable manner. For example, "pair therapy" has been proposed to foster friendships between children and adolescents under adult supervision (Selman, Watts, & Schultz, 2004). Although pair therapy focuses on the quality of the relationship between the friends-to-be, it ignores the role that friends' characteristics may play in influencing children's development (positively or negatively). Another strategy, "buddy pairing," has also been proposed (Hoza, Mrug, Pelham, Greiner, & Gnagy, 2003). This strategy involves pairing potential friends as "buddies" during recreational or learning activities. Buddies are encouraged to interact positively with each other and to help each other to earn privileges. Given the potential for deviancy training and conflict among deviant friends, those adopting this intervention strategy should be sensitive to children's characteristics. Pairing two children with deviant behavioral characteristics may serve only to exacerbate their behavioral problems. Finally, "peer pairing," which consists of simply pairing two children for social interaction with no adult supervision, has also been proposed (Bierman, Greenberg, & the Conduct Problems Prevention Research Group, 1996). The potential for iatrogenic effects of such a procedure are high given that, as in the buddy pairing strategy, two deviant children may be paired and left free to influence each other negatively (Dodge et al., 2006). However, under the right conditions (e.g., a supervised context and competent trainers), these strategies may prove to be important new components for multimodal prevention/intervention programs for children with adjustment problems.

References

Adams, R. E., Bukowski, W. M., & Bagwell, C. (2005). Stability of aggression during early adolescence as moderated by reciprocated friendship status and friend's aggression. *International Journal of Behavioral Development, 29*, 139–145.

Agnew, R. (1991). The interactive effects of peer variables on delinquency. *Criminology, 29*, 47–72.

Aloise-Young, P. A., Graham, J. W., & Hansen, W. B. (1994). Peer influence on smoking initiation during early adolescence: A comparison of group members and group outsiders. *Journal of Applied Psychology, 79*, 281–287.

Archer, J., & Lloyd, B. (2002). *Sex and gender* (2nd ed.). Cambridge, UK: Cambridge University Press.

Bagwell, C. L., & Coie, J. D. (2004). The best friendships of aggressive boys: Relationship quality, conflict management, and rule-breaking behavior. *Journal of Experimental Child Psychology, 88,* 5–24.

Bagwell, C. L., Newcomb, A. F., & Bukowski, W. M. (1998). Preadolescent friendship and peer rejection as predictors of adult adjustment. *Child Development, 69,* 140–153.

Barry, C. M., & Wentzel, K. R. (2006). Friend influence on prosocial behavior: The role of motivational factors and friendship characteristics *Developmental Psychology, 42,* 153–163.

Berndt, T. J. (1996). Exploring the effects of friendship quality on social development. In W. M. Bukowski, A. F. Newcomb, & W. W. Hartup (Eds.), *The company they keep* (pp. 346–365). New York: Cambridge University Press.

Berndt, T. J. (1999). Friends' influence on students' adjustment to school. *Educational Psychologist, 34,* 15–28.

Berndt, T. J. (2002). Friendship quality and social development. *Current Directions in Psychological Science, 11,* 7–10.

Berndt, T. J., Hawkins, J. A., & Jiao, Z. (1999). Influences of friends and friendships on adjustment to junior high school. *Merrill–Palmer Quarterly, 45,* 13–41.

Berndt, T. J., & Keefe, K. (1995). Friends' influence on adolescents' adjustment to school. *Child Development, 66,* 1312–1329.

Bierman, K. L., Greenberg, M. T., & the Conduct Problems Prevention Research Group. (1996). Social skills training in the Fast Track program. In R. D. Peters & R. J. McMahon (Eds.), *Preventing childhood disorders, substance abuse, and delinquency* (pp. 65–89). Thousand Oaks, CA: Sage.

Birch, S. H., & Ladd, G. W. (1996). Interpersonal relationships in the school environment and children's early school adjustment: The role of teachers and peers. In J. Juvonen & K. R. Wentzel (Eds.), *Social motivation: Understanding children's school adjustment* (pp. 199–225). New York: Cambridge University Press.

Boivin, M., Hymel, S., & Hodges, E. (2001). Toward a process view of peer rejection and harassment. In J. Juvonen & S. Graham (Eds.), *Peer harassment in school: The plight of the vulnerable and victimized* (pp. 265–289). New York: Guilford Press.

Boivin, M., & Vitaro, F. (1995). The impact of peer relationships on aggression in childhood: Inhibition through coercion or promotion through peer support. In J. McCord (Ed.), *Coercion and punishment in long-term perspectives* (pp. 183–197). New York: Cambridge University Press.

Boivin, M., Vitaro, F., & Poulin, F. (2005). Peer relationships and the development of aggressive behavior in early childhood. In R. E. Tremblay, W. W. Hartup, & J. Archer (Eds.), *Developmental origins of aggression* (pp. 376–397). New York: Guilford Press.

Bolger, K. E., Patterson, C. J., & Kupersmidt, J. B. (1998). Peer relationships and self-esteem among children who have been maltreated. *Child Development, 69,* 1171–1197.

Bot, S. M., Engels, R. C. M. E., Knibbe, R. A., & Meeus, W. H. (2005). Friend's drinking behaviour and adolescent alcohol consumption: The moderating role of friendship characteristics. *Addictive Behaviors, 30,* 929–947.

Brendgen, M., Bowen, F., Rondeau, N., & Vitaro, F. (1999). Effects of friends' characteristics on social cognitions. *Social Development, 8,* 41–51.

Brendgen, M., Vitaro, F., & Bukowski, W. M. (2000a). Deviant friends and early adolescents' emotional and behavioral adjustment. *Journal of Research on Adolescence, 10,* 173–189.

Brendgen, M., Vitaro, F., & Bukowski, W. M. (2000b). Stability and variability of adolescents' affiliation with delinquent friends: Predictors and consequences. *Social Development, 9,* 205–225.

Buehler, R. E., Patterson, G. R., & Furniss, J. M. (1966). The reinforcement of behavior in institutional settings. *Behaviour Research and Therapy, 4,* 157–167.

Buhrmester, D. (1996). Need fulfillment, interpersonal competence, and the developmental contexts of early adolescent friendship. In W. M. Bukowski, A. F. Newcomb, & W. W. Hartup (Eds.), *The company they keep* (pp. 158–185). Cambridge, UK: Cambridge University Press.

Bukowski, W. M., & Hoza, B. (1989). Popularity and friendship: Issues in theory, measurement, and outcome. In T. Berndt & G. Ladd (Eds.), *Peer relationships in child development* (pp. 15–45). New York: Wiley.

Burk, W. J., & Laursen, B. (2005). Adolescent perceptions of friendship and their associations with individual adjustment. *International Journal of Behavioral Development, 29*, 156–164.

Cairns, R. B., Leung, M.-C., Buchanan, L., & Cairns, B. D. (1995). Friendships and social networks in childhood and adolescence: Fluidity, reliability, and interrelations. *Child Development, 66*, 1330–1345.

Caprara, G. V., & Zimbardo, P. (1996). Aggregation and amplification of marginal deviations in the social construction of personality and maladjustment. *European Journal of Personality, 10*, 79–110.

Cohen, G. L., & Prinstein, M. J. (2006). Peer contagion and health-risk behavior among adolescent males: An experimental investigation of effects on public conduct and private attitudes. *Child Development, 77*, 967–983.

Criss, M. M., Pettit, G. S., Bates, J. E., Dodge, K. A., & Lapp, A. L. (2002). Family adversity, positive peer relationships, and children's externalizing behavior: A longitudinal perspective on risk and resilience. *Child Development, 73*, 1220–1237.

Deptula, D. P., & Cohen, R. (2004). Aggressive, rejected, and delinquent children and adolescents: A comparison of their friendships. *Aggression and Violent Behavior, 9*, 75–104.

Dishion, T. J., & Andrews, D. W. (1995). Preventing escalation in problem behaviors with high-risk young adolescents: Immediate and 1-year outcomes. *Journal of Consulting and Clinical Psychology, 63*, 538–548.

Dishion, T. J., Andrews, D. W., & Crosby, L. (1995). Antisocial boys and their friends in early adolescence: Relationship characteristics, quality, and interactional processes. *Child Development, 66*, 139–151.

Dishion, T. J., Poulin, F., & Burraston, B. (2001). Peer group dynamics associated with iatrogenic effects in group interventions with high-risk young adolescents. In C. Erdley & D. W. Nangle (Eds.), *New directions in child development: The role of friendship in psychological adjustment* (pp. 79–92). San Francisco: Jossey-Bass.

Dishion, T. J., Spracklen, K. M., Andrews, D. W., & Patterson, G. R. (1996). Deviancy training in male adolescent friendships. *Behavior Therapy, 27*, 373–390.

Dodge, K. A., Dishion, T. J., & Lansford, J. E. (Eds.). (2006). *Deviant peer influences in programs for youth.* New York: Guilford Press.

Doyle, A. B., & Markiewicz, D. (1996). Parents' interpersonal relationships and children's friendships. In W. M. Bukowski, A. F. Newcomb, & W. W. Hartup (Eds.), *The company they keep* (pp. 115–136). Cambridge, UK: Cambridge University Press.

Eddy, J. M., & Chamberlain, P. (2000). Family management and deviant peer association as mediator of the impact of treatment condition on youth antisocial behavior. *Journal of Consulting and Clinical Psychology, 68*, 857–863.

Elliott, D. S., Huizinga, D., & Ageton, S. S. (1985). *Explaining delinquency and drug use.* Beverly Hills, CA: Sage.

Engels, R. C. M. E., Knibbe, R. A., De Vries, H., Drop, M. J., & van Breukelen, G. J. P. (1999). Influences of parental and friends' smoking and drinking on adolescent use: A longitudinal study. *Journal of Applied Social Psychology, 29*, 337–361.

Ennett, S. T., Bauman, K. E., Hussong, A., Faris, R., Foshee, V. A., Cai, L., et al. (2006). The peer context of adolescent substance use: Findings from social network analysis. *Journal of Research on Adolescence, 16*, 159–186.

Fergusson, D. M., Wanner, B., Vitaro, F., Horwood, L. J., & Swain-Campbell, N. R. (2003). Deviant peer affiliations and depression: Confounding or causation? *Journal of Abnormal Child Psychology, 31*, 605–618.

Gauze, C., Bukowski, W. M., Aquan-Assee, J., & Sippola, L. (1996). Interactions between family environment and friendship and associations with self-perceived well-being during early adolescence. *Child Development, 67*, 2201–2216.

Hartup, W. W. (1996). The company they keep: Friendships and their development significance. *Child Development, 67*, 1–13.

Hartup, W. W. (2005). Peer interaction: What causes what? *Journal of Abnormal Child Psychology, 33*, 387–394.

Hartup, W. W., & Stevens, N. (1997). Friendships and adaptation in the life course. *Psychological Bulletin, 121*, 355–370.

Hartup, W. W., & Stevens, N. (1999). Friendships and adaptation across the life span. *Current Directions in Psychological Science, 8*, 76–79.

Haynie, D. L., & Osgood, D. W. (2005). Reconsidering peers and delinquency: How do peers matter? *Social Forces, 84*, 1109–1130.

Hodges, E., Boivin, M., Vitaro, F., & Bukowski, W. M. (1999). The power of friendship: Protecting against an escalating cycle of peer victimization. *Developmental Psychology, 35*, 94–101.

Hoza, B., Mrug, S., Pelham, W. E., Jr., Greiner, A. R., & Gnagy, E. M. (2003). A friendship intervention for children with attention-deficit/hyperactivity disorder: Preliminary findings. *Journal of Attention Disorders, 6*, 87–98.

Kupersmidt, J. B., Burchinal, M., & Patterson, C. J. (1995). Developmental patterns of childhood peer relations as predictors of externalizing behavior problems. *Development and Psychopathology, 7*, 825–843.

Ladd, G. W., Kochenderfer, B. J., & Coleman, C. C. (1996). Friendship quality as a predictor of young children's early school adjustment. *Child Development, 67*, 1103–1118.

Ladd, G. W., & Troop-Gordon, W. (2003). The role of chronic peer difficulties in the development of children's psychological adjustment problems. *Child Development, 74*, 1344–1367.

Lamarche, V., Brendgen, M., Boivin, M., Vitaro, F., Dionne, G., & Pérusse, D. (2007). Do friends' characteristics moderate the prospective links between peer victimization and reactive and proactive aggression? *Journal of Abnormal Child Psychology, 35*, 665–680.

Lansford, J. E., Capanna, C., Dodge, K. A., Caprara, G. V., Bates, J. E., Pettit, G. S., et al. (2007). Peer social preference and depressive symptoms of children in Italy and the United States. *International Journal of Behavioral Development, 31*, 274–283.

Laursen, B., Bukowski, W. M., Aunola, K., & Nurmi, J.-E. (2007). Friendship moderates prospective associations between social isolation and adjustment problems in young children. *Child Development, 78*, 1395–1404.

McElhaney, K. B., Immele, A., Smith, F. D., & Allen, J. P. (2006). Attachment organization as a moderator of the link between friendship quality and adolescent delinquency. *Attachment and Human Development, 8*, 33–46.

Mrug, S., Hoza, B., & Bukowski, W. M. (2004). Choosing or being chosen by aggressive–disruptive peers: Do they contribute to children's externalizing and internalizing problems? *Journal of Abnormal Child Psychology, 32*, 53–65.

Nangle, D. W., Erdley, C. A., Newman, J. P., Mason, C. A., & Carpenter, E. M. (2003). Popularity, friendship quantity, and friendship quality: Interactive influences on children's loneliness and depression. *Journal of Clinical Child and Adolescent Psychology, 32*, 546–555.

Newcomb, A. F., & Bagwell, C. L. (1995). Children's friendship relations: A meta-analytic review. *Psychological Bulletin, 117*, 306–347.

Oldenburg, C. M., & Kerns, K. A. (1997). Associations between peer relationships and depressive symptoms: Testing moderator effects of gender and age. *Journal of Early Adolescence, 17*, 319–337.

Parker, J. G., & Asher, S. R. (1993). Friendship and friendship quality in middle childhood: Links with peer group acceptance and feelings of loneliness and social dissatisfaction. *Developmental Psychology, 29*, 611–621.

Parker, J. G., Rubin, K. H., Erath, S. A., Wojslawowicz, J. C., & Buskirk, A. A. (2006). Peer relationships, child development, and adjustment: A developmental psychopathology perspective. In D. Cicchetti & D. J. Cohen (Eds.), *Developmental psychopathology: Vol. 1. Theory and methods* (2nd ed., pp. 96–161). New York: Wiley.

Parker, J. G., & Seal, J. (1996). Forming, losing, renewing, and replacing friendships: Applying temporal parameters to the assessment of children's friendship experiences. *Child Development, 67,* 2248–2268.

Patterson, G. R., Dishion, T. J., & Yoerger, K. (2000). Adolescent growth in new forms of problem behavior: Macro- and micro-peer dynamics. *Prevention Science, 1,* 3–13.

Patterson, G. R., Reid, J. B., & Dishion, T. J. (1992). *A social learning approach: IV. Antisocial boys.* Eugene, OR: Castalia Publishing.

Pedersen, S., Vitaro, F., Barker, E. D., & Borge, A. (2007). The timing of middle childhood peer rejection and friendships: Linking early behavior to adolescent adjustment. *Child Development, 78,* 1037–1051.

Pelkonen, M., Marttunen, M., & Aro, H. (2003). Risk for depression: A 6-year follow-up of Finnish adolescents. *Journal of Affective Disorders, 77,* 41–51.

Piehler, T. F., & Dishion, T. J. (2007). Interpersonal dynamics within adolescent friendships: Dyadic mutuality, deviant talk, and patterns of antisocial behavior. *Child Development, 78,* 1611–1624.

Poulin, F., Dishion, T. J., & Burraston, B. (2001). Three-year iatrogenic effects associated with aggregating high-risk adolescents in cognitive-behavioral preventive interventions. *Applied Developmental Science, 5,* 214–224.

Poulin, F., Dishion, T. J., & Haas, E. (1999). The peer influence paradox: Friendship quality and deviancy training within male adolescent friendships. *Merrill–Palmer Quarterly, 45,* 42–61.

Prinstein, M. J. (2007). Moderators of peer contagion: A longitudinal examination of depression socialization between adolescents and their best friends. *Journal of Clinical Child and Adolescent Psychology, 36,* 1–12.

Rose, A. J. (2002). Co-rumination in the friendship of girls and boys. *Child Development, 73,* 1830–1843.

Scaramella, L. V., Conger, R. D., Spoth, R., & Simons, R. L. (2002). Evaluation of a social contextual model of delinquency: A cross-study replication. *Child Development, 73,* 175–195.

Selfhout, M. H. W., Branje, S. J. T., & Meeus, W. H. J. (2008). The development of delinquency and perceived friendship quality in adolescent best friendship dyads. *Journal of Abnormal Child Psychology, 36,* 471–485.

Selman, R. L., Watts, C. L., & Schultz, L. H. (2004). *Fostering friendship: Pair therapy for treatment and prevention.* New Brunswick, NJ: Transaction.

Snyder, J., Horsch, E., & Childs, J. (1997). Peer relationships of young children: Affiliative choices and the shaping of aggressive behavior. *Journal of Clinical Child Psychology, 26,* 145–156.

Snyder, J., Schrepferman, L., Brooker, M., & Stoolmiller, M. (2007). The roles of anger, conflict with parents and peers, and social reinforcement in the early development of physical aggression. In T. A. Cavell & K. T. Malcolm (Eds.), *Anger, aggression, and interventions for interpersonal violence* (pp. 187–214). Mahwah, NJ: Erlbaum.

Snyder, J., Schrepferman, L., McEachern, A., Barner, S., Johnson, K., & Provines, J. (2008). Peer deviancy training and peer coercion: Dual processes associated with early-onset conduct problems. *Child Development, 79,* 252–268.

Snyder, J., Schrepferman, L., Oeser, J., Patterson, G., Stoolmiller, M., Johnson, K., et al. (2005). Deviancy training and association with deviant peers in young children: Occurrence and contribution to early-onset conduct problems. *Development and Psychopathology, 17,* 397–413.

Stevens, E. A., & Prinstein, M. J. (2005). Peer contagion of depressogenic attributional styles among adolescents: A longitudinal study. *Journal of Abnormal Child Psychology, 33,* 25–37.

Urberg, K. A., Luo, Q., Pilgrim, C., & Degirmencioglu, S. M. (2003). A two-stage model of peer influence in adolescent substance use: Individual and relationship-specific differences in susceptibility to influence. *Addictive Behaviors, 28,* 1243–1256.

Van Lier, P. A. C., Wanner, B., & Vitaro, F. (2007). Onset of antisocial behavior, affiliation with deviant friends and childhood maladjustment: A direct test of the childhood versus adolescent onset model. *Development and Psychopathology, 19,* 167–185.

Vitaro, F., Brendgen, M., Pagani, L. S., Tremblay, R. E., & McDuff, P. (1999). Disruptive behavior, peer association, and conduct disorder: Testing the developmental links through early intervention. *Development and Psychopathology, 11*, 287–304.

Vitaro, F., Brendgen, M., & Tremblay, R. E. (2000). Influence of deviant friends on delinquency: Searching for moderator variables. *Journal of Abnormal Child Psychology, 28*, 313–325.

Vitaro, F., Brendgen, M., & Wanner, B. (2005). Patterns of affiliation with delinquent friends during late childhood and early adolescence: Correlates and consequences. *Social Development, 14*, 82–108.

Vitaro, F., Pedersen, S., & Brendgen, M. (2007). Children's disruptiveness, peer rejection, friends' deviancy, and delinquent behaviors: A process-oriented approach. *Development and Psychopathology, 19*, 433–453.

Vitaro, F., Tremblay, R. E., Kerr, M., Pagani, L. S., & Bukowski, W. M. (1997). Disruptiveness, friends' characteristics, and delinquency: A test of two competing models of development. *Child Development, 68*, 676–689.

Wentzel, K. R. (1996). Social goals and social relationships as motivators of school adjustment. In J. Juvonen & K. R. Wentzel (Eds.), *Social motivation: Understanding children's school adjustment* (pp. 226–247). New York: Cambridge University Press.

Wentzel, K. R., Barry, C. M., & Caldwell, K. A. (2004). Friendships in middle school: Influences on motivation and school adjustment. *Journal of Educational Psychology, 96*, 195–203.

Wentzel, K. R., Filisetti, L., & Looney, L. (2007). Adolescent prosocial behavior: The role of self-processes and contextual cues. *Child Development, 78*, 895–910.

Windle, M. (1994). A study of friendship characteristics and problem behavior among middle adolescents. *Child Development, 65*, 1764–1777.

Zimmerman, M. A., Ramirez-Valles, J., Zapert, K. M., & Maton, K. I. (2000). A longitudinal study of stress-buffering effects for urban African-American male adolescent problem behaviors and mental health. *Journal of Community Psychology, 28*, 17–33.

PART VIII

Translation and Policy

CHAPTER 32

Deviant by Design
Peer Contagion in Development, Interventions, and Schools

THOMAS J. DISHION
TIMOTHY F. PIEHLER

"Peer contagion" describes a mutual influence process that is not intentional, purposeful, or planned, but is initiated and maintained by social dynamics. The term is to be distinguished from a contagious disease process that is the focus in epidemiology (Anthony, 2006). In general, peer contagion emphasizes (often rapid) disinhibition of behavior patterns within a group of children, involving peers, friends, and siblings. The primary focus to date has been peer contagion in problem behavior and, less frequently, the underlying emotion that covaries with problem behavior. As suggested by the definition, peer contagion describes a "contamination" or disruption of a normative developmental process.

This chapter reviews evidence that peer contagion occurs both in the "natural environment" and in interventions and programs designed to benefit youth. The provocative title "Deviant by Design" underscores a critical focus of this chapter: Peer contagion occurs under the supervision of adults, mostly parents, teachers, and other community and family members; that is, we assume that peers are important, but how they are important is largely influenced by the kinds of contexts within which they interact and develop. Developmental researchers working within an ecological framework have often emphasized a broader perspective on the peer group, considering the role of parents in structuring peer interactions and relationships (e.g., Bronfenbrenner, 1979; Dishion, 1990; Youniss, 1980). The chapter emphasizes that the developmental and intervention science literatures are actually quite consistent in emphasizing the importance of adults in structuring peer environments. Thus, by design, some youth are more exposed to peer contagion than are others, whether intentional or not. We offer Figure 32.1 to provide a developmental perspective on the role of adults in general, and parents in particular, in structuring the world of peers. Early in development, attachment relationships form the foundation of parents' efforts to socialize children, which in turn lead to children's selection and success in social settings involving peers.

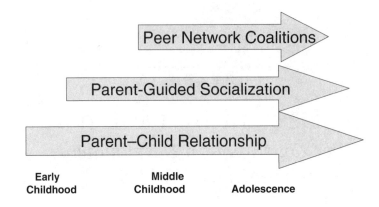

FIGURE 32.1. A developmental perspective on relationship influence.

In this chapter we first review evidence suggesting that adult-organized contexts, such as educational interventions, prevention programs, treatment programs, and even institutionalization, potentially structure peer-group dynamics that contribute to the formation of friendship within which positive and negative influences can be documented. Next, we provide alternative perspectives on peer influence processes that can contribute to contagion and problem behavior, as well as to disruption and emotional adjustment. Third, we examine in depth the idea that the emotional tenor of environments that aggregate children can influence both adjustment and congregation into prosocial and deviant peer groups. Finally, we link research from developmental and intervention science that suggests promising venues for future research to identify key mechanisms of influence and empower adults to structure healthier peer environments.

As suggested in the scholarly and persuasive review by Hartup (1996), we know far more about the dark side than about the positive side of peer relationships. Several years ago, many developmental psychologists would have proposed that peer relationships were more instrumental in influencing development in adolescence than in earlier developmental stages. However, the evidence is clear that peer influence begins early (see Howe & Ross, Chapter 28, this volume) and amplifies during adolescence, and specific behaviors within the context of each developmental phase are more likely to be salient influence factors. It is not surprising that peer influence begins early; developmental scientists have long been aware that children begin spending more time with peers than with adults, as early as ages 3 and 4 (Ellis, Rogoff, & Cromer, 1981).

We address three points in this chapter. The first is related to consequences to the child as a result of peer interaction. For example, there may be two potential outcomes of friendships and peer-group dynamics. One is the emotional well-being of the child. The second is the problem behavior of the child. The form and function of problem behavior varies with development, as in the subsequent review. Finally, as discussed by Oden, Herzberger, Mangione, and Wheeler (1984), peer relationships can be represented on a grid defined by two dimensions: (1) *partnership*, the extent to which there is explicit cooperation in joint activities within the fluid relationship; and (2) *friendship*, which involves an affective state of companionship, liking, and time spent together interacting. We argue herein that most influential to children's social and emotional development are close friendships and acquaintances. It is becoming increasingly clear that the nature and structure of the acquaintanceship network is influential for both friendship formation, and emotional and behavioral adjustment in children.

Early Childhood

The classic study of peer relationships and aggression was published by Dawe in 1934. Dawe directly observed 40 preschoolers and sampled quarrels as they appeared during the free-play period. This was an important study for its descriptive value. As one might expect, boys quarreled 50% more often than did girls. The frequency of quarreling decreased with age, as did the duration of conflict quarrels. Interestingly enough, teachers intervened in only 35% of observable conflicts. Finally, context was seen to be important in children's aggression, in that quarrels tended to be shorter in indoor settings than in outdoor settings. Although important, this work did not clearly delineate which influence mechanism might occur among peer acquaintances in early childhood and play settings. Patterson, Littman, and Bricker (1967) were among the first to identify negative reinforcement as an influence mechanism. In general, they found that children whose potential conflicts escalated and who "won" were more likely to assert themselves aggressively in future peer interactions. This study provided initial support for coercion as a fundamental mechanism in peer groups.

The role of peer reinforcement is widespread and beyond the scope of this chapter. However, a few noteworthy studies shed light on potential mechanisms. Furman and Masters (1980) examined the role of peer reinforcement in children's compliance with normative standards. The investigators were interested in the extent to which preschool peers provided a unique influence on moral development. Looking back on this research almost 30 years later, one cannot help but be impressed by the careful acumen with which influence processes were identified. In general, they found that unpopular young children were the most likely to deviate in their behavior, regardless of who, teachers or peers, promoted the norm. The authors suggested that popularity itself was of little significance in children's adherence to norms. Rather, rejection by peers was a disincentive for norm adherence. These findings suggest that coercive interactions with peers in settings such as schools undermine children's adoption of and compliance with normative standards in those settings.

More recently, Snyder and colleagues have studied two mechanisms relevant to social development among peers. The first is *peer coercion*, which follows up on the earlier work of Patterson et al. (1967), Patterson (1982), and Patterson, Reid, and Dishion (1992). Snyder's work identifies early peer relationships as instrumental in the development of aggressive behaviors in early childhood. He reported that aggressive children tend to select similarly aggressive others as interaction partners, thereby escalating their behavior patterns (Snyder, Horsch, & Childs, 1997). He also studied the tendency for young children to engage in deviancy training in school settings. "Deviancy training" focuses on the actual social interactions that often underlie peer contagion. Peer contagion can occur without social interactions, as is the case in the rapid spread of behaviors based on observations provided by media (suicide, self-mutilation, violent behavior, etc.). The concept of deviance training is discussed in more detail later in the chapter. Suffice it to say that it is a mechanism by which children mutually reinforce one another for deviant, problem behavior.

Reinforcement can take many forms, including positive expressions of laughter or approval; attention and interaction time during deviant talk or behavior bouts; and modeling of deviant behavior. Snyder and colleagues (2005) observed kindergarten children engaging in deviancy training. They found that the tendency for children to mock, engage, and laugh at deviant behavior predicted growth in antisocial behavior over the ensuing 2 years. As early as age 5, some children had learned strategies for obtaining peer reinforcement that were integrally related to growth in problem behavior in the future.

Snyder and colleagues (2008) recently revealed that peer coercion and peer deviancy training have two unique influence outcomes. Peer coercion leads to the development of overt aggression. Peer deviancy training leads to growth in covert patterns of antisocial behavior, related to early distinctions suggested by Loeber and Schmaling (1985). The study is important with respect to appreciating the need for adults to attempt to intervene as early as kindergarten in effecting social and emotional outcomes in children (Snyder et al., 2008).

In summary, the most salient features of peer influence in early childhood come from the kinds of interactions that occur within the larger peer group in relation to conflict and deviancy training. The emotional sequelae of poor adjustment within the larger peer group have not been studied as extensively as has the relevance of the early peer group in the emergence of aggression.

Middle Childhood

New forms of problem behavior that emerge in middle childhood may be particularly relevant to the adjustment of children, including covert antisocial behavior, proactive aggression, relational aggression, and bullying. As in early childhood, aggression and disruptive behavior are associated with peer rejection (e.g., Coie & Kupersmidt, 1983; Dodge, 1983). But it is also the case that peer rejection uniquely predicts later deviant peer involvement (Dishion, Patterson, Stoolmiller, & Skinner, 1991) and gang involvement (Dishion, Nelson, & Yasui, 2005). Therefore, rejection itself can have an indirect influence on later social development.

During middle childhood, relational aggression increases, whereas reactive aggression decreases (Underhill, 2004). Often friendships that are exclusive and intimate promote relational aggression (e.g., Crick & Grotpeter, 1995; Grotpeter & Crick, 1996). Relatedly, research by Poulin and Boivin (2000a, 2000b) suggests that deviant friendships are more influential for proactive than for reactive aggression.

Within schools, research by Kindermann (1993; Sage & Kindermann, 1999) suggests that for academically motivated children, peer approval is a maintaining mechanism. However, Tudge (1992) noted that on occasion peer-group dynamics can lead to decreases in academic competence. This is consistent with Kindermann's finding for low-achieving youth that off-task behavior was rewarded 11:1 when compared with on-task behavior. Thus, in many respects, peer attention seems to be a maintaining condition for high-risk youth to remain disengaged from effortful tasks leading to growth in academic skills.

Adolescence

Although there is considerable continuity in children's peer relations from childhood to adolescence, the general structure of the larger peer group begins to change during the adolescent years. The heterogeneity of the behavioral characteristics associated with peer rejection (Rubin, Bukowski, & Parker, 2006) evolves into a heterogeneity of groups. Within some groups, there is active support for deviant behavior (Stormshak et al., 1999). Furthermore, in early adolescence, many antisocial males are perceived to be popular (Rodkin, Farmer, Pearl, & Van Acker, 2000). In our own recent research, we have found that the conditions conducive to growth in problem behavior, especially drug use, emerge from school environments that both reject and support deviant behavior (Light & Dishion, 2007).

The contagion dynamic in adolescence seems to occur at the level of the friendship. Systematic and longitudinal analyses that control for prior antisocial behavior and family influences reveal that involvement with deviant friends leads to growth in problem behaviors in adolescence (Patterson, 1993). The friendship dyad appears most influential in the emergence of early adolescent substance use (Urberg, Degirmencioglu, & Pilgrim, 1997). Although friendships may be formed among youth with a history of marginal peer relationships, it is clear that the quality of their friendships leaves much to be desired (Brendgen, Little, & Krappmann, 2000). Paradoxically, Poulin, Dishion, and Haas (1999) found that low-quality friendship with a highly deviant friend predicted growth in problem behavior over a 2-year period. Sociological research further suggests that deviant friendships are highly correlated with delinquent behavior for both males and females (e.g., Giordano, Cernkovich, & Pugh, 1986).

Dishion and colleagues (Dishion, Capaldi, Spracklen, & Li, 1995; Dishion, Eddy, Haas, Li, & Spracklen, 1997; Dishion, Spracklen, Andrews, & Patterson, 1996) have examined a process referred to as "deviancy training," which, simply described, may be characterized by give-and-take exchanges between friends that promote both deviant actions (e.g., past stories of deviant acts, future suggestions, and "what if" scenarios) and laughter. A careful analysis of the content of the talk between friends indicates that, for some youth, deviant content is the key mechanism for eliciting positive affective exchanges in the friendship; this positive aspect defines the deviancy training process. Deviancy training in friendship predicted growth in delinquency (Dishion et al., 1996), drug use (Dishion et al., 1995), and violent behavior (Dishion et al., 1997). In addition, Patterson has shown that observed deviancy training mediates the link between involvement in a deviant peer group and drug and alcohol use, and high-risk sexual behavior in early adulthood (Patterson, Dishion, & Yoerger, 2000).

Emerging literature on deviancy training examines the influence process. Granic and Dishion (2003) found that youth comorbid for problems in affect and behavior were more likely to increase the length of their deviant talk bouts throughout a 30-minute laboratory session. Growth in adolescent problem behavior was predicted by the dyadic tendency to have increasingly longer deviant talk bouts. Also, using a dynamic systems framework, Dishion, Nelson, Winter, and Bullock (2004) found that dyads both high in deviant talk and low in entropy were most likely to escalate into antisocial behaviors from age 13 to age 24. "Entropy" in this sense describes a social interaction that is well organized and predictable. Thus, the more practiced one is within the context of a friendship regarding deviant discussions, the more likely one is to continue that trajectory through adulthood.

Extending the organizational focus of entropy toward a somewhat more tangible quality of friendship, Piehler and Dishion (2007) examined the construct of "dyadic mutuality." Friendships high in dyadic mutuality demonstrated responsive and reciprocal exchanges that were marked by a high degree of cooperation and closeness. Supporting the entropy findings, dyads high in both mutuality and deviant talk were especially likely to demonstrate high levels of antisocial behavior. These results lend support to the idea that the most reciprocally engaging and organized friendships may also be the most influential in creating norms for behavior, be they deviant or prosocial.

These findings suggest a psychological adaptation to deviant peer involvement that is highly related to negative influence. Kiesner, Cadinu, Poulin, and Bucci (2002) found that, indeed, those youth who psychologically identified with being in a deviant peer group were more likely to be influenced by members of the group. This study provides some psychological explanation for the powerful influence of gangs. Several researchers have noted that despite deviant youth behavior prior to involvement in the gang, it is gang involvement that leads to increased problem behavior (Craig, Vitaro, Gagnon, & Tremblay, 2002; Lacourse, Nagin, Tremblay, Vitaro, & Claes, 2003; Lahey, Gordon, Loeber, Stouthamer-Loeber, & Farrington, 1999; Thornberry, 1998). Not surprisingly, similarity in problem behaviors creates the initial bonds for gang involvement; however, it is also known that the gang members often have histories of peer rejection and poor academic performance (Dishion et al., 2005).

Several researchers have noted that involvement with deviant peers is not without emotional consequences. Youth heavily involved with deviant peers also tend to experience depression (Brendgen, Vitaro, & Bukowski, 2000). Two possible mechanisms account for high levels of depression among children involved in deviant peer groups or gangs. The first is that poor emotional adjustment may precede gang involvement. Dishion (2000) found evidence to support the predisposition hypothesis. Youth who were comorbid for internalizing and externalizing problems were most intensely engaged in deviant peer groups. When observed interacting with a friend, these youth had longer bouts of deviant talk. The second explanation for the significant association between depression and deviant peer involvement is that these youth do not form warm, close, and intimate relationships (Brendgen, Little, et al., 2000). Connell and Dishion (2006) examined the month-by-month lives of high-risk children and found that months of peer difficulties predicted depressed mood. Interpersonal conflicts and abrasive interactions appear to predict intrapersonal depression (see also Monroe & Harkness, 2005; Vernberg, 1990). Thus, in adolescence there is considerable evidence that peers contribute to growth in problem behavior and are at the core of unhappiness for many teenagers.

There is also evidence that peers can undermine healthy development in other ways. For example, there is a tendency for self-mutilation behaviors to cluster among peer networks in a contagion-like fashion (Rosen & Walsh, 1989). Youth placed in juvenile correction settings develop friendships and networks conducive to learning new forms of crime and strategies for manipulating law enforcement (Clarke-McLean, 1996). A salient and poignant example of learning new ways to behave dysfunctionally derives from iatrogenic effects for programs and contexts designed to prevent problems and promote positive youth development.

Iatrogenic Effects of Interventions

Recently, Dodge, Dishion, and Lansford (2006) reviewed the transdisciplinary literature on intervention programs and strategies involving peer aggregation. Salient examples included the St. Louis Experiment (Feldman, Caplinger, & Wodarski, 1983), the Cambridge Somerville Youth Study (McCord, 2003), and community recreation programs that aggregated youth (Mahony, Schweder, & Stattin, 2002). Interest in this topic was awakened when Dishion and colleagues randomly assigned high-risk youth (average age 12) to cognitive-behavioral interventions delivered to high-risk families in either peer groups (with a focus on self-regulation) or parent groups (with a focus on family management). The good news was that the intervention delivered in peer groups improved adolescent adjustment, as determined by youth reports of skills and observed interactions with parents. The bad news was that the peer intervention also led to increases in reported tobacco use and teacher reports of problem behavior at school over the 3-year follow-up period (Dishion & Andrews, 1995; Poulin, Dishion, & Burraston, 2001).

These findings precipitated additional reports of the possible harm associated with interventions that aggregate high-risk youth (group interventions, summer camps, etc.). Figure 32.2 provides a summary of these studies, as well as of several others, relevant to the issue of whether adults' efforts to improve child and adolescent outcomes can at times be misguided and lead to negative outcomes.

In many ways, the developmental literature on peer contagion and problematic adjustment fits well with the intervention literature on iatrogenic effects. For example, the way in which public schools are organized with respect to the placement of students into classrooms suggests reason for concern. Two intervention studies document that random assignment of youth to classrooms with other aggressive children can escalate problematic behavior (Kellam, Ling, Merisca, Brown, & Ialongo, 1998; Warren, Schoppelrey, Moberg, & McDonald, 2005). Based on the extant data, "selected" interventions are the most problematic. In these interventions, children with a particular psychological profile (high probability of future drug use, delinquency, depression, or eating disorders) are identified; a skills-building curriculum is delivered that putatively protects the children from future harm. This strategy varies from "treatment," in that the youth have yet to show the psychopathology one wishes to prevent. Unfortunately, it appears that these

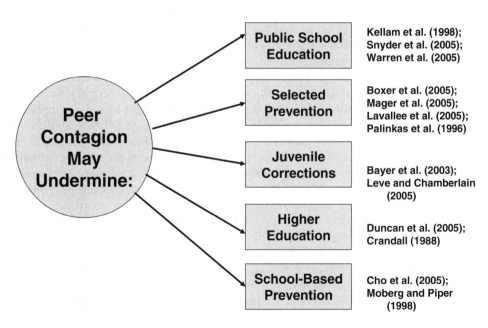

FIGURE 32.2. Research indicating peer contagion undermining intervention goals. Data from Dishion and Dodge (2005).

types of interventions carry the highest risk of either having harmful effects or, more commonly, reducing effect sizes (Lipsey, 2006). Children identified as engaging in delinquent behavior (covert, proactive aggression, etc.) or as using drugs can increase these behaviors within the intervention (Dishion, McCord, & Poulin, 1999; Palinkas, Atkins, Miller, & Ferreira, 1996).

Several researchers suggest that group constitution can be instrumental but complex in nature (e.g., Boxer, Guerra, Huesmann, & Morales, 2005; Mager, Milich, Harris, & Howard, 2005). Dishion, Poulin, and Burraston (2001) found subtle but directly observable dynamics of deviancy training in a group reliably associated with increasing tobacco use and delinquent behavior over a 3-year period. Some youth evoked attention and support for their deviant behavior in the intervention group, and these experiences largely took place during unstructured times, such as prior to the onset of the session, during breaks, and when youth were leaving the group meetings. Similar effects have been observed in the Fast Track social skills training groups delivered in school settings, within which children with escalated aggressive behavior evoked positive responses from peers for their aggressive behavior (Lavallee, Bierman, Nix, & Conduct Problems Prevention Research Group, 2005). It is important to note, however, that we do not mean to suggest that the Fast Track intervention had an overall negative effect. The social skills training group was only one component of a comprehensive prevention strategy (e.g., Conduct Problems Prevention Research Group, 2002).

Schools are often the hosts of interventions to reduce or prevent adolescent problem behaviors and, on occasion, those interventions can fail. For example, interventions to reduce the contraction of HIV infection from unsafe sexual practices have revealed that extensive discussion of these issues in the classroom increased the rate of sexual contact and unsafe sexual practices (Moberg & Piper, 1998). Similarly, creating special high school classrooms for the laudable goal of reconnecting youth who are in the dropout process can, under some circumstances, lead to increases in problem behavior (Cho, Hallfors, & Sanchez, 2005). Often well-intended group leaders, who are likely not well trained in the subtleties of deviancy training, inadvertently reward deviant talk and behavior.

Furthermore, incarcerating problem youth may be harmful given the contagion effects noted earlier. It is easy to imagine that youth leave residential correction settings not only "hardened" with respect to coping with deviant behavior directed toward them, but also with an enhanced repertoire of other problematic behaviors. An unpublished report by Bayer, Pintoff, and Pozen (2003) revealed a statistically reliable tendency for youth to reoffend by committing the crimes of their compatriots in the juvenile correction center. Research that compares group residential placement with an individualized treatment foster care approach indicates that group care leads to deviant peer involvement, which, unsurprisingly, predicts future offending. In contrast, random assignment to treatment foster care, which emphasizes adult monitoring, reduces deviant peer involvement and ultimately translates into fewer arrests and delinquent offenses (Chamberlain & Moore, 1998; Leve & Chamberlain, 2005).

As noted earlier, growth and development are accompanied by increased opportunities for autonomous decision making. Examples include the selection of colleges, friendships, and rooming situations. Duncan, Boisjoly, Kremer, Levy, and Eccles (2005) have suggested that choosing a college roommate is not as mundane as it might otherwise seem. Random assignment of roommates with histories of drinking leads to significant increases in alcohol consumption during the first 2 years of college. In one study, random assignment to programs designed to reduce the risk of eating disorders had the effect of increasing risk (Mann et al., 1997). Most recently, it was reported that obesity may be affected by the weight of one's friends; there is an overall tendency to select friends who are of similar girth, and having an obese friend increases the likelihood of one's own obesity in the future (Christakis & Fowler, 2007).

Three major points can be made about the literature on harmful effects of interventions that aggregate similar youth. First, not all interventions that aggregate result in negative effects; many have positive outcomes (e.g., Weiss et al., 2005). However, it is not generally the rule that published intervention researchers report child and adolescent outcomes that do not support intervention effectiveness.

Second, interventions that aggregate high-risk youth often do so with the implicit goal of improving an educational environment or community by removing the "problem" children (Cook & Ludwig, 2006). Thus, the removal of a child to an alternative school or classroom may improve the educational environment for other students. Similarly, offenders are locked up to prevent future crimes in the community; rehabilitation is perhaps a lesser concern. Yet it is still unknown whether removal from a school or community benefits both the youth and the community (Cook & Ludwig, 2006).

Third, there appears to be some developmental and contextual sensitivity to iatrogenic effects of interventions delivered in peer groups. When interventions target problem behaviors that are of high interest to group members in their particular stage in development, these very behaviors may be most vulnerable to deviant peer contagion (Dishion, Dodge, & Lansford, 2006). It may be that a state of readiness influences the likelihood of peer contagion effects. For example, aggression among elementary school children, or substance use, delinquency, and sexual behavior among adolescents, are examples of behaviors that are of interest to individuals at specific stages of their development. Eating and diet issues are of central importance to adolescents and young adults. College students are often for the first time going to parties at which alcohol is freely available. Perhaps their high level of focus on the opinions of their peers regarding these developmentally relevant behaviors increases susceptibility of youth to contagion effects. Thus, age may be seen as a potentially strong moderating factor for deviant peer contagion.

From developmental research, it is clear that individual differences in youth self-regulation buffer the effect of deviant friendships on subsequent problem behavior (Dishion & Connell, 2007; Goodnight, Bates, Newman, Dodge, & Pettit, 2006). For example, youth with high levels of self-regulation have been found to be less susceptible to the risks of associating with tobacco-using peers. For those adolescents with tobacco-using peers, highly self-regulated youth demonstrated less increase in tobacco use from ages 16 to 19 than did youth with poorer self-regulation (Piehler & Dishion, 2007).

Finally, the context of an intervention may be as important as the content for producing negative effects (Dishion et al., 2006). For example, consider a social skills training intervention conducted in a university or medical setting, involving random assignment and careful attention to youth informally aggregating around the clinic setting. Contrast this with the same intervention offered in a community setting, close to a bus terminal where high-risk youth in the community are "hanging out." Whereas the latter intervention might lead to iatrogenic effects, the former might lead to positive effects. The intervention offered in the community setting does not account for the incidental interactions of a youth with other high-risk youth that might contribute to the development of deviant behavior. Youth may meet after the group and smoke cigarettes at the bus terminal, or steal from the surrounding shopping mall. In this sense, the ecology of a program, intervention, and policy must be considered carefully when determining whether youth will actually benefit from intervention.

Summary and Future Directions

Developmental research on peer contagion in "naturally occurring" peer groups can begin in early childhood and continue through late adolescence. Observational studies of preschool playgrounds, interactions, and dynamics among children in public elementary schools, friendships in adolescence, formation of gangs in community settings, and assignment of roommates in college dorms all have revealed significant negative effects of deviant peer contagion on individual adjustment. In future research, we propose that adults (especially in families and schools) who are highly influential in child and adolescent development play a role in the structuring of day-to-day contacts with peers. Supervision, attention, involvement, positive relationships with youth, and behavior management skills all are integrally related to adults' influence on children's and adolescents' participation in the peer group (Dishion & Stormshak, 2007; Patterson et al., 1992). When family management breaks down, children are often left to raise themselves in the company of friends; in these cases, there is strong potential for becoming entrained in interpersonal styles that support and maintain deviance throughout the early adult years (Dishion, Nelson, & Bullock, 2004; Dishion, Nelson, & Winter, 2004). Dishion, Bullock, and Kiesner (2008) have found that simply counting the number of unsupervised hours per day with peers was the best predictor of growth in drug use among high-risk adolescents. The solution may be as simple as designing programs and environments for children and adolescents that optimize contacts with caring and mindful adults with peer management skills (Dishion et al., 2008).

References

Anthony, J. C. (2006). Deviant peer effects: Perspectives of an epidemiologist. In K. A. Dodge, T. J. Dishion, & J. E. Lansford (Eds.), *Deviant peer influences in programs for youth: Problems and solutions* (pp. 44–66). New York: Guilford Press.

Bayer, P., Pintoff, R., & Pozen, D. (2003). *Building criminal capital behind bars: Social learning in juvenile corrections.* Unpublished manuscript, Yale University.

Boxer, P., Guerra, N. G., Huesmann, L., & Morales, J. (2005). Proximal peer-level effects of a small-group selected prevention on aggression in elementary school children: An investigation of the peer contagion hypothesis. *Journal of Abnormal Child Psychology, 33*(3), 325–338.

Brendgen, M., Little, T. D., & Krappmann, L. (2000). Rejected children and their friends: A shared evaluation of friendship quality? *Merrill–Palmer Quarterly, 46,* 45–70.

Brendgen, M., Vitaro, F., & Bukowski, W. M. (2000). Deviant friends and early adolescents' emotional and behavioral adjustment. *Journal of Research on Adolescence, 10*(2), 173–189.

Bronfenbrenner, U. (1979). *The ecology of human development: Experiments by nature and by design.* Cambridge, MA: Harvard University Press.

Chamberlain, P., & Moore, K. J. (1998). Models of community treatment for serious offenders. In J. Crane (Ed.), *Social programs that really work* (pp. 258–276). Princeton, NJ: Russell Sage Foundation.

Cho, H., Hallfors, D. D., & Sanchez, V. (2005). Evaluation of a high school peer group intervention for at-risk youth. *Journal of Abnormal Child Psychology, 33*(3), 363–374.

Christakis, N. A., & Fowler, J. H. (2007). The spread of obesity in a large social network over 32 years. *New England Journal of Medicine, 357,* 370–379.

Clarke-McLean, J. G. (1996). Social networks among incarcerated juvenile offenders. *Social Development, 5,* 203–217.

Coie, J. D., & Kupersmidt, J. B. (1983). A behavioral analysis of emerging social status in boys groups. *Child Development, 54,* 1400–1416.

Conduct Problems Prevention Research Group. (2002). The implementation of the Fast Track program: An example of a large-scale prevention science efficacy trial. *Journal of Abnormal Child Psychology, 30,* 1–17.

Connell, A. M., & Dishion, T. J. (2006). The contribution of peers to monthly variation in adolescent depressed mood: A short-term longitudinal study with time-varying predictors. *Development and Psychopathology, 18*(1), 1–16.

Cook, P. J., & Ludwig, J. (2006). Assigning youths to minimize total harm. In K. A. Dodge, T. J. Dishion, & J. E. Lansford (Eds.), *Deviant peer influences in programs for youth: Problems and solutions* (pp. 67–89). New York: Guilford Press.

Craig, W. M., Vitaro, F., Gagnon, C., & Tremblay, R. E. (2002). The road to gang membership: Characteristics of male gang and nongang members from ages 10 to 14. *Social Development, 11,* 53–68.

Crandall, C. S. (1988). Social contagion of binge eating. *Journal of Personality and Social Psychology, 55,* 588–598.

Crick, N. R., & Grotpeter, J. K. (1995). Relational aggression, gender, and social-psychological adjustment. *Child Development, 66,* 710–722.

Dawe, H. C. (1934). An analysis of two hundred quarrels of preschool children. *Child Development, 5,* 139–157.

Dishion, T. J. (1990). The family ecology of boys' peer relations in middle childhood. *Child Development, 61,* 874–892.

Dishion, T. J. (2000). Cross-setting consistency in early adolescent psychopathology: Deviant friendships and problem behavior sequelae. *Journal of Personality, 68*(6), 1109–1126.

Dishion, T. J., & Andrews, D. (1995). Preventing escalations in problem behaviors with high-risk young adolescents: Immediate and 1-year outcomes. *Journal of Consulting and Clinical Psychology, 63,* 538–548.

Dishion, T. J., Bullock, B. M., & Kiesner, J. (2008). Vicissitudes of parenting adolescents: Daily variations in parental monitoring and the early emergence of drug use. In M. Kerr, H. Stattin, & R. C. M. E. Engels (Eds.), *What can parents do? New insights into the role of parents in adolescent problem behavior* (pp. 113–133). Chichester, UK: Wiley.

Dishion, T. J., Capaldi, D., Spracklen, K. M., & Li, F. (1995). Peer ecology of male adolescent drug use. *Development and Psychopathology, 7,* 803–824.

Dishion, T. J., & Connell, A. M. (2007). Adolescents' resilience as a self-regulatory process: Promising themes for linking intervention with developmental science. In B. M. Lester, A. Masten, & B. McEwen (Eds.), *Resilience in children* (pp. 125–138). Boston: New York Academy of Sciences.

Dishion, T. J., Dodge, K. A., & Lansford, J. E. (2006). Findings and recommendations: A blueprint to minimize deviant peer influence in youth interventions and programs. In K. A. Dodge, T. J. Dishion, & J. E. Lansford (Eds.), *Deviant peer influences in programs for youth: Problems and solutions* (pp. 366–394). New York: Guilford Press.

Dishion, T. J., Eddy, J. M., Haas, E., Li, F., & Spracklen, K. (1997). Friendships and violent behavior during adolescence. *Social Development, 6,* 207–223.

Dishion, T. J., McCord, J., & Poulin, F. (1999). When interventions harm: Peer groups and problem behavior. *American Psychologist, 54*(9), 755–764.

Dishion, T. J., Nelson, S. E., & Bullock, B. M. (2004). Premature adolescent autonomy: Parent disengagement and deviant peer process in the amplification of problem behavior [Special issue]. *Journal of Adolescence, 27,* 515–530.

Dishion, T. J., Nelson, S. E., Winter, C., & Bullock, B. M. (2004). Adolescent friendship as a dynamic system: Entropy and deviance in the etiology and course of male antisocial behavior. *Journal of Abnormal Child Psychology, 32*(6), 651–663.

Dishion, T. J., Nelson, S. E., & Yasui, M. (2005). Predicting early adolescent gang involvement from middle school adaptation. *Journal of Clinical Child and Adolescent Psychology, 34*(1), 62–73.

Dishion, T. J., Patterson, G. R., Stoolmiller, M., & Skinner, M. S. (1991). Family, school, and behavioral antecedents to early adolescent involvement with antisocial peers. *Developmental Psychology, 27*, 172–180.

Dishion, T. J., Poulin, F., & Burraston, B. (2001). Peer group dynamics associated with iatrogenic effects in group interventions with high-risk young adolescents. In C. Erdley & D. W. Nangle (Eds.), *New directions in child development: The role of friendship in psychological adjustment* (pp. 79–92). San Francisco: Jossey-Bass.

Dishion, T. J., Spracklen, K. M., Andrews, D. W., & Patterson, G. R. (1996). Deviancy training in male adolescent friendships. *Behavior Therapy, 27*, 373–390.

Dishion, T. J., & Stormshak, E. A. (2007). *Intervening in children's lives: An ecological, family-centered approach to mental health care.* Washington, DC: American Psychological Association.

Dodge, K. A. (1983). Behavioral antecedents: A peer social status. *Child Development, 54*, 1386–1399.

Dodge, K. A., Dishion, T. J., & Lansford, J. E. (Eds.). (2006). *Deviant peer influences in programs for youth: Problems and solutions.* New York: Guilford Press.

Duncan, G. J., Boisjoly, J., Kremer, M., Levy, D. M., & Eccles, J. (2005). Peer effects in drug use and sex among college students. *Journal of Abnormal Child Psychology, 33*(3), 375–385.

Ellis, S., Rogoff, B., & Cromer, C. (1981). Age segregation in children's interactions. *Developmental Psychology, 17*, 399–407.

Feldman, R. A., Caplinger, T. E., & Wodarski, J. S. (1983). *The St. Louis conundrum.* Englewood Cliffs, NJ: Prentice-Hall.

Furman, W., & Masters, J. C. (1980). Peer interactions, sociometric status, and resistance to deviation in young children. *Developmental Psychology, 16*, 229–236.

Giordano, P. C., Cernkovich, S. A., & Pugh, M. D. (1986). Friendships and delinquency. *American Journal of Sociology, 91*, 1170–1202.

Goodnight, J. A., Bates, J. E., Newman, J. P., Dodge, K. A., & Pettit, G. S. (2006). The interactive influences of friend deviance and reward dominance on the development of externalizing behavior during middle adolescence. *Journal of Abnormal Child Psychology, 34*, 573–583.

Granic, I., & Dishion, T. J. (2003). Deviant talk in adolescent friendships: A step toward measuring a pathogenic attractor process. *Social Development, 12*, 314–334.

Grotpeter, J. K., & Crick, N. R. (1996). Relational aggression, overt aggression, and friendship. *Child Development, 67*, 2328–2338.

Hartup, W. W. (1996). The company they keep: Friendships and their developmental significance. *Child Development, 67*, 1–13.

Kellam, S., Ling, X., Merisca, R., Brown, H., & Ialongo, N. (1998). The effect of the level of aggression in the first grade classroom on the course of malleability of aggressive behavior into the middle school. *Development and Psychopathology, 10*(2), 165–185.

Kiesner, J., Cadinu, M., Poulin, F., & Bucci, M. (2002). Group identification in early adolescence: Its relation with peer adjustment and its moderator effect on peer influence. *Child Development, 73*, 196–208.

Kindermann, T. A. (1993). Natural peer groups as contexts for individual development: The case of children's motivation in school. *Developmental Psychology, 29*, 970–977.

Lacourse, E., Nagin, D., Tremblay, R. E., Vitaro, F., & Claes, M. (2003). Developmental trajectories of boys' delinquent group membership and facilitation of violent behaviors during adolescence. *Development and Psychopathology, 15*, 183–197.

Lahey, B. B., Gordon, R. A., Loeber, R., Stouthamer-Loeber, M., & Farrington, D. P. (1999). Boys who join gangs: A prospective study of predictors of first gang entry. *Journal of Abnormal Child Psychology, 27,* 261–276.

Lavallee, K. L., Bierman, K. L., Nix, R. L., & Conduct Problems Prevention Research Group. (2005). The impact of first-grade "friendship group" experiences on child social outcomes in the Fast Track program. *Journal of Abnormal Child Psychology, 33,* 307–324.

Leve, L. D., & Chamberlain, P. (2005). Association with delinquent peers: Intervention effects for youth in the juvenile justice system. *Journal of Abnormal Child Psychology, 33*(3), 339–347.

Light, J. M., & Dishion, T. J. (2007). Early adolescent antisocial behavior and peer rejection: A dynamic test of a developmental process. In P. C. Rodkin & L. D. Hanish (Eds.), *Social network analysis and children's peer relationships* (pp. 77–89). San Francisco: Jossey-Bass.

Lipsey, M. (2006). The effects of community-based group treatment for delinquency: A meta-analytic search for cross-study generalizations. In K. A. Dodge, T. J. Dishion, & J. E. Lansford (Eds.), *Deviant peer influences in programs for youth: Problems and solutions* (pp. 162–184). New York: Guilford Press.

Loeber, R., & Schmaling, K. B. (1985). Empirical evidence for overt and covert patterns of antisocial conduct problems: A meta-analysis. *Journal of Abnormal Child Psychology, 13,* 337–352.

Mager, W., Milich, R., Harris, M. J., & Howard, A. (2005). Intervention groups for adolescents with conduct problems: Is aggregation harmful or helpful? *Journal of Abnormal Child Psychology, 33*(3), 349–362.

Mahoney, J. L., Schweder, A. E., & Stattin, H. (2002). Structured after-school activities as a moderator of depressed mood for adolescents with detached relations to their parents. *Journal of Community Psychology, 30*(1), 69–86.

Mann, T., Nolen-Hoeksema, S., Huang, K., Burgard, D., Wright, A., & Hanson, K. (1997). Are two interventions worse than none? Joint primary and secondary prevention of eating disorders in college females. *Health Psychology, 16*(3), 215–225.

McCord, J. (2003). Cures that harm: Unanticipated outcomes of crime prevention programs. *Annals of the American Academy of Political and Social Science, 587,* 16–30.

Moberg, D. P., & Piper, D. L. (1998). The Healthy for Life project: Sexual risk behavior outcomes. *AIDS Education and Prevention, 10,* 128–148.

Monroe, S. M., & Harkness, K. L. (2005). Life stress, the "kindling" hypothesis, and the recurrence of depression: Considerations from a life stress perspective. *Psychological Review, 112*(2), 417–445.

Oden, S., Herzberger, S. D., Mangione, P. L., & Wheeler, V. A. (1984). Children's peer relationships: An examination of social processes. In J. C. Masters & K. Yarkin-Levin (Eds.), *Boundary areas in social and developmental psychology* (pp. 131–158). New York: Academic.

Palinkas, L. A., Atkins, C. J., Miller, C., & Ferreira, D. (1996). Social skills training for drug prevention in high-risk female adolescents. *Preventive Medicine, 25,* 692–701.

Patterson, G. R. (1982). *Coercive family process.* Eugene, OR: Castalia.

Patterson, G. R. (1993). Orderly change in a stable world: The antisocial trait as a chimera. *Journal of Consulting and Clinical Psychology, 61,* 911–919.

Patterson, G. R., Dishion, T. J., & Yoerger, K. (2000). Adolescent growth in new forms of problem behavior: Macro- and micro-peer dynamics. *Prevention Science, 1,* 3–13.

Patterson, G. R., Littman, R. A., & Bricker, W. (1967). Assertive behavior in children: A step toward a theory of aggression. *Monographs for the Research in Psychology and Child Development, 32,* 1–43.

Patterson, G. R., Reid, J. B., & Dishion, T. J. (1992). *Antisocial boys.* Eugene, OR: Castalia.

Piehler, T. F., & Dishion, T. J. (2007). Interpersonal dynamics within adolescent friendship: Dyadic mutuality and deviant talk and patterns of antisocial behavior. *Child Development, 78*(5), 1611–1624.

Poulin, F., & Boivin, M. (2000a). Proactive and reactive aggression: Evidence of a two-factor model. *Psychological Assessment, 12,* 115–122.

Poulin, F., & Boivin, M. (2000b). The role of proactive and reactive aggression: The formation and development of friendships in boys. *Developmental Psychology, 36*, 1–8.

Poulin, F., Dishion, T. J., & Burraston, B. (2001). Three-year iatrogenic effects associated with aggregating high-risk adolescents in cognitive–behavioral preventive interventions. *Applied Development Science, 5*(4), 214–224.

Poulin, F., Dishion, T. J., & Haas, E. (1999). The peer influence paradox: Relationship quality and deviancy training within male adolescent friendships. *Merrill–Palmer Quarterly, 45*, 42–61.

Rodkin, P. C., Farmer, T. W., Pearl, R., & Van Acker, R. (2000). Heterogeneity of popular boys: Antisocial and prosocial configurations. *Development Psychology, 36*, 14–24.

Rosen, P. M., & Walsh, D. S. W. (1989). Patterns of contagion in self-mutilation epidemics. *American Journal of Psychiatry, 146*(5), 656–658.

Rubin, K. H., Bukowski, W., & Parker, J. (2006). Peer interactions, relationships, and groups. In N. Eisenberg (Ed.), *Handbook of child psychology: Social, emotional, and personality development* (6th ed., pp. 571–645). New York: Wiley.

Sage, N. A., & Kindermann, T. A. (1999). Peer networks, behavior contingencies, and children's engagement in the classroom. *Merrill–Palmer Quarterly, 45*(1), 143–171.

Snyder, J., Horsch, E., & Childs, J. (1997). Peer relationships of young children: Affiliative choices and the shaping of aggressive behavior. *Journal of Child Clinical Psychology, 26*(2), 145–156.

Snyder, J., Schrepferman, L., McEachern, A., Barner, S., Johnson, K., & Provines, J. (2008). Peer deviancy training and peer coercion: Dual processes associated with early-onset conduct problems. *Child Development, 79*(2), 252–268.

Snyder, J., Schrepferman, L., Oeser, J., Patterson, G., Stoolmiller, M., Johnson, K., et al. (2005). Deviancy training and association with deviant peers in young children: Occurrence and contribution to early-onset conduct problems. *Development and Psychopathology, 17*(2), 397–413.

Stormshak, E. A., Bierman, K. L., Bruschi, C., Dodge, K. A., Coie, J. D., & Conduct Problems Prevention Research Group. (1999). The relation between behavior problems and peer preference in different classroom contexts. *Child Development, 70*, 169–182.

Thornberry, T. P. (1998). Membership in youth gangs and involvement in serious and violent offending. In R. Loeber & D. P. Farrington (Eds.), *Serious and violent juvenile offenders: Risk factors and successful interventions* (pp. 147–166). Newbury Park, CA: Sage.

Tudge, J. R. H. (1992). Processes and consequences of peer collaboration: A Vygotskian analysis. *Child Development, 63*, 1364–1379.

Underhill, P. (2004). *Call of the mall.* New York: Simon & Schuster.

Urberg, K. A., Degirmencioglu, S. M., & Pilgrim, C. (1997). Close friend and group influence on adolescent cigarette smoking and alcohol use. *Developmental Psychology, 33*, 834–844.

Vernberg, E. M. (1990). Psychological adjustment and experiences with peers during early adolescence: Reciprocal, incidental, or unidirectional relationships. *Journal of Abnormal Child Psychology, 18*, 187–198.

Warren, K., Schoppelrey, S., Moberg, D. P., & McDonald, M. (2005). A model of contagion through competition in the aggressive behaviors of elementary school students. *Journal of Abnormal Child Psychology, 33*(3), 283–292.

Weiss, B., Caron, A., Ball, S., Tapp, J., Johnson, M., & Weisz, J. R. (2005). Iatrogenic effects of group treatment for antisocial youths. *Journal of Consulting and Clinical Psychology, 73*(6), 1036–1044.

Youniss, J. (1980). *Parents and peers in social development: A Sullivan–Piaget perspective.* Chicago: University of Chicago Press.

CHAPTER 33

Social Skills Training to Improve Peer Relations

KAREN L. BIERMAN
C. J. POWERS

Based on empirical demonstrations that children who are unable to function adequately with peers are at risk for several forms of concurrent and subsequent maladjustment, clinically oriented peer researchers have recognized the need for the development of intervention strategies. Beginning in the late 1970s, social skill training (SST) programs, originally intended to remediate the deficits of clinic populations, were adapted to improve the social behaviors of children who were unaccepted by their peers. For a period of about 15 years, SST studies targeting unaccepted or rejected children flourished. Innovations in SST program design were linked closely with the rapidly evolving empirical literature on the developmental features, interpersonal dynamics, and longitudinal course of poor peer relations. Intervention research designs tested the short-term effects of alternative SST components and thereby provided a rich "feedback loop" to developmental theory, functioning as short-term experimental studies testing the hypotheses generated by naturalistic longitudinal studies. As research accumulated on the behavioral features and interpersonal dynamics associated with the most serious and chronic forms of peer rejection, however, the belief that short-term, stand-alone SST programs could change the long-term trajectories of the most high-risk children faded.

About the same time, the emergence of prevention science as a formal field of inquiry dramatically affected the design of preventive strategies. By the 1990s, SST was increasingly incorporated into epidemiologically based, long-term, multicomponent interventions targeting children with significant behavior problems (e.g., emerging conduct disorders, attention-deficit/hyperactivity disorder [ADHD]). In many of these intervention studies, the focus of SST continued to be the promotion of positive peer relations, but the nature of the multicomponent research designs made it impossible to detect the specific contribution or impact of the SST programs on child peer relations. Accordingly, SST intervention studies migrated toward the more "applied" end of the research spectrum, and the close, transactional relationship with developmental research on peer relations dissipated.

Since 2000, SST research has focused primarily on promoting behavior change in special needs populations; very few SST studies have targeted the improved peer relations of disliked children as a proximal outcome. Although innovations in SST have continued, they have often been embedded in disorder-specific, multicomponent intervention models. Insofar as these projects have not been well integrated with each other or with the broader literature on peer relations, SST intervention research has not continued to develop in a programmatic way. New peer intervention targets have emerged (e.g., bullying), but a comprehensive framework that fosters the identification of theoretical and methodological "common ground" across SST studies is currently lacking, creating an increasingly disparate empirical literature on peer interventions.

In this chapter, we review the "rise and fall" of research on SST interventions intended to improve the peer relations of unaccepted and rejected children, and we discuss the issues challenging this field of inquiry. Much of our discussion concerns the importance of the traditional transaction between developmental and intervention research on poor peer relations. A goal of this chapter is to consider whether and how a mutually enriching transaction between these domains of research might be recaptured.

Central Issues and Key Studies

Early Years (1970s to Early 1980s): Emergence of the SST "Coaching" Model

In the late 1970s, several landmark longitudinal studies demonstrated that poor peer relations in childhood predict serious adjustment difficulties in adolescence and early adulthood (Cowen, Pedersen, Babigian, Izzo, & Trost, 1973; Kohlberg, LaCross, & Ricks, 1972). This research prompted an intense interest in the development of preventive interventions among researchers studying peer relations. The hope was that timely interventions that focused on improving childhood peer relations could reduce exposure to the risks associated with rejection and isolation, promote healthy peer socialization, and thereby foster positive long-term outcomes (Bierman, 2004; LaGreca, 1993).

At this same time clinical research relied primarily on behavioral management strategies to address the social behavior problems of young children. Several studies had demonstrated that contingency management could be employed in social settings to reinforce positive child behaviors (using contingent attention, token reinforcement, or primary reinforcements) or to decrease undesirable child behaviors (using time-out, response–cost, and differential reinforcement programs; see Elliott & Gresham, 1993). For example, a number of studies demonstrated that teachers could increase the rate at which socially isolated children approached peers by prompting them to initiate social interaction, then providing selective attention and praise (Strain, Shores, & Kerr, 1976). Although these operant techniques effectively increased the performance of behaviors within a child's repertoire, it quickly became clear that contingency management alone could not produce sustained improvements in child social behavior, nor did these strategies improve the quality of children's peer relations.

By the end of the 1970s, the SST intervention approach, which emerged originally as an intervention for adult clinical populations, was being applied to children, with the explicit goal of improving their peer relations by fostering socially competent behavior

(Ladd & Mize, 1983). The premise of the SST model was that social skills deficits make it difficult for children to engage effectively in mutually enjoyable social exchanges with peers. The model assumes that these skills can be taught, and that the remediation of skill deficits will result in improved social behavior that, in turn, will elicit positive peer responding and acceptance (Ladd & Mize, 1983; Elliott & Gresham, 1993). Coaching programs begin by presenting target skills concepts to participants using a combination of modeling, instruction, and discussion, often with exposure to both positive and negative examples. The purpose of SST is to enhance children's skills knowledge and understanding, providing information about the purpose, form, and functional value of the target skills (Ladd & Mize, 1983). Next, to promote their abilities to perform the skills comfortably and flexibly, children are provided with opportunities for behavioral rehearsal, practicing the skills with peer partners under supportive conditions. Finally, children receive performance feedback and reinforcement. In addition to helping the child adjust his or her social behavior, the purpose of this feedback is to strengthen the child's attention to his or her own behavior and awareness of its interpersonal impact. By enhancing the child's self-monitoring and social awareness, the goal is to promote socially responsive behavioral flexibility (Bierman, 2004). The majority of SST training studies (then and now) target clinical or special needs populations and focus on changing social behavior. The coaching studies that emerged in the late 1970s focused on improving children's peer relations as well, and utilized developmental research on peer relations in new ways to inform intervention design and evaluation.

Research-Based Adaptations of the SST Model

During the 1980s, developmental research on peer relations informed the methods used to define target skills, as well as the standards used to assess intervention effectiveness. Initial SST programs focused primarily on increasing children's rate of peer interaction or social behaviors selected on the basis of face validity (greeting behaviors, eye contact; Elliott & Gresham, 1993). Developmental research, however, had demonstrated that discrete social behaviors rarely had "absolute" value in social situations. Instead, their impact on others often depended upon factors such as context, timing, and partners (Rubin, Bukowski, & Parker, 2006). Social competence was redefined in terms of a child's capacity to affect the social responses of others (elicit positive responses and avoid negative responses) in a manner consistent with prevailing social conventions and morals (Dodge & Murphy, 1984). Methodologically, researchers began to use the "competence correlates" approach to identify skills targets for SST. In this strategy, behavioral response classes, such as "cooperation," were targeted for intervention based on empirical evidence of correlation with peer acceptance (LaGreca, 1993). Parallel to this change, sociometric measures became the "gold standard" for assessing intervention impact on social competence and peer relations.

Initial SST Studies Promoting Peer Relations

One of the first studies to use a randomized, controlled group comparison approach to evaluate the sociometric impact of coaching was conducted by Oden and Asher (1977). Relative to a peer play condition and no-treatment condition, unaccepted third and fourth graders who received five coaching sessions showed significant gains in "play with" sociometric ratings at posttreatment, although no behavioral improvements were documented. Following this initial project, several other studies used SST to enhance the prosocial behavior and peer acceptance of children selected on the basis of low peer acceptance scores. Gresham and Nagle (1980) compared the impact of SST components (e.g., coaching only, modeling only, coaching and modeling). LaGreca and Santogrossi (1980) varied the timing of coaching sessions, using longer sessions held after school.

In general, the results from these studies were promising but mixed. Some studies produced significant improvements on peer ratings (Gresham & Nagle, 1980; Oden & Asher, 1977), whereas others reported no significant impact (LaGreca & Santogrossi, 1980). Most demonstrated some behavioral changes (Gresham & Nagle, 1980; LaGreca & Santogrossi, 1980), but some did not (Oden & Asher, 1977). Overall, these studies demonstrated a "proof of concept" for the SST approach to improving peer relations but suggested that further refinements were needed to strengthen the consistency and size of effect, as well as to promote generalized maintenance of behavioral and sociometric gains.

Refining the Coaching Method

As the coaching model evolved during the 1980s, several new innovations increased the effectiveness of this approach. First, developmental research revealed considerable behavioral heterogeneity among children with low peer acceptance, as well as evidence that nonbehavioral characteristics contributed to the low acceptance of some children. Given that SST improves peer acceptance by remediating the skills deficits associated with peer problems, it followed that SST would be most effective for the subset of children who showed preintervention deficits in the targeted skills. Hence, researchers began to use a dual screen process, selecting participants based upon both low sociometric ratings and observed deficits in the targeted social skills. In addition, the typical SST program increased in length (from 4–5 sessions to 8–12 sessions). Finally, a greater emphasis was placed on the involvement of peers in the intervention sessions, with the goal of enhancing the generalization of intervention effects to classroom peer interactions and peer evaluations.

For example, in both Ladd (1981) and Bierman and Furman (1984), children were chosen based on evidence from sociometric ratings indicating low peer acceptance, along with observations indicating deficits in conversation skills. Each of these SST programs included 12 sessions, essentially doubling the amount of instructional time used by Oden and Asher (1977), and including more naturalistic practice opportunities. Both of these studies also incorporated peer partners into coaching sessions in new ways, in the hope of increasing the magnitude and sustainability of program impact on peer attitudes and evaluations. Although the SST model assumes that improvements in child social behavior will promote changes in peer responses and attitudes, developmental research had also documented an array of other factors affecting peer evaluations, including negative reputational biases (Coie, 1990; Hymel, Wagner, & Butler, 1990). There was no guarantee that improved behavior would secure positive peer inclusion or evaluation. Furthermore, nonresponsive peers could effectively "extinguish" behavioral gains made in SST, making a focus on peer responses a central issue for SST design (see also Bierman, 2004).

To strengthen peer involvement in SST, Ladd (1981) built upon the peer-pairing idea introduced by Oden and Asher (1977). In his SST program, he conducted six SST sessions with pairs of socially isolated children, then added two sessions with "rotating" peer partners, focused on promoting skills generalization to interactions with classmates.

Children in both the coached and the attention-control group improved in "play with" sociometric ratings collected immediately after the intervention, but only the coached children showed sustained improvements at the 4-week follow-up assessment.

The Bierman and Furman (1984) study compared SST conducted in the context of a small peer group (including one low-accepted child and two accepted classmates) with SST conducted individually or in a peer-group experience without SST. Similar to the Ladd (1981) study, children who interacted in play sessions with peers (with or without SST) received higher sociometric play ratings at the posttreatment assessment than the children who did not have the peer experience. The children who took part in the play sessions also rated themselves as more socially competent and showed higher rates of lunchtime peer interaction than children who did not have the peer experience. In this study, only children who received SST with peers showed enduring gains in conversation skills and improved social interaction, along with improved peer acceptance at the 6-week follow-up. Interestingly, a follow-up analysis of the intervention session videotapes showed that peer partners who participated in the SST sessions showed a higher rate of contingent positive responding to the positive behaviors of target children in the group coaching condition compared with the peers who were involved in groups that did not receive SST (Bierman, 1986). In other words, exposure to SST increased the positive responsivity of peers to the positive social behaviors of the low-accepted target children, thereby enhancing peer support for sustained behavior change.

A few critical conclusions can be reached based on these studies. Certainly, the studies from the 1970s to early 1980s established the potential of SST to enhance positive peer relations. SST began with a straightforward model that anticipated coaching would remediate the social skills deficits of socially isolated and unaccepted children, resulting in improved social behavior and enhanced peer acceptance. Although positive impact emerged, the desire to produce stronger, more consistent, and well-generalized effects led to several critical developments in intervention design, including extensions in program length, selective focus on behaviorally defined subgroups of unaccepted children, and inclusion of peer partners in intervention. Peer relations research informed these developments, documenting the behavioral heterogeneity among unaccepted children and the multidetermined nature of peer responses.

Middle Years (Mid-1980s to Mid-1990s)

Initial SST studies focused on promoting the prosocial behavior of "socially isolated" children with low levels of peer acceptance. However, by the early 1980s, peer relation research was beginning to document important differences between "neglected" and "rejected" children, both of whom tend to receive low ratings on roster-rating scales of peer acceptance (Coie, Dodge, & Coppotelli, 1982). Whereas neglected children were ignored and not well-liked by peers, they were not actively disliked. In contrast, rejected children not only were not well-liked, they were also actively disliked by classmates (Coie et al., 1982). Across studies, rejected children were more likely than neglected children to exhibit aggressive–disruptive behavioral problems, to be socially anxious and withdrawn, to experience psychological distress and to express loneliness, and to have cross-situational and stable adjustment difficulties (for a review, see Rubin et al., 2006). Rejected children were also more likely to experience ostracism and victimization by peers that contributed to feelings of resentment, frustration, and social anxiety over time (Coie, 1990; Rubin, Burgess, Kennedy, & Stewart, 2003). Indeed, evidence from landmark longitudinal studies suggested that rejected children (rather than neglected children) accounted for the strong predictive relations between childhood peer problems and adult mental health and adjustment difficulties (Cowen et al., 1973).

Developmental research documenting the particular characteristics of rejected children had important implications for SST design. Emergent research suggested that different skills were needed to avoid rejection than were needed to obtain acceptance (Rubin et al., 2006). Whereas the primary determinants of peer liking were positive social behaviors, including conversation skills and cooperative behaviors, the factors that led to peer dislike were aggressive–disruptive, hyperactive–inattentive, and anxious–avoidant behaviors (Bierman, Smoot, & Aumiller, 1993; Coie, Dodge, & Kupersmidt, 1990; Rubin et al., 2003). Correspondingly, interventions aimed at reducing rejection needed to focus both on promoting positive social behaviors to enhance peer liking and on reducing problem behaviors contributing to peer disliking.

To reduce problem behaviors, SST programs for rejected children began to incorporate intervention strategies used in cognitive-behavioral therapy that were linked theoretically with self-regulation and aggression control. Cognitive-behavioral models of child psychopathology, which were also emerging in the late 1970s and early 1980s, theorized that information-processing skills played a central role in the development of self-regulation. In particular, it was hypothesized that cognitive distortions and information-processing deficits contributed to dysregulated behavior problems, particularly ADHD and aggression (Abikoff, 1979; Kendall, 1985). The application of cognitive training models to improve peer relations first emerged in "universal," school-based social problem-solving programs. These models, with their emphasis on self-regulation, were then incorporated into SST interventions for rejected children.

School-Based Social Problem-Solving Interventions

School-based social problem-solving curricula, originally developed as "universal" primary prevention programs, emerged in the late 1970s, parallel to initial SST programs (Weissberg & Allen, 1986). Unlike behavioral management or modeling approaches, the social problem-solving method emphasized the importance of the thinking skills that regulate effective social interaction. The premise of these programs was that children's cognitive capacities to recognize and accurately assess social problems, as well as their ability to generate and evaluate multiple potential responses, to set goals, and to self-monitor their behavioral performance in light of those goals, provided the critical building blocks for flexible, responsive, and adaptive social behavior (Allen, Chinsky, Larcen, Lochman, & Selinger, 1976; Weissberg & Allen, 1986). Whereas initial SST programs promoted specific prosocial interaction strategies, initial social problem-solving programs emphasized covert thinking processes (e.g., generating alternative solutions, anticipating consequences) thought to foster regulatory control, particularly in interpersonal conflict situations (Spivack & Shure, 1974; Weissberg & Allen, 1986). These programs shared the goal of improving peer relations, albeit via different pathways

Weissberg and colleagues (1981) were among the first to assess the impact of a universal, classroom-based social problem-solving program on sociometric outcomes. The program, taught by teachers, utilized videotaped modeling, class discussions, and teacher-led role playing to foster social problem-solving skills development. Teachers were asked to foster students' generalized use of the skills by mediating peer conflicts using the social problem-solving steps. With this program, Weissberg et al. documented increases among children in intervention classes, compared with those in control classrooms, in areas of perceived social competence and teacher ratings of shy–anxious behaviors, general school adjustment, and global ratings of likability. Measures of changes in acceptance, as assessed by sociometric scores, however, showed no intervention effects.

Developmental research on rejected children suggested that the information-processing and self-regulatory skills targeted in social problem-solving interventions might address deficits that characterized many rejected children. Specifically, asocial goals, negatively biased social perceptions and interpretations, and a reliance on domineering approaches to social problem solving had emerged in developmental research on the social-cognitive processing skills of both aggressive and rejected children (Dodge, 1989). Based on these observations, social-cognitive intervention techniques designed to reduce child aggression by teaching children to inhibit their initial responses, and to think more carefully about the causes and effects of their social behavior, appeared particularly appropriate (Lochman & Lenhart, 1993).

Interventions that adapted social problem-solving skills training specifically for aggressive children began to emerge. For example, Lochman, Burch, Curry, and Lampron (1984) developed the Anger Coping program. This 12-session group program included coaching in self-control procedures, anger coping strategies, and interpersonal problem-solving skills. In addition, teachers monitored classroom behavior, providing contingent reinforcement for the inhibition of aggressive behaviors and the display of positive behaviors. The program was shown to be effective at reducing aggressive behavior according to both parent and youth reports. Peer ratings of aggression, however, were not affected by the program (Lochman et al., 1984).

Similarly, Hudley and Graham (1993) developed an attributional reframing intervention designed to reduce hostile attributions among aggressive African American boys in grades 4–5. The 12-session attributional intervention was designed to train boys to detect intentionality accurately, to make attributions of nonhostile intent when intentionality was unclear, and to develop decision rules to guide decision making when facing ambiguous causation. Relative to boys randomly assigned to attention or to no-treatment control groups, aggressive boys in the attribution training condition showed decreases in hostile attribution in laboratory and hypothetical situations, and were rated by teachers as less aggressive than at pretreatment. No changes were observed, however, in teacher ratings of prosocial behavior.

Considered together, the results of both universal and indicated intervention programs suggested that cognitive interventions (targeting social information-processing and social problem-solving skills) might support positive behavioral improvements among aggressive children. Used alone, however, neither of them appeared to be sufficient to promote positive social engagement or improve the peer relations of rejected children.

Expanding SST Programs for Rejected Children

In recognition of the need for continued efforts to build the prosocial skills of rejected children, expanded multicomponent SST models began to emerge. These new projects emphasized the promotion of positive behaviors to promote peer liking (with SST) in addition to the self-regulatory skills needed to reduce aggressive and insensitive social behaviors, and the use of contingency management procedures to reduce aggression.

In support of this general approach, Bierman, Miller, and Stabb (1987) found that aggressive–rejected boys in grades 1–3 who received a coaching program that included a joint focus on increasing positive behaviors along with inhibiting negative (aggressive) behaviors showed greater sociometric and behavioral improvements than boys who received a program that focused on only one of these aspects of behavior change.

Lochman, Coie, Underwood, and Terry (1993) developed and tested the effects of an ambitious, comprehensive SST program for aggressive–rejected fourth graders. They used an extended period of individual sessions (26 sessions, lasting 30 minutes each) followed by eight small-group sessions designed to promote practice of adaptive social behavior in naturalistic peer interactions. Sessions focused on both positive skills (cooperative play skills and group entry) and self-regulatory social-cognitive skills (dealing effectively with negative feelings and social problem-solving skills). Multiple intervention strategies were used to support both social-cognitive and behavior change, including modeling videotapes, discussion, role playing, instruction in self-talk, cooperative activities (including group video making), feedback, and goal setting. Postintervention and 1-year follow-up data showed reductions in observed aggression and peer-nominated rejection for coached children compared with the no-treatment group. The length and structure of the program, with multiple instructional strategies, graduated and extended opportunities to practice and consolidate skills, and the dual focus on both prosocial interaction strategies and self-regulatory skills may have contributed to the effectiveness of this program for aggressive–rejected children.

Addressing the Academic Deficits of Rejected Children

As SST programs expanded to include a broader set of intervention strategies targeting a broader array of skills (prosocial and self-regulatory), emerging evidence also suggested that the academic deficits that characterized many rejected children might also (in addition to their behavior) disrupt their peer relations. An innovative SST study conducted by Coie and Krehbiel (1984) targeted peer-rejected children who also exhibited significant academic difficulties in reading or math. Their study compared the effects of (1) academic skills training alone, (2) SST alone, (3) the combination of academic skills and SST, and (4) no treatment. Children who received academic skills training improved in multiple domains, showing more increases in on-task behavior in the classroom, higher achievement scores, and higher social preference scores than untreated children. In contrast, SST alone produced only transitory improvements in sociometric ratings and no changes in classroom behavior. Coie and Krehbiel suggested that the academic delays led to student frustration and high rates of disruptive, off-task behaviors in the classroom that in turn alienated peers. They hypothesized that the academic improvements promoted improved classroom behavior that in turn enhanced peer relations. In addition, tutoring was conducted in the context of positive, one-to-one relationships with adults, which may have provided children with a source of social–emotional support in the school setting, positively influencing their affect and social behavior.

Additional evidence emerged from studies of children with learning disabilities, suggesting that, for children with academic difficulties, interventions targeting academic skills also improve peer relations. Indeed, a meta-analytic review of such studies by Wanzek, Vaugh, Kim, and Cavanaugh (2006) suggests that academic interventions for students with learning disabilities consistently produce small benefits on teacher-rated and sociometric measures of peer relations.

Meta-Analyses

Two meta-analyses conducted in the early 1990s summarized the impact of SST and social problem-solving interventions on children's social competence and peer relations (Beelman, Pfingsten, & Losel, 1994; Schneider, 1992). Beelman et al. (1994) found strong effects on social cognitions, such as responses to hypothetical social problem-solving vignettes (Cohen's $d = 0.83$). Program effects on targeted behaviors, assessed via direct observations, showed moderate effect sizes ($d = 0.49$), as did peer, parent, and teacher reports of child behavior (d's ranging from 0.40 to 0.47). Sociometric measures of peer status and reputation, however, appeared particularly difficult to change (Beelman et al., 1994), and many studies showed limited generalization and maintenance of effects (Gresham, 1994).

Summary

In many ways, the 1980s represented the "heyday" of SST research focused on improving peer relations, both in terms of the number of SST studies and the pace of innovation (Beelman et al., 1994; LaGreca, 1993). Intervention models utilized cognitive-behavioral change techniques drawn from clinical psychology, but design innovations were fueled primarily by developmental research on peer relations. Rapid advancements were made in validating the criteria used to identify children in need of peer interventions, as well as in the measurement of outcomes (behavior change and improved peer relations). The effectiveness of various intervention components was tested in short-term studies that compared intervention components, contributing to increasingly complex and multifaceted interventions. By the end of the decade, there was considerable optimism about the power of SST programs to improve peer relations, reflected in meta-analyses that showed generally positive effects. However, there was also increasing concern about the potential of SST programs to alter the peer relations and developmental trajectories of rejected children, who often experienced risk factors in multiple domains (prosocial behavior, self-regulation, academic adjustment), complicating the challenge of improving their peer relations, and compounding their developmental risk.

Later Years (Mid-1990s to Mid-2000s)

As developmental research progressed, it confirmed that serious, concurrent behavior problems, attentional and academic deficits, and family risk factors often accompanied and contributed to chronic peer rejection. At the same time, studies of clinical populations, including children with ADHD, oppositional defiant disorder, and conduct disorder, revealed that significant social adjustment problems, including peer rejection, often accompanied the disorder and exacerbated children's behavioral and emotional adjustment difficulties (Parker, Rubin, Erath, Wojslawowicz, & Buskirk, 2006). For example, longitudinal research demonstrated that peer rejection increased the stability and negative outcomes associated with aggressive behavior problems (Cillessen, van IJzendoorn, van Lieshout, & Hartup, 1992; Miller-Johnson, Coie, Bierman, Maumary-Gremaud, & the Conduct Problems Prevention Research Group, 2002).

At the beginning of the 1990s, three factors significantly influenced the emerging shape of SST interventions. First, among peer intervention researchers, there was a growing concern that short-term, "stand alone" SST programs were unlikely to improve the peer relations of the most high-risk, chronically rejected children, who often had significant concurrent conduct problems (Bierman, 2004; LaGreca, 1993). Reviews of SST research called for intervention models that incorporated a broader perspective on the socializing influences that affected children's social behavior and peer relations (e.g., parents and teachers, as well as peers) (Coie & Koeppl, 1990; LaGreca, 1993; McFadyen-Ketchum & Dodge, 1998).

Second, clinical researchers developing prevention and early intervention programs targeting childhood behavior disorders such as ADHD and conduct disorder were increasingly interested in expanding traditionally parent-focused interventions focused on compliance training with intervention components that addressed social skills deficits and problematic peer relations (Coie & Dodge, 1998). As SST interventions increasingly targeted the highest-risk rejected children, their target populations began to overlap to an increasing extent with populations of interest to clinical researchers studying clinical (or subclinical) levels of ADHD and conduct problems.

A third important factor was the emergence of the field of prevention science in the early 1990s (Coie et al. 1993). Defined as a new research discipline "forged at the interfaces of psychopathology, criminology, psychiatric epidemiology, human development, and education" (p. 1013), a goal was to set standards for and to promote advances in preventive intervention research to address more effectively the complex biomedical and social processes associated with the development of mental health and related disorders. Central to the theoretical framework was a recognition that interdependent risk factors operate at the level of the individual, family, school, peers, and community contexts to affect the development of disorder, and that prevention program designs needed, in a corresponding fashion, to include more complex, multilevel intervention approaches. In addition, a goal was to improve the methodological rigor associated with prevention research, particularly in areas of representative sampling and statistical modeling.

Due to these three strands of influence, the 1990s witnessed the emergence of multicomponent prevention research programs that combined social competence coaching with parent training, school-based interventions, and/or academic tutoring to meet the needs of children with (or at high risk for) specific disorders. Several large prevention trials mounted during the 1990s tested the effectiveness of multifaceted programs that included SST to improve peer relations, along with parent-focused and school-based interventions. For example, Tremblay and his colleagues (1992) designed a comprehensive prevention program to improve the behaviors and social adjustment of aggressive boys by combining behavior management training for parents with SST for youth. Similarly, SST was embedded in the collaborative, multisite Multimodal Treatment Study of Children with Attention-Deficit/Hyperactivity Disorder (MTA Study; MTA Cooperative Group, 1999). SST was also embedded in three large-scale prevention trials focused on community-based samples of children at risk for the development of conduct problems: the Early Alliance study (Dumas, Lynch, Laughlin, Smith, & Prinz, 2001), the Metropolitan Area Child Study (MACS; Metropolitan Area Child Study Research Group, 2002), and the Fast Track program (Conduct Problems Prevention Research Group [CPPRG], 1992). Although a full description of these studies is beyond the scope of this chapter, the innovations included in their SST programs to improve peer relations are of central relevance. Due to the multicomponent design of these intervention studies, the impact on peer relations cannot be attributed uniquely to SST, but the design innovations and findings are worth examination.

Within these multicomponent prevention trials, SST incorporated innovative design features based upon prior developmental and SST research, including (1) extended and intensive interventions, typically lasting for a year or more; (2) the use of multiple, nested layers of intervention, including classroom-level "universal" interventions to foster a positive peer climate, as well as specialized SST groups for target children with behavior problems; (3) a joint focus on prosocial skills and self-regulatory skills, targeting cognitive, affective, and behavioral features of social competence; and (4) strategies to foster affiliations with nonproblem peers.

The MTA Study

The six-site MTA Study (MTA Coooperative Group, 1999) examined the effectiveness of well-monitored medication and psychosocial intervention (alone or in combination) for children ages 7–10 with ADHD. The multicomponent, 14-month psychosocial intervention included parent training, teacher consultation, and classroom behavioral management support provided by paraprofessionals (see Wells et al., 2000). SST was provided during an intensive summer camp program, which included daily skills presentation lessons focused on social problem-solving skills, fair play and good sportsmanship skills, and following rules. Cooperative tasks, superordinate goals, and nonproblem peer buddies were included to create a positive peer learning environment. The camp program was conducted for 3 hours per day, over a period of 8 weeks. In addition to SST, the camp utilized contingency management to support positive social behavior (point system, time-out), provided behavioral feedback (daily report card), and included academic skills support. To promote generalized change, teacher consultation and a structured behavioral management plan were used in the classroom to reduce off-task and disruptive–aggressive behavior problems. The SST program also included follow-up "booster" sessions held biweekly on Saturdays during the school year. Despite the thoughtful and comprehensive design of the intervention, no intervention effects emerged on the sociometric outcomes. After intervention, children in all three of the intervention groups (medication alone, psychosocial intervention alone, or the combination) continued to show significant impairments in their social functioning.

The MACS

The MACS targeted children in two urban contexts who were at-risk for conduct disorders based upon high rates of aggressive behavior. The multicomponent intervention utilized both universal (classroom) and selective (SST groups) levels of intervention. The SST intervention included 28 sessions, spread over 2 years. Children met in groups of six, with a leader and coleader of matched ethnicity. The universal intervention was conducted weekly for 1-hour sessions. Parallel programs were undertaken with young elementary children (grades 2–3) and older elementary children (grades 5–6) to determine whether developmental level affected response to SST. The SST program targeted social cognitions (e.g., emotional understanding, social perception, normative beliefs about aggression, social problem-solving skills) and social behaviors (e.g., inhibitory control, communication skills, and cooperation skills). The research design compared the outcomes of children who received one (universal classroom intervention), two (universal plus SST groups), or three intervention components (the two levels of SST with parent training). Moderated effects emerged, with child age, school/community context, and intervention condition all affecting outcome. The most comprehensive intervention reduced aggressive behavior for the younger children in the less-resource-poor urban community. In contrast, in the very poorly resourced intercity context, aggression levels were more likely to decrease for young children in the control condition than for young children who received the comprehensive intervention (Metropolitan Area Child Study Research Group, 2002).

Fast Track

The Fast Track project (CPPRG, 1992) also involved a multicomponent prevention program initiated for children screened as highly aggressive at school entry, and included parent training, academic tutoring, and home visiting, as well as SST programming. The SST components included a "universal" classroom program, SST sessions for high-risk children, and an in-school peer-pairing program (see Bierman, Greenberg, & the Conduct Problems Prevention Research Group, 1996). Classroom teachers taught the Promoting Alternative THinking Strategies (PATHS) curriculum (Greenberg & Kusche, 1993; CPPRG, 1999b), targeting emotional understanding, friendship skills, self-regulation, problem-solving skills, and a positive peer climate. Prior to its inclusion in the Fast Track program, the PATHS curriculum demonstrated positive effects on students' emotion knowledge, social problem-solving skills, and teacher-rated social behavior when used as a stand-alone program (Greenberg & Kusche, 1993; Greenberg, Kusche, Cook, & Quamma, 1995). Fast Track SST "friendship groups" used comprehensive coaching methods and cooperative practice activities to target the same skills during extracurricular sessions for groups of five to six high-risk youth. Friendship group sessions occurred weekly in grade 1, biweekly in grade 2, and monthly in grades 3–5. Finally, a peer-pairing program was used to enhance skills generalization from extracurricular friendship group sessions to the school setting, and to build friendships with classmates, by providing high-risk children with supportive play opportunities with rotating classroom partners.

At the end of the first 3 years of Fast Track prevention services, high-risk children in the intervention group, compared with those in the nontreated group, showed improved social-cognitive skills and reduced levels of aggressive–oppositional behaviors at home and school (CPPRG, 1999a). At the end of first grade, school observations revealed higher rates of positive peer exchange and sociometric interviews produced higher social preference scores for children who received the intervention compared with those in the control condition. When the high-risk children who received additional intervention were removed from the analysis, the intervention also had a positive impact on peer sociometrics for other children in the intervention classrooms (e.g., lower levels of peer-nominated aggressive and disruptive behavior, and higher classroom mean levels of positive peer nominations; CPPRG, 1999b), reflecting positive intervention impact at both the classroom and individual levels. However, when high-risk children were followed longitudinally, although reduced aggression was still evident at the end of third grade, peer sociometric nominations did not show sustained intervention effects (CPPRG, 2002).

Summary

During the mid-1990s to mid-2000s, SST research on children with special needs continued, directed at improving behavior. However, SST programs that focused specifically on improving peer relations declined precipitously. The contribution of developmental research on peer relations to SST models was most evident in the large, multicomponent prevention trials undertaken to improve the life trajectories of children with clinical or subclinical levels of behavior problems (ADHD or aggression) who were at high-risk for peer rejection. The SST programs embedded in these multicomponent prevention programs were characterized by innovations in design that stemmed directly from peer relations research. Compared with earlier SST models, these interventions moved from a limited focus on specific social behaviors or social skills response classes, to a conceptualization of social competence as an "organizational" construct (Sroufe, 1990) with multifaceted affective, cognitive, and behavioral determinants. Moving beyond the view that peer rejection is a child characteristic that can be addressed by changing child social behavior alone, these SST interventions targeted peers by including classroom-level programs to enhance positive peer-responding and peer-pairing programs, cooperative activities, and superordinate goals to promote friendly relationships. Despite the significant increases in SST program breadth and depth, however, and the integration with teacher- and parent-focused interventions, these multicomponent programs produced an inconsistent pattern of effects across and within studies, with some evidence of very positive impact, yet ongoing difficulties demonstrating consistent and sustained gains on measures of social behavior and peer relations.

Challenges and Future Directions

The Institute of Medicine (1994) has described the development of preventive interventions as a multiphased cycle. First, designed intervention programs are based upon empirical research and developmental theory that identify risk and protective factors, as well as potentially effective intervention strategies. Then, these interventions are tested in carefully controlled pilot studies to demonstrate program impact and efficacy. Finally, effective programs are transferred to the field and tested under "real-world" conditions, with implementation conducted by community-based service agencies. Ideally, the results of efficacy and effectiveness studies provide a feedback loop to developmental theory and clinical methods that fuel the "next generation" of prevention efforts.

In some ways, the first 20 years of SST research to promote positive peer relations was characterized by "efficacy" trials designed for the rapid testing of theoretical models of change. The dismantling designs and short-term programs commonly used in those years also contributed in a feedback loop to developmental research, fostering an enriched understanding of peer relation dynamics. In the past 10 years, SST research to promote positive peer relations moved toward the applied "effectiveness trial" phase of inquiry, focused primarily on determining whether large-scale, multicomponent interventions could make substantial life changes for the highest-risk youth. Although an important direction, this general trend resulted in the lack of process-oriented studies that tested mechanisms of change. In large-scale trials of this kind, it becomes difficult to analyze the reasons for intervention success or failure, because program impact is heavily affected by features such as implementation fidelity, portability and sustainability across contexts, and generalizability across a heterogeneous set of participants. Ongoing efforts to understand and improve the functioning of SST programs in "real-world" settings are needed. At the same time, the field could benefit from efforts to complete the "feedback loop" and use information from these large studies to inform process-oriented studies that look inside the "black box" at the components and organization of SST programs. Several specific areas of inquiry are especially needed to understand better (1) the mechanisms and processes of change underlying effective treatments; (2) the way variations in peer inclusion or group experiences affect peer outcomes, with a broad perspective examining acceptance, rejection, victimization, and friendship; and (3) the impact of intervention targets and methods that expand beyond the behavior change orientation of the SST model.

Understanding Change Processes

Research is needed to clarify better the active mechanisms underlying effective coaching programs. Initial program design was based upon a behaviorally oriented social learning theory model, and informed by cognitive-behavioral therapy. Hence, there has been a primary focus on social-cognitive variables and behavior shaping as key mechanisms of change. The fundamental assumption is that SST fosters improved social behavior that, in turn, fosters peer acceptance. Yet children may benefit from social competence interventions via other mechanisms (Furman & Gavin, 1989). For example, recent developmental research on peer relations has emphasized self-system processes that affect social behavior and adjustment, including rejection sensitivity, self-efficacy, and emotionally laden response patterns. Motivational features may be important to enhance child engagement in SST interventions, and intervention experiences may affect motivational and related self-system processes, such as self-perceptions (perceived control, as well as feelings of psychological distress) and stress reactivity in peer contexts. Experiential, as well as instructional, aspects of coaching programs may be important influences in this regard. In other words, models of change processes in SST interventions need to expand beyond the behavioral focus that first informed the intervention to assess more clearly impact on the organizational components of child social competence as they are emerging in developmental research. This kind of expansion may enhance our understanding of why some programs have more enduring effects than others.

Exploring Peer Involvement and Peer Affiliations

Early SST programs tried to enhance generalization of intervention effects to naturalistic peer interactions by giving homework assignments, designing intervention sessions to include more naturalistic peer interaction practice opportunities, and including selected peer partners in coaching sessions (Gresham, 1985). However, the resistance to change in peer sociometric ratings even in the context of documented improvements in child behavior (LaGreca & Santogrossi, 1980; Prinz, Blechman, & Dumas, 1994) suggests that greater attention to generalization issues in general, and to peer responding and reputational biases in particular, might strengthen the impact of coaching programs. The most recent multicomponent prevention programs included peers in new ways, nesting targeted SST programs within classroom-level programs, and utilizing extended peer-pairing strategies. These efforts were designed both to enhance the generalized use of skills by target children and to increase positive peer responding and foster friendships with peers. However, because these innovations were studied in the context of multicomponent programs, it is not clear how effectively the various strategies changed peer behavior and evaluations.

In addition, although there is reason to believe that groups of children who share aggressive–disruptive behavior problems may be iatrogenic in some cases (Dishion & Piehler, Chapter 32, this volume; Dishion, Poulin, & Burraston, 2001), it is not clear which peers might make optimal peer partners. On the one hand, highly skilled and well-liked children might be good partners, providing outstanding models of socially skillful behavior, and possibly providing entree into mainstream peer groups. On the other hand, popular children may have many friends and be less likely than more "average" children to be open to new friendships. One recent SST program utilized a "mixed category" approach, including peer-rejected, victimized, and socially anxious students together in SST groups with positive results (DeRosier & Marcus, 2005). It may be that grouping students who share a need and desire to make friends, but have complementary social deficits, may be a viable intervention strategy. In general, the relative impact on coaching success of different partner characteristics has yet to be studied.

Changing negative peer reputations and improving peer responding may be critical in eliciting sustained improvements in social behavior from rejected or victimized children, yet it is not clear yet how best to accomplish this goal. Peer relations are multifaceted, and multiple dimensions of peer relations warrant closer attention in interventions, including the facilitation of high-quality friendships, the control of victimization, and the promotion of niches of opportunity for positive affiliations in adaptive peer networks, along with reduction of deviant peer partnerships and rejection by mainstream peers.

In addition, the degree of malleability in children's attraction to different peers warrants exploration. Particularly among rejected–aggressive children, attraction to other aggressive children contributes to deviant partnerships that support problematic social behaviors, and may buffer children against a need or desire to change.

Expanding Beyond a Cognitive-Behavioral Focus

Reflecting their roots in social learning theory and cognitive-behavioral therapy, SST programs utilize a coaching method that emphasizes the value of instruction, practice, and feedback. This approach has proven to be successful yet limited. Expanding upon the length and intensity of SST sessions, as was done in the large-scale, multicomponent prevention programs, did not appear to magnify impact in the manner that was expected. Hence, exploratory efforts to expand beyond a cognitive-behavioral focus are warranted to determine whether SST impact can be strengthened.

Research on social development is becoming increasingly "translational"—incorporating measures of biological processes associated with social responding into studies of socialization and intervention. A particular emphasis has been the study of emotion regulation, focusing on the role of developing executive functions and inhibitory control on effective social development and peer relations (Eisenberg & Fabes, 1992; Hubbard, 2001). One promising direction for future intervention innovation might involve a closer incorporation of intervention strategies derived from developmental research on emotional functioning (Izard, 2002) and executive function development (Bierman, Nix, Greenberg, Blair, & Domitrovich, in press; Greenberg, 2006).

Summary

The past 30 years have witnessed the extensive development and refinement of SST interventions to promote positive peer relations and social adjustment. Fueled by developmental research elucidating the behavioral, cognitive, and affective characteristics associated with problematic peer relations and the dynamics of rejection processes, SST interventions have become increasingly multifaceted. The technology for producing improvements in social relationships has expanded in notable ways. Across studies, there is substantial evidence for the effectiveness of SST, with moderate size of effects. SST programs have been integrated into in multicomponent prevention programs, paired with parent training, and nested within universal, school-based social competence promotion efforts. These are all positive developments reflecting vibrant research on SST interventions to foster positive peer relations.

At the same time, the growing diversity in the children targeted for intervention and in the methodology used to evaluate intervention effects has resulted in a dissipated empirical literature. The transactional relationship between SST studies and developmental research on peer relations that characterized the 1980s has eroded. Despite intensive efforts, intervention researchers face the sobering realization that SST has not yet produced the substantive and sustained changes in social functioning needed to help the most high-risk youth avoid the long-term negative effects of their social difficulties.

In many ways, we stand at an important precipice in SST research. As a field, we cannot go "backwards" to the self-contained and coherent intervention designs of the 1980s when we optimistically expected 10- to 12-week programs fundamentally to shift the problematic social development trajectories of peer-rejected children. On the other hand, when SST research is fully embedded in disorder-specific prevention models, the impact is fragmented innovation, reduced opportunities for cross-fertilization and development of the change technologies, and little transactional input from or influence on developmental research on peer relations. Hence, the time has come for a new rapprochement and, we hope, a new generation of peer intervention research and SST studies.

References

Abikoff, H. (1979). Cognitive training interventions in children: Review of a new approach. *Journal of Learning Disabilities, 12*, 65–77.

Allen, G. J., Chinsky, J. M., Larcen, S. W., Lochman, J. E., & Selinger, H. V. (1976). *Community psychology and the schools: A behaviorally oriented multilevel preventive approach.* Hillsdale, NJ: Erlbaum.

Beelmann, A., Pfingsten, U., & Losel, F. (1994). Effects of training social competence in children: A meta-analysis of recent evaluation studies. *Journal of Clinical Child Psychology, 23*, 260–271.

Bierman, K. L. (1986). Process of change during social skills training with preadolescents and its relation to treatment outcome. *Child Development, 57*, 230–240.

Bierman, K. L. (2004). *Peer rejection: Developmental processes and intervention strategies.* New York: Guilford Press.

Bierman, K. L., & Furman, W. (1984). The effects of social skills training and peer involvement on the social adjustment of preadolescents. *Child Development, 55*, 151–162.

Bierman, K. L., Greenberg, M. T., & the Conduct Problems Prevention Research Group. (1996). Social skills training in the Fast Track program. In R. D. Peters & R. J. McMahon (Eds.), *Preventing childhood disorders, substance abuse, and delinquency* (pp. 65–89). Thousand Oaks, CA: Sage.

Bierman, K. L., Miller, C. M., & Stabb, S. (1987). Improving the social behavior and peer acceptance of rejected boys: Effects of social skill training with instructions and prohibitions. *Journal of Consulting and Clinical Psychology, 55*, 194–200.

Bierman, K. L., Nix, R. L., Greenberg, M. T., Blair, C., & Domitrovich, C. E. (in press). Executive functions and school readiness intervention: Impact, moderation, and mediation in the Head Start REDI Program. *Development and Psychopathology.*

Bierman, K. L., Smoot, D. L., & Aumiller, K. (1993). Characteristics of aggressive-rejected, aggressive (nonrejected), and rejected (nonaggressive) boys. *Child Development, 64*, 139–151.

Cillessen, A. H. N., van IJzendoorn, H. W., van Lieshout, C. F. M., & Hartup, W. W. (1992). Heterogeneity of peer rejected boys. *Child Development, 63*, 893–905.

Coie, J. D. (1990). Toward a theory of peer rejection. In S. R. Asher & J. D. Coie (Eds.), *Peer rejection in childhood* (pp. 365–401). Cambridge, UK: Cambridge University Press.

Coie, J. D., & Dodge, K. A. (1998). Aggression and antisocial behavior. In W. Damon (Series Ed.) & N. Eisenberg (Vol. Ed.), *Handbook of child psychology: Vol. 3. Social, emotional, and personality development* (5th ed., pp. 779–862). New York: Wiley.

Coie, J. D., Dodge, K. A., & Coppotelli, H. (1982). Dimensions and types of status: A cross-age perspective. *Developmental Psychology, 18*, 557–570.

Coie, J. D., Dodge, K. A., & Kupersmidt, J. B. (1990). Peer group behavior and social status. In S. R. Asher & J. D. Coie (Eds.), *Peer rejection in childhood* (pp. 17–59). Cambridge, UK: Cambridge University Press.

Coie, J. D., & Koeppl, G. K. (1990). Adapting intervention to the problems of aggressive and disruptive rejected children. In S. R. Asher & J. D. Coie (Eds.), *Peer rejection in childhood* (pp. 309–337). Cambridge, UK: Cambridge University Press.

Coie, J. D., & Krehbiel, G. (1984). Effects of academic tutoring on the social status of low-achieving, socially rejected children. *Child Development, 55*, 1465–1478.

Coie, J. D., Watt, N. F., West, S. G., Hawkins, J. D., Asarnow, J. R., Markman, H. J., et al. (1993). The science of prevention: A conceptual framework and some directions for a national research program. *American Psychologist, 48*, 1013–1022.

Conduct Problems Prevention Research Group. (1992). A developmental and clinical model for the prevention of conduct disorders: The Fast Track program. *Development and Psychopathology, 4*, 505–527.

Conduct Problems Prevention Research Group. (1999a). Initial impact of the Fast Track prevention trial for conduct problems: I. The high-risk sample. *Journal of Consulting and Clinical Psychology, 67*, 631–647.

Conduct Problems Prevention Research Group. (1999b). Initial impact of the Fast Track prevention trial for conduct problems: II. Classroom effects. *Journal of Consulting and Clinical Psychology, 67*, 648–657.

Conduct Problems Prevention Research Group. (2002). Evaluation of the first 3 years of the Fast Track prevention trial with children a high risk for adolescent conduct problems. *Journal of Abnormal Child Psychology, 30*, 19–35.

Cowen, E. L., Pedersen, A., Babigian, H., Izzo, L. D., & Trost, M. A. (1973). Long-term follow-up of early detected vulnerable children. *Journal of Consulting and Clinical Psychology, 41*, 438–446.

DeRosier, M. E., & Marcus, S. R. (2005). Building friendships and combating bullying: Effectiveness of S.S. GRIN at one-year follow-up. *Journal of Clinical Child and Adolescent Psychology, 34*, 140–150.

Dishion, T. J., Poulin, F., & Burraston, B. (2001). Peer group dynamics associated with iatrogenic effects in group interventions with high-risk young adolescents. In C. Erdley & D. W. Nangle (Eds.), *Damon's new directions in child development* (pp. 79–91). San Francisco: Jossey-Bass.

Dodge, K. A. (1989). Problems in social relationships. In E. Mash & R. Barkley (Eds.), *Treatment of childhood disorders* (pp. 222–244). New York: Guilford Press.

Dodge, K. A., & Murphy, R. R. (1984). The assessment of social competence in adolescents. *Advances in Child Behavior Analysis and Therapy, 3*, 61–96.

Dumas, J. E., Lynch, A. M., Laughlin, J. E., Smith, E. P., & Prinz, R. J. (2001). Promoting intervention fidelity: Conceptual issue, methods, and preliminary results from the Early Alliance Prevention Trial. *American Journal of Preventive Medicine, 20*, 38–47.

Eisenberg, N., & Fabes, R. A. (1992). Emotion, regulation, and the development of social competence. In M. S. Clark (Ed.), *Review of personality and social psychology: Vol. 14. Emotion and social behavior* (pp. 119–150). Newbury Park, CA: Sage.

Elliott, S. N., & Gresham, F. M. (1993). Social skills interventions for children. *Behavior Modification,* *17*, 287–313.

Furman, W., & Gavin, L. A. (1989). Peers' influence on adjustment and development: A view from the intervention literature. In T. J. Berndt & G. W. Ladd (Eds.), *Peer relationships in child development* (pp. 319–340). Oxford, UK: Wiley.

Greenberg, M. T. (2006). Promoting resilience in children and youth: Preventive interventions and their interface with neuroscience. *Annals of the New York Academy of Sciences, 1094*, 139–150.

Greenberg, M. T., & Kusche, C. A. (1993). *Promoting social and emotional development in deaf children: The PATHS project.* Seattle: University of Washington Press.

Greenberg, M. T., Kusche, C. A., Cook, E. T., & Quamma, J. P. (1995). Promoting emotional competence in school-aged deaf children: The effects of the PATHS curriculum. *Development and Psychopathology, 7*, 117–136.

Gresham, F. M. (1985). Utility of cognitive-behavioral procedures for social skills training with children: A critical review. *Journal of Abnormal Child Psychology, 13*, 411–423.

Gresham, F. M. (1994). Generalization of social skills: Risks of choosing form over function. *School Psychology Quarterly, 9*, 142–144.

Gresham, F. M., & Nagle, R. J. (1980). Social skills training with children: Responsiveness to modeling and coaching as a function of peer orientation. *Journal of Consulting and Clinical Psychology, 48*, 718–729.

Hubbard, J. A. (2001). Emotion expression processes in children's peer interaction: The role of peer rejection, aggression, and gender. *Child Development, 72*, 1426–1438.

Hudley, C., & Graham, S. (1993). An attributional intervention to reduce peer-directed aggression among African-American boys. *Child Development, 64*, 124–138.

Hymel, S., Wagner, E., & Butler, L. J. (1990). Reputational bias: View from the peer group. In S. R. Asher & J. D. Coie (Eds.), *Peer rejection in childhood* (pp. 156–186). Cambridge, UK: Cambridge University Press.

Institute of Medicine. (1994). *Reducing risks for mental disorders: Frontiers for preventive intervention research.* Washington, DC: National Academy Press.

Izard, C. (2002). Translating emotion theory and research into preventive interventions. *Psychological Bulletin, 128*, 796–824.

Kendall, P. C. (1985). Toward a cognitive-behavioral model of child psychopathology and a critique of related interventions. *Journal of Abnormal Child Psychology, 13*, 357–372.

Kohlberg, L., LaCross, J., & Ricks, D. (1972). The predictability of adult mental health from childhood behavior. In B. Wolman (Ed.), *Manual of child psychopathology* (pp. 1217–1284). New York: McGraw-Hill.

Ladd, G. W. (1981). Effectiveness of a social learning method for enhancing children's social interaction and peer acceptance. *Child Development, 52*, 171–178.

Ladd, G. W., & Mize, J. (1983). A cognitive-social learning model of social skill training. *Psychological Review, 90*, 127–157.

LaGreca, A. M. (1993). Social skills training with children: Where do we go from here? *Journal of Clinical Child Psychology, 22*, 288–298.

LaGreca, A. M., & Santogrossi, D. S. (1980). Social skills training with elementary school students: A behavioral group approach. *Journal of Consulting and Clinical Psychology, 48*, 220–227.

Lochman, J. E., Burch, P. R., Curry, J. F., & Lampron, L. B. (1984). Treatment and generalization effects of cognitive-behavioral and goal setting interventions with aggressive boys. *Journal of Consulting and Clinical Psychology, 52*, 915–916.

Lochman, J. E., Coie, J. D., Underwood, M. K., & Terry, R. (1993). Effectiveness of a social relations intervention program for aggressive and nonaggressive, rejected children. *Journal of Consulting and Clinical Psychology, 61*, 1053–1058.

Lochman, J. E., & Lenhart, L. A. (1993). Anger coping intervention for aggressive children: Conceptual models and outcome effects. *Clinical Psychology Review, 13*, 785–805.

McFadyen-Ketchum, S. A., & Dodge, K. A. (1998). Problems in social relationships. In E. J. Mash & R. A. Barkley (Eds.), *Treatment of childhood disorders* (2nd ed., pp. 338–368). New York: Guilford Press.

Metropolitan Area Child Study Research Group. (2002). A cognitive-ecological approach to preventing aggression in urban settings: Initial outcomes for high-risk children. *Journal of Consulting and Clinical Psychology, 70,* 179–194.

Miller-Johnson, S., Coie, J. D., Bierman, K., Maumary-Gremaud, A., & the Conduct Problems Prevention Research Group. (2002). Peer rejection and aggression and early-starter models of conduct disorder. *Journal of Abnormal Child Psychology, 30,* 217–230.

MTA Cooperative Group. (1999). A 14-month randomized clinical trial of treatment strategies for attention deficit hyperactivity disorder (ADHD). *Archives of General Psychiatry, 56,* 1073–1086.

Oden, S. L., & Asher, S. R. (1977). Coaching children in social skills for friendship making. *Child Development, 48,* 495–506.

Parker, J., Rubin, K. H., Erath, S., Wojslawowicz, J. C., & Buskirk, A. A. (2006). Peer relationships and developmental psychopathology. In D. Cicchetti & D. Cohen (Eds.), *Developmental psychopathology: Risk, disorder, and adaptation* (2nd ed., Vol. 2, pp. 419–493). New York: Wiley.

Prinz, R. J., Blechman, E. A., & Dumas, J. E. (1994). An evaluation of peer coping skills training for childhood aggression. *Journal of Clinical Child Psychology, 23,* 193–203.

Rubin, K. H., Bukowski, W., & Parker, J. (2006). Peer interactions, relationships, and groups. In N. Eisenberg (Ed.), *Handbook of child psychology: Social, emotional, and personality development* (6th ed., pp. 571–645). New York: Wiley.

Rubin, K. H., Burgess, K., Kennedy, A. E., & Stewart, S. (2003). Social withdrawal and inhibition in childhood. In E. Mash & R. Barkley (Eds.), *Child psychopathology* (2nd ed., pp. 372–406). New York: Guilford Press.

Schneider, B. H. (1992). Didactic methods for enhancing children's peer relations: A quantitative review. *Clinical Psychology Review, 12,* 363–382.

Spivack, G., & Shure, M. B. (1974). *Social adjustment of young children: A cognitive approach to solving real-life problems.* San Francisco: Jossey-Bass.

Sroufe, L. A. (1990). An organizational perspective on the self. In D. Cicchetti & M. Beeghly (Eds.), *The self in transition: Infancy to childhood* (pp. 281–307). Chicago: University of Chicago Press.

Strain, P. S., Shores, R. E., & Kerr, M. M. (1976). An experimental analysis of "spillover" effects on the social interaction of behaviorally handicapped preschool children. *Journal of Applied Behavior Analysis, 9,* 31–40.

Tremblay, R. E., Vitaro, F., Bertrand, L., LeBlanc, M., Beauchesne, H., Boileau, H., et al. (1992). Parent and child training to prevent early onset of delinquency: The Montreal Longitudinal Study. In J. McCord & R. E. Tremblay (Eds.), *Preventing antisocial behavior: Interventions from birth through adolescence* (pp. 117–138). New York: Guilford Press.

Wanzek, J., Vaughn, S., Kim, A., & Cavanaugh, C. L. (2006). The effects of reading interventions on social outcomes for elementary students with reading difficulties: A synthesis. *Reading and Writing Quarterly, 22,* 121–138.

Weissberg, R. P., & Allen, J. P. (1986). Promoting children's social skills and adaptive behavior. In B. Edelstein & L. Michelson (Eds.), *Handbook of prevention* (pp. 153–175). New York: Plenum Press.

Weissberg, R. P., Gesten, E. L., Carnrike, C. L., Toro, P. A., Rapkin, B. D., Davidson, E., et al. (1981). Social problem-solving skills training: A competence building intervention with second- to fourth-grade children. *American Journal of Community Psychology, 9,* 411–423.

Wells, K. C., Pelham, W. E., Kotkin, R. A., Hoza, B., Abikoff, H. B., Abramowitz, A., et al. (2000). Psychosocial treatment strategies in the MTA Study: Rationale, methods, and critical issues in design and implementation. *Journal of Abnormal Child Psychology, 28*(6), 483–505.

Author Index

Subject Index

St. Louis Experiment, 594
Stability
  of friendships, 221, 281, 397
  of groups, 109, 199
  of peer groups, 365
  of peer reputations, 548
Standardization method in
    sociometric studies, 89–90
Status
  academic achievement and,
    534–535
  aggressive behavior and,
    289–291
  bullying and, 327–329, 331
  cliques, crowds, and, 367
  conflict and, 278–279
  constructs of, 550
  depressive symptoms and,
    561–562
  ethnicity and, 395
  group and, 333–334
  negative emotion and, 479
  in network context, 106
  peer groups and, 370–371
  self-regulation, impulsivity, and,
    476–477
  sociometric, 83–84
  temperament, competence,
    and, 474–475
Stereotypes, 403
Structural balance theory, 106
Structural descriptions of
    transactions
  affiliation, 199–203
  dominance, 203–206
  integrating affiliation and
    dominance, 207–209
  overview of, 195–199
  social ethology and, 197–199
Structure
  of peer groups, 364–365
  of peer relationships, and sex
    differences, 382
Structured activities
  adjustment and, 416–418,
    419–420
  definition of, 415
  theories of, 416
  youth choice of, 420–422
Substance abuse
  alcohol drinking, and team
    sports, 417
  college roommates, assignment
    of, and, 596
  peer reputation and, 558–560
Success in peer relationships,
    440–441
Sullivanian theory
  overview of, 9, 306
  romantic relationships and,
    344–345

Symbolic interactionism
  overview of, 306
  peer groups and, 369
  romantic relationships and,
    345–346
  See also Social identity theory
Symbolic play, 148
Symbolic thought, 6–7

Teachers, relationships with, 540,
    541–542
Team sports, and alcohol
    drinking, 417
Technology
  measurement of interactional
    patterns using, 58
  wireless transmission, 243–244
Temperament
  activity level, adaptability, and,
    483–484
  choice of activities and, 421
  competence, status, and,
    474–475
  conflict and, 276
  definition of, 473
  early peer relations and,
    132–133
  effortful control and, 476–479
  formation of friendship in
    preschool years and, 184–185
  future study of, 484–485
  model of, 473–474
  negative emotionality and,
    479–481
  positive emotionality, 481–482
  sociability and behavioral
    inhibition, 482–483
  See also Self-regulation
Theories
  of behavioral-genetics method,
    456–457
  of bullying, 326–329
  on development of sex
    differences, 379–381
  of early peer relations, 122–
    126
  of friendships, 181–182, 223
  of neighborhood contexts, 416
  of peer groups, 369–370
  of peer relations of aggressive
    children, 288–289, 296–297
  of peer reputations, 551–553
  of social withdrawal, 305–307
  See also specific theories, such as
    Cognitive theories
Theory of mind development
  play and, 152
  social–emotional competence
    and, 171
Tobacco use, and peer reputation,
    558–559

Toddlers
  aggressive behavior in,
    128–129, 134
  group interaction in, 130,
    136–137
  relationships between, 129–130
  See also Friendship in preschool
    years; Preschool years
Transactional model of peer
    reputations, 552–553, 555, 559
Transactional nature of social–
    emotional competence,
    164–165, 174–175
Transactions within groups
  affiliation and affiliative
    structures, 199–203
  dominance structures, 203–206
  integrating affiliation and
    dominance, 207–209
  overview of, 195–199
Translational relationship
  between social skills training
    and developmental research,
    617–618
Travails, definition of, 21
Trend, definition of, 21
Turning point in research
  definition of, 21
  on friendships and friendship
    relations, 28–32
  on peer-group rejection, 32–38
Two worlds/cultures framework of
    sex differences, 385–386

Unilateral friendships, 70–71
Unlimited nominations, 87
Unoccupied behavior, 144, 145
Unsociable, definition of, 304–305
Unstructured activities
  adjustment and, 418–420
  definition of, 415
  deviant behavior and, 425–426
  theories of, 416
  youth choice of, 420–422
  youth recreation centers,
    422–425, 426–428

Validation and friendship,
    223–224
Verbal aggression
  cliques and, 292
  friendship and, 294–296
  perceived popularity and,
    290–291
  social preference and, 289–290
Victimization
  academic competence and,
    537–538
  behavioral-genetics method
    and, 463–464
  consequences of, 335